Swine Diseases: A Veterinarian’s Guide

Swine Diseases: A Veterinarian's Guide

Editor: Anna Hunt

STATES
ACADEMIC PRESS
www.statesacademicpress.com

States Academic Press,
109 South 5th Street,
Brooklyn, NY 11249, USA

Visit us on the World Wide Web at:
www.statesacademicpress.com

ISBN: 978-1-63989-504-5 (Hardback)

Cataloging-in-Publication Data

Swine diseases : a veterinarian's guide / edited by Anna Hunt.
p. cm.
Includes bibliographical references and index.
ISBN 978-1-63989-504-5
1. Swine--Diseases. 2. Veterinary medicine. I. Hunt, Anna.
SF971 .S95 2022
636.408 96--dc23

Table of Contents

Preface

This book has been an outcome of determined endeavour from a group of educationists in the field. The primary objective was to involve a broad spectrum of professionals from diverse cultural background involved in the field for developing new researches. The book not only targets students but also scholars pursuing higher research for further enhancement of the theoretical and practical applications of the subject.

A veterinarian protects and improves the health of animal species by preventing, controlling and eliminating diseases, and at the same time monitoring and promoting animal health. Swine production is an important component of agricultural economies and global food security. Swine are also known as pigs, and can harbor a range of parasites and pathogens that can be transmitted to humans. African swine fever, classical swine fever, swine brucellosis, pseudo rabies, influenza virus in swine are some of the major threat to the health of both swine and mankind. These diseases are highly contagious and infectious. A veterinarian uses medicines like antibiotics, vaccines, supplements, analgesics and parasecticides to improve the health of swine. This book provides comprehensive insights into the field of swine diseases. Its aim is to present researches that have transformed this discipline and aided its advancement. This book will prove to be immensely beneficial to students and researchers in this field.

It was an honour to edit such a profound book and also a challenging task to compile and examine all the relevant data for accuracy and originality. I wish to acknowledge the efforts of the contributors for submitting such brilliant and diverse chapters in the field and for endlessly working for the completion of the book. Last, but not the least; I thank my family for being a constant source of support in all my research endeavours.

Editor

Preface

1

A longitudinal study on the performance of in vivo methods to determine the osteochondrotic status of young pigs

Christian P. Bertholle[1], Ellen Meijer[1], Willem Back[2,3], Arjan Stegeman[1], P. René van Weeren[2] and Arie van Nes[1*]

Abstract

Background: In today's porcine industry, lameness has a major welfare and economic impact, and is often caused by osteochondrosis (OC). The etiological factors of the disease have been studied in depth, however, to this day, little is known about the natural course of the disorder and how it can be detected at an early stage in pigs. The aim of this pilot study was to assess the potential of three non-invasive techniques for the detection and monitoring of early OC processes in piglets. A group of weaned piglets ($n = 19$) were examined longitudinally using radiographs, a visual lameness scoring scheme and a quantitative pressure-mat based locomotion analysis system to detect OC in the humeroradial, femoropatellar and tarsocrural joints. At several time points, a selection of animals was euthanized for post-mortem examinations, including histology, which was the gold standard.

Results: In this study, clear signs of subclinical signs of OC were observed, however, we were unsuccessful in producing clinical OC. Lesions were observed to be commonly bilaterally symmetric in the joints examined in 80 % of cases. The radiographic examinations showed a clear correlation with the gold standard, particularly when subclinical lesions were of a high histological score. Moreover, radiography was also able to detect the early repair processes, which appeared to take place at least until 14 weeks of age. Both visual scoring and pressure mat analyses showed good intra-assay reproducibility, with the pressure mat showing intra-class correlation values between 0.44 and 0.6 and the inter-observer agreement of visual scoring method was between 88 and 96 %, however their correlation to OC lesions detected by histology was very weak, with only 2 out of 12 traits for the visual scoring method showing significant and biologically logical relations to a specific joint having histological OC lesions. For the pressure mat, only a maximum of 5 associations for specific joints with histological OC lesions were found out of a possible 8.

Conclusion: All tested in-vivo methods showed good reproducibility. Radiography was the most reliable technique to detect and monitor longitudinally the earliest signs of OC in these piglets. It also demonstrated that the "Point of No Return" (PNR) of the disease, when repair processes end, might be later than anticipated, after 13 weeks of age. All in all, our study shows that the timing of the use of these in-vivo methods is critical to detect and monitor OC, especially in the early phases of the disease. It also shows the difficulty in producing OC regardless of the optimization of the experimental settings in relation to the etiological factors known to induce OC.

Keywords: Pig health, Osteochondrosis, Lameness, Gait analysis, Radiography, Histology, Early detection

* Correspondence: A.vanNes@uu.nl
[1]Department of Farm Animal Health, Faculty of Veterinary Medicine, Utrecht University, Yalelaan 7, NL-3584 CL Utrecht, The Netherlands
Full list of author information is available at the end of the article

Background

Osteochondrosis has often been reported to be the main cause of lameness in pigs [1–3] and is still currently causing substantial economic losses and alarming welfare concerns for both sows and slaughter pigs [4]. It is estimated that 80 % of the pigs in today's porcine industry show superficial to mild signs of OC [1]. OC has been defined as a multi-focal disturbance in the endochondral ossification process that occurs during skeletal growth, leading to lesions in both the articular and physeal cartilage [1, 5]. Many advances have been achieved in the understanding of the disease process, for example with respect to the identification of etiological factors. However, little is known still on the natural course of the disease and especially on the early stages [5]. Nevertheless, the fact that the molecular and cellular structure of epiphyseal cartilage and that the mechanism of disruption of the endochondral ossification process are similar in different species, lead us to believe that these early stages could also be comparable in the pig [6–8]. This means that recent findings in equine medicine on OC, where it is suggested now that there is a dynamism of the interplay process between lesion initiation and early repair, could be extrapolated to porcine OC [9, 10]. Additionally, the existence of a Point of No Return (PNR) has also been discovered in the horse. In the pig, this PNR is anticipated to be before 13 weeks of age, after which lesions can no longer be repaired, as vascularization of the cartilage tissue has disappeared [11, 12]. The understanding of OC has for a long time principally relied on data that was acquired by either radiography or post-mortem analysis [13], however more recent techniques have also shown promising results, such as micro-CT [14, 15]. In the pig, good correlations have been reported between radiographic results and post-mortem macroscopic and microscopic data, although this was in animals showing more the later clinical stages of the disease [13], than the early stages or subclinical signs of OC. In spite of the valuable performance of radiography, there is a need in the field to have other effective in-vivo detection methods able to detect the early signs of OC in a higher through-put way. In other species, such as the horse, the dog and cattle, the development of locomotion in relation to leg and claw disorders has been studied successfully using modern gait analysis techniques [16–18]. In this pilot study, we investigated the frequency of OC in our pigs and per joint. We studied also the bilateral symmetry of OC, and the efficacy and suitability of three non- invasive techniques to detect early signs of OC, by comparing them to the gold standard (histological examination). These in-vivo techniques included the visual scoring of the conformation and gait of the animals, the use of a pressure mat to quantify gait and radiographic screening.

Results

Health-prevalence of OC-bilateral symmetrical aspect

Average daily weight gain of the 19 pigs was 253 g/day (+/− 246 g) and average body weight was 6.5 kg (stdev. +/− 0.64) and 34.2 kg (stdev. +/− 0.79), at 4 and 14 weeks of age respectively. At necropsy, no macroscopic OC lesions were detected in any of the joints in any of the pigs. At histology, most of the lesions were observed in the femoropatellar joint, which featured the most severe lesions (Fig. 1). The OC status appeared to be highly symmetrical in left and right joints for all three joints with an identical histological score (H score) or an H score differing only by one unit in over 80 % of cases (Table 1).

In-vivo versus post-mortem gold standards (Radiographic versus Histological examination)

The comparison between histology and radiography was done using the data from both techniques from the 10 radiographed pigs at the last time point. Fig. 2 shows a receiver operating characteristic (ROC) curve describing the sensitivity/specificity of radiographic results for all joints with different cut-offs of histology, considered as the gold standard, Table 2 shows the statistical difference in sensitivity and specificity between the radiographs and histology. Results show that the sensitivity increases and the specificity decreases, as the threshold setting for histology increases.

When examining the different areas under the curve (AUC), which measure the general accuracy of the test, for each threshold setting, the range is chronological from 72.3 % (for H and R scores >1) to 89.1 % (for scores above 3). This demonstrates a good overall specificity and sensitivity of radiographs compared to the gold standard, which appears to increase as the histological lesions become more severe. Concerning the correct identification of negative joints for OC, radiography has

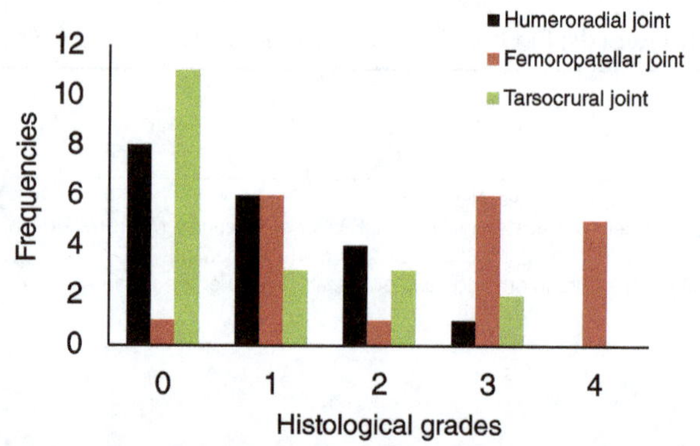

Fig. 1 Histology scores for $n = 19$ pigs (using both left and right sides of the joint were combined and the overall worst score from all investigated locations within the joints)

Table 1 Left/right comparison of OC histological status ($n = 19$)

	Humeroradial ($n = 32^a$)	Femoropatellar ($n = 39^a$)	Tarsocrural ($n = 25^a$)
Bilateral lesions (both scores >1)	9.4 %	33.4 %	8.0 %
Bilateral no lesions (both scores 0)	56.3 %	23.1 %	68.0 %
1 side score 0, the other score >1	31.3 %	25.6 %	12.0 %
1 side score 0, the other score >2	3.1 %	18.0 %	12.0 %

[a]Only the outcomes where left and right histology scores were available for each location

a good specificity from R score 0 up to R score 2, but is accompanied by a low sensitivity.

Above R score 2 (R scores 3–4) the opposite occurs: the sensitivity dramatically increases up to 81.2 % compared to 67.8 % (for R score 2), and specificity decreases, demonstrating that radiography identifies positive histological joints better from R score 3 onwards (Table 2). Overall, from these results we can establish that there is a good relation between histology and radiography and additionally both sensitivity and specificity vary with the cut-off. Figure 3 shows typical examples of histological lesions with the corresponding radiographs.

Longitudinal radiographic monitoring

Our results showed that lesions remained stable (80–95 % of lesions) except for the femoropatellar joint, where progression, regression and even resolution of lesions were apparent (Table 3). Resolution occurred in all joints after the hypothetical timing of the PNR (7 weeks of age < PNR < 13 weeks of age).

Visual scoring reproducibility

Inter-observer agreement was good to excellent (88–96 %) for all scored parameters but one: (sickled-buckled fore, Table 4).

Pressure mat reproducibility

Table 5 gives intra-class correlation (ICC) data on the pressure mat kinetic factors showing overall excellent reproducibility (ICC values $0.44 < x < 0.6$).

Comparison of visual scoring and histology

When considering visual scoring and histology, 12 pigs were selected on the basis that they were the only ones showing the highest number of results present for both techniques, in a total of 9 joint locations (2 in the humeroradial joint, 4 in the femoropatellar joint and 3 in the tarsocrural joint). This comparison showed that the hind pasterns was the only element that showed a significant relationship at joint level, once the Benjamini

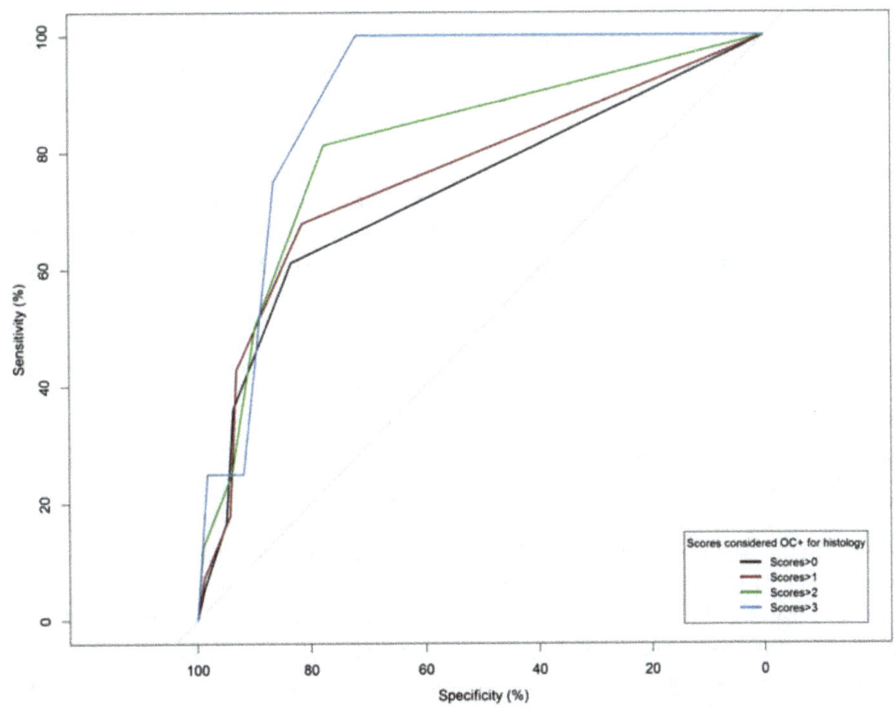

Fig. 2 ROC curves showing the difference in sensitivity and specificity of radiography versus the gold standard, histology using various thresholds

Table 2 Description of the sensitivity and specificity of radiography for the detection of OC as defined by the gold standard, histology ($n = 10$)

	Specificity (%)	Sensitivity (%)	AUC	Confidence interval
Roc 1 (Both H&R scores >0)	83.3	61.1	72.3	63.61–82.22 %
Roc 2 (Both H&R scores >1)	81.4	67.8	75.3	65.66–85.79 %
Roc 3 (Both H&R scores >2)	77.5	81.2	80.9	69.49–92.24 %
Roc 4 (Both H&R scores >3)	71.8	100.0	89.1	79.9 %–98.2 %

R scores radiographic scores, *H scores* histological scores, *AUC* area under the curve, *ROC*

and Hochberg false discovery rate correction was applied to all the Spearman correlation test results (Table 6).

Comparison of pressure mat and histology

Using the same set of pigs as for the visual scoring/histology comparison, four comparisons between the ASIs (Asymmetry Indexes) and histology were tested. The first two were based on the ASIs and the transformed H scores. Only Fore/Hind ASIs showed relations with Animal and Femoropatellar levels (Table 7).

Thirdly, an "ASI animal level score" (sum of all ASI absolute values) was compared to the H score on animal level, but no associations were found (results not shown). Finally, a direct comparison between ASIs of severe histologically OC Positive joints (H scores >3) and those of OC negative joints was tested. Only ASI Pmax fore (Right/Left setting) showed a significant link with the presence and absence of severe histological OC lesions (results not shown).

Discussion

Frequency, severity of and bilateral symmetrical aspect of OC lesions

In the present study, 64.9 % of the animals showed microscopic signs of OC, with 24.6 % having histologically severe lesions (H scores > 3; Fig. 1). The femoropatellar joint had the highest incidence of lesions and the highest number of high grade lesions. Nevertheless, in clinical terms, only 7 % of animals lesions of a high grade radiographically (R scores > 3) and at necropsy, no lesions were macroscopically visible in any of the pigs. We were therefore unexpectedly unsuccessful in creating clinically OC, despite using environmental conditions (slippery flooring) and nutritional regimens (high protein diets fed ad-libitum) designed to promote the development of the disorder [5]. The advantage of this situation was that we were able to assess our non-invasive methods under challenging conditions. Few studies have looked at the the frequency of OC in pigs on a longitudinal scale and in the early subclinical phases of OC. Some studies reported frequencies from 41.4 % using macroscopic evaluation to 78 % using microscopy [18]. There are also large differences with respect to the frequency per joint, with some studies reporting the tarsocrural joint as the joint to be most commonly affected [19], while others mention the medial condyles of the femur and humerus [13]. The techniques used to detect OC were similar in nature, thus these differences are most likely linked to the multifactorial aspect of this diseases, which can affect one population of identical genetic pigs differently if they were exposed to different environmental conditions for example. Regarding the bilateral symmetrical effect, the humeroradial joint was the most consistent in showing this effect in our study (Table 1). OC is generally seen as a multifocal disease with a relatively strong bilateral occurrence of lesions [5, 20, 21]. This finding has even prompted some studies to analyse solely one side of the animal [13]. Our results confirm these previous findings.

In-vivo radiography as a diagnostic tool for OC detection compared to histology

Unsurprisingly, the different AUC results measuring the accuracy of radiographs versus histology showed that radiography performed best for detecting the most severe histological lesions (Table 2). Additionally, in terms of specificity, radiography showed that all histological lesions from H score 2, 1 and 0 were identified as OC negative. This was expected, as these lesions are mostly mild subclinical ones and would be therefore challenging to visualize with a clinical tool, such as radiography. All things considered, from these results, we can conclude that the most reliable threshold for radiography, to identify correctly the OC status of these joints, is situated around H score 3, when lesions are at high score histologically. This observation is important, as it demonstrates the ability of radiography to detect only the more severe subclinical OC lesions in pigs reliably. Although radiography is considered currently as the standard imaging method to diagnose clinical OC [22], and most studies have investigated OC in other species [7, 21–23], not many have focused on pigs [24, 25]. Other studies have also shown significant correlations between both methods, which were joint dependent [13, 26], however these studies were performed on older pigs and foals. Our results show a similar relevant correlation between both methods. In terms of monitoring, the results showed that lesions occur already at 7 weeks of age, and

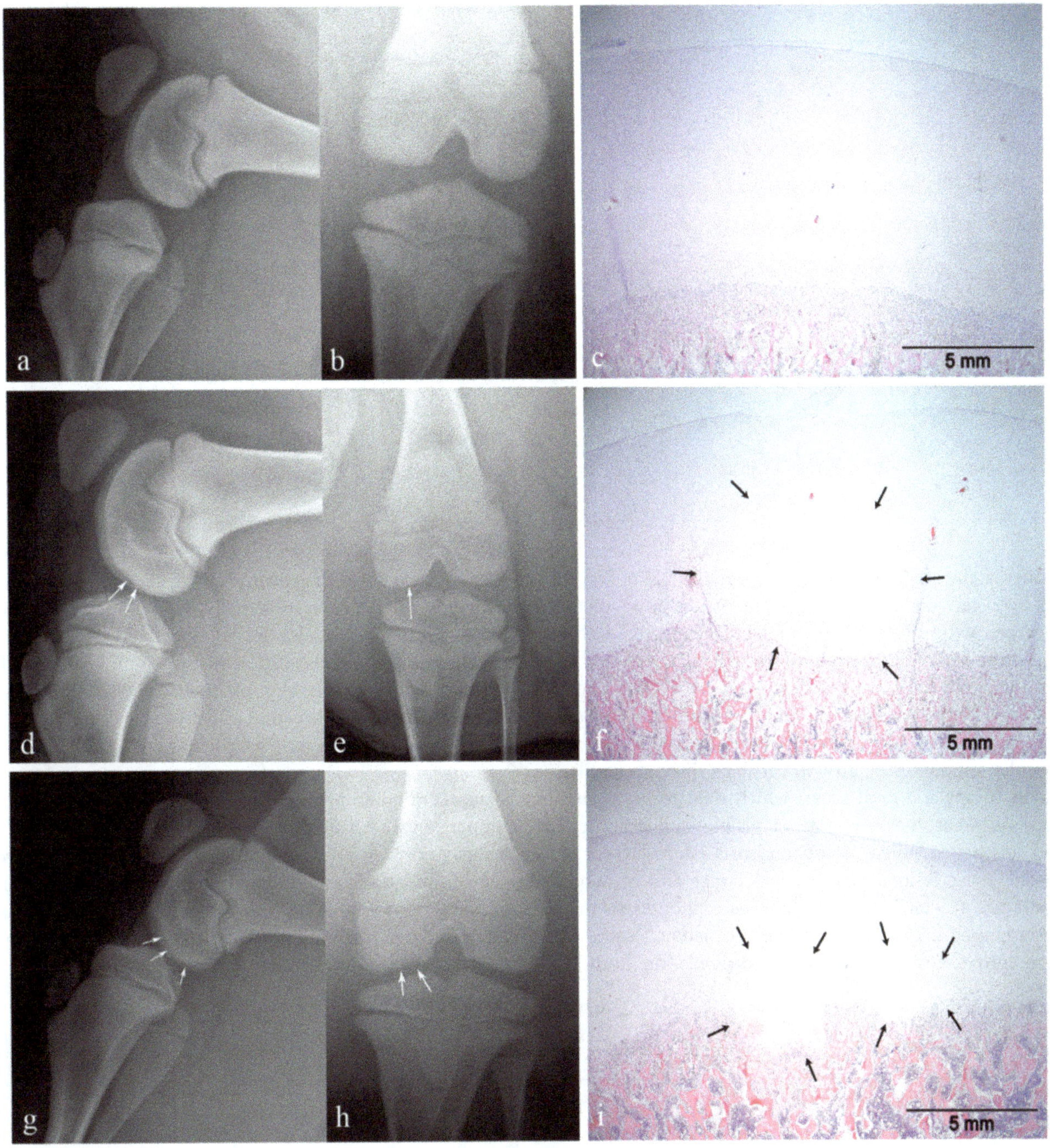

Fig. 3 a–**i**. Typical images of the histological grades with corresponding radiographic findings. Photo pairs **a**, **b**, **d**, **e** and **g**, **h** are radiographic images taken of 3 different respective pigs at 14 weeks of age. Pictures C, F and I are the corresponding histological slides in chronological order to the radiographic paired images. All stained with hematoxylin and eosin. All pictures depict assessments of the femoropatellar joint with G/H/I being from the left limb only. **a**–**c** represent the lateral side and **d**–**f** and **g**–**i** represent the medial side of the distal femoral condyle. All three pairs represent animals with no OC lesions present (**a**–**c**), with mild OC lesions ($R = 2$ and $H = 3$, **d**–**f**) and with severe OC lesions ($R = 4$ and $H = 4$, **g**–**i**)

are mostly of a low grade nature for radiological standards (R scores <3). Although OC lesions progressed, as expected, between 11 to 14 weeks of age, mostly in the humeroradial and femoropatellar joints, simultaneous repair processes were also taking place. This means that the PNR, which was anticipated to be before 13 weeks of age, is probably situated somewhat later in time. In horses, OC is known to be a very dynamic disease in which lesions appear, but then may, to a large extent, resolve spontaneously afterwards as a repair process starts

Table 3 Frequencies of lesion development detected radiographically at 7, 11 and 14 weeks of age ($n = 20$, for 10 pigs and 2 sides for each joint)

	Grade	Lesions present	Stationary	Progression	Regression	Resolution
7–11 weeks						
Humeroradial	0	13	13	0	0	0
	1–4	7	4	0	0	3
Femoropatellar	0	11	3	0	0	0
	1–4	9	2	11	0	4
Tarsocrural	0	18	17	0	0	0
	1–4	2	0	1	0	2
11–14 weeks						
Humeroradial	0	16	14	0	0	0
	1–4	4	2	2	0	2
Femoropatellar	0	7	3	0	0	0
	1–4	13	7	5	2	3
Tarsocrural	0	19	19	0	0	0
	1–4	1	0	0	0	1

immediately after occurrence of a lesion [27]. For the pig, we can conclude that a similar dynamic picture emerges, with differences per joint. Unexpectedly, there does not seem be a straightforward relation with the time window until 7–13 weeks of age, when the growth cartilage is still vascularized [11, 12]. The current paradigm is that OC is very likely caused by a failure of the vascular supply of the growth cartilage through cartilage canals in specific focal areas, which then leads to small necrotic areas that are not yet visible radiographically and are hence called osteochondrosis latens. If not resolved, these lesions may become larger and of clinical relevance, at which stage the term osteochondrosis manifesta is used [27]. Whether or not OC latens lesions will turn into OC manifesta lesions depends on both the initial size of the lesions and the repair capacity of the cartilage, which decreases rapidly with time, as the animal gets older [28]. This latter aspect is influenced by the changes in vascularization of the epiphyseal growth cartilage due to the ongoing process of endochondral ossification that will ultimately lead to the mature state in which there is only avascular articular cartilage left.

Visual scoring and pressure mat reproducibility and comparison with histology

In this study, visual scoring of lameness and the pressure mat showed both a good reproducibility within session measurements (Tables 4 and 5). Only one relationship was found between the hind pasterns and the femoropatellar joint. In the literature, visual assessment as a

Table 4 Percentages of the frequencies of all visual scoring categories scored (VS scores) by both raters for all pigs measured at all time points

Traits	Agreement (%)	Disagreement (%)	Missing scores (%)
O or X shape fore legs	95	4	1
Sickled or Buckled fore legs	46	54	0
Steep/Low angled Pasterns fore	94	6	0
Claw size fore	99	0	1
O or X shape hind legs	88	11	1
Straight or Sickled hind legs	94	5	1
Steep/Low angled Pasterns hind	91	8	1
Claw size hind	99	0	1
Ham	91	8	1
Gait pattern	93	6	1
Twisting hocks	99	0	1
Swaying hind	95	4	1

Table 5 Intra-class correlation data for the pressure mat parameters

	Average FMAX	Average VI	Average CA	Average Pmax
ICC(1)	0.58	0.60	0.56	0.44
F-Test	5.51	5.75	4.98	3.50
P value	<0.05	<0.05	<0.05	<0.05

potential indication of OC has only been compared with macroscopic joint assessments thus far [19, 29]. Some reports claim no relationship [30, 31], or weak associations [13], whereas others claim to have found positive associations when lesions were severe [32], or even strong associations between leg weakness and OC macroscopic scores, at joint level only [33], or animal and joint level [29]. Our results hence seem to reflect the current contradictory position in the literature regarding this relation. Until recently, quantifying lameness was usually performed by a force plate system, measuring the ground reaction forces. However, our more recent pressure mat system is able to provide information on the pressure distribution pattern of the foot or claw, and has already been used successfully in recent studies in horses, cattle, dogs and pigs [16–18, 34], however never in this study format for detecting OC. For the pressure mat, very few associations with histological data were established in this study, mostly with hind limb and animal level parameters. Other more direct comparisons between the two methods were unsuccessful. The reason for this could be the low number of pigs having clinical OC, and the presence of only sub clinical OC. This would be the reason why conformational changes, in terms of lameness, are not occurring due to OC, or that if there are conformational changes taking place, that they are actually occurring but they are not linked to OC. This makes it difficult to appreciate the full potential of the pressure mat in detecting the earliest signs of OC in-vivo, as intended in this study, and requires more testing to be performed on larger populations with more clinical OC present.

Conclusions

Whereas the frequency of clinical OC lesions in this study was much lower than expected, histological prevalence of OC lesions was relatively high, especially in the femoropatellar joint, providing a good opportunity to assess the potential value of the in-vivo measuring systems under scrutiny for the detection of subclinical porcine OC. Moreover, as in other studies, the strong bilateral character of OC was confirmed. From the positive correlations found between radiological and histological findings in all joints and especially in the femoropatellar joint, we can conclude that in-vivo radiography performs well in terms of diagnosing and monitoring OC only at high radiographic scores and works safely in pigs at a young age. Lesions were already radiographically detected at 7 weeks of age and progression and regression/resolution of lesions continued until 14 weeks of age, which suggests that the PNR may occur later in time, than previously expected. Both visual scoring of lameness and pressure mat measurements appeared to be repeatable and well feasible in a logistical sense, but their relationship to the gold standard was weak and they are not apt to detect subclinical OC. Nevertheless, further development of the pressure mat approach seems to show potential for high-throughput assessments of joint disorders in pigs, even at a very young age and warrants further exploration in more heavily affected populations and over a longer timescale.

Methods

Animals and experimental set-up

Nineteen "Topigs 20" piglets at weaning age (4 weeks of age, Van Beek BV, Lelystad, NL) were used for this study. Male-female numbers were close to a 50/50 ratio with 10 males and 9 females to have a good gender distribution. The animals were housed in three groups in relatively equal size pens (153 cm × 256 cm) equipped with toys and smooth wooden plates covering half of the floor to increase slipperiness and the chance of developing OC [20]. An 18 h light-dark cycle was used and stall temperature was set at 24 °C. Pigs were fed ad libitum with a customised diet with a high concentration of proteins (20 % feed) including a high volume of lysine (14.0 g/kg feed) and without cartilage residues (Research Diet Services B.V., Wijk bij Duurstede, NL) and had constant access to water. The pigs were housed for 1 week on arrival for adaptation and training purposes, and were 14 weeks old at the end of the study. The study was divided into four periods of three weeks, separated by weekly in-vivo measuring time-points. Every week, all pigs were weighed using a standard scale (Schippers BV, Bladel, NL). At each period, randomly selected pigs were euthanized and the humeroradial, femoropatellar and tarsocrural joints were examined macroscopically and histologically at specific locations for the presence of OC lesions. All joints were examined

Table 6 Associations between visual scoring and histology (9 joint locations - $n = 12$)

Visual scoring element	Animal or Joint level	Spearman's rank correlation test	Benjamini and Hochberg correction
Pasterns hind	Femoropatellar	−.786 ($P = 0.00$)	0.01

Table 7 Associations between pressure mat and histology data (9 joint locations - $n = 12$)

Pressure mat ASIs of kinetic factors		Histology OC score level (Joint or animal level)	Spearman's test	Benjamini and Hochberg correction
Fore/Hind ASIs	ASI CA Right	Animal	−0.772 ($p = 0.00$)	0.05
	ASI Pmax Right	Femoropatellar	0.822 ($p = 0.00$)	0.03
	ASI Pmax Left	Femoropatellar	0.751 ($p = 0.00$)	0.05

specifically at specific sites known to develop osteochondrotic lesions (24 total). The list of sites is based on a previous study for macroscopic evaluations in pigs that originated from horses [19]. Three pigs were euthanized at the first three time points and ten at the last one. The ten pigs, of the last time point, were the only ones to be radiographed. Radiographic monitoring of these pigs took place at the last 3 time points (Additional file 1).

Visual scoring

The method used to score the pigs was derived from a scoring system previously devised by Van Steenbergen [35] and used in a previous study on OC [29]. Briefly, nine anatomical and three mobility categories were scored each with two opposing traits. In this study, due to the small number and young age of the pigs, we regrouped the 1–9 category scale system into a three-point scale (Additional file 2).

Pressure mat analysis

The claw pressures were measured using a Footscan 3D 2 m-system (RsScan International, Olen, Belgium) containing 16 384 force pressure sensors operating at a frequency of 126 Hz. The mat was protected by a 0.5 mm thick mat (shore value 65° ± 5) and was set into a "runway" system so the pigs could "strike" the mat precisely (Fig. 4). Pigs were trained in the first week to perform "successful runs", in which they trotted smoothly, in straight line and with their heads staying horizontal. To avoid any influence of velocity and other interfering parameters (e.g. growth) on the results, asymmetry indexes (ASI's) of the Peak Vertical Force (Fmax in N), Peak Vertical Pressure (Pmax in N/cm^2), Contact Area (CA in cm^2) and Vertical Impulse (VI in Ns) were used as outcome parameters, as previously described in Meijer et al. [31]. The ASIs were calculated using the following formula: [(Left parameter − Right parameter)/ 0.5X (Left parameter + Right parameter)]X100.

Radiographical analysis

Radiographs were taken of the ten pigs that were euthanized at the end of the study, at 8, 11 and 14 weeks of age. The images were taken with a two-view setting for all three joints on both sides (Left and Right): a lateromedial view and cranial/dorsal view, using a Philips Optimus full radiography digital system with flat panel detectors (FPDs). Settings for the contrast (mA) and density (kVp) were for pigs at 8 weeks of age: 55 kV and 5.5mAs for all joints (no grid used) using medial/lateral and cranial caudal views. The settings for the larger pigs (11 weeks and 14 weeks old) medial/lateral views (no grid) were used with 60 kV and 8mAs settings for the

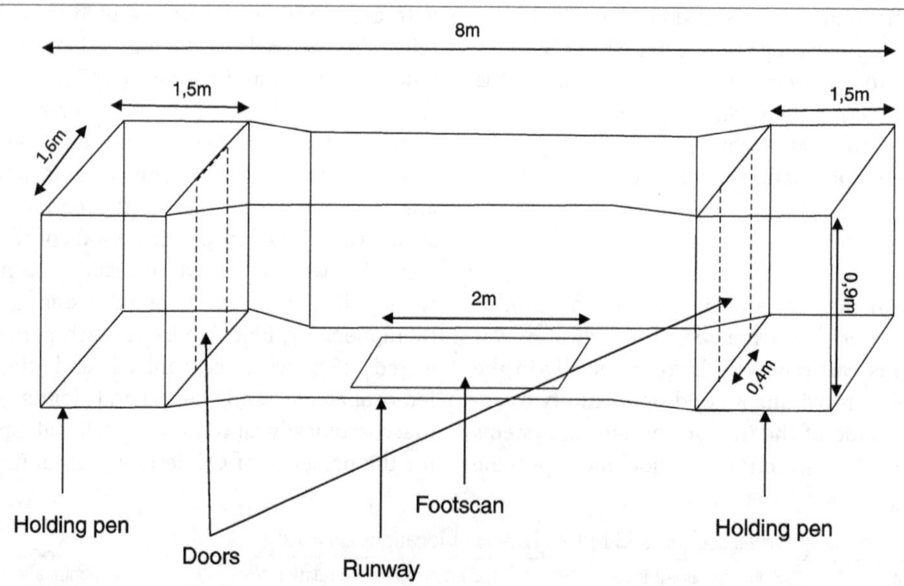

Fig. 4 Schematic drawing of the custom-built runway with a pressure mat for quantitative gait assessment

Table 8 Radiography grading (from Dik et al. [9])

Grade	Classification	Bone contour	Subchondral bone texture	Fragment
0	Normal	Rounded	Diffuse density	Absent
1	Minimal	Smoothly flattened	Obscure lucency	Absent
2	Mild	Irregularly flattened	Obvious, ill-bordered local lucency	Absent
3	Moderate	Small, rounded/irregular concavity	Obvious, well-bordered local lucency	Small fragment(s)
4	Severe	Large, rounded/irregular concavity	Obvious, well-defined extensive lucency	Large fragment(s)

humeroradial and femoropatellar joints. These 2 joints had also a caudal cranial view taken (with grid) at 60–63 kV and 10–12.5mAs. For the tarsocrural joint we used a plantar/dorsal and medial/lateral view (no grid) with a 55–60 kV and 5-10mAs setting. The variations in the settings are due to the fact settings had to be adapted due to the growth of the animals during the study. Prior to radiography, the pigs were sedated using Stresnil (azaperone 40 mg/ml-Janssen Animal Health Benelux) intramuscularly, in a dose of 1 ml/10 kg. X-rays were assessed independently by 2 veterinary radiologists, using a 0–4 scale adapted from a grading system previously used in horses [9]. To allow a better comparison between radiography and histology, the joints were imaged in such a way that they would encompass the same locations that were assessed with histology. The grading is detailed in Table 8.

Macroscopic grading of joints

At 5, 8 and 11 weeks of age, three pigs were euthanized at each time point and at 14 weeks of age for the remaining ten pigs were euthanized. Euthanasia was carried out using pentobarbital (200 mg/kg) injected intracardially (Euthanimal, Alfasan, Woerden, NL) after they had been previously sedated with Stresnil (azaperone 40 mg/ml-Janssen Animal Health Benelux) intramuscularly, in a dose of 1 ml/10 kg. At necropsy, all three joints were scored using a 0–4 scale, as described by van Grevenhof et al. [19] with 0 meaning OC-free, and 1–4 representing minimal, mild, moderate and severe lesions. The scoring was carried out independently by both researchers involved in the study.

Histology

After necropsy, all joints were cut into 0.3 cm thick slices using a band saw, in a sagittal approach in order to visualise cartilage and subchondral bone (except for the right side samples of the pigs from the 2nd time point, which were cut in a frontal plane). Samples were directly processed for histology, except for the left side samples for the 3 pigs of the 3rd time point and the ten pigs from the last time point. Only few samples from these ten pigs were selected for logistical reasons, as it was technically too difficult to be able to analyse all samples. This selection was made using a simple visual examination of the cut tissue and first took place on the cut samples that showed OC lesions on radiographs during any one of the radiograph imaging time points. Two locations of that same joint (medial and lateral) were selected, to obtain an OC positive and negative sample (as normally only either the medial or lateral side is affected). If both sides were OC positive, then control samples were selected on the contralateral joint. Controls were randomized by selecting samples blindly from the list of samples which had corresponding negative radiographs for OC. From all the other radiographically negative joint locations random samples were chosen as control samples. All these pre-selected samples were examined by a veterinary clinician. All samples from this study were fixated in formalin, decalcified in 10 % EDTA and embedded in paraffin before being cut into 3 μm slices and stained with haematoxylin and eosin, and then scored on a 0–4 scale (Table 9).

Table 9 Schematic overview of the histological grading system used in this study

Grade	Classification	Signs
0	Normal	Vessels with erythrocytes, No necrotic areas, No irregularities on ossification front, Normal thickness of cartilage
1	Normal-Mod	Vessels with erythrocytes, Few to no very small necrotic areas, Some irregularities on ossification front, Some mild focal thickening of cartilage
2	Moderate	Vessels with/without erythrocytes, Some mild necrotic areas (not large), Mild irregularities on ossification front, Moderate focal thickening of cartilage
3	Mod-Severe	Vessels mostly without erythrocytes, Some large necrotic areas, Distinct irregularities on ossification front, areas of thickened cartilage
4	Severe	Vessels without or with extremely few erythrocytes, very large necrotic areas, Very severe irregularities of ossification front, Severe thickening of cartilage areas

Statistical analysis

All statistical analyses were performed using the statistical program R (R: A Language and Environment for Statistical Computing, R Core Team, R Foundation for Statistical Computing, Vienna, Austria) and IBM SPSS Statistics 22 (IBM Corp. Released 2013. IBM SPSS Statistics for Windows, Version 22.0. Armonk, NY: IBM Corp).

Bilaterally symmetrical aspect of OC

The degree of bilateral occurrence of presence and absence of lesions was examined by calculating the percentages of occurrences of total, partial or no bilateralism of histological findings between Left and Right joints.

Radiography versus histology

The agreement strength between both methods was assessed using a receiver operating characteristic (ROC) curve that generates an area under the curve (AUC) statistic. This was performed on the histological and radiographic data from all examined joints from the last ten pigs of the study, where results for both techniques were available (Additional file 3).

Visual scoring and pressure mat reproducibility

The frequencies of agreement and disagreement between both raters for all visual scoring aspects were counted and transformed into percentages (Table 4). For the pressure mat, an ICC (inter class correlation) was calculated using a one-way system, to measure the intra-assay variation of all four kinetic parameters from three successful runs each pig performed at all time points. The pressure mat software rating the subjects was considered as the constant and the pigs' runs during one session as the random effects (Table 5). ICC outcomes were deduced using the Landis and Koch's agreement scale [36].

Visual scoring and pressure mat versus histology

Categorical H scores were transformed into continuous ones using the liability model used by van Grevenhof et al. for all joint locations [37, 38] to be able to compare them to the in-vivo method results which measure according to joint or animal level. Joint locations H scores were added up into joint level H scores and these were added up to make animal level H scores. A Spearman's correlation test was used and a Benjamini and Hochberg false discovery rate was applied to $p = 0.05$ to determine significant p-values for individual tests. This study was approved by the Ethical committee of Utrecht University (DEC N. 2011.III.08.092.).

Additional files

Additional file 1: Description: Illustration of the timeline of the analysis. (PDF 112 kb)

Additional file 2: Description: Visual scoring characteristics and scoring categories for anatomical and mobility traits (PDF 86 kb)

Additional file 3: Description: Final data set obtained for all pigs for histology and radiography Table 4a. Radiographic and histological joint assessments for the right side Table 4b. Radiographic and histological joint assessments for the left side. (PDF 186 kb)

Abbreviations

ASI: asymmetry index; AUC: area under the curve; CA: contact area; Fmax: peak vertical force; FPD: flat panel detector; ICC: intra-class correlation; OC: osteochondrosis; Pmax: peak vertical pressure; PNR: point of no return; ROC: receiver operating characteristic; VI: vertical impulse.

Competing interests

There are no present financial, professional, or personal conflicting interests from any of the authors involved in the writing of this article.

Authors' contributions

CPB was involved in devising the aim and the experimental design of this study, in generating and analysing the data and the writing of this manuscript. EM contributed to the planning of the study and the gathering and analysis of the data. AvN and AS assisted in the analysis of the data. RvW and WB provided assistance in designing the study, and assisted in the analysis of the data. All the authors assisted in the reviewing of this manuscript during the writing process and have read and accepted the final version of this manuscript. All authors read and approved the final manuscript.

Acknowledgments

The authors would like to thank the animal caretakers of our department for caring for the animals and for their help designing and building the runway system and the pens. We are also very grateful for the insights and expertise provided by Nancy Rietbroek and Leo van Leengoed, on the practical, scientific and medical aspects of the study. We would like to thank Andrea Gröne for her advice and support to enable the analysis of the histological samples and Guy Grinwis for his assistance with making the pictures of the histological slides. This work is funded by the Technology Foundation STW (grant number 11116), by the Institute for Pig Genetics BV (IPG) and by the Product Board Animal Feed (PDV).

Author details

[1]Department of Farm Animal Health, Faculty of Veterinary Medicine, Utrecht University, Yalelaan 7, NL-3584 CL Utrecht, The Netherlands. [2]Department of Equine Sciences, Faculty of Veterinary Medicine, Utrecht University, Yalelaan 112-114, NL-3584 CM Utrecht, The Netherlands. [3]Department of Surgery and Anaesthesia of Domestic Animals, Ghent University, 17 Salisburylaan 133, B-9820 Merelbeke, Belgium.

References

1. Crenshaw TD. Arthritis or OCD-identification and prevention. Adv Pork Prod. 2006;17:199.
2. Jørgensen B. Osteochondrosis/osteoarthrosis and claw disorders in sows, associated with leg weakness. Acta Vet Scand. 2000;41:123–38.
3. Nakano T, Brennan JJ, Aherne FX. Leg weakness and osteochondrosis in swine: a review. Can J Anim Sci. 1987;67:883–901.
4. Jørgensen B, Sorensen MT. Different rearing intensities of gilts: II. Effects on subsequent leg weakness and longevity. Livest Prod Sci. 1998;54:167–71.
5. Ytrehus B, Carlson CS, Ekman S. Etiology and Pathogenesis of Osteochondrosis. Vet Pathol Online. 2007;44:429–48.
6. Thorp BH, Farquharson C, Kwan APL, Loveridge N. Osteochondrosis/dyschondroplasia: failure of chondrocyte differentiation. Equine Vet J. 1993; 25:13–8.

7. Olstad K, Ytrehus B, Ekman S, Carlson CS, Dolvik NI. Early lesions of articular osteochondrosis in the distal femur of foals. Vet Pathol Online. 2011;48(6):1165–75.
8. Olstad K, Ytrehus B, Ekman S, Carlson CS, Dolvik NI. Epiphyseal cartilage canal blood supply to the tarsus of foals and relationship to osteochondrosis. Equine Vet J. 2008;40(1):30–9.
9. Dik KJ, Enzerink E, Weeren PR. Radiographic development of osteochondral abnormalities, in the hock and stifle of Dutch Warmblood foals, from age 1 to 11 months. Equine Vet J. 1999;31:9–15.
10. Laverty S, Girard C. Pathogenesis of epiphyseal osteochondrosis. Vet J. 2013; 197(1):3–12.
11. Ytrehus B, Carlson CS, Lundeheim N, Mathisen L, Reinholt FP, Teige J, Ekman S. Vascularisation and osteochondrosis of the epiphyseal growth cartilage of the distal femur in pigs—development with age, growth rate, weight and joint shape. Bone. 2004;34:454–65.
12. Ytrehus B, Ekman S, Carlson CS, Teige J, Reinholt FP. Focal changes in blood supply during normal epiphyseal growth are central in the pathogenesis of osteochondrosis in pigs. Bone. 2004;35:1294–306.
13. Jørgensen B, Arnbjerg J, Aaslyng M. Pathological and Radiological Investigations on Osteochondrosis in Pigs, Associated with Leg Weakness. J Vet Med Ser A. 1995;42:489–504.
14. Olstad K, Kongsro J, Grindflek E, Dolvik NI. Consequences of the natural course of articular osteochondrosis in pigs for the suitability of computed tomography as a screening tool. BMC Vet Res. 2014;10:212.
15. Olstad K, Cnudde V, Masschaele B, Thomassen R, Dolvik N. Micro-computed tomography of early lesions of osteochondrosis in the tarsus of foals. Bone. 2008;43(3):574–83.
16. Van der Tol PPJ, Metz JHM, Noordhuizen-Stassen EN, Back W, Braam CR, Weijs WA. The vertical ground reaction force and the pressure distribution on the claws of dairy cows while walking on a flat substrate. J Dairy Sci. 2003;86:2875–83.
17. Oosterlinck M, Bosmans T, Gasthuys F, Polis I, Van Ryssen B, Dewulf J, Pille F. Accuracy of pressure plate kinetic asymmetry indices and their correlation with visual gait assessment scores in lame and nonlame dogs. Am J Vet Res. 2011;72:820–5.
18. Oosterlinck M, Pille F, Back W, Dewulf J, Gasthuys F. Use of a stand-alone pressure plate for the objective evaluation of forelimb symmetry in sound ponies at walk and trot. Vet J. 2010;183:305–9.
19. Van Grevenhof EM, Ott S, Hazeleger W, van Weeren PR, Bijma P, Kemp B. The effects of housing system and feeding level on the joint-specific prevalence of osteochondrosis in fattening pigs. Livest Sci. 2011;135:53–61.
20. Dewey CE, Friendship RM, Wilson MR. Clinical and postmortem examination of sows culled for lameness. Can Vet J. 1993;34:555.
21. van Grevenhof EM, Ducro BJ, van Weeren PR, van Tartwijk JM, van Den Belt AJ, Bijma P. Prevalence of various radiographic manifestations of osteochondrosis and their correlations between and within joints in Dutch Warmblood horses. Equine Vet J. 2009;41:11–6.
22. Bourzac C, Alexander K, Rossier Y, Laverty S. Comparison of radiography and ultrasonography for the diagnosis of osteochondritis dissecans in the equine femoropatellar joint. Equine Vet J. 2009;41:685–92.
23. Biezyński J, Skrzypczak P, Piatek A, Kościółek N, Drozdzyńska M. Assessment of treatment of Osteochondrosis dissecans (OCD) of shoulder joint in dogs–the results of two years of experience. Pol J Vet Sci. 2012;15:285–90.
24. Eibed M, Zimmermann W. The radiographic diagnosis of osteochondrosis in pigs: A retrospective study. Swine Health Prod. 1998;6:121–5.
25. Devine DV, VanPelt SR, Boileau MJ. What Is Your Diagnosis? J Am Vet Med Assoc. 2011;238:39–40.
26. Van Weeren PR, van Oldruitenborgh-Oosterbaan MMS, Barneveld A. The influence of birth weight, rate of weight gain and final achieved height and sex on the development of osteochondrotic lesions in a population of genetically predisposed Warmblood foals. Equine Vet J. 1999;31:26–30.
27. Van Weeren PR. Chapter 88 - Osteochondrosis. In: Auer JA, Stick JA, editors. Equine Surg. Fourthth ed. Saint Louis: W.B. Saunders; 2012. p. 1239–55.
28. Ekman S, Carlson CS, van Weeren PR. Third International Workshop on Equine Osteochondrosis, Stockholm, 29-30th May 2008. Equine Vet J. 2009;41:504–7.
29. de Koning DB, van Grevenhof EM, Laurenssen BFA, Ducro BJ, Heuven HCM, de Groot PN, Hazeleger W, Kemp B. Associations between osteochondrosis and conformation and locomotive characteristics in pigs. J Anim Sci. 2012;90:4752–63.
30. Goedegebuure SA, Rothschild MF, Christian LL, Ross RF. Severity of osteochondrosis in three genetic lines of Duroc swine divergently selected for front-leg weakness. Livest Prod Sci. 1988;19:487–98.
31. Carlson CS, Hilley HD, Henrikson CK, Meuten DJ. The ultrastructure of osteochondrosis of the articular-epiphyseal cartilage complex in growing swine. Calcif Tissue Int. 1986;38:44–51.
32. Lundeheim N. Genetic analysis of osteochondrosis and leg weakness in the Swedish pig progeny testing scheme. Acta Agric Scand. 1987;37:159–73.
33. Stern S, Lundeheim N, Johansson K, Andersson K. Osteochondrosis and leg weakness in pigs selected for lean tissue growth rate. Livest Prod Sci. 1995; 44:45–52.
34. Meijer E, Bertholle CP, Oosterlinck M, van der Staay FJ, Back W, van Nes A. Pressure mat analysis of the longitudinal development of pig locomotion in growing pigs after weaning. BMC Vet Res. 2014;10.
35. Van Steenbergen EJ. Description and evaluation of a linear scoring system for exterior traits in pigs. Livest Prod Sci. 1989;23:163–81.
36. Landis JR, Koch GG. The measurement of observer agreement for categorical data. Biometrics. 1977;33:159–74.
37. Falconer DS. The inheritance of liability to certain diseases, estimated from the incidence among relatives. Ann Hum Genet. 1965;29:51–76.
38. Van Grevenhof EM, Heuven HCM, van Weeren PR, Bijma P. The relationship between growth and osteochondrosis in specific joints in pigs. Livest Sci. 2012;143:85–90.

2

Evaluation of an accelerated hydrogen peroxide disinfectant to inactivate porcine epidemic diarrhea virus in swine feces on aluminum surfaces under freezing conditions

Kimberlee L. Baker[1], Paul R. Thomas[2,3], Locke A. Karriker[1,3], Alejandro Ramirez[1,3], Jianqiang Zhang[1], Chong Wang[1] and Derald J. Holtkamp[1*]

Abstract

Background: Since its emergence in 2013, porcine epidemic diarrhea virus (PEDV) spread rapidly throughout the country due, in part, to contaminated livestock trailers. The objective of this study was to test the efficacy of an accelerated hydrogen peroxide (AHP) disinfectant for inactivating PEDV in swine feces on metal surfaces under freezing conditions. One 15.24 X 15.24 X 2.54 cm aluminum coupon, contaminated with swine feces, and randomly matched to one pig was the experimental unit. Eight treatment groups representing two AHP concentrations (1:16 and 1:32) in a 10% propylene glycol solution, two contact times in a -10 °C freezer (40 min and 60 min), and two levels of fecal contamination (5 mL and 10 mL) in addition to negative and positive control groups were evaluated. Forty 3-week-old pigs, intragastrically inoculated with the contents of the coupons after treatment, were used as a bioassay to determine the infectivity of PEDV after treatment. Infectivity was determined by detection of virus with a nucleocapsid (N) gene-based quantitative real-time reverse transcription polymerase chain reaction (RT-qPCR) on rectal swabs collected from the inoculated pigs on days three and seven post-inoculation.

Results: All post-treatment swabs from the negative control coupons were negative for PEDV via RT-qPCR. All post-treatment swabs collected from coupons in the AHP disinfectant treatment groups and the positive control group were positive for PEDV via RT-qPCR. For the bioassay, no rectal swabs from pigs in the negative control (0 of 4) or the AHP disinfectant treatment groups (0 of 32) were positive for PEDV. Rectal swabs from all pigs within the positive control group (4 of 4) were positive for PEDV by RT-qPCR.

Conclusions: Under the conditions of this study, 1:16 and 1:32 dilutions of the AHP disinfectant successfully inactivated PEDV in swine feces on metal surfaces when applied at -10 °C with 40 or 60 min of contact time. This study also suggests that a positive RT-qPCR result for PEDV on an environmental sample should be expected when the AHP disinfectant is applied under freezing conditions, but does not necessarily indicate that an infectious dose of PEDV remains after disinfection.

Keywords: Swine, PEDV, Disinfection, Temperature, Accelerated hydrogen peroxide

* Correspondence: holtkamp@iastate.edu
[1]Department of Veterinary Diagnostic and Production Animal Medicine, Iowa State University College of Veterinary Medicine, 1809 S Riverside Dr, Ames, IA, USA
Full list of author information is available at the end of the article

Background

Porcine epidemic diarrhea (PED) was first described in 1971 as cases of profuse, watery diarrhea affecting all ages of pigs in England [1]. In 1978, a novel coronavirus, porcine epidemic diarrhea virus (PEDV), was determined to be the causative agent [2, 3]. The first cases of PEDV in the United States were confirmed during May 2013 from farms in Iowa and Indiana [4]. PEDV spread rapidly throughout the United States after its introduction mainly due to the ease of transmission via fecal-oral and pig-to-pig contact [5]. Livestock trailers that haul pigs to and from collection points such as livestock auctions or harvest facilities have been implicated as mechanical vectors for PEDV [6]. Contaminated livestock trailers likely pose a significant risk for PEDV transmission and movement throughout the country.

This risk has historically been mitigated through trailer sanitation and decontamination procedures developed for porcine reproductive and respiratory syndrome virus (PRRSV) when high pressure washing alone was found insufficient to inactivate PRRSV [7–10]. Because disinfection and drying are more effective when applied to a clean trailer with little or no remaining organic matter, the industry standard for sanitation and decontamination of livestock trailers includes trailer washing, disinfection, and drying, either naturally or with a thermo-assisted drying and decontamination (TADD) system [7–9]. Similar research on PEDV demonstrated that the industry standard wash, disinfection, and dry successfully inactivated PEDV on metal surfaces when detergent and a combination of quaternary ammonium and glutaraldehyde disinfect were used [11].

The industry standard wash, disinfect, and dry is always the best method for livestock trailer sanitation and decontamination. For this reason, swine producers should always strive to use the industry standard sanitation and decontamination protocols on all livestock trailers between loads. However, a complete wash, disinfect, and dry requires an investment in time, logistics, and specialized facilities which deters some swine producers and contract haulers from performing the industry standard protocols between every load of pigs hauled. Consequently, a significant number of pigs, especially market pigs, are hauled on trailers that are not subjected to any sanitation or decontamination procedures between loads, posing a significant risk. Successfully decreasing the risk of PEDV transmission from contaminated livestock trailers may depend on the development of cost-effective sanitation procedures, as an alternative to doing nothing, which can be completed in a short period of time without specialized facilities. In addition, identification of disinfectants and other decontamination processes that work in the presence of some organic matter may decrease the risk of viral transmission from livestock trailers that are washed, but sanitation and decontamination procedures are not closely monitored or performed poorly.

Recent PEDV research demonstrated that holding a metal surface contaminated with PEDV positive feces at 71 °C for 10 min or 20 °C for 7 days was efficacious at inactivating PEDV [12]. An accelerated hydrogen peroxide® (AHP®) disinfectant (Intervention®, Virox Technologies Inc., Oakville, Ontario, Canada) successfully inactivated PEDV in the presence of fecal contamination on metal surfaces with a 30-min contact time at 20 °C. The concentrated form of the AHP disinfectant was efficacious at dilutions of 1:16 and 1:32 in the presence of feces [13]. Intervention® is labeled as virucidal at dilution rates of 1:16 to 1:64 in the presence of 200 ppm hard water and 5% serum load with a 5-min contact time. It contains anionic surfactants, nonionic surfactants, and stabilizers that help improve the stability and microbicidal action of hydrogen peroxide [14, 15]. PEDV outbreaks, however, tend to be more prevalent in the cooler winter months where a complete wash, disinfect, and dry is more difficult to complete due to freezing temperatures. Water along with most aqueous disinfectants freeze around 0 °C; making trailer sanitation and decontamination difficult. It has been previously demonstrated that diluting a quaternary ammonium and glutaraldehyde combination disinfectant (Synergize; Preserve International, Atlanta, Georgia) in either a 10% propylene glycol (PG) or 40% methanol solution prevented freezing and allowed the disinfectant to inactivate PRRSV at temperatures below 0 °C [10].

The objective of this study was to evaluate two concentrations of an AHP disinfectant in a 10% PG solution to determine if the mixture was sufficient to inactivate PEDV in the presence of swine feces on metal surfaces at -10 °C. Conditions were chosen to mimic those found in commercial livestock trailers in winter months after most of the fecal and organic matter has been removed by scraping and a traditional wash is unavailable.

Methods

Experimental design

The experimental unit was a single aluminum coupon contaminated with swine feces matched to an individual 3-week old pig. The pig was intragastrically inoculated with the contents of the coupon post treatment, as a bioassay to determine if the treatment applied to the contaminated coupon effectively inactivated PEDV. Three-week old pigs were used in this study because they are relatively susceptible to infection with PEDV, but mortality is rare. Previous work reported that 100% of 21-day-old pigs inoculated with 10 mL of a virulent PEDV prototype isolate with titers of 5.6–560 $TCID_{50}$/ml were infected, but pigs inoculated with lower titers (0.0056–0.56 $TCID_{50}$/ml) of PEDV were not infected [16].

The primary outcome variable was the proportion of pigs in each treatment group that were PEDV-positive by bioassay to determine if infectious PEDV was present after the disinfectant treatment. The null hypothesis was that there was no difference between the positive control group and the disinfectant treatment groups in the proportion of pigs infected with PEDV after being inoculated with the material collected from the coupons. The bioassay result was determined by nucleocapsid (N) gene-based quantitative real-time reverse transcription polymerase chain reaction (RT-qPCR) performed at the Iowa State University Veterinary Diagnostic Laboratory (ISU VDL) on rectal swabs collected from each pig on days three and seven post-inoculation. The primers and probe of the PEDV RT-qPCR were previously described [6, 16, 17]. Each PCR was set up and performed in accordance with previously described procedures [13, 16, 17]. Current viral culture methods make it difficult to culture wild-type PEDV outside of an animal model. Therefore, to determine if live infectious PEDV is present in a sample, a bioassay using an animal model remained the best alternative. The use of a bioassay also eliminated questions about the cytotoxic impact feces and disinfectant may have had on the outcome of virus isolation.

Personnel performing disinfectant treatments, necropsies, and collecting samples were not blinded to the treatment groups. Blinding these individuals was not possible because all procedures were performed in a specific order, starting with the negative control group and ending with the positive control group, to minimize the risk of transmitting PEDV between treatment groups. Laboratory personnel that performed the RT-qPCR testing for PEDV and personnel performing the statistical analyses were blinded to the treatment groups.

Coupons

Forty 15.24 cm X 15.24 cm X 2.54 cm aluminum coupons were manufactured using aluminum with a material thickness of 0.32 cm, resembling the type of material found in livestock trailers. These coupons were used in previous studies evaluating the efficacy of other sanitation and decontamination procedures for PEDV inactivation [11–13]. To simulate the cleaning action of the AHP disinfectant and runoff seen in commercial livestock trailers as the AHP disinfectant is transformed from foam to a liquid, six 8 mm diameter holes were drilled at the junction of the bottom and sidewall of the coupon.

Treatment groups

Two volumes of fecal contamination (5 mL and 10 mL); two concentrations of AHP disinfectant (1:16 and 1:32) prepared in a solution that was 10% PG by volume; and two contact times (40 min and 60 min) were evaluated. A positive control and negative control group were also included (Table 1). Forty minutes of contact time was chosen by applying the Arrhenius equation which in previous work led to the conclusion that for every 10 °C decrease in temperature the contact time of a disinfectant doubles [18]. PEDV-positive feces were used to contaminate coupons in the positive control group (B) and all treatment groups (C through J). PEDV negative feces were used to contaminate coupons in the negative control group (A). The negative (A) and positive (B) control groups were not sham disinfected. The AHP disinfectant used in this study was applied as a thick foam which persisted for the duration of the contact time and had minimal rinsing and diluting effects. The best candidate for a sham disinfectant would be a non-disinfecting solution that produced a persistent foam similar to that of the AHP disinfectant; however, after extensive research and pre-trial work, a suitable non-disinfecting foam was not identified by the investigators. Using a non-foam liquid for sham disinfection would result in a greater rinsing and diluting effect as the liquid would run out of the holes in the coupons at a faster rate than the persistent foam produced by the AHP disinfectant would; therefore, sham disinfection was not done. Four replicates of aluminum coupons were included for each treatment group.

Contamination and disinfection procedures

The feces used to contaminate the coupons were obtained from a previous experiment where 3-week-old pigs were inoculated with PEDV isolate US/Iowa/18984/2013 [17]. Feces were collected from pigs, confirmed to be positive for PEDV by RT-qPCR, 7 days post inoculation, which was within the peak viral shedding timeframe [17]. After collection, feces from individual pigs were stored at -80 °C. On study day 0, the feces from individual pigs were thawed and pooled into a single fecal homogenate to ensure that the amount of PEDV and composition of the feces was uniform for each replicate. Samples from each replicate were tested at the ISU VDL by RT-qPCR. The quantitative genomic copies/mL ranged from $10^{8.00}$ to $10^{9.06}$ genomic copies/mL across all replicates (Table 2 and Additional file 1). PEDV negative feces were obtained from the negative control pigs in a previous study [13]. Fecal collection and storage

Table 1 Description of treatment groups (4 replicates per treatment group)

Treatment group	Volume and PEDV status of feces	Disinfectant and concentration	Contact time at -10 °C
(A) Negative Control	5 mL PEDV-negative feces	None	None
(B) Positive Control	5 mL PEDV-positive feces	None	40 min
(C) Light, 1:32, 40 min	5 mL PEDV-positive feces	AHP at 1:32	40 min
(D) Heavy, 1:32, 40 min	10 mL PEDV-positive feces	AHP at 1:32	40 min
(E) Light, 1:16, 40 min	5 mL PEDV-positive feces	AHP at 1:16	40 min
(F) Heavy, 1:16, 40 min	10 mL PEDV-positive feces	AHP at 1:16	40 min
(G) Light, 1:32, 60 min	5 mL PEDV-positive feces	AHP at 1:32	60 min
(H) Heavy, 1:32, 60 min	10 mL PEDV-positive feces	AHP at 1:32	60 min
(I) Light, 1:16, 60 min	5 mL PEDV-positive feces	AHP at 1:16	60 min
(J) Heavy, 1:16, 60 min	10 mL PEDV-positive feces	AHP at 1:16	60 min

Table 2 Summary of PEDV RT-qPCR results for the pre-treatment and post-treatment swabs

Treatment group	Pre-treatment Ct Value and (genomic copies/mL)	Percentage positive or suspect for PEDV	Post-treatment Ct Value and (genomic copies/mL)	Percentage positive or suspect for PEDV
(A) Neg Control	>35 (0) >35 (0) >35 (0) >35 (0)	0% (0 of 4)	>35 (0) >35 (0) >35 (0) >35 (0)	0% (0 of 4)
(B) Pos Control	18.2 ($10^{8.56}$) 19.0 ($10^{8.32}$) 19.5 ($10^{8.17}$) 19.2 ($10^{8.26}$)	100% (4 of 4)	18.6 ($10^{8.44}$) 17.1 ($10^{8.88}$) 18.8 ($10^{8.38}$) 18.8 ($10^{8.38}$)	100% (4 of 4)
(C) Light, 1:32, 40 mins	17.2 ($10^{8.85}$) 17.4 ($10^{8.79}$) 17.9 ($10^{8.64}$) 17.6 ($10^{8.73}$)	100% (4 of 4)	27.1 ($10^{5.94}$) 21.0 ($10^{7.73}$) 29.1 ($10^{5.35}$) 28.6 ($10^{5.49}$)	100% (4 of 4)
(D) Heavy, 1:32, 40 mins	16.8 ($10^{8.97}$) 18.0 ($10^{8.61}$) 17.8 ($10^{8.67}$) 18.1 ($10^{8.58}$)	100% (4 of 4)	24.6 ($10^{6.67}$) 19.2 ($10^{8.26}$) 24.0 ($10^{6.85}$) 20.6 ($10^{7.85}$)	100% (4 of 4)
(E) Light, 1:16, 40 mins	18.7 ($10^{8.41}$) 17.9 ($10^{8.64}$) 18.2 ($10^{8.56}$) 18.7 ($10^{8.41}$)	100% (4 of 4)	33.6 ($10^{4.02}$) 31.1 ($10^{4.76}$) 28.9 ($10^{5.41}$) 30.7 ($10^{4.88}$)	100% (4 of 4)
(F) Heavy, 1:16, 40 mins	17.2 ($10^{8.85}$) 17.8 ($10^{8.67}$) 18.5 ($10^{8.47}$) 18.2 ($10^{8.56}$)	100% (4 of 4)	26.1 ($10^{6.23}$) 23.0 ($10^{7.14}$) 23.9 ($10^{6.88}$) 23.0 ($10^{7.14}$)	100% (4 of 4)
(G) Light, 1:32, 60 mins'	18.0 ($10^{8.61}$) 17.6 ($10^{8.73}$) 17.0 ($10^{8.91}$) 18.2 ($10^{8.56}$)	100% (4 of 4)	27.5 ($10^{5.82}$) 26.1 ($10^{6.23}$) 23.6 ($10^{6.97}$) 27.3 ($10^{5.88}$)	100% (4 of 4)
(H) Heavy, 1:32, 60 mins	17.6 ($10^{8.73}$) 17.9 ($10^{8.64}$) 18.7 ($10^{8.41}$) 17.0 ($10^{8.91}$)	100% (4 of 4)	26.1 ($10^{6.23}$) 23.7 ($10^{6.94}$) 21.5 ($10^{7.59}$) 24.8 ($10^{6.61}$)	100% (4 of 4)
(I) Light, 1:16, 60 mins	17.6 ($10^{8.73}$) 17.5 ($10^{8.76}$) 17.8 ($10^{8.67}$) 17.9 ($10^{8.64}$)	100% (4 of 4)	34.5 ($10^{3.76}$) 33.4 ($10^{4.08}$) 34.7 ($10^{3.70}$) 32.3 ($10^{4.40}$)	100% (4 of 4)
(J) Heavy, 1:16, 60 mins	16.5 ($10^{9.06}$) 18.0 ($10^{8.61}$) 17.3 ($10^{8.82}$) 20.1 ($10^{8.00}$)	100% (4 of 4)	28.0 ($10^{5.67}$) 24.9 ($10^{6.58}$) 24.7 ($10^{6.64}$) 24.9 ($10^{6.58}$)	100% (4 of 4)

procedures were the same as those for the PEDV positive feces. Prior to freezing, a sample of the PEDV negative feces was submitted to the ISU VDL to confirm its PEDV negative status. Diagnostic testing confirmed that the sample was negative for PEDV by RT-qPCR.

The in-vivo portion of the study was initiated on study day 0. Prior to contamination and treatment of the coupons, 2 mm thick plastic sheeting was placed on the floor. The plastic sheeting was changed and the floor under the plastic sheeting was disinfected with Virkon™ S disinfectant (Lanxess, Wilmington, DE, USA) between each treatment group to reduce the risk of cross contamination. For the negative control group (A), 5 mL of PEDV negative feces were applied to four aluminum coupons. Five mL of PEDV positive feces was applied to all coupons in groups B, C, E, G, and I. Ten mL of PEDV positive feces were applied to all coupons in groups D, F, H, and J (Fig. 1). For all study groups (A through J), contamination of the coupons with feces was performed using a disposable hard plastic spreader sold in hardware stores to spread adhesive on floors. A new adhesive spreader was used on each coupon to prevent cross-contamination between replicates. Five mL and 10 mL of feces, when spread evenly over the floor of each coupon, resulted in an even layer that was ≤2 mm and were chosen to reflect the range of organic matter remaining in the interior of a commercial livestock trailer after it has been manually scraped to remove bedding and feces. Following contamination with feces, all coupons were individually sampled using a commercial swab and transport system. The pre-treatment swabs were submitted to the ISU VDL to test for the presence of PEDV by RT-qPCR.

Following fecal contamination, coupons, except those assigned to the negative control group A, were pre-cooled in a commercial refrigerator, set to 4 °C for 30 min. This pre-cooling period was designed to mimic conditions in a scraped livestock trailer after transporting pigs during the winter months. Plastic sheeting was placed on the refrigerator's shelves and changed between each treatment group to prevent cross-contamination.

After the pre-cooling period, AHP disinfectant solution was applied to the contaminated coupons in the treatment groups C through J. The AHP disinfectant was prepared by diluting a 4.25% concentrate of the AHP disinfectant (Intervention®, Virox Technologies Inc., Oakville, Ontario, Canada) with tap water from a municipal water source and PG. The final AHP disinfectant solution contained 10% PG and a ratio of AHP concentrate to final solution of 1:16 for treatment groups E, F, I, and J and 1:32 for treatment groups C, D, G, and H. PG is an organic solvent that can be used as a safe anti-freezing agent when mixed with phenol, quaternary ammonium, and quaternary ammonium formaldehyde disinfectants without reducing their efficacy [19]. Coupons in the negative control (A) and positive control (B) groups were not sham disinfected. A liquid volume of approximately 30 mL of AHP disinfectant solution was applied as a foam to all 4 coupons in each treatment group (C through J) using a 5.7 L pump-up foamer (model #A8020A, Ogena Solutions, LLC, Stoney Creek, ON, Canada). To disinfect a 15.8 m double-decked livestock trailers, 189 L of AHP disinfectant would be applied over a 10-min period using a proportioning foamer with a flow rate of 18.9 L per minute. Based on the area of the coupons used in this study, 30 mL of AHP disinfectant was determined proportionally equivalent to the 189 L used on livestock trailers. Using the same 5.7 L foamer, a series of timed applications were performed prior to study initiation to establish that a 3 s application time was required to apply the 30 mL of AHP disinfectant solution.

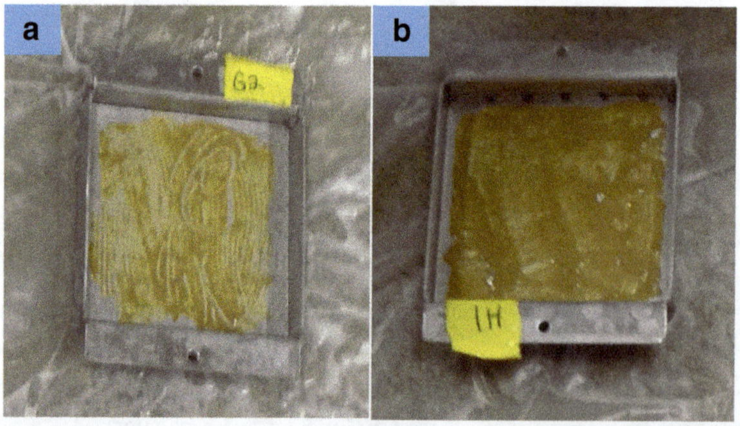

Fig. 1 Fecal contamination of aluminum coupons. Feces were applied in an even layer to aluminum coupons using an adhesive spreader. Five mL of feces were applied to coupons in treatment groups **A**, **B**, **C**, **E**, **G**, and **I**. Ten mL of feces were applied to coupons in treatment groups **D**, **F**, **H**, and **J**. One representative coupon in group G (**a**) and group H (**b**) is shown

Following treatment with AHP disinfectant solution, the coupons were placed in a freezer set at −10 °C for their allotted contact time as described in Table 1. To prevent cross contamination between treatments, the freezer drawers were lined with 2 mm plastic sheeting and a folded bath towel was placed on top of the plastic to absorb any liquid runoff from the coupons. To prevent replicates within the treatment group from cross-contaminating each other, each coupon was placed into a 16 cm X 16 cm X 3 cm pan crafted from aluminum foil. New plastic, towels and aluminum foil pans were used for every treatment group. Coupons in the positive control group (B) were also placed in the freezer for 40 min to confirm that the time at -10 °C alone was not responsible for PEDV inactivation. Coupons in the negative control group (A) were not placed in the freezer.

Ten minutes after contamination of the coupons in the negative control group (A), a post-treatment swab was taken using a commercial swab and transport system. For all other study groups (B through J), the swabs were collected following the treatment described in Table 1. All swabs collected post-treatment were submitted to the ISU VDL and tested for the presence of PEDV RNA by RT-qPCR.

After the post-treatment swab was collected, the coupon was tipped away from the holes and 10 mL of sterile 0.9% sodium chloride (saline) solution was added using a new 12 mL syringe for each coupon. A coupon dedicated toothbrush was used to re-suspend the feces/AHP disinfectant/PG/saline mixture; creating a homogenate sample suitable for recollection as inoculum. The resultant homogenate was collected using a 20-mL syringe (Fig. 2). During recollection of the inoculum sample, nitrile gloves were changed between each coupon to prevent cross contamination between replicates and 2 mm plastic sheeting was placed under the coupons and changed between treatment groups to prevent cross-contamination between treatments.

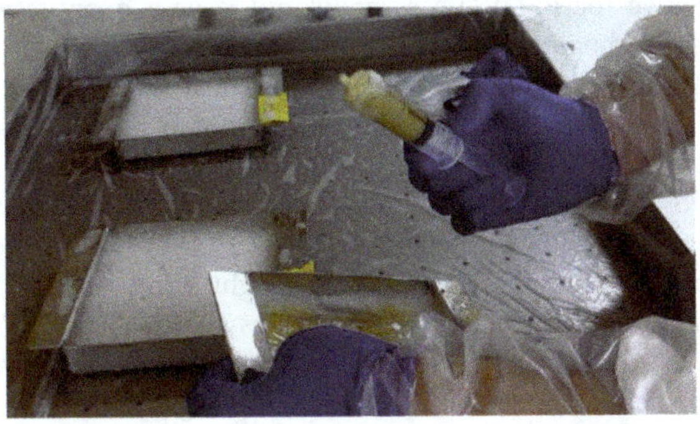

Fig. 2 Collection of feces/AHP disinfectant homogenate used to inoculate a pig for the bioassay. A mixture of feces, AHP disinfectant, PG, and saline was recollected from the coupon using a 20 mL syringe. This syringe was labeled with the coupon identification number and matched to a single pig for the bioassay

Swine bioassay

Source of animals and housing

The experimental protocol was approved by the Iowa State University Institutional Animal Care and Use Committee (Log Number: 11–14-7904-S) and the Iowa State University Institutional Biosafety Committee (Log Number 14-I-0040-A) prior to initiation of any experimental activity. Forty 3-week-old commercial pigs, 17 barrows and 23 gilts, were obtained from WeSearch, LLC in Iowa and housed in the Iowa State University Veterinary Medical Research Institute for the duration of the study. Upon delivery (study day −4), all pigs (40/40) were individually identified with a unique ID number on a plastic ear tag and weighed. Pigs were blocked by weight and then randomly assigned within each weight group to one of the 10 treatment groups (Table 1) using the RAND function in Microsoft Excel (version 2010).

On study day −1, serum and rectal swabs were collected from the pigs to confirm their PEDV negative status. Eight mL of whole blood was collected from each pig via jugular venipuncture and transferred to an 8.5 mL serum separator tube and centrifuged at 3100 g for 8 min. Serum was submitted to the ISU VDL for diagnostic testing. Serum samples were pooled (5 samples per pool) and tested for porcine reproductive and respiratory virus (PRRSV) via RT-qPCR. Individual serum samples were tested for antibodies to PRRSV using a commercial PRRS X3 Ab Test (IDEXX Laboratories, Inc., Westbrook, Maine), and for antibodies to transmissible gastroenteritis virus (TGEV) and porcine respiratory corona virus (PRCV) by a commercial TGEV/PRCV-Ab differential enzyme-linked immunosorbent assay (ELISA, SVANOVA Biotech AB, Uppsala, Sweden). Individual serum samples were also screened for antibodies to PEDV by indirect fluorescent antibody (IFA) assay following previously described procedures [16]. Rectal swabs were obtained via the same commercial swab and transport system used to swab the coupons. Individual rectal swabs were tested for TGEV, porcine rotaviruses (groups A, B and C), and PEDV by real time RT-PCRs at the ISU VDL.

Each treatment group was designated one room. The four pigs in each group were housed individually in a raised tub described in detail in previous studies [12, 13]. Individual housing was accomplished using solid transparent dividers, creating four compartments within one tub. The transparent dividers allowed visual and auditory contact between the pigs, but prevented nose-to-nose and fecal-oral contact. Urine and feces fell through a grate at the bottom of the tub and drained into a bucket to minimize the risk of contaminating the room's floor. Each section of the tub had designated water and feed sources. During the study, each pig was assigned its own bag of feed and feed cup to minimize cross contamination. Previous studies demonstrated that this housing method successfully prevented transmission of PEDV between pigs in a group [12]. Pigs were fed an age appropriate, pelleted, starter diet ad libitum. The diet consisted primarily of corn and soybean meal and did not contain porcine derived products.

Inoculation of pigs with contents of coupon post-treatment
On study day 0, the homogenate of feces, AHP disinfectant, PG and saline, collected from each coupon as described above, was immediately used to inoculate pigs for the bioassay via oral gastric gavage with a 14 French rubber catheter as previously described [12]. Each pig was inoculated with the contents of its designated coupon, with PEDV RT-qPCR results ranging from $10^{3.70}$–$10^{8.88}$ genomic copies/mL for coupons assigned to treatment groups B – J (Table 2 and Additional file 1). To prevent cross contamination between treatment groups and replicates within the same treatment, study personnel followed a strict biosecurity protocol used successfully in previous work [12]. Disposable Tyvek coveralls (DuPont, USA) and respirators were worn by personnel at all times and were changed between each treatment group. Coveralls were inspected after each inoculation and were changed between pigs if inoculum or fecal material was present. Furthermore, nitrile gloves and arm-length disposable obstetrical sleeves were worn and changed between each pig to prevent cross-contamination between replicates.

Pigs were monitored daily, on study days 0 through 7, for clinical signs consistent with PEDV by the same study investigator. On days 3 and 7 post-inoculation, rectal swabs were collected from each pig using a commercial swab and transport system. To avoid cross contamination between replicates, pigs were not removed from their compartment and personnel used the same biosecurity procedures as previously described for inoculation. A bioassay was considered positive if the rectal swab was PEDV-positive by RT-qPCR (Ct value less than 35) on study day 3 or study day 7. A bioassay was considered negative if both rectal swabs (study days 3 and 7) were PEDV-negative by RT-qPCR (Ct > 35).

On study day 7, all pigs were humanely euthanized using a penetrating captive bolt gun and necropsied. During necropsy, all organ systems were evaluated and any gross lesions or abnormal pathology was noted. Fresh and 10% formalin-fixed samples of mesenteric lymph nodes, ileum, and jejunum and fresh cecal and spiral colon contents were collected from each pig. All fresh samples were placed in a -80 °C freezer and all samples were held in the event further testing might be required to confirm the results of the swine bioassay.

All statistical analyses were performed using SAS® (Enterprise Guide 5.1; SAS Institute, Cary, NC, USA). A Fisher's Exact Test was used to evaluate pairwise differences in the proportion of pigs positive by bioassay between all 10 treatment groups. Ct values were analyzed using two way analyses of variance (ANOVA) models with treatment, time (pre versus post) and their interaction. Pre-treatment Ct values were compared between groups using an F-test. Differences in Ct values between pre- and post-treatment were assessed for each study group using a two-sided T-Test. A p value <0.05 was considered statistically significant.

Results

Pre-trial diagnostic screening

Serum and fecal samples obtained on study day −1 confirmed that all 40 pigs were negative for PEDV by RT-qPCR as well as negative for antibodies to PEDV via IFA. Additionally, all pigs were negative for PRRSV, porcine rotaviruses (groups A, B, and C), and TGEV by RT-qPCR and for antibodies to TGEV via differential ELISA. Fifteen pigs were positive, 23 were suspect, and 2 were negative for antibodies to PRCV by differential ELISA. Three pigs were positive for antibodies to PRRSV via ELISA.

Coupon swabs

PEDV RT-qPCR results from swabs taken from fecal contaminated aluminum coupons before and after treatment with AHP disinfectant are displayed in Table 2 and Additional file 1. In the negative control (A), all pre-treatment swabs, taken immediately after PEDV negative feces were applied to the four coupons, were negative for PEDV RNA by RT-qPCR. All pre-treatment swabs, taken immediately after PEDV positive feces were applied to coupons, from the positive control (B) were positive for PEDV RNA by RT-qPCR with quantitative results ranging from $10^{8.17}$–$10^{8.56}$ genomic copies/mL. Likewise, all swabs obtained after fecal contamination but prior to treatment from the coupons in groups C – J were PEDV-positive via RT-qPCR with quantitative results from $10^{8.00}$–$10^{9.06}$ genomic copies/mL. There were no significant differences in pre-treatment Ct values from the coupons assigned to the eight disinfectant (C – J) and the positive control (B) groups (p-value = 0.9435).

Post-treatment swabs (4 of 4) from the negative control (A) coupons, taken 10 min after PEDV negative feces were applied to the coupon, were negative for PEDV RNA by RT-qPCR. All (4 of 4) post-treatment swabs from the positive control (B) coupons, taken after pre-cooling and 40 min in a -10 °C freezer, were positive for PEDV RNA via RT-qPCR with quantitative results ranging from $10^{8.38}$–

$10^{8.88}$ genomic copies/mL. All (32 of 32) post-treatment swabs collected from coupons in the AHP disinfectant treatment groups C – J were positive for PEDV RNA via RT-qPCR with quantitative results ranging from $10^{3.76}$–$10^{8.26}$ genomic copies/mL. The difference in Ct values between pre- and post-treatment were significantly different than zero (*p* value <0.0001) for all of the AHP disinfectant treatment groups (C – J).

Swine bioassay

PEDV RT-qPCR results for rectal swabs taken 3 and 7 days post inoculation and the final swine bioassay results by treatment group are displayed in Table 3 and Additional file 1. Rectal swabs collected from all pigs in the negative control (A) and AHP disinfectant treatment groups C – J on study days 3 and 7 were negative for PEDV by RT-qPCR. Rectal swabs from all four pigs in the positive control (B) collected on study days 3 and 7 were positive for PEDV by RT-qPCR. The proportion of pigs positive by bioassay for the negative control (A) and all of the AHP disinfectant treatment groups (C – J) were significantly different than proportion of pigs positive in the positive control (B) group via Fishers Exact Test (*p*-value <0.05).

Discussion

Under freezing conditions (−10 °C) an AHP disinfectant prepared in a 10% PG solution inactivated PEDV in the

Table 3 Post-inoculation rectal swab PEDV N-gene RT-qPCR and swine bioassay results

Treatment Group	Day 3 Rectal Swab; Individual CT results (genomic copies / mL)	Day 3 Rectal Swab; Percentage positive for PEDV RNA	Day 7 Rectal Swab; Individual CT Results (genomic copies / mL)	Day 7 Rectal Swab; Percentage positive for PEDV RNA	Swine Bioassay Result; Percentage positive for PEDV RNA
(A) Negative Control	>35 (0) >35 (0) >35 (0) >35 (0)	0% (0 of 4)	>35 (0) >35 (0) >35 (0) >35 (0)	0% (0 of 4)	0% (0 of 4)[a]
(B) Positive Control	16.2 ($10^{9.14}$) 15.1 ($10^{9.46}$) 16.8 ($10^{8.96}$) 15.0 ($10^{9.49}$)	100% (4 of 4)	22.2 ($10^{7.37}$) 15.2 ($10^{9.43}$) 19.3 ($10^{8.23}$) 17.4 ($10^{8.79}$)	100% (4 of 4)	100% (4 of 4)[b]
(C) Light, 1:32, 40 mins	>35 (0) >35 (0) >35 (0) >35 (0)	0% (0 of 4)	>35 (0) >35 (0) >35 (0) >35 (0)	0% (0 of 4)	0% (0 of 4)[a]
(D) Heavy, 1:32, 40 mins	>35 (0) >35 (0) >35 (0) >35 (0)	0% (0 of 4)	>35 (0) >35 (0) >35 (0) >35 (0)	0% (0 of 4)	0% (0 of 4)[a]
(E) Light, 1:16, 40 mins	>35 (0) >35 (0) >35 (0) >35 (0)	0% (0 of 4)	>35 (0) >35 (0) >35 (0) >35 (0)	0% (0 of 4)	0% (0 of 4)[a]
(F) Heavy, 1:16, 40 mins	>35 (0) >35 (0) >35 (0) >35 (0)	0% (0 of 4)	>35 (0) >35 (0) >35 (0) >35 (0)	0% (0 of 4)	0% (0 of 4)[a]
(G) Light, 1:32, 60 mins	>35 (0) >35 (0) >35 (0) >35 (0)	0% (0 of 4)	>35 (0) >35 (0) >35 (0) >35 (0)	0% (0 of 4)	0% (0 of 4)[a]
(H) Heavy, 1:32, 60 mins	>35 (0) >35 (0) >35 (0) >35 (0)	0% (0 of 4)	>35 (0) >35 (0) >35 (0) >35 (0)	0% (0 of 4)	0% (0 of 4)[a]
(I) Light, 1:16, 60 mins	>35 (0) >35 (0) >35 (0) >35 (0)	0% (0 of 4)	>35 (0) >35 (0) >35 (0) >35 (0)	0% (0 of 4)	0% (0 of 4)[a]
(J) Heavy, 1:16, 60 mins	>35 (0) >35 (0) >35 (0) >35 (0)	0% (0 of 4)	>35 (0) >35 (0) >35 (0) >35 (0)	0% (0 of 4)	0% (0 of 4)[a]

[a,b] Different superscripts indicate statistically significant differences (*p*-value <0.05) by a Fishers Exact Test

presence of feces on metal surfaces. Both AHP disinfectant dilutions (1:16 and 1:32), and contact times (40 min and 60 min) evaluated were sufficient to inactivate PEDV at either fecal load (5 mL and 10 mL), under the conditions of this study. Bioassay results from this study support previous work where the same AHP disinfectant successfully inactivated PEDV in swine feces on metal surfaces at 20 °C [13]. Findings from this study demonstrate that manually removing the organic material from a trailer via scraping and then applying an AHP disinfectant may be an effective alternative to doing nothing between loads, year round. Additionally, mixing the AHP disinfectant in a 10% PG solution prevented the disinfectant solution from freezing during 40 or 60 min of contact time in a freezer set to -10 °C, supporting previously published data on utilizing PG as an antifreezing agent [10, 19].

In contrast to previous work [13], all post-treatment swabs (32 of 32), from the coupons contaminated with PEDV positive feces and then subjected to one of eight AHP disinfectant treatments (groups C-J) at -10 °C, were positive for the presence of PEDV RNA by RT-qPCR. However, none of the coupons (0 of 32) contained infectious virus as demonstrated by swine bioassay. While swine veterinarians sometimes use RT-PCR to evaluate the success of sanitation and decontamination protocols in practice, its major limitation is that it does not differentiate between infectious virus and noninfectious fragments of PEDV RNA. These results indicate that the AHP disinfectant inactivated the virus while leaving a sufficient amount of genetic material intact to interact with the primers used in the RT-qPCR assay. Hydrogen peroxide is an oxidizing agent that inactivates viruses by denaturing viral proteins, lipids and nucleic acids [20, 21]. These results suggest that denaturation of nucleic acid by the AHP disinfectant occurred to a lesser degree at lower temperatures than at higher temperatures, but this difference did not affect its ability to inactivate PEDV as demonstrated by the swine bioassay results. These results are consistent with those from previous studies where disinfection of contaminated metal surfaces with oxidizing disinfectants inactivated PEDV but did not consistently produce negative PEDV RT-qPCR results after disinfection [22, 23]. Therefore, PEDV-positive RT-qPCR results on environmental samples should be expected when the AHP disinfectant is utilized under freezing conditions, but this does not necessarily indicate that an infectious dose of PEDV remains in the trailer.

Livestock trailers have many non-smooth surfaces and are more complex than the coupons utilized in this study. Trailers contain many channels, grooves, rough surfaces, hinges, latches, and corners that organic material can build up on and provide areas for a virus to be missed by a disinfectant. While, it was understood the smooth aluminum coupons do not replicate all of the surfaces found within livestock trailers, performing a study of this magnitude would not have been feasible with full-size trailers, so the coupons were utilized as a model. The ease with which the 15.24 X 15.24 X 2.54 cm aluminum coupons could be handled made it possible to contaminate the coupons, perform the treatments, collect the inoculum and inoculate pigs for the bioassay for all study groups in less than 1 day. The model also enabled the investigators to stagger the start time for each treatment group so that the pigs could be inoculated immediately after the inoculum was collected, thereby eliminating the need to attempt to neutralize the AHP disinfectant after the 40 min or 60 min contact time.

Livestock trailers are frequently bedded with wood shavings prior to transporting pigs. Incorporation of wood shavings into the model was considered however, the size and type of shavings used for bedding varies widely across the industry and previous work demonstrated that some wood has virucidal properties [24]. Therefore, the aluminum coupons were contaminated with swine feces alone to avoid the possibility of confounding the results with the effect of choice of wood shavings.

While the AHP disinfectant utilized in this study is labeled as virucidal in 5 min with dilutions of 1:16 to 1:64, this study only evaluated two dilutions (1:16 and 1:32) and used considerably longer contact times (40 and 60 min). The longer contact times were chosen because the conditions in this study were less favorable than those used in determining the label and in a previous study which evaluated its efficacy at 20 °C [13]. Further research on the efficacy of an AHP disinfectant under other adverse conditions such as shorter contact times, greater dilution rates, and on perpendicular surfaces to simulate trailer sidewalls is warranted.

Conclusions

In cold weather months when a complete wash, disinfection, and dry cannot be accomplished, due to lack of resources or other logistical constraints, the results of this study suggest that scraping livestock trailers to remove as much organic material as possible followed by disinfection with at minimum a 1:32 concentration of AHP disinfectant in a solution with 10% PG with at least 40 min of contact time, may be used, as an alternative to doing nothing, to reduce the risk of PEDV transmission associated with livestock trailers.

The results also suggest that a PEDV-positive RT-qPCR result on an environmental sample should be expected after 60 min of contact time when the AHP disinfectant is applied under freezing conditions, but does not necessarily indicate that an infectious dose of PEDV remains in the trailer. Obtaining a negative real-time RT-qPCR result on an environmental sample after disinfection is largely dependent on the type of disinfectant used and the conditions under which it was applied.

Additional file

Additional file 1: Results of PEDV N-gene RT-qPCR tests on environmental samples from coupons and rectal swabs from pigs used for bioassay. Results from all diagnostic tests conducted for the study are reported for each replicate, one row for each replicate. Test results, Ct value and genomic copies are reported for PCR tests on pre and post treatment environmental samples from coupons. Test result and Ct values are reported for PCR tests on rectal swabs from pigs 3 and 7 days post inoculation for the bioassay. (XLSX 12 kb)

Abbreviations

AHP: Accelerated hydrogen peroxide; ANOVA: Analyses of variance; ELISA: Enzyme-linked immunosorbent assay; IFA: Indirect fluorescent antibody; ISU VDL: Iowa State University Veterinary Diagnostic Laboratory; N: Nucleocapsid; NPB: National Pork Board; PED: Porcine epidemic diarrhea; PEDV: Porcine epidemic diarrhea virus; PG: Propylene glycol; PRCV: Porcine respiratory corona virus; PRRSV: Porcine reproductive and respiratory syndrome virus; RT-qPCR: Real-time reverse transcription quantitative polymerase chain reaction; TADD: Thermo-assisted drying and decontamination; TGEV: Transmissible gastroenteritis virus

Acknowledgements

The authors would like to thank the Swine Medicine Education Center as well as the Iowa State University College of Veterinary Medicine Department of Veterinary Diagnostic and Production Animal Medicine faculty, staff, and students for assistance with live animal work.

Funding

Funding for this study was provided by the National Pork Board (NPB#14–272).

Authors' contributions

KLB, DJH, PRT, LAK, AR designed, organized and conducted the trial. JZ assisted with study design and performed the diagnostic testing. CW conducted the statistical analysis. KLB drafted the manuscript with significant contributions from DJH. All authors read, revised, and approved the final manuscript.

Consent for publication

Not Applicable

Competing interests

All authors declare that they have no competing interests.

Author details

[1]Department of Veterinary Diagnostic and Production Animal Medicine, Iowa State University College of Veterinary Medicine, 1809 S Riverside Dr, Ames, IA, USA. [2]AMVC Management Services, 1786 190th St, Audubon, IA, USA. [3]Swine Medicine Education Center, Iowa State University College of Veterinary Medicine, 1809 S Riverside Dr, Ames, IA, USA.

References

1. Oldham J. Epidemic diarrhea - how it all began. Pig Farming. 1972;(Suppl):72–3.
2. Pensaert MB, de Bouck P. A new coronavirus-like particle associated with diarrhea in swine. Arch Virol. 1978;58:243–7.
3. Chasey D, Cartwright SF. Virus-like particles associated with porcine epidemic diarrhea. Res Vet Sci. 1978;25:255–6.
4. Stevenson GW, Hoang H, Schwartz KJ, Burrough ER, Sun D, Madson D, Cooper VL, Pillatzki A, Gauger P, Schmitt BJ, Koster LG, Killian ML, Yoon KJ. Emergence of porcine epidemic diarrhea virus in the United States: clinical signs, lesions, and viral genomic sequences. J Vet Diag Invest. 2013;25(5):649–54.
5. Pospischil A, Stuedli A, Kiupel M. Update on porcine epidemic diarrhea. J Swine Health Prod. 2002;10(2):81–5.
6. Lowe J, Gauger P, Harmon K, Zhang J, Connor J, Yeske P, Loula T, Levis I, Dufresne L, Main R. Role of transportation in spread of porcine epidemic diarrhea virus infection, United States. Emerg Infec Dis. 2014;20(5):872–4.
7. Dee SA, Deen J, Otake S, Pijoan C. An experimental model to evaluate the role of transport vehicles as a source of transmission of porcine reproductive and respiratory syndrome virus to susceptible pigs. Can J Vet Res. 2004a;68(2):128–33.
8. Dee S, Deen J, Burns D, Douthit G, Pijoan C. An assessment of sanitation protocols for commercial transport vehicles contaminated with porcine reproductive and respiratory syndrome virus. Can J Vet Res. 2004b;68(3):208–14.
9. Dee S, Torremorell M, Thompson B, Deen J, Pijoan C. An evaluation of thermo-assisted drying and decontamination for the elimination of porcine reproductive and respiratory syndrome virus from contaminated livestock transport vehicles. Can J Vet Res. 2005a;69(1):58–63.
10. Dee S, Burns D, Douthit G, Pijoan C. An evaluation of disinfectants for the sanitation of porcine reproductive and respiratory syndrome virus-contaminated transport vehicles at cold temperatures. Can J Vet Res. 2005b; 69(1):64–70.
11. Holtkamp D, Thomas P, Gerardy K, Karriker L, Ramirez A, Zhang J, Bates J. Review of PEDV disinfectant research. In: Proc. 47th American Association of Swine Veterinarians Annual Meeting. LA: New Orleans; 2016. p. 146–50.
12. Thomas P, Karriker L, Ramirez A, Zhang J, Ellingson J, Holtkamp DJ. Evaluation of time and temperature sufficient to inactivate PEDV in swine feces on metal surfaces. J Swine Health Prod. 2015;23(2):84–90.
13. Holtkamp DJ, Myers J, Thomas PR, Karriker LA, Ramirez A, Zhang J, Wang C. Efficacy of an accelerated hydrogen peroxide disinfectant to inactivate porcine epidemic diarrhea virus in swine feces on metal surfaces. Can J Vet Res. 2017;81(2):100–7.
14. Omidbakhsh N, Sattar S. Broad-spectrum microbicidal activity, toxicologic assessment, and materials compatibility of a new generation of accelerated hydrogen peroxide-based environmental surface disinfectant. An J Infect Control. 2006;34(5):251–7.
15. Omidbakhsh N. A new peroxide-based flexible endoscope-compatible high-level disinfectant. Am J Infect Control. 2006;34(9):571–7.
16. Thomas JT, Chen Q, Gauger PC, Giménez-Lirola LG, Sinha A, Harmon KM, Madson DM, Burrough ER, Magstadt DR, Salzbrenner HM, Welch MW, Yoon KJ, Zimmerman J, Zhang J. Effect of porcine epidemic diarrhea virus infectious doses on infection outcomes in Naïve conventional neonatal and weaned pigs. PLoS One. 2015; doi: 10.1371/journal.pone.0139266.
17. Madson DM, Magstadt DR, Arruda PHE, Hoang H, Sun D, Bower LP, Bhandari M, Burrough ER, Gauger PC, Pillatzki AE, Stevenson GW, Wilberts BL, Brodie J, Harmon KM, Wang C, Main RG, Zhang J, Yoon KJ. Pathogenesis of porcine epidemic diarrhea virus isolate (US/Iowa/18984/2013) in 3-week-old weaned pigs. Vet Microbiol. 2014;174(1–2):60–8.
18. Thrash RJ, Robert RR. Physical factors influencing the activity of antimicrobial agents. In: Block SS, editor. Disinfection, sterilization, and preservation. Philadelphia: Lippincott Williams and Wilkins; 2001. p. 57–64.
19. Davison S, Benson CE, Ziegler AF, Eckroade RJ. Evaluation of disinfectants with the addition of antifreezing compounds against nonpathogenic H7N2 avian influenza virus. Avian Dis. 1999;43(3):533–7.
20. Dvorak G. Disinfection 101. Iowa State Center for Food Security and Public Health. 2008. http://www.cfsph.iastate.edu/Disinfection/Assets/Disinfection101.pdf. Accessed 06 Mar 2015.
21. Block SS. Peroxygen compounds. In: Block SS, editor. Disinfection, sterilization, and preservation. Philadelphia: Lippincott Williams and Wilkins; 2001. p. 185–204.

22. Bowman AS, Nolting JM, Nelson SW, Bliss N, Stull JW, Wang Q. Premanandan. Effects of disinfection on the molecular detection of porcine epidemic diarrhea virus. Vet Microbiol. 2015;179:213–8. doi: 10.1016/j.vetmic.2015.05.027.
23. Huss AR, Schumacher LL, Cochrane RA, Poulsen E, Bai J, Woodworth JC, Dritz SS, Stark CR, Jones CK. Elimination of porcine epidemic diarrhea virus in an animal feed manufacturing facility. PLoS One. 2017;12(1):e0169612. doi: 10.1371/journalpone.0169612.
24. Greatorex JS, Digard P, Curran MD, Moynihan R, Wensley H, Wreghitt T, Varsani H, Garcia F, Enstone J, Nguyen-Van-Tam JS. Survival of influenza a(HINI) on materials found in households: implications for infection control. PLoS One. 2011;6(11):e27932. doi: 10.1371/journal.pone.0027932.

3

The biomedical piglet: establishing reference intervals for haematology and clinical chemistry parameters of two age groups with and without iron supplementation

Domenico Ventrella, Francesco Dondi*, Francesca Barone, Federica Serafini, Alberto Elmi, Massimo Giunti, Noemi Romagnoli, Monica Forni and Maria L. Bacci

Abstract

Background: The similarities between swine and humans in physiological and genomic patterns, and the great correlation in size and anatomy, make pigs extremely useful in preclinical studies. New-born piglets can represent a model for congenital and genetic diseases in new-born children. It is known that piglets may have significant differences in clinicopathological results compared to adult pigs. Therefore, adult laboratory reference intervals cannot be applied to piglets. The aim of this study was to compare haematological and chemical variables in piglets of two ages and determinate age-related reference intervals for commercial hybrid young pigs.
Blood samples were collected under general anaesthesia from 130 animals divided into five- (P5) and 30- (P30) day-old piglets. Only P30 animals were treated with parenteral iron after birth. Samples were analysed using automated haematology (ADVIA 2120) and chemistry analysers, and age-related reference intervals were calculated.

Results: Significant higher values of RBC, Hb and HCT were observed in P30 animals when compared to P5, with an opposite trend for MCV. These results were associated with a reduction of the RBC regeneration process and the thrombopoietic response. The TSAT and TIBC were significantly higher in P30 compared to P5; however, piglets remained iron deficient compared to adult reference intervals reported previously.

Conclusions: In conclusion, this paper emphasises the high variability occurring in clinicopathological variables between new-born and 30-day-old pigs, and between piglets and adult pigs. This study provides valuable reference data for piglets at precise ages and could be used in the future as historical control improving the Reduction in animal experiments, as suggested by the 3Rs principle.

Keywords: ADVIA 2120, Clinical chemistry, Haematology, Reference intervals, Swine

* Correspondence: f.dondi@unibo.it
Department of Veterinary Medical Sciences, Alma Mater Studiorum, University of Bologna, Via Tolara di Sopra 50, 40064 Ozzano dell'Emilia, BO, Italy

Background

The interest in the pig as an animal model for experimental medicine can be traced back to Galen, in 1586 [1]. One reason for this interest is the strong similarities between the pig and the human in both physiological [2] and genomic [3] patterns. In addition, size and anatomy can be easily related to the development stages of people, making the pig the perfect preclinical model for human diseases [4, 5], surgical techniques and, more recently, for transplantation research [6–8]. When compared to other models such as mice or rats, the pig has a longer lifespan of 10–15 years [9], so disease progression is more similar to that seen in humans [1]. Furthermore, in the neonatal period, pigs represent an accurate model for studying congenital and genetic diseases in humans [10]. Piglets can even represent a good model for the preterm neonate, as they show similar anthropometric and physiological characteristics [11].

However, age differences, even within the same species, significantly affect the comparison of some developmental patterns, especially in extremely young subjects. Therefore, these processes need to be thoroughly investigated in order to create an accurate and standardised preclinical model and to help reduce and refine experimental protocols. As an important example, iron deficiency, which is one of the most common nutritional defects during the neonatal period in mammals [12, 13], is extremely common in swine, due to the high reproductive performance required of these animals. Unless given iron supplements, piglets may develop iron-deficiency a few days after birth [14, 15]. This condition occurs regardless of the breed and management system, and is the result of interactions of several factors including low levels of iron stores, increased requirements, poor exogenous supply and immaturity of absorption mechanisms [15, 16]. Similarly, iron requirements cannot be completely fulfilled by hepatic reserves and milk consumption due to the constant request for larger litter sizes, higher birth weights and faster growth that result in a greater blood volume and red blood cell (RBC) count [17]. It is therefore mandatory to supplement piglets with exogenous iron to prevent dangerous deficiency [18]. This procedure may interfere with several clinical chemistry parameters [19] and is the reason why it is very inaccurate to evaluate piglets based on the clinicopathological findings of older pigs. Therefore, it is extremely important to have specific age-related reference intervals for both haematological and chemical variables for piglets. Some values have been described in a single litter of Duroc x Jersey piglets [20], but the small number of animals and the lack of information about iron supplementation make them hard to rely on.

The aim of this study was to evaluate haematological and chemical variables in two groups of healthy hybrid piglets of different ages. Secondary objectives were to establish age-related reference intervals (RI) for both haematology and clinical chemistry variables and to evaluate the iron profile in new-born piglets without exogenous supplementation (5 days old) and young pigs administered with exogenous iron within 3 days after birth (30 days old).

Methods

Animals

All of the animals were Italian Large White x Duroc x Landrace commercial hybrids used in our facility. We only selected control and/or pre-treated animals previously enrolled in other experimental protocols and approved by the local ethical committee to be part of this study. The above mentioned protocols included blood tests to evaluate the animals, and we decided to work on the obtained data set of blood values.

We analysed piglets at two different time points: P5 were five-day-old piglets born in our facility that had not received any iron supplementation before blood sampling and were not neutered; P30 were 30-day-old pigs that were transferred to our piggery on the day of weaning (28th day of life) and were administered a single iron injection (100 mg IM; Endofer, FATRO, Italy) within the first 72 h after birth, and males were neutered. None of the animals was included in both age groups. In order to rule out any possible variation in genetic line and management, both pregnant sows and pigs were born and raised in the same farm. All of the animals were housed in multiple stalls and fed with a standard swine diet; P5 were housed in the farrowing crate with the sow until weaning. Body weight (kg) was measured in P5 and P30 and recorded.

A total of one hundred-thirty animals were included in the study; 74/130 (57%) were females, while 56/130 (43%) were males. Body weight was 2.3 (1.2–3.8) kg in P5 and 8.0 (5.3–11.2) kg in P30. For haematologicalal analyses, samples from 130 animals were available: 66 P5 and 64 P30. For chemistry evaluations, samples from 119 animals were available: 56 P5 and 63 P30.

Blood sample collection and analyses

Blood samplings were performed on day 5 (P5) or 30 (P30) under general anaesthesia, using an advanced anaesthesia delivery unit (Datex-Ohmeda ADU S/5, GE Healthcare, USA), achieved by inhalation induction with sevoflurane (Sevoflo, Abbott Laboratories, Chicago, USA). No premedication was performed in order to avoid blood alterations due to injected drug adsorption. After oro-tracheal intubation, anaesthesia was maintained with $4 \pm 0.5\%$ sevoflurane in a 1:1 oxygen/air mixture. Samples were obtained from the femoral artery using a 21 G butterfly needle and a vacuum system;

tubes with K_3EDTA anticoagulant, citrate and clot activator were used. The total volume of withdrawn blood was approximately 10 ml, which was considered completely safe and negligible for these animals.

Blood samples (K_3EDTA tubes) were analysed within 30 min from collection; serum (clot activator tubes) and citrate plasma (citrate tubes) were obtained by centrifugation (10 min at 3000 × g) within 1 h and analysed or stored at −80 °C until analysis.

Complete blood count (CBC) was performed with a new automated haematology analyser (ADVIA 2120, Siemens Healthcare Diagnostics, Tarrytown NY, USA) that combines classic haematological variables with individual cell indices. The variables evaluated in our study were haematocrit value (HCT), haemoglobin concentration (Hb), cellular haemoglobin content (CH), cellular haemoglobin content of mature red blood cells (CHm), red blood cells count (RBC), mean corpuscular volume (MCV), mean corpuscular volume of mature RBCs (MCVm), mean corpuscular haemoglobin concentration (MCHC), mean corpuscular haemoglobin (MCH), corpuscular haemoglobin concentration mean (CHCM), corpuscular haemoglobin concentration mean of mature RBCs (CHCMm), haemoglobin concentration distribution width (HDW), haemoglobin concentration distribution width of mature RBC (HDWm), RBC distribution width (RDW) and mature RBC distribution width (RDWm). Total white blood cell (WBC) count and differential WBC count were also performed. Platelet indices were analysed and included platelet count (PLT), mean platelet volume (MPV), PLT volume distribution width (PDW), plateletcrit (PCT), mean PLT component (MPC), platelet component distribution width (PCDW), mean PLT mass (MPM) and platelet mass distribution width (PMDW).

In addition to the above mentioned variables, we evaluated the following reticulocyte indices: absolute reticulocyte count (Retic), percentage of reticulocytes (%Retic), average size of reticulocytes (MCVr), average cell haemoglobin concentration (CHCMr), average haemoglobin content (CHr), distribution width of reticulocyte cell size (RDWr), distribution width of CHCMr (HDWr), percentage of microcytic reticulocytes (%Micro-r), percentage of macrocytic reticulocytes (%Macro-r), percentage of hypochromic reticulocytes (%Hypo-r), percentage of hyperchromic reticulocytes (%Hyper-r), percentage of reticulocytes with a low CH (%LowCHr), percentage of reticulocytes with a high CH (%HighCHr), CHr-CHm (CH delta), CHCMr-CHCMm (CHCM delta), CHDWr-CHDWm (CHDW delta), HDWr-HDWm (HDW delta), MCVr-MCVm (MCV delta), and RDWr-RDWm (RDW delta). The haematologicalal evaluation was completed by a blood smear microscopic examination using Romanovsky staining.

All chemistry analyses were carried out on an automated chemistry analyser (Olympus AU 400, Beckman Coulter/Olympus) and included aspartate transaminase (AST), alanine transaminase (ALT), alkaline phosphatase (ALP), creatinine, urea, glucose, total proteins (TP), albumin, albumin to globulin ratio (A/G), sodium, potassium, total iron (TI), unsaturated iron binding capacity (UIBC), total iron binding capacity (TIBC) and TIBC saturation (TSAT). Total iron and UIBC were measured using colorimetric methods (Iron Ferene, KAL 002, Olympus/Sentinel Diagnostics, Milan, Italy; UIBC OSR61205, Olympus/Beckman Coulter, O'Callaghan's Mills, Ireland). Total iron binding capacity and TSAT were calculated as follows: TIBC = TI + UIBC; TSAT = (TI × 100)/TIBC.

ADVIA 2120 erythrocytes, reticulocytes and platelet indices, and other variables evaluated in the study are reported in the Additional file 1, including their abbreviations.

Statistical analyses

Statistical analyses were performed using MedCalc statistical software (version 15.6; MedCalc Software, Ostend, Belgium). The D'Agostino-Pearson test was used to assess normal distribution of data. Data were reported as mean ± SD or median (minimum-maximum) based on their distribution. Comparisons between the two age groups were performed using the Mann-Whitney *U* test due to the non-Gaussian distribution of the majority of the data. Reference intervals were obtained using the 2.5th – 97.5th percentiles method following the Clinical and Laboratory Standards Institute (CLSI) guidelines for estimating percentiles and their 90% confidence intervals [21]. Outliers were identified with the Tukey test. Differences were considered to be statistically significant with $P < 0.05$.

Results and discussion

For the haematological and chemical analyses, the number of samples available for each analyses, descriptive statistics, differences between groups and estimated RI in P5 and P30 are reported in Tables 1, 2 and 3. A significant increase in the circulating erythrocyte mass was detected in P30 compared to P5 as demonstrated by the higher values of Hb, HCT and RBC count. This finding was associated with a significant reduction in volume (MCV, MCVm) and a significant increase in anisocytosis (RDW, RDWm). Erythrocyte haemoglobin content indices (CH, CHm, MCH) were significantly lower in P30 compared to P5 with the exception of CHCM which was significantly higher in P30, while MCHC and CHCMm were not significantly different between groups (Table 1). Absolute reticulocyte count and percentage of reticulocytes were significantly lower in P30 compared to P5.

Table 1 Descriptive statistics, differences between groups and estimated reference intervals for haematological variables. Data are expressed as mean ± SD or median (minimum-maximum)

Variable	P5 Descriptive data	P5 Reference Interval	P5 *n*	P30 Descriptive data	P30 Reference Interval	P30 *n*	*P*-value
Hb (g/dL)	6.03 ± 1.02	3.56-7.74	61	8.84 ± 2.0	4.32-13.31	64	<0.0001
HCT (%)	20 ± 3	13-25	61	29 ± 6	16-41	64	<0.0001
CH (pg)	16.85 (14.10–22.30)	14.30–21.82	66	14.0 (9.0–19.0)	9.3–18.9	64	<0.0001
CHm (pg)	18.3 (16.1–22.4)	16.27–22.01	50	15.4 ± 1.5	12.7–18.8	33	<0.0001
CHDW (pg)	3.72 (2.90–5.84)	3.01–5.71	66	3.99 ± 0.66	2.66–5.33	64	0.3541
CHDWm (pg)	3.36 (2.82–5.47)	2.83–5.34	50	4.78 (2.61–5.55)	2.61–5.50	33	<0.0001
RBC (10^6/μL)	3.26 ± 0.52	1.88–4.11	61	6.08 ± 0.93	4.08–8.17	64	<0.0001
MCV (fL)	61.97 ± 5.39	51.41–73.65	61	48.5 (32.4–61.5)	34.2–61.3	64	<0.0001
MCVm (fL)	65.9 ± 4.5	56.4–74.9	50	52.9 ± 3.9	45.3–60.5	33	<0.0001
MCHC (g/dL)	30.0. ± 1.6	26.1–32.7	61	29.9 ± 1.59	26.5–33.6	63	0.9606
MCH (pg)	18.50 ± 1.36	15.45–21.54	61	14.8 (9.1–20.2)	9.4–19.8	64	<0.0001
CHCM (g/dL)	27.35 ± 1.11	24.84–29.13	66	28.35 ± 1.60	25.13–31.62	64	0.0003
CHCMm (g/dL)	28.2 (26.7–30.8)	26.8–30.8	50	28.6 (26.8–30.9)	26.8–30.9	33	0.5389
RDW (%)	18.8 (15.8–25.7)	15.9–25.7	56	26.5 (13.5–38.5)	13.5–38.0	64	<0.0001
RDWm (%)	15.9 (14.2–25.7)	14.2–25.1	50	25.5 (12.7–32.2)	12.7–32.0	33	<0.0001
HDW (g/dL)	2.89 (2.28–4.13)	2.29–3.93	66	2.63 ± 0.40	2.02–3.50	64	<0.0001
HDWm (g/dL)	2.60 (2.14–3.68)	2.16–3.63	50	2.73 ± 1.99–3.28	1.99–3.28	33	0.1685
WBC (10^3/μL)	7.47 (4.39–12.58)	4.50–12.55	58	11.6 ± 3.2	5.6–18.5	58	<0.0001
neutrophil (%)	44.71 ± 9.66	22.77–61.33	60	35.3 ± 15.0	10.8–70.6	63	0.0001
lymphocyte (%)	49.30 ± 9.49	33.45–70.86	60	57.9 ± 14.5	26.2–82.9	64	0.0005
monocyte (%)	3.11 ± 1.13	1.10–5.85	59	4.4 ± 1.5	1.4–8.3	64	<0.0001
eosinophil (%)	0.5 (0.1–3.1)	0–2.3	57	0.6 (0.1–7.6)	0–1.9	64	0.5699
basophil (%)	0.41 ± 0.16	0–0.79	60	0.4 (0.2–1.2)	0–0.9	63	0.1183
neutrophil (10^3/μL)	3.17 ± 0.98	1.15–5.43	54	3.5 (0.8–9.9)	0.8–9.7	61	0.1472
lymphocyte (10^3/μL)	3.85 ± 1.11	1.91–6.45	58	6.6 ± 2.4	2.7–12.8	60	<0.0001
monocyte (10^3/μL)	0.23 (0.07–0.7)	0.075–0.68	59	0.4 (0.1–1.1)	0.1–1.1	59	<0.0001
eosinophil (10^3/μL)	0.04 (0.01–0.48)	0–0.28	60	0.07 (0.01–0.38)	0.00–0.20	63	0.0014
basophil (10^3/μL)	0.03 (0.01–0.2)	0–0.08	60	0.05 (0.02–0.33)	0.00–0.13	63	<0.0001
PLT (10^3/μL)	594 (219–1142)	253–1286	61	503 ± 141	192–832	63	<0.0001
MPV (fL)	17.84 ± 3.78	9.99–25.32	61	8.5 (6.2–13.0)	6.5–12.7	63	<0.0001
PDW (%)	84.22 ± 8.32	69.17–100.30	61	60.40 (17.90–106.60)	18.59–101.98	64	<0.0001
PCT (%)	1.20 ± 0.50	0.29–2.52	61	0.40 (0.12–0.94)	0.18–0.91	62	<0.0001
MPC (g/dL)	24.5 (17.2–26.3)	17.81–26.30	61	24.09 ± 0.96	21.69–26.50	64	0.0182
MPM (pg)	2.84 ± 0.34	2.10–3.44	61	1.96 ± 0.22	1.58–2.45	63	<0.0001
PCDW (g/dL)	4.6 (4.0–5.7)	4.0–5.6	66	4.6 (3.8–5.9)	3.9–5.9	64	0.4354
PMDW (pg)	1.45 (0.99–1.62)	0.99–1.61	66	0.87 (0.61–1.55)	0.62–1.54	64	<0.0001

Many other reticulocyte indices were significantly different between age groups (Table 2).

Circulating platelet number (PLT, PCT) was significantly decreased in P30 compared to P5; these results were associated with a significant reduction in platelet volume and mass (MPV, MPM) in P30 animals.

In the chemistry analysis, P5 subjects had significantly lower values of creatinine, urea, ALT, albumin and A/G and significantly higher ALP and potassium compared to P30 animals. Total iron concentration and TSAT % were significantly higher in P30 piglets compared to P5 (Table 3).

Table 2 Descriptive statistics, differences between groups and estimated reference intervals for reticulocyte indices. Data are expressed as mean ± SD or median (minimum-maximum)

Variable	P5 Descriptive data	P5 Reference Interval	P5 *n*	P30 Descriptive data	P30 Reference Interval	P30 *n*	*P*-value
Retic (10^9cell/L)	369.3 ± 101.1	152.2–547.9	45	148.2 (53.4–554.5)	53.4–554.5	33	<0.000001
%Retic (%)	11.8 ± 3.8	4.6–20.7	49	2.5 (0.8–9.2)	0.8–9.2	33	<0.000001
MCVr (fL)	74.5 ± 7.3	60.7–89.4	48	56.5 ± 6.8	43.0–71.1	33	<0.000001
CHCMr (g/dL)	24.9 ± 0.9	23.4–27.0	48	26.1 ± 1.0	24.2–28.0	33	0.000008
CHr (pg)	18.1 (16.0–24.3)	16.2–23.8	48	14.6 ± 1.4	12.1–18.0	33	<0.000001
CHDWr (pg)	3.7 ± 0.3	3.1–4.4	48	3.5 (2.4–4.6)	2.4–4.6	33	0.166288
RDWr (%)	17.6 ± 2.1	14.2–20.7	48	19.5 (13.0–33.0)	13.0–33.0	33	0.055130
HDWr (g/dL)	3.36 ± 0.36	2.66–3.84	48	3.9 ± 0.62	2.7–5.1	33	0.000003
%Micro-r (%)	0.05 (0–0.8)	0.0–0.45	48	0.7 (0.0–15.5)	0.0–15.5	33	0.000005
%Macro-r (%)	26.5 (4.8–71.9)	6.7–70.7	48	2.6 (1.0–17.4)	1.0–17.4	33	<0.000001
%Hypo-r (%)	83.0 (62.8–94.3)	62.2–92.2	48	76.4 (57.2–85.8)	57.2–85.8	33	0.000036
%Hyper-r (%)	0.1 (0.0–0.3)	0.0–0.3	48	0.3 (0.0–2.7)	0.0–2.7	33	<0.000001
%LowCHr (%)	10.9 (0.5–35.4)	0.5–32.1	48	57.3 (6.0–76.8)	6.0–76.8	33	<0.000001
%HighCHr (%)	22.6 (9.2–76.3)	10.1–74.9	48	7.1 ± 2.5	3.3–13.0	33	<0.000001
CH delta (pg)	−0.1 ± 1.6	−3.3–2.1	48	−0.7 ± 0.7	−2.4–0.7	33	0.012741
CHCM delta (g/dL)	−3.4 ± 0.9	−5.2–(−1.8)	48	−2.6 ± 1.7	−5.3–0.8	33	0.075
CHDW delta (pg)	0.38 (−0.54–0.86)	−0.33–0.67	48	−1.0 ± 0.6	−2.19–(−0.05)	33	<0.000001
HDW delta (g/dL)	0.66 ± 0.27	0.12–1.07	48	1.26 ± 0.46	0.18–2.06	33	<0.000001
MCV delta (fL)	8.9 ± 6.6	−3.4–18.3	48	3.6 ± 4.4	−3.8–12.5	33	0.000255
RDW delta (%)	1.4 (−7.4–5.2)	−6.3–4.2	48	−3.8 ± 4.3	−12.6–3.0	33	<0.000001

Table 3 Descriptive statistics, differences between groups and estimated reference intervals for clinical chemistry. Data are expressed as mean ± SD or median (minimum-maximum)

Variable	P5 Descriptive data	P5 Reference Interval	P5 *n*	P30 Descriptive data	P30 Reference Interval	P30 *n*	*P*-value
Glucose (mg/dL)	124 (69–200)	71–196	49	111 ± 26	34–159	62	0.0016
Urea (mg/dL)	12.4 (4.9–31.7)	5.0–30.8	55	17 (4–40)	4–39	59	0.0002
Creatinine (mg/dL)	0.65 (0.30–0.88)	0.38–0.85	56	1.09 (0.31–1.41)	0.51–1.39	62	<0.0001
AST (U/L)	29 ± 7	10–47	56	31 (11–68)	13–65	62	0.9915
ALT (U/L)	23 ± 6	5–38	56	30 (11–58)	14–54	60	<0.0001
ALP (U/L)	3773 ± 1017	1324–6031	56	770 ± 270	110–1292	61	<0.0001
TP (g/dL)	5.0 ± 0.5	3.7–6.2	54	4.8 (1.2–6.7)	2.5–6.6	59	0.4464
Albumin (g/dL)	1.8 ± 0.3	1.0–2.6	55	3.0 (1.8–4.0)	1.9–4.0	59	<0.0001
A/G	0.56 (0.36–0.99)	0.37–0.98	53	1.5 ± 0.3	0.7–2.2	60	<0.0001
TI (µg/dL)	15 (9–31)	9–30	49	34 (7–157)	7–151	60	<0.0001
UIBC (µg/dL)	338 ± 72	218–524	44	326 (40–1058)	63–980	62	0.2031
TIBC (µg/dL)	354 ± 72	230–542	44	397 (128–882)	142–877	60	0.0031
TSAT (%)	4.2 ± 1.2	1.3–6.7	42	8.6 (0.8–55.6)	0.9–54	61	0.0058
Potassium (mEq/L)	4 ± 0.5	2.8–5.1	54	3.7 ± 0.4	2.9–4.6	63	0.0252
Sodium (mEq/L)	135 (126–140)	126–140	53	136 ± 4.7	125–147	63	0.2448

Swine are probably one of the most important models for translational medicine [7], and therefore a complete and accurate knowledge of their physiology should be mandatory. This kind of knowledge would represent a big improvement when it comes to refinement of animal experiments. When using commercial hybrids for scientific purposes, it is important to acknowledge that those animals are the products of strong zootechnical manipulation that constantly requires higher breeding and production performance [18]. Moreover, very young piglets (first month of age) present high variability in many clinical and clinicopathological variables due to rapid growth, nutrition and other metabolic conditions, some which are potentially related to iron status [15, 20]. As in other species, new-born and young piglets are extremely different than adult animals regarding laboratory results [20], thus, the determination of reliable age-related reference intervals for both haematology and chemistry variables in 5- and 30-day-old piglets is warranted. It is important to acknowledge the fact that our results may not perfectly translate to every other pigs' breeds, but still represent a valid and robust general reference especially because obtained by one of the most common hybrid cross in Europe. Another important issue to address, before the discussion of the results, is the feeding protocol: P5 only received milk from the sows, while P30 were weaned at 28 days of life, therefore only ate solid feed for 2 days before blood sampling. This difference in alimentation may have contributed to some of the differences alongside with evolution of the gastro-intestinal system.

The results reported in this study showed high variability in the blood profiles among P5 and P30 animals. Unfortunately, it is hard to compare our data with the ones previously described in the literature mainly because of the poor or absent age distinction and the different types of animals used. However, our P5 and P30 animals had lower Hb, HCT, RBC, MCV and MCH values compared to animals of similar ages (days 6 and 36 from birth, respectively) [20].

In our study, P5 animals had a RBC regenerative response that was significantly reduced in P30, as further demonstrated by the results of reticulocyte indices (significantly higher Retic, %Retic, MCVr, %Macro-r and MCV delta). Similar findings have been reported previously and could represent a physiological response in the new-born pigs [15, 20]. However, a condition of iron deficiency could not be excluded in our piglets. It is well known that piglets can suffer from iron deficiency due to many causes such as immature iron metabolism, decreased iron intake or absorption and rapid growth. Iron deficiency can be associated with reduced weight gain, anaemia and even with increased mortality in these animals [22]. For these reasons, iron supplementation is highly recommended and the benefit of this treatment is well documented [18]. The role of iron deficiency in P5 animals, although suspected based on haematological results, could not be demonstrated with the current study design. In the initial phase, iron deficiency is characterised by enhanced erythropoiesis and even a regenerative anaemia, while microcytosis and hypochromasia (reduction of MCV and MCHC) are late findings associated with iron deficiency in animals and humans [23, 24]. The P30 animals that were supplemented with parenteral iron within the first 72 h after birth had a decreased reticulocyte response compared to the new-born animals. In addition, the results of iron profile parameters, particularly TI and TSAT, supported the potential role of iron deficiency in the piglets included in the present study. Total iron and TSAT values in P5 and even P30 animals were extremely decreased compared to the adult pig values reported in the literature [25]. However, TI and TSAT values were significantly higher at 30 days after birth, compared to new-born piglets. A previous study, using a different schedule of iron treatment, reported different results with particular regard to the iron profile parameters, compared to our study [15]. In our study, the upper limit for TI in P30 animals was five times higher than the P5 upper limit, however the lower limit was similar; the same happened for TSAT. The TIBC showed a slightly different trend, with a wider interval and both lower and higher values in P30 compared to P5. The overall pattern shown by iron-related parameters indicated that circulating iron was very low in these healthy animals. For this reason iron deficiency is hard to investigate in piglets and the determination of other iron-related variables such as ferritin, which is considered the main iron storage protein, may be helpful. Further studies on non-treated animals should be performed in order to investigate and quantify the physiological erythroid response of growing pigs. However, it is possible that an enhanced erythropoiesis accompanied by a relative iron deficiency may be considered a paraphysiological condition for this type of piglet in the first month after birth.

Swine are known to have an elevated platelet count compared to other animals, with frequent platelet clumping upon blood smear examination [20]. Although the total platelet count at both experimental times was comparable to adult animal values available in the literature, PLT, volume and mass were significantly reduced in P30 pigs compared to the new-born piglets. Similar data for young pigs are lacking in veterinary medicine to the best of our knowledge. Analogous to erythropoiesis, an enhanced thrombocytopoiesis that decreases shortly after birth could be explained by the increased need for platelets due to rapid growth or even iron deficiency. Iron deficiency, in fact, is recognised as a stimulus for the bone marrow to produce and release platelets, leading to thrombocytosis in small animals and humans [26].

The P5 and P30 total WBC count results in our study were consistent with the literature: neutrophil percentage decreased from P5 to P30 while the neutrophil total number did not differ significantly. On the contrary, the lymphocyte count and percentage were significantly increased in older animals, as previously reported [20].

Many chemistry variables evaluated were significantly different between the two age groups. These differences may impact the RI definition, however, it is difficult to clarify the exact physiological significance of these changes from an observational study. Interestingly, new-born swine may have a very low concentration of albumin that was significantly higher in 30-day-old animals, while TP concentration did not differ significantly between groups. As supported by the increase in A/G in P30 piglets, albumin concentration increased with the growth of these animals and this process was associated with a progressive reduction in the globulin fraction. Similar findings are lacking in previous studies.

Creatinine and urea values were significantly higher in P30 animals compared to P5, however both values were fully comparable to the adult values available in the veterinary literature [27]. In the authors' opinion, this is the result of the fast growing rate of pigs leading to a rapid increase in muscle mass, helped by the gradual supplementation of enriched solid diet throughout the lactation period.

Another significant difference can be noticed in the ALP concentration, which was extremely higher in younger animals. The literature suggests that this finding is related to higher osteoblast activity in young, growing animals; nevertheless the exact role of ALP in swine in poorly understood, and its clinicopathological usefulness needs to be clarified in further studies [28, 29].

Age-related reference intervals for haematological and biochemical variables in wild boars have been recently published [30]. Although a similar automated haematology system (ADVIA 120) was used in that study, animals from zero to six months were referred to as piglets, and therefore a comparison of their data with our results would not be accurate or reliable. This different stratification of the population in their study design reflects changes in chemical variables as well, and their data seem to be more comparable to our P30 results.

Conclusions

In conclusion, this paper highlights the high variability in haematological and chemistry variables between new-born and 30-day-old pigs, and between these animals and adult pigs. Moreover, our study provides specific age-related reference intervals for healthy commercial hybrid piglets that can be used as physiological standards for both translational and swine medicine. Age-related reference intervals will help in the correct interpretation of experimental results and should be considered an important step towards a more in-depth knowledge and standardisation of the swine animal model.

Acknowledgements

The authors would like to thank the personnel of the veterinary clinical pathology service, and in particular Dr Elisa Brini and Dr Marta Gruarin, for their technical assistance in the use of the ADVIA 2120 haematology system.

Funding

The study was supported by RFO 60% Ateneo di Bologna.

Authors' contributions

DV drafted the manuscript, conceived and designed the study, organized the data and performed statistical analyses. FD drafted the manuscript, helped designing the study, carried out the laboratory analyses and helped organizing and interpreting the data. FB helped handling the animals and collecting blood samples, organized and interpreted the data and review the draft. FS helped acquiring the data and carrying out the laboratory and statistical analyses. AE helped collecting blood samples and organizing the data, performed and reviewed the statistical analyses. MG helped handling the animals and collecting blood samples and critically reviewed the results and the entire draft. NR coordinated the activities performed on the animals and helped drafting the manuscript. MF co-funded the study and helped conceiving and designing the study. MLB funded and conceived the study, coordinated the work team and finally approved the manuscript. All authors read and approved the manuscript.

Competing interests

The authors declare that they have no competing interests.

Consent for publication

Not applicable.

References

1. Kuzmuk KN, Schook LB. Pigs as a model for biomedical Sciences. In: Rothschild MF, Ruvinsky A, editors. The Genetics of the Pig. 2nd ed. Wallingford: CAB International; 2011. p. 426–44.
2. Tumbleson ME, Schook LB. Advances in Swine in Biomedical Research. New York: Plenum Press; 1996.
3. Humphray SJ, Scott CE, Clark R, Marron B, Bender C, Camm N, et al. A high utility integrated map of the pig genome. Genome Biol. 2007;8:R139.
4. Forni M, Mazzola S, Ribeiro LA, Pirrone F, Zannoni A, Bernardini C, et al. Expression of endothelin-1 system in a pig model of endotoxic shock. Regul Pept. 2005;131:89–96.
5. Busnelli M, Froio A, Bacci ML, Giunti M, Cerrito MG, Giovannoni R, et al. Pathogenetic role of hypercholesterolemia in a novel preclinical model of vascular injury in pigs. Atherosclerosis. 2009;207:384–90.
6. Lavitrano M, Bacci ML, Forni M, Lazzereschi D, Di Stefano C, Fioretti D, et al. Efficient production by sperm-mediated gene transfer of human decay accelerating factor (hDAF) transgenic pigs for xenotransplantation. Proc Natl Acad Sci U S A. 2002;99:14230–5.
7. Swanson KS, Mazur MJ, Vashisht K, Rund LA, Beever JE, Counter CM, et al. Genomics and clinical medicine: rationale for creating and effectively evaluating animal models. Exp Biol Med (Maywood). 2004;229:866–75.
8. Smolenski RT, Forni M, Maccherini M, Bacci ML, Slominska EM, Wang H, et al. Reduction of hyperacute rejection and protection of metabolism and function in hearts of human decay accelerating factor (hDAF)-expressing pigs. Cardiovasc Res. 2007;73:143–52.
9. Hau J, Van Hoosier GL. Handbook of Laboratory Animal Science. Boca Raton: CRC Press; 2003.
10. Flamm EG. Neonatal animal testing paradigms and their suitability for testing infant formula. Toxicol Mech Methods. 2013;23:57–67.
11. Eiby YA, Wright LL, Kalanjati VP, Miller SM, Bjorkman ST, Keates HL, et al. A pig model of the preterm neonate: anthropometric and physiologicalal characteristics. PLoS One. 2013;8:e68763.

10. Flamm EG. Neonatal animal testing paradigms and their suitability for testing infant formula. Toxicol Mech Methods. 2013;23:57–67.
11. Eiby YA, Wright LL, Kalanjati VP, Miller SM, Bjorkman ST, Keates HL, et al. A pig model of the preterm neonate: anthropometric and physiologicalal characteristics. PLoS One. 2013;8:e68763.
12. Cook JD, Skikne BS, Baynes RD. Iron deficiency: the global perspective. Adv Exp Med Biol. 1994;356:219–28.
13. Clark SF. Iron deficiency anemia: diagnosis and management. Curr Opin Gastroenterol. 2009;52:122–8.
14. Venn JA, Davies ET. Piglet anaemia. Vet Rec. 1965;77:1004–5.
15. Starzyński RR, Laarakkers CM, Tjalsma H, Swinkels DW, Pieszka M, Styś A, et al. Iron supplementation in suckling piglets: how to correct iron deficiency anemia without affecting plasma hepcidin levels. PLoS One. 2013;8:e64022.
16. Venn JA, McCance RA, Widdowson EM. Iron metabolism in piglet anaemia. J Comp Pathol Ther. 1947;57:314–25.
17. Csapó J, Martin TG, Csapó-Kiss ZS, Házas Z. Protein, fats, vitamin and mineral concentrations in porcine colostrum and milk from parturition to 60 days. Int Dairy J. 1995;6:881–902.
18. Lipinski P, Starzyński RR, Canonne-Hergaux F, Tudek B, Oliński R, Kowalczyk P, et al. Benefits and risks of iron supplementation in anemic neonatal pigs. Am J Pathol. 2010;177:1233–43.
19. Egeli AK, Framstad T, Morberg H. Clinical biochemistry, haematology and body weight in piglets. Acta Vet Scand. 1998;39:381–93.
20. Thorn CE. Hematology of the pig. In: Weiss DJ, Wardrop KJ, editors. Schalm's Veterinary Hematology. 6th ed. Ames: Wiley-Blackwell; 2010. p. 843–51.
21. Kjelgaard-Hansen M, Jensen AL. Reference intervals. In: Weiss DJ, Wardrop KJ, editors. Schalm's Veterinary Hematology. 6th ed. Ames: Wiley-Blackwell; 2010. p. 1034–8.
22. Svoboda M, Drabek J. Iron deficiency in suckling piglets: etiology, clinical aspects and diagnosis. Folia Vet. 2005;49:104–11.
23. Stockham SL, Scott MA. Erythrocytes. In: Fundamentals of Veterinary Clinical Pathology. 2nd ed. Ames: Wiley-Blackwell; 2008. p. 107–222.
24. Weiss DJ. Iron and copper deficiencies and disorders of iron metabolism. In: Weiss DJ, Wardrop KJ, editors. Schalm's Veterinary Hematology. 6th ed. Ames: Wiley-Blackwell; 2010. p. 167–71.
25. Harvey JW. Iron metabolism and its disorders. In: Kaneko JJ, Harvey JW, Bruss ML, editors. Clinical Biochemistry of Domestic Animals. 6th ed. Philadelphia: Elsevier; 2008. p. 259–85.
26. Stockham SL, Scott MA. Platelets. In: Fundamentals of Veterinary Clinical Pathology. 2nd ed. Ames: Wiley-Blackwell; 2008. p. 223–58.
27. Kaneko JJ, Harvey JW, Bruss ML. Appendix VII. In: Kaneko JJ, Harvey JW, Bruss ML, editors. Clinical Biochemistry of Domestic Animals. 6th ed. Philadelphia: Elsevier; 2008. p. 882–8.
28. Hoffmann WE, Dorner JL. Separation of isoenzymes of canine alkaline phosphatase by cellulose acetate electrophoresis. J Am Anim Hosp Assoc. 1975;11:283–5.
29. Tennant BC, Center SA. Hepatic function. In: Kaneko JJ, Harvey JW, Bruss ML, editors. Clinical Biochemistry of Domestic Animals. 6th ed. Philadelphia: Elsevier; 2008. p. 379–412.
30. Casas-Diaz E, Closa-Sebastià F, Marco I, Lavin S, Bach-Raich E, Cuenca R. Hematologic and biochemical reference intervals for wild boar (Sus Scrofa) captured by cage trap. Vet Clin Pathol. 2015;44:215–22.

4

Estimating the scale of adverse animal welfare consequences of movement restriction and mitigation strategies in a classical swine fever outbreak

Shankar Yadav[1,2] and Hsin-Yi Weng[1*]

Abstract

Background: The study aim was to quantify the impact of movement restriction on the well-being of pigs and the associated mitigation responses during a classical swine fever (CSF) outbreak. We developed a stochastic risk assessment model and incorporated Indiana swine industry statistics to estimate the timing and number of swine premises that would encounter overcrowding or feed interruption resulting from movement restriction. Our model also quantified the amount of on-farm euthanasia and movement of pigs to slaughter plants required to alleviate those conditions. We simulated various single-site (i.e., an outbreak initiated from one location) and multiple-site (i.e., an outbreak initiated from more than one location) outbreak scenarios in Indiana to estimate outputs.

Results: The study estimated that 14% of the swine premises in Indiana would encounter overcrowding or feed interruption due to movement restriction implemented during a CSF outbreak. The number of premises that would experience animal welfare conditions was about 2.5 fold of the number of infected premises. On-farm euthanasia needed to be performed on 33% of those swine premises to alleviate adverse animal welfare conditions, and more than 90% of on-farm euthanasia had to be carried out within 2 weeks after the implementation of movement restriction. Conversely, movement of pigs to slaughter plants could alleviate 67% of adverse animal welfare conditions due to movement restriction, and only less than 1% of movement of pigs to slaughter plants had to be initiated in the first 2 weeks of movement restrictions. The risk of secondary outbreaks due to movement of pigs from movement restriction areas to slaughter plants was low and only seven pigs from each shipment needed to be tested for CSF infection to prevent a secondary outbreak.

Conclusions: We found that the scale of adverse animal welfare consequences of movement restriction during a CSF outbreak in Indiana was substantial, and controlled movement of pigs to slaughter plants was an efficient and low-risk alternative mitigation response to on-farm euthanasia. The output estimates generated from this study provide empirical evidence for decision makers to properly incorporate required resources for mitigating adverse animal welfare conditions in CSF outbreak management strategic planning.

Keywords: Classical swine fever, Movement restriction, Pigs, Swine, Outbreak control, Animal welfare, Overcrowding, Risk assessment

* Correspondence: weng9@purdue.edu
[1]Department of Comparative Pathobiology, Purdue University, 625 Harrison Street, West Lafayette, IN 47907, USA
Full list of author information is available at the end of the article

Background

After the confirmation of a foreign animal disease (FAD) outbreak in the United States, different countermeasures must be initiated immediately, including designation of control zones, depopulation of infected and contact premises, implementation of movement restrictions, and disease surveillance. Movement restriction is an essential step in containing an outbreak, based on both historical outbreak data [1] and epidemiological simulations [2–5]. According to the FAD outbreak response plan in the United States, no movement of live animals, animal products, vehicles, or people is allowed in a movement restriction area until 28 days after disinfection of the last infected premises [6].

A prolonged period of movement restriction may greatly affect the well-being of pigs. During the 1997–1998 classical swine fever (CSF) outbreaks in the Netherlands, seven million healthy pigs were euthanised due to adverse animal welfare conditions, such as overcrowding and feed interruption, which comprised more than 50% of the total direct costs of the overall outbreak-control initiative [7, 8]. Adverse animal welfare consequences of movement restriction during a CSF outbreak can be particularly problematic in modern intensive pork production systems where pigs are often raised utilising the maximum allowed space of swine premises. Overcrowding may emerge quickly in swine premises if pigs are not moved after reaching their harvest/transition age. Overcrowding may suppress pigs' biological functioning (e.g., normal growth) and expression of natural behaviours [9, 10]. Obstruction in expression of pigs' natural behaviours (e.g., exploration or chewing of objects) may trigger tail-biting, ear-chewing, aggression, and fighting [11, 12]. In addition to overcrowding, restricting vehicles into movement restriction areas may interrupt feed supply for swine premises, which can have an immediate impact on the well-being of pigs [13, 14]. Pork producers might also decide to discontinue feed purchases and euthanise the pigs to reduce economic losses during an outbreak.

Despite the significance of this issue, only limited studies have directly assessed animal welfare implications during an FAD outbreak [15, 16]. To address this knowledge gap, our research team initiated a series of studies to quantitatively assess the impacts of movement restriction on the well-being of pigs using CSF as a disease outbreak model [17, 18]. Here we reported the results of a study that integrated the findings from our previous models and Indiana swine industry statistics to estimate the timing and number of swine premises that would encounter adverse animal welfare conditions resulting from movement restriction, and to quantify the frequency of associated mitigation strategies.

Methods

The study started with a roundtable discussion bringing together experts in epidemiology, immunology, animal welfare science, swine veterinary medicine, and pork production to construct a conceptual framework (Fig. 1). During the meeting, we selected overcrowding and feed interruption as the adverse animal welfare consequences of movement restriction for investigation and controlled movement to slaughter plants and on-farm euthanasia as the mitigation strategies for these adverse conditions. We then developed a stochastic risk assessment model based on that conceptual framework and incorporated Indian swine industry statistics to estimate the time elapsed between implementation of movement restriction and onset of overcrowding or feed interruption, the number of swine premises that would encounter adverse animal welfare conditions, and the risk of moving pigs to slaughter plants as a mitigation strategy during a CSF outbreak.

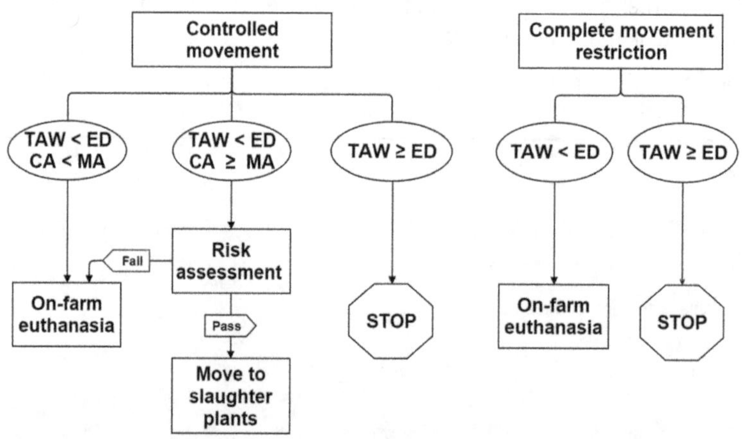

Fig. 1 Conceptual framework for the animal welfare mitigation plans under two movement restriction strategies. (*CA*: current age of pigs when animal welfare concerns emerge, *MA*: market-age of pigs, *ED*: epidemic duration, *TAW*: time to adverse animal welfare conditions)

Conceptual framework

We compiled expert opinions obtained from the roundtable discussion to construct a conceptual framework (Fig. 1) that presented model parameters and decision points for initiating different mitigation responses. Two movement restriction strategies were evaluated: (a) complete movement restriction and (b) controlled movement. Complete movement restriction is the currently recommended CSF control measure in the United States [6], whereas controlled movement is the proposed alternative to be evaluated in this study. Under complete movement restriction, all movement of pigs, people, and vehicles in a designated movement restriction area was prohibited. Under controlled movement, market-age pigs were allowed to be moved to a slaughter plant after a pre-movement risk assessment. The time elapsed between the onset of an outbreak and the emergence of animal welfare conditions such as overcrowding or feed interruption (*TAW*) was compared to epidemic duration (*ED*) to determine the corresponding actions. If $TAW \geq ED$, no overcrowding or feed interruption emerged during an outbreak and no further action was initiated. If $TAW < ED$, overcrowding or feed interruption emerged before an outbreak ended and further mitigation responses must be initiated. Under complete movement restriction, on-farm euthanasia was the only option for alleviating these adverse conditions. Under controlled movement, either on-farm euthanasia or movement of pigs to slaughter plants would be initiated to alleviate animal welfare conditions, depending on the current age of the pigs at the time when overcrowding or feed interruption emerged (*CA*). If the pigs had not reached the market age (i.e., $CA < MA$), on-farm euthanasia was initiated; otherwise (i.e., $CA \geq MA$) the pigs were moved to a slaughter plant after passing the pre-movement risk assessment. If the pre-movement risk assessment identified potential exposure to an infection, on-farm euthanasia was initiated.

Risk assessment model

We took different steps to develop a novel risk assessment model to estimate the parameters presented in the conceptual framework. In the first step, we established a risk metric to select the most likely CSF outbreak scenarios in Indiana for model simulations in order to estimate *ED* as well as the daily number of newly infected premises during an outbreak. Second, we developed and implemented algorithms to estimate *TAW* and CA. Third, we developed the second set of algorithms to integrate *ED*, *TAW*, and *CA* with Indiana swine industry statistics to estimate the number of swine premises in Indiana that would encounter overcrowding or feed interruption due to movement restrictions during a CSF outbreak and the frequency of different mitigation responses. Fourth, we used the risk assessment model to estimate the number of pigs that needed to be tested from each shipment to prevent a secondary outbreak due to movement to slaughter plants. We modeled nursery (19 to 65 days of age) and finisher (40 to 165 days of age) pork production operations separately. Simulations were run with 100,000 iterations each unless otherwise stated.

Simulation of the most likely CSF outbreak scenarios to estimate ED

We developed a risk metric for selecting the most likely CSF outbreak scenarios in Indiana using different data sources, including the 2012 Indiana State Swine Premise Identification Database (USAHERDS), United States Census data, and 2013 Indiana State Natural Resources data. Based on the risk metric, we selected 19 single-site (i.e., outbreaks initiated from one location) and 15 multiple-site (i.e., outbreaks initiated from more than one location) CSF outbreak scenarios for the simulations to estimate probability distributions of *ED*. We performed the simulations using the North American Animal Disease Spread Model (NAADSM), a stochastic, temporal, and spatial state transition disease spread model [19]. Details on the development of the risk metric, the selection of outbreak scenarios, and the estimations of *ED* can be found in a previous study [17].

The simulation results of single-site outbreaks revealed a bimodal distribution of *ED* [17]. Therefore, we assigned two triangular distributions [denoted as Triangle (minimum, most likely, maximum)], Triangle (24, 50, 100) and Triangle (100, 224, 343), to present the two clusters of *ED* for a single-site CSF outbreak. In addition, we assigned a Bernoulli distribution [denoted as Bernoulli (probability of event)], Bernoulli (0.3) for Triangle (24, 50, 100). We randomly selected four multiple-site outbreak scenarios from the 15 scenarios to estimate the study outputs. Table 1 presents different triangular distributions for the *ED* for the sampled multiple-site outbreaks.

Risk assessment model to estimate TAW and CA

In this study, we defined overcrowding as a condition in which the total weight of pigs on premises exceeds 100–115% of the maximum capacity of that premises. The maximum capacity of premises was quantified by the total weight of pigs at the harvest/transition age on that premises. We implemented algorithms to compute the daily total weight of pigs on premises and compared it to the threshold weight that defined overcrowding. The model implemented those algorithms to flag the time at which the total weight exceeded the threshold (i.e., when overcrowding occurred).

Table 1 Probability distributions for epidemic duration in different classical swine fever outbreak scenarios in Indiana, USA

Outbreak scenario	Probability distribution
Single-site outbreak[a]	Cluster 1: Triangle (24, 50, 100) Cluster 2: Triangle (100, 224, 343) Probability of cluster 1: Bernoulli (0.3)
Multiple-site outbreak with 4 index premises[b]	Triangle (29, 203, 514)
Multiple-site outbreak with 17 index premises[b]	Triangle (138, 185, 341)
Multiple-site outbreak with 20 index premises[b]	Triangle (142, 187, 440)
Multiple-site outbreak with 26 index premises[b]	Triangle (146, 197, 311)

The results were generated from the simulation with 500 iterations using the North American Animal Disease Spread Model
[a]The results are for four single-site outbreak scenarios combined
[b]Index premises are infected premises when an outbreak starts

We modeled feed interruption to emerge shortly after a swine producer decided to discontinue feed supply and euthanise the pigs on premises in order to reduce economic losses due to a CSF outbreak. We implemented three decision attributes in the algorithms that would increase the probability for a producer to discontinue feed supply: (a) when the estimated epidemic duration was longer than a producer's tolerance level; (b) when the time interval between the age of pigs at the onset of the outbreak and the harvest/transition age was longer than a producer's tolerance level; and (c) when the progression of an ongoing outbreak lasted longer than a producer's tolerance level. The tolerance level of a producer was modeled by the uniform distributions between 14 and 46 days and between 30 and 125 days for nursery and finisher operations, respectively. For simplicity, we assigned the probability for a producer to discontinue feed supply to high [Bernoulli (0.3)] or low [Bernoulli (0.05)] depending these three decision attributes. High probability was implemented when any of the three decision attributes exceeded a producer's tolerance level; otherwise low probability was implemented.

We quantified *TAW* as the number of days between the implementation of movement restriction and the onset of overcrowding or feed interruption, whichever occurred first. We then computed *CA* as the age of pigs at the onset of an outbreak plus *TAW*. In the model we assumed that (a) movement restriction would be implemented within 24 h of the detection of an outbreak and (b) the age of pigs represented the oldest age among pigs on the same premises. With the latter assumption, the simulations returned the shortest *TAW* for that premises. Based on the results, we assigned Triangle (2, 14, 59) and Triangle (2, 17, 59) for *TAW* in nursery operations in single-site outbreaks and multiple-site outbreaks, respectively [18]. Triangle (2, 14, 260) and Triangle (2, 14, 253) were assigned for *TAW* in finisher operations in single-site outbreaks and multiple-site outbreaks, respectively [18]. Details of the model algorithms for estimating *TAW* are described in a previous study [18].

Estimation of the scale of adverse animal welfare conditions and mitigation responses

In this final step of model building, we implemented 2012 Indiana swine industry statistics compiled in USAHERDS in the risk assessment model, incorporating the input parameters generated in the previous steps. We did so to estimate the number of swine premises in Indiana that would encounter overcrowding or feed interruption during a CSF outbreak, the scope of corresponding mitigation responses, and the risk of secondary outbreaks due to movements of pigs from movement restriction areas to slaughter plants. The data compiled in USAHERDS included identification number, herd size, operation type, and geolocation of premises.

Based on the United States CSF response plan, a movement restriction area was designated as a circular area 7 km away from the perimeter of an infected zone. We identified the locations of infected premises at the onset of an outbreak for a sample of four single-site and six multiple-site most likely CSF outbreak scenarios. Movement restriction areas were mapped for each infected premises and the number of unique swine premises in movement restriction areas was determined. We used those results to derive a logarithmic regression equation (Table 2) to estimate the number of unique swine premises that fell under movement restrictions given the number of infected premises. In addition to the four multiple-site outbreak scenarios described previously (Table 1), two scenarios with the number of index premises of 23 and 32 were included in the computation of regression equation. The regression line had an $R^2 = 0.945$, indicating a good fit to the data.

We simulated the selected eight CSF outbreak scenarios using NAADSM to estimate the number of daily new infections. Five hundred iterations were simulated for each outbreak scenario, and the average daily number of new infections and standard error were computed for all single-site outbreak scenarios combined and for individual multiple-site outbreak scenarios. We implemented the estimates of number of new infections in the regression equation to estimate the number of unique swine premises that fell under movement restrictions. We also modeled standard errors for the number of new infections and regression residuals to account for variations. The model algorithms then computed *TAW* for premises under movement restrictions on a particular day and compared it to *ED* to identify premises that would encounter overcrowding or feed interruption before an outbreak ended (i.e., $TAW < ED$). Among them, the

Table 2 Parameters for estimating the number of premises encountering animal-welfare conditions during a CSF outbreak

Parameter	Description	Distribution and algorithm
Number of daily new infections (*N_inf*)	This parameter was derived from the simulations of four single-site and four multiple-site CSF outbreak scenarios in Indiana (500 iteractions each). The mean and standard error (SE) of number of daily new infections were computed. Normal (0,1) represnted the distribution for number of SE. Thus, the estimates of *N_inf* varied around an overall mean by different numbers of SE.	$N\_inf_i = \text{Mean}_i + \text{Normal}\ (0,1) \times \text{SE}_i$ on day *i*
Number of premises under movment restriction (*N_MR*)	This parameter was estimated as a function of the number of infected premises. Logarithmic regression equation was derived from the simulations of four single-site and six multiple-site CSF outbreak scenarios in Indiana. Normal (17,36) was dedrived from the regression residuals.	$N\_MR_i = 201.5 \times \text{LN}\left(\sum_{t=0}^{t=i} N\_inf_t\right) + \text{Normal}\ (17{,}36)$ on day *i*
Index for *TAW* < *ED* (*Index*)	The probability distributions for *TAW* and *ED* were published in previous studies [17, 18]. A binary index was created to flag *TAW* < *ED* (i.e., *Index* = 1; else *Index* = 0), indicating that animal-welfare conditions occurred before an outbreak ended.	Number of premises that encountered animal-welfare consequencs of movement restriction on day $i = N\_MR_i \times Index_i$

TAW The time elapsed between the onset of an outbreak and the emergence of animal welfare conditions, *ED* Epidemic duration

model compared *CA* to *MA* to determine whether on-farm euthanasia (i.e., $CA < MA$) or movement of pigs to slaughter plants (i.e., $CA \geq MA$) should be initiated to alleviate the adverse animal welfare conditions on that premises (Fig. 1). Using the risk assessment model, we estimated the total number of swine premises that would encounter overcrowding or feed interruption and the amount of on-farm euthanasia and movement of pigs to slaughter plants to be initiated during a CSF outbreak in Indiana. Table 2 presents details on model input parameters and algorithms for this step of risk assessment.

The final step of model building was to estimate the maximum threshold risk that would not trigger a secondary outbreak due to movement of pigs from movement restriction areas to slaughter plants. We then used that maximum threshold risk to estimate the number of pigs that had to be sampled and tested for CSF from each shipment to detect an infection. To accomplish this objective, we included all listed slaughter plants in USAHERDS as potential receipting sites in the disease spread simulations using NAADSM. To determine the maximum threshold risk, we simulated various levels of within-premises CSF prevalence of subclinical infections to manipulate the disease transmission rate of direct contact in NAADSM. The model assumed that pigs were held at a slaughter plant for no more than 24 h before being processed. With this assumption and the assumption that pigs showing clinical signs of CSF would be inevitably identified, only pigs that were at the subclinical stage of CSF infection on premises before movement had the chance to spread the disease while at a slaughter plant. This was because the average latent and subclinical periods of CSF were 4 days and 6 days, respectively [20]. In NAADSM, infected pigs were assumed to start shedding the virus at the subclinical stage of CSF. The rate of disease transmission through indirect contact was adopted from a previous study [17].

Sensitivity analyses

We performed sensitivity analyses to identify influential input parameters. In the first step, we used Spearman's correlation to identify parameters that were associated with the target output (e.g., number of premises that would encounter adverse animal welfare conditions). We further investigated the parameters that showed a correlation coefficient ≥ 0.3 using simulations of different input values to quantify their influences on output estimates.

Results

There were 8631 swine premises listed in Indiana USAHERDS in 2012; 86% of them were small operations (herd size range: 1–699) and 14% were commercial (herd size range: 200–20,000). The estimated *TAW* was similar between the single-site and multiple-site outbreak scenarios, with a median (25th, 75th percentiles) of 19 days (10, 29) in nursery operations and 57 days (13, 93) in finisher operations [18].

The median (25th and 75th percentiles) numbers of infected swine premises and swine premises that would encounter animal welfare consequences of movement restriction for all four single-site CSF outbreak scenarios combined were 466 (443, 488) and 1169 (603, 1224), respectively (Table 3). The median numbers of infected swine premises ranged from 468 to 614 in the four multiple-site outbreak scenarios, and the median numbers of swine premises that would encounter animal welfare consequences of movement restriction ranged from 1170 to 1293 (Table 3). Among them, approximately 5% were nursery and 95% were finisher operations. On-farm euthanasia would need to be initiated for

Table 3 Numbers of infected swine premises and premises with animal welfare conditions during a CSF outbreak

Outbreak scenario	Infected premises	Premises with animal welfare conditions
Single-site outbreak[a]	466 (443, 488)	1169 (603, 1224)
Multiple-site outbreak with 4 index premises[b]	467 (446, 488)	1182 (1016, 1231)
Multiple-site outbreak with 17 index premises[b]	590 (575, 606)	1277 (1233, 1307)
Multiple-site outbreak with 20 index premises[b]	609 (596, 621)	1293 (1259, 1321)
Multiple-site outbreak with 26 index premises[b]	614 (602, 625)	1289 (1248, 1319)

Numbers are the median (25th and 75th percentiles)
[a]The results are for four single-site (i.e., an outbreak starts with one infected premises) CSF outbreak scenarios in Indiana combined
[b]Index premises are infected premises when an outbreak starts

about 33% of the swine premises that encountered adverse animal welfare conditions, whereas movement of pigs to slaughter plants could be initiated for about 67% of the swine premises to alleviate adverse animal welfare conditions (Fig. 2). On-farm euthanasia was carried out for all nursery operations and for approximately 28% of finisher operations that encountered adverse animal welfare conditions, and about 90% of the on-farm euthanasia was initiated within the first 2 weeks of the implementation of movement restriction (Fig. 3). In comparison, only 1% of movement of pigs to slaughter plants was initiated within the first 2 weeks of movement restriction (Fig. 4).

Using the risk assessment model, we found that the risk of secondary outbreaks due to movement of pigs from movement restriction areas to slaughter plants was very low. Such movements would not trigger a secondary outbreak even with the within-premises prevalence of CSF as high as 50%. We further estimated that each swine premises was allowed to have a maximum of five

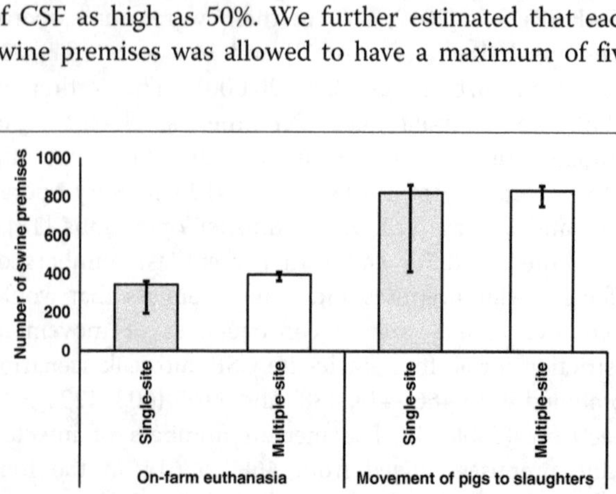

Fig. 2 Number of premises that required mitigation of animal welfare conditions during a CSF outbreak in Indiana. (The *bar chart* represents the median and *error bars* at the 25th and 75th percentiles. The results were generated from simulations of four single-site (i.e., an outbreak initiated from one location) and four multiple-site (i.e., an outbreak initiated from more than one location) outbreak scenarios in Indiana)

movements during an outbreak, and seven pigs should be sampled and tested for CSF before each shipment to detect an infection with a confidence level of 99%.

In the initial sensitivity analyses, we identified that *TAW* for finisher operations was negatively, and *ED* positively, correlated with the estimate of number of premises experiencing adverse animal welfare consequences of movement restriction. In further investigations, a ± 10% margin of the original input probability distributions of those two input parameters resulted in a less than 1% change in the output estimates.

Discussion

The aim of this study was to estimate the scale of adverse animal welfare consequences of movement restriction and associated mitigation responses during a foreign animal disease outbreak that affects swine. We simulated different CSF outbreak scenarios combining with Indiana swine industry data to estimate outputs. Using the risk assessment model, we estimated that approximately 14% of the swine premises in Indiana would encounter adverse animal welfare conditions that resulted from movement restrictions imposed as one of the countermeasures for outbreak control. According to the 2012 U.S. Census of Agriculture, Indiana produced about 11 million pigs in 2012 [21], and, therefore, 1.5 million pigs would need to be euthanised on-farm or moved to slaughter plants as a mitigation of adverse animal welfare conditions due to movement restrictions during a CSF outbreak. The estimates varied depending on the characteristics of an outbreak, with a multiple-site outbreak resulting in slightly more swine premises with animal welfare consequences compared to a single-site outbreak. However, the differences in the estimates of the total number of both infected premises and premises with animal welfare consequences between the two types of outbreak were negligible (Table 3). The number of premises that would encounter animal welfare conditions was approximately 2.5 fold of the number of infected premises. These estimates provide valuable information for decision makers to develop proper strategic plans for alleviating animal welfare consequences of movement restrictions during a CSF outbreak. Although we used the Indiana swine industry data to simulate the estimates, the finding that the scale of animal welfare consequences of movement restrictions was substantial and greater than the number of infections agreed with findings based on historical CSF outbreaks in Europe [1, 22, 23]. Our risk assessment model could be easily adapted by other states in the United States that have a similar pork production system to generate state-specific estimates.

The timing of initiating on-farm euthanasia or movement of pigs to slaughter plants to alleviate animal welfare conditions is also a critical parameter for planning CSF outbreak management. Our model showed that about 90% of on-

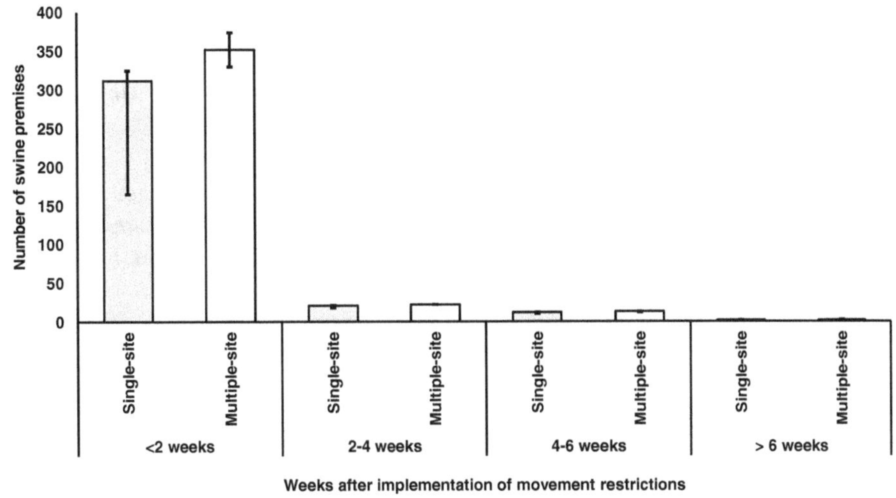

Fig. 3 Timing of on-farm euthanasia to alleviate animal welfare conditions during a CSF outbreak in Indiana. (The *bar chart* represents the median and *error bars* at the 25th and 75th percentiles. The results were generated from simulations of four single-site (i.e., an outbreak initiated from one location) and four multiple-site (i.e., an outbreak initiated from more than one location) outbreak scenarios in Indiana)

farm euthanasia had to be initiated within 2 weeks of movement restrictions. This finding suggested a competing resource for depopulating infected and contact premises in an infected zone that was required to be completed as soon as possible after the identification of an infection. It could greatly hinder outbreak control efforts if the high demand of animal welfare alleviation response activities was not properly considered in outbreak response plans. For example, during the 2001 ft-and-mouth disease outbreaks in the United Kingdom, slaughter staff, labor, and carcass

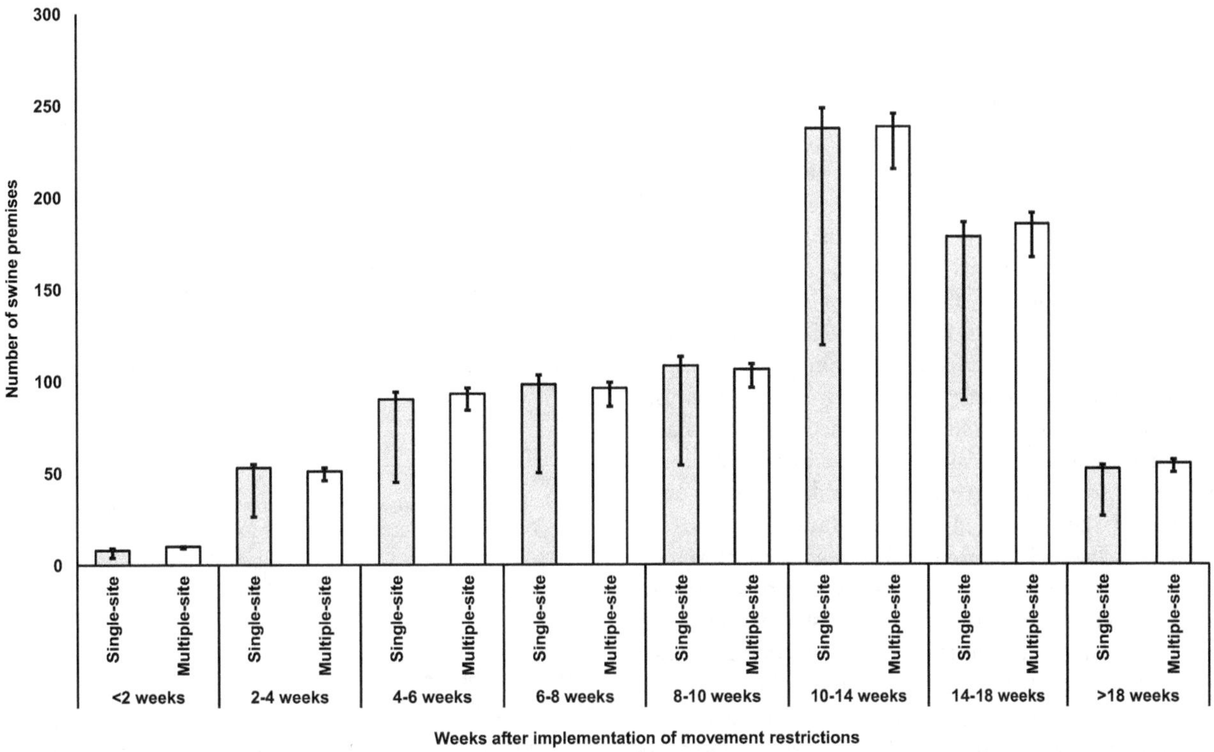

Fig. 4 Timing of movement to slaughter as an animal welfare mitigation during a CSF outbreak in Indiana. (The *bar chart* represents the median and *error bars* at the 25th and 75th percentiles. The results were generated from simulations of four single-site (i.e., an outbreak initiated from one location) and four multiple-site (i.e., an outbreak initiated from more than one location) outbreak scenarios in Indiana)

disposal sites were found to be insufficient mainly due to inadequate consideration of animal welfare implications [24]. In the 1997–1998 CSF outbreaks in the Netherlands, the number and capacity of rendering plants were insufficient to dispose of the large volume of swine carcasses that were mostly from the euthanasia of pigs for alleviating adverse-welfare conditions [22, 25, 26]. In contrast to on-farm euthanasia, our model showed that only less than 1% of movement of pigs to slaughter plants would need to be initiated within 2 weeks of movement restrictions. This mitigation strategy could greatly reduce pressure from competing limited resources for outbreak controls.

Movement of pigs to slaughter plants may also help moderate food insecurity concerns due to discontinuation of the pork supply chain [27, 28]. Consequently, it can significantly reduce the economic losses of pork producers. Furthermore, euthanasia of a large number of animals, particularly healthy animals, may affect livestock owners, their families, and people involved in executing mass depopulation not only economically but also psychologically [29–31]. Mass euthanasia could pose negative public and social perception of the agriculture industry, detrimental effects on the local tourist industry, and delayed recovery and resumption of normal reproduction of livestock. In their study, Thompson et al. [30] showed that inappropriate carcass disposal of euthanised animals during the 2001 FMD outbreak in UK may have contributed substantially to an estimated $3.2 billion in losses to the country's tourist industry. We demonstrated that movement of pigs to slaughter plants can greatly reduce the amount of on-farm euthanasia for mitigating adverse animal welfare conditions during a CSF outbreak. Based on the study model, movement of pigs to slaughter plants could be initiated to alleviate approximately 67% of pigs that experienced adverse-welfare conditions in Indiana.

During a CSF outbreak, all swine premises that are under movement restrictions are under surveillance for potential infection. A detection of infections will prompt the designation of new control zones surrounding infected premises. However, even with ongoing surveillance it is still vital to conduct pre-movement risk assessment to prevent a subclinical pig from carrying disease outside a control zone. Our model showed that a limited number of controlled movements (i.e., ≤5 per premises) of pigs from movement restriction areas to slaughter plants posed very low risk for secondary outbreaks. With such a low risk, only seven pigs have to be sampled and tested for CSF infection from each shipment to detect an infection with a 99% confidence level. This amount of pre-movement risk assessment is considered practicable during a CSF outbreak, owing to the advances in CSF diagnostic tests. The World Organisation of Animal Health (OIE) recommends different diagnostic techniques for CSF infections or exposures in pigs, such as conventional reverse transcription polymerase chain reaction (RT-PCR), antigen enzyme linked immune-sorbent assay (ELISA), fluorescence antibody test (FAT), and virus neutralization [32]. Among them, RT-PCR is considered the most sensitive and reliable test for quick CSF diagnosis during an outbreak [33–35]. Studies have shown that infected pigs could be detected as early as 2 days post-infection and 3 to 4 days before onset of clinical signs using RT-PCR [36, 37]. In addition, RT-PCR could generate test results in 2 h [37]. Therefore, we recommend applying RT-PCR in pre-movement risk assessment for the mitigation strategy of movement of pigs to slaughter plants during a CSF outbreak.

Conclusions

The scale of animal welfare consequences of movement restrictions during a CSF outbreak in Indiana was substantial. Movement of pigs to slaughter plants was an efficient and low-risk alternative to on-farm euthanasia to alleviate adverse animal welfare conditions. Our risk assessment model estimated that movement of pigs to slaughter plants could be used to alleviate approximately 67% of the animal welfare consequences of movement restrictions in Indiana. Seven pigs needed to be tested for CSF infection in the pre-movement risk assessment to ensure the prevention of a secondary outbreak.

Abbreviations

CA: Current age of pigs at the onset of animal welfare conditions; CSF: Classical swine fever; ED: Epidemic duration; FAD: Foreign animal disease; MA: Market-age of pigs; NAADSM: North American Animal Disease Spread Model; TAW: The time elapsed between the onset of an outbreak and the emergence of animal welfare conditions

Acknowledgements

The authors thank Dr. Marianne Ash and Dr. Maria Cooper at the Indiana State Board of Animal Health for querying selected information on farm locations in Indiana. We also thank Dr. Marianne Ash, Dr. Anna Butters-Johnson, Dr. Maria Cooper, Dr. Candace Croney, Mr. Jim Erickson, Dr. Megan Inskeep, Dr. Donald Lay, Jr., Mr. Mark Legan, Dr. Karen Lehe, Dr. Jeremy Marchant-Forde, Dr. Max Rodibaugh, Dr. Sandra San Miguel, Mr. Josh Trenary, Dr. Ramesh Vemulapalli, Dr. Nicole J. Olynk Widmar, and Dr. Amy Woods for their participation in the roundtable discussion in June of 2014.

Funding

This material is based upon work that is supported by the National Pork Board (Project # 13-153) and the USDA National Institute of Food and Agriculture, Hatch project 230919. The funding bodies do not play a role in the design of the study and collection, analysis, and interpretation of data and in writing the manuscript.

Authors' contributions

SY developed the risk metric for selecting most likely CSF outbreak scenarios, simulated NAADSM to estimate ED and daily newly infected premises, mapped and identified swine premises in movement restriction areas, and was a major contributor in writing the manuscript. HYW designed the study, developed the risk assessment model, simulated and interpreted the results, and prepared the manuscript. Both authors read and approved the final manuscript.

Competing interests
The authors declare that they have no competing interests.

Consent for publication
Not applicable.

Author details
[1]Department of Comparative Pathobiology, Purdue University, 625 Harrison Street, West Lafayette, IN 47907, USA. [2]Plum Island Animal Disease Center Research Participation Program (ORISE fellow), Orient Point, NY 11957, USA.

References

1. Elbers AR, Stegeman A, Moser H, Ekker HM, Smak JA, Pluimers FH. The classical swine fever epidemic 1997-1998 in the Netherlands: descriptive epidemiology. Prev Vet Med. 1999;42(3–4):157–84.
2. Thulke HH, Eisinger D, Beer M. The role of movement restrictions and pre-emptive destruction in the emergency control strategy against CSF outbreaks in domestic pigs. Prev Vet Med. 2011;99(1):28–37.
3. Nielen M, Jalvingh AW, Meuwissen MP, Horst SH, Dijkhuizen AA. Spatial and stochastic simulation to evaluate the impact of events and control measures on the 1997-1998 classical swine fever epidemic in the Netherlands. II. Comparison of control strategies. Prev Vet Med. 1999;42(3–4):297–317.
4. Jalvingh AW, Nielen M, Maurice H, Stegeman AJ, Elbers AR, Dijkhuizen AA. Spatial and stochastic simulation to evaluate the impact of events and control measures on the 1997-1998 classical swine fever epidemic in the Netherlands. I. Description of simulation model. Prev Vet Med. 1999;42(3–4):271–95.
5. Mangen MJ, Nielen M, Burrell AM. Simulated effect of pig-population density on epidemic size and choice of control strategy for classical swine fever epidemics in the Netherlands. Prev Vet Med. 2002;56(2):141–63.
6. USDA. APHIS foreign animal disease framework response strategies. In: FAD preparedness and response plan manual 2-0. Animal and plant health inspection service (APHIS), veterinary services, United States Department of Agriculture (USDA). 2012. http://www.aphis.usda.gov/fadprep. Accessed 21 Jan 2013.
7. De Vos CJ, Saatkamp HW, Huirne RB. Cost-effectiveness of measures to prevent classical swine fever introduction into the Netherlands. Prev Vet Med. 2005;70(3–4):235–56.
8. Saatkamp HW, Berentsen PB, Horst HS. Economic aspects of the control of classical swine fever outbreaks in the European Union. Vet Microbiol. 2000;73(2–3):221–37.
9. Keeling LJ. Healthy and happy: animal welfare as an integral part of sustainable agriculture. Ambio. 2005;34(4):316–9.
10. Fraser D, Duncan IJH, Edwards SA, Grandin T, Gregory NG, Guyonnet V, Hemsworth PH, Huertas SM, Huzzey JM, Mellor DJ, et al. General principles for the welfare of animals in production systems: the underlying science and its application. Vet J. 2013;198(1):19–27.
11. Anil L, Anil S, Deen J. Effects of allometric space allowance and weight group composition on grower-finisher pigs. Can J Anim Sci. 2007;187:139–51.
12. Moinard C, Mendl M, Nicol CJ, Green LE. A case control study of on-farm risk factors for tail biting in pigs. Appl Anim Behav Sci. 2003;81:333–55.
13. Crispin SM, Roger PA, O'Hare H, Binns SH. The 2001 foot and mouth disease epidemic in the United Kingdom: animal welfare perspectives. Rev Sci Tech. 2002;21(3):877–83.
14. Galli ME. Movement restriction implications on potential welfare slaughter for texas high plains feedlots. College Station: Master thesis. Texas A & M Univerisity; 2011.
15. Bargen LL, Whiting TL. Time to critical overcrowding of Manitoba swine barns in the event of restriction on animal movement. Can Vet J. 2002;43(11):855–62.
16. East IJ, Roche SE, Wicks RM, de Witte K, Garner MG. Options for managing animal welfare on intensive pig farms confined by movement restrictions during an outbreak of foot and mouth disease. Prev Vet Med. 2014;117(3–4):533–41.
17. Yadav S, Olynk Widmar NJ, Weng H-Y. Modeling classical swine fever outbreak-related outcomes. Front Vet Sci. 2016;3:7. doi:10.3389/fvets.2016.00007.
18. Weng HY, Yadav S, Olynk Widmar NJ, Ash M, Cooper M, Croney C. Modelling the time at which overcrowding and feed shortage emerge on the swine premises under movement restrictions during a classical swine fever outbreak. Animal 11:493-9.
19. NAADSM. North American Animal Disease Spread Model (NAADSM). In: NAADSM version 33. 2013. http://www.naadsm.org. Accessed 13 Aug 2013.
20. Martinez-Lopez B, Ivorra B, Ramos AM, Sanchez-Vizcaino JM. A novel spatial and stochastic model to evaluate the within- and between-farm transmission of classical swine fever virus. I. General concepts and description of the model. Vet Microbiol. 2011;147(3–4):300–9.
21. USDA. USDA census of agriculture. In: 2012 census of agriculture. United State Department of Agriculture (USDA). 2012. https://www.agcensus.usda.gov/Publications. Accessed 07 Jul 2016.
22. Stegeman A, Elbers A, de Smit H, Moser H, Smak J, Pluimers F. The 1997-1998 epidemic of classical swine fever in the Netherlands. Vet Microbiol. 2000;73(2–3):183–96.
23. Edwards S, Fukusho A, Lefevre PC, Lipowski A, Pejsak Z, Roehe P, Westergaard J. Classical swine fever: the global situation. Vet Microbiol. 2000;73(2–3):103–19.
24. Scudamore JM, Trevelyan GM, Tas MV, Varley EM, Hickman GA. Carcass disposal: lessons from great Britain following the foot and mouth disease outbreaks of 2001. Rev Sci Tech. 2002;21(3):775–87.
25. Pluimers FH, de Leeuw PW, Smak JA, Elbers AR, Stegeman JA. Classical swine fever in the Netherlands 1997-1998: a description of organisation and measures to eradicate the disease. Prev Vet Med. 1999;42(3–4):139–55.
26. Roche SE, Garner MG, Wicks RM, East IJ, de Witte K. How do resources influence control measures during a simulated outbreak of foot and mouth disease in Australia? Prev Vet Med. 2014;113(4):436–46.
27. Domenech J, Lubroth J, Eddi C, Martin V, Roger F. Regional and international approaches on prevention and control of animal transboundary and emerging diseases. Ann N Y Acad Sci. 2006;1081:90–107.
28. Otte M, Nugent R, McLeod A. Transboundary animal diseases: Assessment of socio-economic impacts and institutional responses. In: Livestock policy discussion paper number 9. Food and Agriculture Organization (FAO). 2004. http://www.fao.org/3/a-ag273e.pdf. Accessed 15 Jul 2016.
29. Nusbaum KE, Wenzel JG, Everly Jr GS. Psychologic first aid and veterinarians in rural communities undergoing livestock depopulation. J Am Vet Med Assoc. 2007;231(5):692–4.
30. Thompson D, Muriel P, Russell D, Osborne P, Bromley A, Rowland M, Creigh-Tyte S, Brown C. Economic costs of the foot and mouth disease outbreak in the United Kingdom in 2001. Rev Sci Tech. 2002;21(3):675–87.
31. Driijfhout A, De Leeuw J. The mental health status of local veterinarians, 2 years after the foot and mouth disease crisis in their practice. Tijdschr Diergeneeskd. 2005;130(3):82.
32. OIE. Manual of diagnostic tests and vaccines for terrestrial animals 2015. In: classical swine fever. World Organization for Animal Health (OIE). 2015. http://www.oie.int/en/international-standard-setting/terrestrial-manual/access-online. Accessed 15 Jul 2016.
33. Dewulf J, Koenen F, Mintiens K, Denis P, Ribbens S, de Kruif A. Analytical performance of several classical swine fever laboratory diagnostic techniques on live animals for detection of infection. J Virol Methods. 2004;119(2):137–43.
34. Leifer I, Blome S, Beer M, Hoffmann B. Development of a highly sensitive real-time RT-PCR protocol for the detection of classical swine fever virus independent of the 5' untranslated region. J Virol Methods. 2011;171(1):314–7.
35. McGoldrick A, Lowings J, Ibata G, Sands J, Belak S, Paton D. A novel approach to the detection of classical swine fever virus by RT-PCR with a fluorogenic probe (TaqMan). J Virol Methods. 1998;72(2):125–35.
36. Zhao J-J, Cheng D, Li N, Sun Y, Shi Z, Zhu Q-H, Tu C, Tong G-Z, Qiu H-J. Evaluation of a multiplex real-time RT-PCR for quantitative and differential detection of wild-type viruses and C-strain vaccine of classical swine fever virus. Vet Microbiol. 2008;126(1):1–10.
37. Risatti GR, Callahan JD, Nelson WM, Borca MV. Rapid detection of classical swine fever virus by a portable real-time reverse transcriptase PCR assay. J Clin Microbiol. 2003;41(1):500–5.

5

Curcumin is a promising inhibitor of genotype 2 porcine reproductive and respiratory syndrome virus infection

Taofeng Du[1,2†], Yunpeng Shi[1,2†], Shuqi Xiao[1,2], Na Li[1,2], Qin Zhao[1,2], Angke Zhang[1,2], Yuchen Nan[1,2], Yang Mu[1,2], Yani Sun[1,2], Chunyan Wu[1,2], Hongtao Zhang[3] and En-Min Zhou[1,2*]

Abstract

Background: Porcine reproductive and respiratory syndrome virus (PRRSV) could lead to pandemic diseases and huge financial losses to the swine industry worldwide. Curcumin, a natural compound, has been reported to serve as an entry inhibitor of hepatitis C virus, chikungunya virus and vesicular stomatitis virus. In this study, we investigated the potential effect of curcumin on early stages of PRRSV infection.

Results: Curcumin inhibited infection of Marc-145 cells and porcine alveolar macrophages (PAMs) by four different genotype 2 PRRSV strains, but had no effect on the levels of major PRRSV receptor proteins on Marc-145 cells and PAMs or on PRRSV binding to Marc-145 cells. However, curcumin did block two steps of the PRRSV infection process: virus internalization and virus-mediated cell fusion.

Conclusions: Our results suggested that an inhibition of genotype 2 PRRSV infection by curcumin is virus strain-independent, and mainly inhibited by virus internalization and cell fusion mediated by virus. Collectively, these results demonstrate that curcumin holds promise as a new anti-PRRSV drug.

Keywords: PRRSV, Curcumin, Binding, Internalization, Virus-mediated cell fusion

Background

Porcine reproductive and respiratory syndrome (PRRS), a serious pandemic disease, causes huge economic losses to the swine industry. Clinically, PRRS causes fetal abortion in pregnant sows and respiratory disease in pigs of all ages [1, 2]. The etiological agent, PRRS virus (PRRSV), is an enveloped single-stranded positive-sense RNA virus belonging to the *Arteriviridae* family [3]. PRRSV strains belong to two major genotypes, the European (type 1) and North American (type 2) genotypes, with distinct genetic profiles and geographic distributions [4–6]. Highly pathogenic PRRSV (HP-PRRSV) isolates from China belong to the type 2 genotypic group [7].

* Correspondence: zhouem@nwsuaf.edu.cn
†Equal contributors
[1]Department of Preventive Veterinary Medicine, College of Veterinary Medicine, Northwest A&F University, Yangling, Shaanxi 712100, China
[2]Experimental Station of Veterinary Pharmacology and Veterinary Biotechnology, Ministry of Agriculture, Yangling, Shaanxi 712100, China
Full list of author information is available at the end of the article

Although PRRSV was discovered over twenty years ago, an effective vaccine still has not been developed for the following reasons: (1) Infection of pigs can occur during every phase of production; (2) The semen of boars is a hiding place for virus; (3) The virus is passed between pig farms through multiple routes; (4) High virus mutation frequency is observed; (5) Persistence of infection is observed; (6) Immunosuppression induced by infection prevents virus control [8, 9]; and (7) Although, attenuated PRRSV vaccines can induce weak humoral and cell-mediated immune responses, but have less protection against heterologous strains [10]. Therefore, development of new antiviral drugs or vaccine adjuvants is needed to control PRRSV.

Curcumin, 1,7-bis(4-hydroxy-3-methoxyphenyl)-1,6-heptadiene-3,5-dione), also known as diferuloylmethane, is a natural bioactive polyphenolic compound isolated from *Curcuma longa* rhizomes. The main components of *C. longa* include diferuloylmethane (65–80%), demethoxycurcumin (15–25%) and bisdemethoxycurcumin

(5–15%). Curcumin accounts for most of the biological and pharmacological effects of *C. longa* including immunomodulating, anti-tumor, anti-inflammatory, antioxidant, antimutagenic, antibacterial, antifungal and antiviral activities [11–14]. Notably, curcumin inhibits entry of several types of viruses into cells, including hepatitis C virus (HCV), chikungunya virus (CHIKV) and vesicular stomatitis virus (VSV) [13, 15]. To our knowledge, no potential anti-PRRSV effect of curcumin has yet been reported. Therefore, we evaluated curcumin as an anti-PRRSV agent in Marc-145 cells and PAM and found it inhibited PRRSV infection by preventing virus internalization and virus-mediated cell fusion.

Methods

Viruses, cells and compounds

Four North American PRRSV strains were tested, including highly pathogenic strains PRRSV GD-HD (HP-PRRSV/GD-HD) (GenBank ID: **KP793736**), HP-PRRSV/JXA1 (GenBank ID: **EF112445**), classic PRRSV VR-2332 (GenBank ID: **EF442771**) and a low pathogenic strain, PRRSV CH-1a (GenBank ID: **AY032626**). All strains were propagated and titrated in Marc-145 cells grown in Dulbecco's modified Eagle's medium (DMEM) (Gibco, USA) supplemented with 3% heat-inactivated fetal bovine serum (HI-FBS; Biological Industries, CT, USA). Marc-145 cells were cultured in DMEM with 10% HI-FBS, 100 units/ml penicillin and 100 μg/ml streptomycin (Gibco) at 37 °C in 5% CO_2 incubator. PAMs were obtained from healthy 6-week-old PRRSV-negative pigs using modified lung lavage collection method as previously described [16]. PAMs were maintained in RPMI-1640 medium (Gibco) supplemented with 10% HI-FBS and 1% penicillin-streptomycin-amphotericin B (100×) (Life Technologies Corp., CA, USA). Curcumin (Sigma-Aldrich, St. Louis, MO, USA) was dissolved in dimethyl sulphoxide (DMSO) to make 5, 10, and 15 mM/L as the stock solution and was used at 1/1000 dilution.

Cell viability assay

To evaluate curcumin cytotoxicity, a Cell Counting Kit-8 (CCK8) (Sigma-Aldrich) was used [17]. Briefly, Marc-145 cells and PAMs were seeded into 96-well plates at densities of 1×10^4/well or 1×10^5/well in the presence of various curcumin concentrations for 48 h. 10 μL/well of CCK-8 reagent was added before incubation for 2 h. Absorbance was measured at 450 nm.

Virus inhibition assay

To examine curcumin antiviral activity during early infection stages, Marc-145 cells or PAMs were treated with various curcumin concentrations at 37 °C for 1 h before, during or after GD-HD infection at a multiplicity of infection (MOI: 0.1). The inoculum was discarded and cells were washed three times with PBS and maintained in DMEM containing 3% HI-FBS at 37 °C. After incubation for 36 h, supernatants and cells were harvested to measure virus titers, PRRSV N protein levels and ORF7 mRNA levels. Chloroquine (20 μM) was used as the positive control.

Virus binding assay

Marc-145 cells were seeded into 24-well plates, incubated for 24 h at 37 °C, then treated with curcumin using the following three distinct methods: (i) Virus pretreatment: The virus GD-HD strain (MOI: 100) was incubated with curcumin for 10 min at 37 °C and the mixture was cooled to 4 °C before infection. Then, Marc-145, cells, after prechilling at 4 °C for 1 h, were infected with pretreated virus at 4 °C for 1 h. (ii) Cell pretreatment: Marc-145 cells were treated with curcumin for 1 h at 37 °C and GD-HD was added to cells for 1 h at 4 °C. (iii) Co-treatment: Marc-145 cells were prechilled at 4 °C for 1 h and infected with GD-HD in the presence of curcumin at 4 °C for 1 h. After incubation, cells were washed with ice-cold PBS and harvested to detect PRRSV ORF7 gene using qRT-PCR.

Virus internalization assay

Marc-145 cells were prechilled for 1 h at 4 °C then incubated for 1 h at 4 °C with GD-HD (MOI: 0.1). After virus attachment, cells were washed three times with ice-cold PBS and incubated at 37 °C for 1 h in DMEM with curcumin or chloroquine. Next, cells were washed three times with PBS and incubated with proteinase K (Sigma) for 45 min at 4 °C to get rid of non-internalized viruses. A cocktail (Roche, Meylan, France) was used to inactivate proteinase K. And then the cells were washed thrice with PBS plus 0.2% BSA and maintained in medium without curcumin at 37 °C. At 36 h post infection, supernatants and cells were harvested to measure virus titers and PRRSV N protein levels.

Virus post-internalization assay

After internalization of GD-HD (MOI: 0.1), Marc-145 cells were washed three times with PBS and treated with curcumin in DMEM containing 3% HI-FBS. After incubation at 37 °C for 36 h, culture medium and cells were harvested to measure virus titers and PRRSV N protein levels, respectively. Chloroquine (20 μM) was used as the positive control. Meanwhile, a low pH-dependent cell fusion assay was used to examine whether curcumin inhibited virus-mediated cell fusion in PRRSV-infected Marc-145 cells [18]. Briefly, Marc-145 cells were infected with GD-HD (MOI: 5) at 37 °C. After incubation for 36 h, cells were treated with curcumin at 37 °C for 2 h, washed with PBS, then incubated with fusion medium [10 mM Na_2HPO_4, 10 mM NaH_2PO_4, 150 mM NaCl,

10 mM 2-(N-morpholino) ethanesulfonic acid, adjusted to pH 5.6 with HCl] for 2 min at room temperature. Cells were washed after fusion medium was discarded, incubated with 3% DMEM for 2 h at 37 °C, then fixed with 70% ethanol, stained with fuchsine solution and viewed using light microscopy (Motic AE31, Xiamen, China).

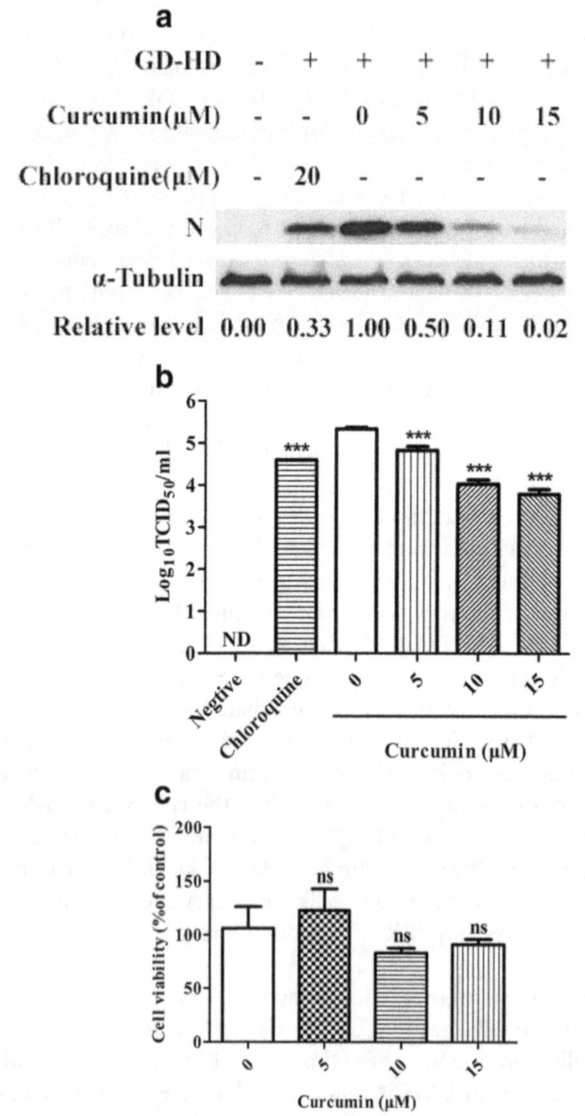

Fig. 1 Effects of curcumin on PRRSV infection of Marc-145 cells. Marc-145 Cells were co-incubated with GD-HD (MOI: 0.1) and various curcumin concentrations at 37 °C for 1 h. Cells were washed and incubated at 37 °C for 36 h in medium without curcumin. PRRSV N protein expression levels were analyzed using western blot with α-tubulin as a control for sample loading (**a**). Virus titers in the supernatants were determined using $CCID_{50}$ (**b**). Curcumin cytotoxicity was determined in Marc-145 cells using a CCK8 assay and is presented as experimental cell viability relative to cell viability of untreated control (100%) (**c**). Each value represents the mean ± SD from three independent experiments (*, $p < 0.05$; **, $p < 0.01$; ***, $p < 0.001$; ND means non-detectable)

Quantitative reverse transcription-PCR (qRT-PCR)

Total RNA was extracted from Marc-145 cells using Total RNA Kit (OMEGA Bio-Tek, GA, USA) using the manufacturer's instructions. Reverse transcription of RNA to cDNA was performed using a Primescript RT reagent Kit (TaKaRa, Dalian, China). Reverse-transcribed products were analyzed using a StepOnePlus Real-Time PCR System (Applied Biosystems, CA, USA) and FastStart Universal SYBR Green Master (Roche, Basel, Switzerland). Specific primer sequences were as follows: Forward primer, PRRSV ORF-7: 5′-AGATCATCA TCGCCCAACAAAAC-3′ and Reverse primer, PRRSV ORF-7: 5′-GACACAATTGCCGCTCACTA-3′; Forward primer, monkey β-actin: 5′-TCCCTGGAGAAGAGC TACGA-3′ and Reverse primer, monkey β-actin: 5′-AGCACTGTGTTGGCGTACAG-3′. β-actin was used as an internal control.

Western blot

Cells were lysed with NP-40 lysis buffer containing 1 mM PMSF (Beyotime, Beijing, China). Whole cell lysates were electrophoresed on 12% glycine SDS-PAGE gels, transferred to PVDF membranes, and membranes

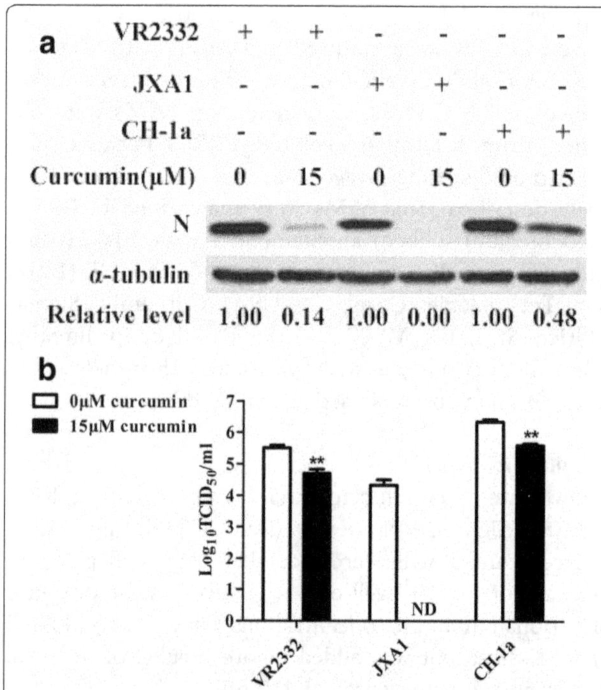

Fig. 2 Assessment of virus strain-dependence of curcumin anti-PRRSV activity. Marc-145 cells were co-treated with PRRSV (MOI: 0.1) and 15 μM curcumin at 37 °C for 1 h. Cells were washed and incubated in medium without curcumin at 37 °C for 36 h. N protein (**a**) and PRRSV production (**b**) were analyzed by western blot and virus titration assay, respectively. Each value represents the mean ± SD from three independent experiments (*, $p < 0.05$; **, $p < 0.01$; ***, $p < 0.001$; ND means non-detectable)

were incubated with one of the following primary antibodies: mouse anti-PRRSV-N monoclonal antibody 6D10 (1 µg/ml, produced in our laboratory), mouse anti-non-muscle myosin heavy chain II-A monoclonal anti-idiotypic antibody Mab2-5G2 [19], mouse anti-CD163 polyclonal antibody (1:3000, produced in our laboratory), anti-vimentin (Santa Cruz Biotechnology, CA, USA), rabbit anti-CD169 polyclonal antibody (Proteintech Group, Inc., China) or anti-α-tubulin antibody (Sigma) at dilutions recommended by the manufacturers. HRP-conjugated goat anti-mouse IgG or HRP-conjugated goat anti-rabbit IgG (1:2000, Jackson Labs, ME, USA) was used as secondary antibody. Protein signals were visualized using ECL reagent (Pierce, Rockford, IL, USA).

Virus titration

Virus progeny were titrated as described previously [20]. Briefly, Marc-145 cells were seeded into 96-well plates, incubated for 24 h at 37 °C then incubated with 100 µL/well of 10-fold serial dilutions of virus supernatants. After a 6-day incubation, the 50% cell culture infection dose ($CCID_{50}$) was calculated using the Reed-Muench method.

Statistical analysis

All experiments were performed independently at least three times. Western blots were analyzed using Image Lab 5.1 software (Bio-Rad Laboratories Inc., CA, USA). Virus titers and virus RNA levels were analyzed using GraphPad Prism software (GraphPad Software Inc., San Diego, CA, USA). Statistical significance was determined using Student's t-test for comparison of two groups or by one-way analysis of variance (ANOVA) for comparison of more than two groups. A value of $P < 0.05$ was considered statistically significant.

Results

Curcumin treatment inhibited PRRSV infection of Marc-145 cells

The ability of curcumin to inhibit PRRSV infection was evaluated in Marc-145 cells by detection of PRRSV N protein and virus production. Chloroquine served as the positive control by inhibiting the necessary initial stage of virus infection, endosome acidification, in a pH-dependent manner [21]. Co-incubation of Marc-145 cells for 1 h with curcumin and PRRSV (GD-HD) significantly reduced N protein (Fig. 1a) and PRRSV progeny titers (Fig. 1b) and 5 to 15 µM curcumin reduced N protein levels in a dose-dependent manner from 50 to 98%, respectively. Moreover, using 15 µM curcumin, virus titers deceased by 1.55 log relative to supernatants with PRRSV alone. CCK-8 testing of Marc-145 cells with added curcumin indicated that curcumin exhibited no significant cytotoxic effects (Fig. 1c).

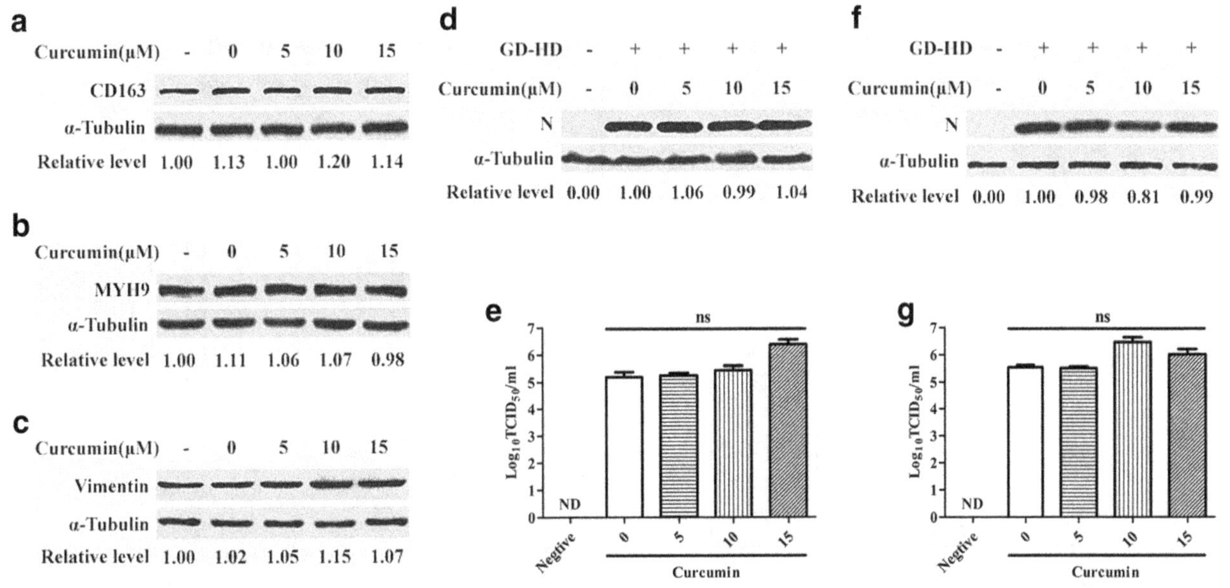

Fig. 3 PRRSV receptors and infectivity analysis of Marc-145 cells treated with curcumin before or after infection. Marc-145 cells were incubated with various curcumin concentrations at 37 °C for 1 h. CD163 (**a**), MYH9 (**b**) and vimentin (**c**) protein levels were measured by western blot. Marc-145 cells were incubated with curcumin before addition of GD-HD (MOI: 0.1, **d**, **e**) or after infection (**f**, **g**) with indicated curcumin concentrations. After incubation at 37 °C for 1 h, cells were maintained in medium without curcumin for 36 h. Next, PRRSV N protein expression levels (**d** and **f**) and viral production (**e** and **g**) were determined by western blot and virus titration assay, respectively. Each value represents the mean ± SD from three independent experiments (*, $p < 0.05$; **, $p < 0.01$; ***, $p < 0.001$; ND means non-detectable)

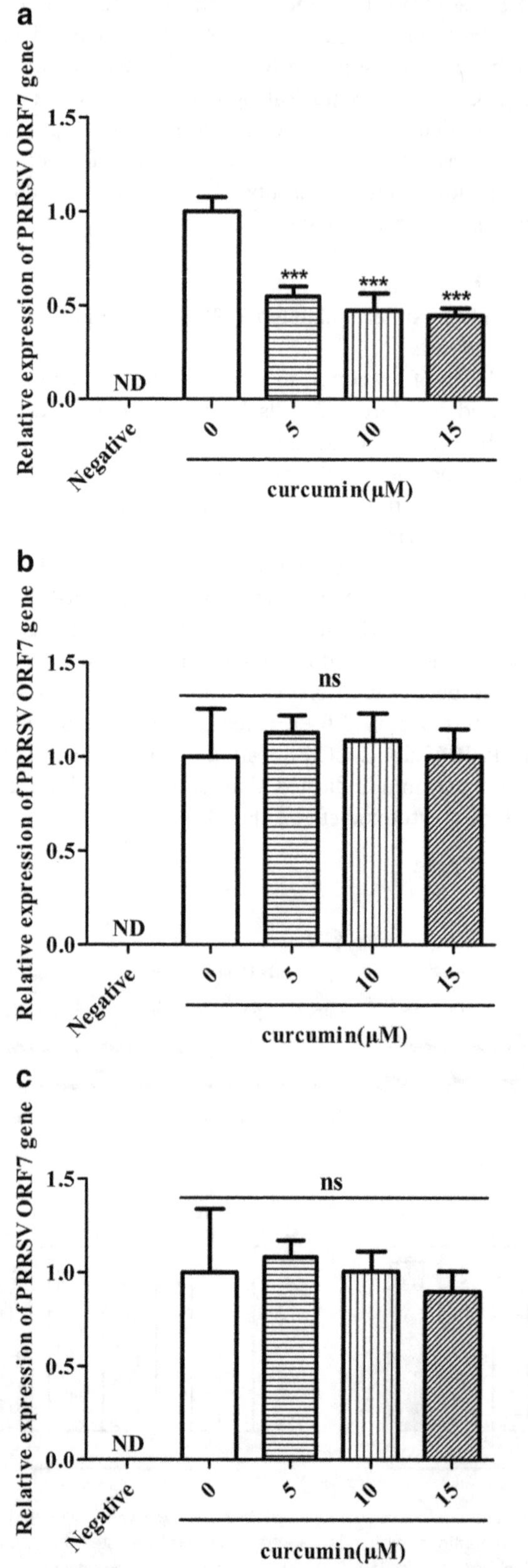

Fig. 4 Measurement of a curcumin effect on PRRSV absorption in Marc-145 cells. Marc-145 cells were pre-chilled at 4 °C for 1 h followed by incubation with curcumin-pretreated GD-HD (MOI: 100) (**a**), or a mixture of GD-HD (MOI: 100) and curcumin (**c**) at 4 °C for 1 h. For pretreatment of cells, Marc-145 cells were pre-incubated with curcumin at 37 °C for 1 h. After incubating cells at 4 °C for 1 h, both GD-HD (MOI: 100) and curcumin were added and incubated for 1 h at 4 °C (**b**). After washing out unbound virus, total RNA was extracted from the cells and the relative cell-bound PRRSV RNA levels were measured using qRT-PCR

Curcumin inhibited the infection of different genotype 2 PRRSV strains

To assess whether curcumin inhibits infection of Marc-145 cells by various genotype 2 PRRSV strains, classic strains PRRSV VR-2332 and HP-PRRSV/JXA1, and a low pathogenic strain, PRRSV CH-1a, were studied in the same way as the pathogenic GD-HD strain described above. Using 15 μM curcumin, relative N protein levels for VR-2332, JXA1 and CH-1a were 0.14, 0.00 and 0.48, respectively, as compared to PRRSV-only control (Fig. 2). Likewise, virus

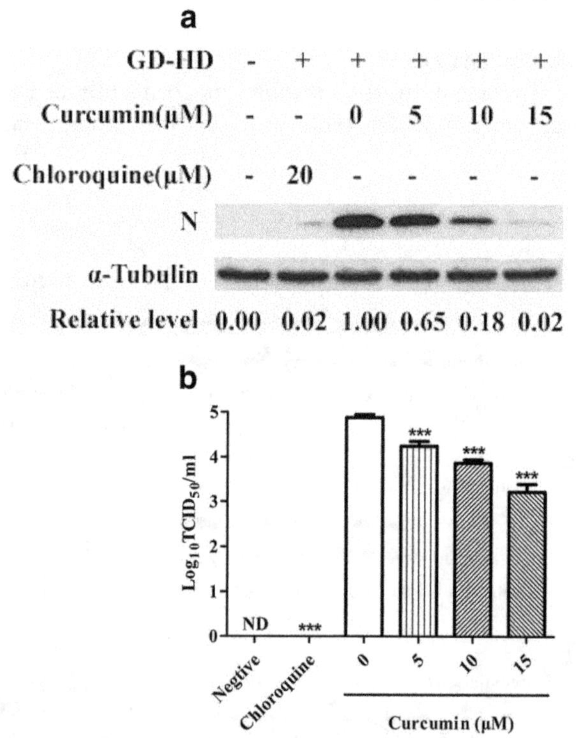

Fig. 5 Analysis of curcumin treatment effect on PRRSV internalization in Marc-145 cells. Pre-chilled Marc-145 cells were infected with GD-HD (MOI: 0.1) at 4 °C for 1 h then incubated with indicated curcumin concentrations at 37 °C for 1 h. After incubation, non-internalized viruses were removed and maintained in medium without curcumin for 36 h. Cells and culture supernatants were harvested to analyze PRRSV N protein expression levels (**a**) and viral production (**b**). Each value represents the mean ± SD from three independent experiments (*, $p < 0.05$; **, $p < 0.01$; ***, $p < 0.001$; ND means non-detectable)

titers of curcumin-treated groups were decreased by varying log values (VR2332, 0.54 log; JXA1, 4.32 log; CH-1a, 0.75 log) vs. PRRSV-only controls (Fig. 2b).

Curcumin had no effect on PRRSV receptor expression, but inhibited PRRSV infection during the inoculation phase of virus infection

To investigate whether curcumin downregulated known PRRSV receptors, CD163 [22], non-muscle myosin heavy chain 9 (MYH9) [19] and vimentin [23] expression levels in Marc-145 cells were tested using western blot analysis. Curcumin did not cause downregulation of cellular PRRSV receptors (Fig. 3a-c).

We next assessed curcumin antiviral effect upon addition to Marc-145 cells before or after PRRSV infection. As shown in Fig. 3d-g, N protein expression levels and progeny titers were not reduced by either of these treatment methods. Therefore, curcumin does not render Marc-145 cells more susceptible to PRRSV infection, but does interfere with PRRSV infection during the inoculation period of infection.

Curcumin did not affect PRRSV binding to Marc-145 cells

PRRSV binding to Marc-145 cells is considered a first step in infection. Thus, a virus binding assay was performed to determine if curcumin inhibits this binding. Virus RNA was collected and relative PRRSV ORF7 gene levels were analyzed using qRT-PCR. When virus was pretreated with curcumin, PRRSV ORF7 gene levels decreased in a dose-dependent manner (Fig. 4a). However, pretreatment of cells with curcumin or treatment with curcumin during virus adsorption did not affect PRRSV ORF7 gene levels (Fig. 4b, c). Therefore, curcumin has the potential to affect the infectivity of PRRSV at 37 °C, but did not inhibit virus attachment to Marc-145 cells.

Curcumin inhibited PRRSV internalization

After PRRSV attachment to Marc-145 cells, the next step of infection would be clathrin-mediated internalization [21]. Therefore, we examined virus endocytosis by treating Marc-145 cells with 5–15 μM curcumin. N protein expression decreased in a dose-dependent manner, demonstrating prevention of virus internalization (Fig. 5a). Moreover, N protein levels were reduced by factors of 0.65 to 0.02 of untreated controls, while PRRSV progeny titers deceased by 0.63 to 1.65 log compared to PRRSV infection without curcumin (Fig. 5b). Therefore, curcumin inhibits PRRSV internalization by Marc-145 cells.

Curcumin inhibits PRRSV uncoating by blocking virus-mediated cell fusion

After internalization and transport of PRRSV particles to endosomes, virus glycoprotein conformational changes occur and virus membranes fuse with endosome membranes, resulting in uncoating of virus particles [24]. To establish if curcumin affects PRRSV uncoating in Marc-145 cells, post-internalization and low pH-dependent

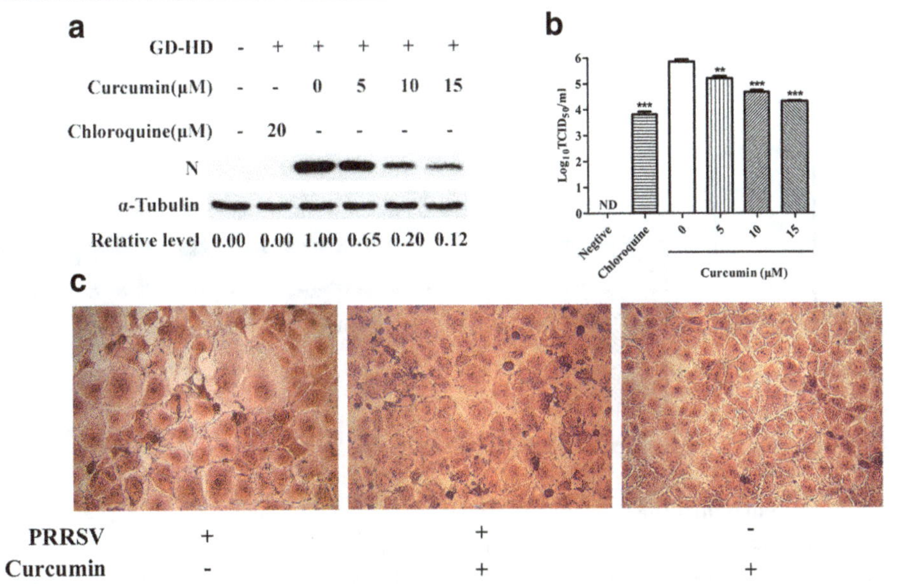

Fig. 6 Assessment of the effect of curcumin on post-internalization and cell fusion in PRRSV-infected Marc-145 cells. Marc-145 cells were infected with GD-HD (MOI: 0.1) and subjected to a virus post-internalization assay. PRRSV N protein levels (**a**) and virus titers in cell supernatants (**b**) were detected using western blot and $CCID_{50}$ assay, respectively. Each value represents the mean ± SD from three independent experiments (*, $p < 0.05$; **, $p < 0.01$; ***, $p < 0.001$; ND means non-detectable). For the observation of cell fusion, Marc-145 cells were subjected to the low pH-dependent cell fusion assay. Cell changes were observed under light microscope (**c**)

cell fusion assays were conducted. Treatment using 5–15 μM curcumin led to a dose-dependent reduction in N protein levels (Fig. 6a). Furthermore, a dose-dependent increase in curcumin concentration correlated with reduced PRRSV progeny titers (Fig. 6b). Therefore, curcumin inhibited post-internalization events of PRRSV infection of Marc-145 cells, including virus uncoating. Additionally, in the low pH-dependent cell fusion assay, curcumin markedly blocked cell fusion (Fig. 6c) with subsequent inhibition of virus uncoating.

Curcumin inhibition of PRRSV infection in PAMs

In addition to cell lines, to evaluate whether curcumin inhibits infection of primary cells, we isolated PAMs and tested these cells as conducted for Marc-145 cells above. As expected, 15 μM curcumin blocked PRRSV infection in PAMs and reduced ORF7 mRNA levels (Fig. 7a) and virus production (a 2.02 log decrease) (Fig. 7b). Additionally, CCK-8 assays ruled out curcumin cytotoxic effects as the cause of inhibition of viral infection (Fig. 7c).

To determine whether curcumin inhibition of PRRSV infection was due to downregulation of the known major PRRSV receptors, the expression levels of CD163, MYH9, vimentin and sialoadhesin (CD169) [25] were detected after 1 h of curcumin treatment of PAMs. The results in Fig. 7d showed that curcumin did not downregulate the expression levels of these receptors.

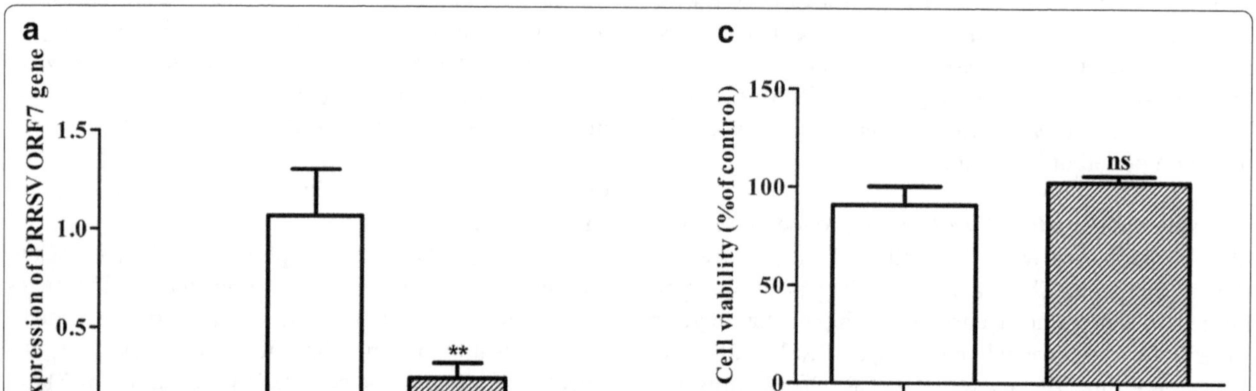

Fig. 7 Evaluation of the effect of curcumin on PRRSV entry and levels of receptors in PAMs. Treatment of PAMs was performed as in Fig. 1. After incubation for 36 h, total cellular RNA was extracted and PRRSV ORF7 RNA levels were detected by qRT-PCR (**a**). Culture supernatants were tested for virus titers (**b**). Curcumin cytotoxicity was detected in PAMs using a CCK8 assay and is presented as experimental cell viability relative to cell viability of untreated control (100%) (**c**). PAMs were incubated with curcumin (15 μM) at 37 °C for 1 h and CD163, MYH9, vimentin, and CD169 protein levels were detected by western blot. In addition, PAMs were incubated with curcumin at 37 °C for 1 h and then the cells were infected with PRRSV GD-HD strain (MOI: 0.1). After 36 h, PRRSV N protein expression levels were determined by western blot (**d**). Each value represents the mean ± SD from three independent experiments (*, $p < 0.05$; **, $p < 0.01$; ***, $p < 0.001$; ND means non-detectable)

Moreover, this treatment had no effect on PRRSV infection in PAMs (Fig. 7d).

Discussion

PRRSV remains a major threat to the swine industry worldwide because effective measures for preventing and treating PRRS do not yet exist. Therefore, anti-PRRSV drugs are urgently needed to eradicate PRRS. In this study, we studied the mechanism of action of curcumin underlying inhibition of PRRSV infection.

Curcumin is a broad-spectrum antiviral agent, it inhibits entry of lentiviral vectors pseudotyped with HCV and CHIKV envelope proteins into hepatocytes and 293 T cells, respectively [13, 15]. Because our data suggest that curcumin inhibits different strains of genotype 2 PRRSV infection in Marc-145 (Figs. 1, 2) and PAMs (Fig. 7a, b), we systematically elucidated curcumin's antiviral mechanism of action.

To investigate curcumin inhibition of PRRSV infection, the effect of curcumin on virus binding was first tested. Our results showed that expression levels of major PRRSV receptors (Figs. 3a-c and 7d) and susceptibility of target cells to virus (Figs. 3d, e and 7d) were unaffected by curcumin. In contrast, after incubation directly with virus at 37 °C, curcumin inhibited PRRSV attachment to Marc-145 cells (Fig. 4b), suggesting that curcumin reduced the infectivity of PRRSV particles. It has been reported that curcumin could affect membrane fluidity [26]. A previous study found that curcumin reduced the infectivity of HCV particles through decreasing the fluidity of viral envelopes, not rupturing virus particles [13]. PRRSV particles are comprised of an isometric core surrounded by a lipid-containing envelope. Moreover, our data showed that curcumin could inhibit PRRSV-mediated cell fusion (Fig. 6c). We therefore speculate that curcumin attenuated the infectivity of PRRSV by affecting the membrane fluidity of viral envelopes, not inactivating virus particles. After virus binding, curcumin also inhibited subsequent infection steps, virus internalization (Fig. 5) and uncoating (Fig. 6), in agreement with another study, where curcumin inhibited HCV binding and fusion [13].

The in vivo effect of curcumin has been studied in many animal disease models using multiple delivery strategies [27], but no studies of curcumin effects on PRRSV infection in vivo have been reported. One study investigated curcumin's antiviral role against HCV in primary human hepatocytes in vitro, demonstrating that the α,β-unsaturated ketone groups of curcumin were largely responsible for antiviral activity [13]. Another study reported that 200 mg/kg dietary curcumin had no effect on animal well-being or immune status [28]. Thus, curcumin shows promise as an antiviral agent and is well tolerated in pigs with minimal detrimental effects.

Conclusions

In summary, this research demonstrated the effect of curcumin, a natural compound, to prevent infection by several PRRSV strains. Curcumin affected PRRSV internalization and uncoating during the early virus infection stage and shows promise as an inhibitor of PRRSV infection in vitro. Further studies are needed to evaluate curcumin for prevention of PRRSV infection in vivo.

Abbreviations

ANOVA: Analysis of variance; $CCID_{50}$: 50% cell culture infection dose; CCK8: Cell Counting Kit-8; CHIKV: Chikungunya virus; DMEM: Dulbecco's modified Eagle's medium; HCV: Hepatitis C virus; HP-PRRSV: Highly pathogenic PRRSV; MOI: Multiplicity of infection; MYH9: Non-muscle myosin heavy chain 9; PAMs: Porcine alveolar macrophages; PRRS: Porcine reproductive and respiratory syndrome; PRRSV: Porcine reproductive and respiratory syndrome virus; qRT-PCR: Quantitative reverse transcription-PCR; VSV: Vesicular stomatitis virus

Acknowledgements

We would like to thank our funding sources.

Funding

This work was supported by National Natural Science Foundation of China (31,402,178, 31,430,084), Shaanxi Science and Technology Coordination and Innovation Project (2014KTCL02–11), Fundamental Research Funds for the Central Universities of Ministry of Education of China (2014YB013), Funds for International Scientific and Technological Cooperation of Northwest A&F University (A213021504) and Scientific Research Staring Foundation for Doctor (2013BSJJ011).

Authors' contributions

TFD and EMZ conceived and designed the experiments. TFD and YPS performed theexperiments. SQX, NL, QZ, AZ, YM, YNS and CYW contributed reagents, materials and analysis tools. TFD, YCN and EMZ analyzed the data. TFD drafted the manuscript. HTZ and EMZ revised the manuscript. All of the authors read and approved the final manuscript.

Consent for publication

Not applicable.

Competing interests

The authors declare that they have no competing interests.

Author details

[1]Department of Preventive Veterinary Medicine, College of Veterinary Medicine, Northwest A&F University, Yangling, Shaanxi 712100, China. [2]Experimental Station of Veterinary Pharmacology and Veterinary Biotechnology, Ministry of Agriculture, Yangling, Shaanxi 712100, China. [3]Department of Pathology and Lab Medicine, University of Pennsylvania Perelman School of Medicine, 3620 Hamilton Walk, Philadelphia, PA 19104, USA.

References

1. Wongyanin P, Buranapraditkun S, Chokeshai-Usaha K, Thanawonguwech R, Suradhat S. Induction of inducible CD4+CD25+Foxp3+ regulatory T lymphocytes by porcine reproductive and respiratory syndrome virus (PRRSV). Vet Immunol Immunopathol. 2010;133(2–4):170–82.
2. Neumann EJ, Kliebenstein JB, Johnson CD, Mabry JW, Bush EJ, Seitzinger AH, Green AL, Zimmerman JJ. Assessment of the economic impact of porcine reproductive and respiratory syndrome on swine production in the United States. J Am Vet Med Assoc. 2005;227(3):385–92.

3. Cavanagh D. Nidovirales: a new order comprising Coronaviridae and Arteriviridae. Arch Virol. 1997;142(3):629–33.
4. Murtaugh MP, Stadejek T, Abrahante JE, Lam TT, Leung FC. The ever-expanding diversity of porcine reproductive and respiratory syndrome virus. Virus Res. 2010;154(1–2):18–30.
5. Shi M, Lam TT, Hon CC, Hui RK, Faaberg KS, Wennblom T, Murtaugh MP, Stadejek T, Leung FC. Molecular epidemiology of PRRSV: a phylogenetic perspective. Virus Res. 2010;154(1–2):7–17.
6. Yun SI, Lee YM. Overview: replication of porcine reproductive and respiratory syndrome virus. J Microbiol. 2013;51(6):711–23.
7. Zhou L, Yang H. Porcine reproductive and respiratory syndrome in China. Virus Res. 2010;154(1–2):31–7.
8. Butler JE, Lager KM, Golde W, Faaberg KS, Sinkora M, Loving C, Zhang YI. Porcine reproductive and respiratory syndrome (PRRS): an immune dysregulatory pandemic. Immunol Res. 2014;59(1–3):81–108.
9. Murtaugh MP, Xiao Z, Zuckermann F. Immunological responses of swine to porcine reproductive and respiratory syndrome virus infection. Viral Immunol. 2002;15(4):533–47.
10. Du T, Nan Y, Xiao S, Zhao Q, Zhou EM. Antiviral strategies against PRRSV infection. Trends Microbiol. doi:10.1016/j.tim.2017.06.001.
11. Anand P, Kunnumakkara AB, Newman RA, Aggarwal BB. Bioavailability of curcumin: problems and promises. Mol Pharm. 2007;4(6):807–18.
12. Pulido-Moran M, Moreno-Fernandez J, Ramirez-Tortosa C, Ramirez-Tortosa M. Curcumin and health. Molecules. 2016;21(3):264.
13. Anggakusuma, Colpitts CC, Schang LM, Rachmawati H, Frentzen A, Pfaender S, Behrendt P, Brown RJ, Bankwitz D, Steinmann J, et al. Turmeric curcumin inhibits entry of all hepatitis C virus genotypes into human liver cells. Gut. 2014;63(7):1137–49.
14. Saleheen D, Ali SA, Ashfaq K, Siddiqui AA, Agha A, Yasinzai MM. Latent activity of curcumin against leishmaniasis in vitro. Biol Pharm Bull. 2002;25(3):386–9.
15. von Rhein C, Weidner T, Henss L, Martin J, Weber C, Sliva K, Schnierle BS. Curcumin and Boswellia Serrata gum resin extract inhibit chikungunya and vesicular stomatitis virus infections in vitro. Antivir Res. 2016;125:51–7.
16. Xiao S, Zhang A, Zhang C, Ni H, Gao J, Wang C, Zhao Q, Wang X, Ma C, Liu H, et al. Heme oxygenase-1 acts as an antiviral factor for porcine reproductive and respiratory syndrome virus infection and over-expression inhibits virus replication in vitro. Antivir Res. 2014;110:60–9.
17. Du Y, Du T, Shi Y, Zhang A, Zhang C, Diao Y, Jin G, Zhou EM. Synthetic toll-like receptor 7 ligand inhibits porcine reproductive and respiratory syndrome virus infection in primary porcine alveolar macrophages. Antivir Res. 2016;131:9–18.
18. Luo Z, Tian D, Zhou M, Xiao W, Zhang Y, Li M, Sui B, Wang W, Guan H, Chen H, et al. Lambda-carrageenan P32 is a potent inhibitor of rabies virus infection. PLoS One. 2015;10(10):e0140586.
19. Gao JM, Xiao SQ, Xiao YH, Wang X, Zhang C, Zhao Q, Nan Y, Huang B, Liu H, Liu N, et al. MYH9 is an essential factor for porcine reproductive and respiratory syndrome virus infection. Sci Rep-Uk. 2016;6:25120. doi:10.1038/srep25120.
20. Xiao S, Wang Q, Gao J, Wang L, He Z, Mo D, Liu X, Chen Y. Inhibition of highly pathogenic PRRSV replication in MARC-145 cells by artificial microRNAs. Virol J. 2011;8:491.
21. Kreutz LC, Ackermann MR. Porcine reproductive and respiratory syndrome virus enters cells through a low pH-dependent endocytic pathway. Virus Res. 1996;42(1–2):137–47.
22. Calvert JG, Slade DE, Shields SL, Jolie R, Mannan RM, Ankenbauer RG, Welch SK. CD163 expression confers susceptibility to porcine reproductive and respiratory syndrome viruses. J Virol. 2007;81(14):7371–9.
23. Kim JK, Fahad AM, Shanmukhappa K, Kapil S. Defining the cellular target(s) of porcine reproductive and respiratory syndrome virus blocking monoclonal antibody 7G10. J Virol. 2006;80(2):689–96.
24. Snijder EJ, Kikkert M, Fang Y. Arterivirus molecular biology and pathogenesis. J Gen Virol. 2013;94(Pt 10):2141–63.
25. Vanderheijden N, Delputte PL, Favoreel HW, Vandekerckhove J, Van Damme J, van Woensel PA, Nauwynck HJ. Involvement of sialoadhesin in entry of porcine reproductive and respiratory syndrome virus into porcine alveolar macrophages. J Virol. 2003;77(15):8207–15.
26. Barry J, Fritz M, Brender JR, Smith PE, Lee DK, Ramamoorthy A. Determining the effects of lipophilic drugs on membrane structure by solid-state NMR spectroscopy: the case of the antioxidant curcumin. J Am Chem Soc. 2009;131(12):4490–8.
27. Epstein J, Sanderson IR, MacDonald TT. Curcumin as a therapeutic agent: the evidence from in vitro, animal and human studies. Brit J Nutr. 2010;103(11):1545–57.
28. Ilsley SE, Miller HM, Kamel C. Effects of dietary quillaja saponin and curcumin on the performance and immune status of weaned piglets. J Anim Sci. 2005;83(1):82–8.

6

Classical swine fever virus replicated poorly in cells from MxA transgenic pigs

Yicheng Zhao[1,2*], Tiedong Wang[2], Li Yao[1], Bo Liu[2,3], Chunbo Teng[1] and Hongsheng Ouyang[2*]

Abstract

Background: In addition to their value as livestock, pigs are susceptible to classical swine fever virus (CSFV) and can serve as reservoirs for CSFV, allowing it to develop into an epizootic. CSFV, a pestivirus of the Flaviviridae family, has a single-stranded RNA genome. Recent research has indicated that the human MxA protein inhibits the life cycles of certain RNA viruses, such as members of the Bunyaviridae family, the Flaviviridae family and others.

Results: To produce pigs with antiviral protection against CSFV, transgenic pigs expressing human MxA were generated by nuclear transplantation. Cells from three MxA transgenic piglets were used to investigate in vitro antiviral activity of MxA aganist CSFV, and the results of in vitro indirect immunofluorescence assays, virus titration and real-time PCR indicated that the MxA transgenic pig has an antiviral capacity against CSFV.

Conclusions: Transgene with human MxA on pigs is feasible. High levels of MxA expression do inhibit CSFV in vitro at early time points post-infection at 60-96dpi.

Keywords: Classical swine fever virus, MxA, Nuclear transplantation, Transgenic pig

Abbreviations: CSFV, Classical swine fever virus; EF1a, Elongation factor 1 alpha; H5N1, Influenza A virus subtype H5N1; MXA, Myxovirus resistance gene A; NLS, Nuclear localization signal; NT, Nuclear transfer; ORF, Open reading frame

Background

Human MxA has been shown to exhibit a wide antiviral capacity against small RNA viruses. This interferon-induced protein is one of the best-studied determinants of innate immunity to viral infection [1]. MxA belongs to the dynamin superfamily of large GTPases and has a C-terminal stretch of basic amino acids that constitutes a nuclear localization signal (NLS). This NLS mediates the nuclear accumulation of MxA, whereas the swine Mx1 protein is not located inside nucleus for lack of NLS. At present, the known MxA-sensitive viruses include members of the bunyaviruses, orthomyxoviruses, paramyxoviruses, rhabdoviruses and togaviruses, along with Hepatitis B virus [2–7].

Classical swine fever virus (CSFV) is a pestivirus of the Flaviviridae family [8] with an enveloped virion incorporating glycosylated membrane proteins. The CSFV genome has a single strand of positive-sense RNA [9] and a single open reading frame (ORF) that encodes a large protein that is cleaved and modified into several smaller proteins, including N^{pro}, C, E0, E1, E2, P7, NS2-3, NS4A, NS4B, NS5A and NS5B. CSFV infects pigs and replicates predominantly in myeloid cells, causing classical swine fever (CSF), a severe disease that is characterized by fever, leukopenia and hemorrhage [9–11].

The expression of porcine Mx1 was absent from CSFV-infected pigs because of the Interferon-blocking effects of N^{pro} [12, 13]. Moreover, our earlier study concluded that highly expressed MxA inhibits CSFV in vitro [14]. As the inherently wide antiviral capacity of MxA, we sought to generate a transgenic pig model that would express a high level of MxA under the control of the EF1a promoter to protect swine against CSF. In this study, three MxA transgenic pigs were generated by Nuclear transplantation (NT), and we determined the levels at which CSFV replicated in cells from different tissues of these transgenic clone piglets.

* Correspondence: yichengzhao@live.cn; oyhs64@hotmail.com
[1]College of Life Science, Northeast Forestry University, Harbin, China
[2]College of Animal Sciences, Jilin University, Changchun, China
Full list of author information is available at the end of the article

Methods

DNA transfection and the establishment of stable cell lines

The plasmid pGKneotAloxp2MxA, which expresses human MxA in eukaryotic cells, was constructed in our previous study [14]. Porcine fetal fibroblasts (large white) cultured in Dulbecco's modified Eagle's medium (GIBCO) with 20 % fetal bovine serum (PAA) were seeded in a 60-mm dish prior for transfection. Then, the linearized plasmid was transfected into the porcine fetal fibroblasts using Fugene HD Transfection Reagent (Roche). After 14-36 h, the cells were split into 6-well dishes and cultured in selective medium containing 300 ng/mL of G418 antibiotic (Amresco) for 7-12 days. The surviving cell colonies were selected for further analysis.

The generation of transgenic pigs by nuclear transplantation

Positive cell clones were used to construct transgenic pigs by Nuclear transplantation (NT). The details of the method of porcine NT used were described in our earlier work [15]. Briefly, oocytes were washed three times and then matured in maturation medium at 39 °C. In vitro-matured metaphase II oocytes were harvested by the removal of their polar bodies and the associated metaphase plates. An electrical pulse was used to fuse the donor cells and the oocytes. The reconstructed oocytes were electrically activated to initiate cell division and subsequent development. The embryos were cultured for 20 h following activation and were surgically transferred into the oviducts of surrogate pigs.

DNA extraction, RNA extraction, PCR analysis and Integration site analysis

Genomic DNA from different tissues and cells was extracted and purified using a QIAamp DNA Mini Kit (QIAGEN). RNA was extracted with TRIzol reagent (Invitrogen) and purified using an RNeasy column (QIAGEN). The sites of transgene integration were assessed using high-efficiency thermal asymmetric interlaced PCR (hiTAIL-PCR) [16]. Primers specific to the transgenic vectors (pMl1, pMl2 and pMl3) were designed using Vector NTI 10 software (Invitrogen). The detailed method has been previously described [17].

All the primers used in our research and their sequences are listed below:

- MxAq1 GAGAGGAAACTGTAGGGGAG
- MxAq2 GGAAACATCTGTGAAAGCAA
- Neo1 TGAAGTAACTGCAGGACGAG
- Neo2 AATATCACGGGTAGCCCACG
- β-actin1 GAACCCCAAAGCCAACCGT
- β-actin2 CCTCGTAGATGGGCACCGT
- rFPprimer GGGATGATGGTCTCCTGATCAC
- rRPprimer CATCAAATTGGTAGGCCACTTTC
- Prob5B FAM-CCTTGCTCGCGAATTTCTCACC GATAMRA (TaqMan)
- Vs1 TCGCCCTTATTCCCTTTTTT
- Vs2 AGCAGCCGATTGTCTGTTGT
- pMl1 TCGGTGATGACGGTGAAAAC
- pMl2 CGGAGACGGTCACAGCTTGT
- pMl3 AGAGCAGATTGTACTGAGAG
- LAD1 ACGATGGACTCCAGAGCGGCCGC (G/C/A) N (G/C/A)NNNGGAA
- LAD2 ACGATGGACTCCAGAGCGGCCGC (G/C/T) N (G/C/T)NNNGGTT
- LAD3 ACGATGGACTCCAGAGCGGCCGC (G/C/A) (G/C/A) N(G/C/A) NNNCCAA
- LAD4 ACGATGGACTCCAGAGCGGCCGC (G/C/T) (G/A/T) N (G/C/T) NNNCGGT

Viral infections, virus titration, the indirect immunofluorescence assay (IFA) and real-time PCR

These assays were performed according to Xu et al. [18]. CSFV (SM) from the Institute of Veterinary Drug Control, China, was used in this study. Positive anti-CSFV serum was kindly provided by Dr. CC Tu. To determine the viral titer, cells were infected with CSFV for 60 h, and samples of the medium were collected, serially diluted 10-fold from 10^{-1} to 10^{-6} and inoculated onto PK-15 cells. Each dilution was examined for viral proliferation using IFA. The $TCID_{50}$ values were calculated using the Kärber method. For IFA, cells were infected with CSFV for 72 h, fixed in precooled 80 % acetone, and incubated with the positive anti-CSFV serum. A FITC-conjugated rabbit anti-pig IgG (Sigma) was used as the secondary antibody, and the cells were examined using an ECLIPSE TE2000-V (Nikon). Real-time PCR was performed with an iQ^{tm}5 Multicolor Real-time PCR Detection System (Bio-Rad) using a QuantiTect™ Probe PCR Kit (QIAGEN). The special primers (rFPprimer, rRPprimer and Prob5B) for the CSFV NS5B gene have been previously described [14].

Western blotting

The cells were washed with PBS and a hypotonic cell lysis buffer containing morpholinepropanesulfonic acid-buffered saline with Triton X-100 (15ul for 10^6 cells). The cell extract was centrifuged at 12,000 x *g* to remove the cellular debris. Detailed methods regarding separating the sample by SDS-PAGE, transferring proteins to nitrocellulose membranes, and immunostaining will be described elsewhere. As a control, a monoclonal mouse anti-β-actin antibody (human/mouse, 1:1000, kangchen) was used. The MxA protein was immunostained with a mouse monoclonal anti-MxA (p78) antibody (human/mouse, 1:500 Novus Biologicals).

Southern blotting

The sample was digested overnight with EcoRI at 36 °C (1.5ul for 1ug, NEB). Then, the gDNA was electrophoresed for 22 h in a 1 % agarose gel at 13 V and transferred to a Hybond þ nylon membrane (GE Healthcare) for 12 h. A DIG-labeled probe was generated using a PCR DIG Probe Synthesis Kit (Roche) with primers Vs1 and Vs2. Hybridization was performed overnight at 55 ° C using a DIG Easy Hyb Kit (Roche).

Results

To select supporting donor cells, several stable MxA-positive clones were constructed, infected with CSFV and analyzed (data not shown). The No. 34 clone (Fig. 1a) was chosen for NT, about 500 SCNT embryos were transferred into 3 surrogate mothers that exhibited natural estrus and three male transgenic piglets were obtained by natural delivery on day 119 post-implantation (Fig. 1b) and one piglet died before birth, the other three live transgenic piglets displayed no obvious weight differences comparing to a normal male piglet born at the same day (Fig. 1c).

The results of PCR detection of the neomycin resistance gene (Neo) from tail DNA and RT-PCR detection of MxA from blood RNA were both positive (Fig. 2a and b). The amplification of template genomic DNA with nested PCR primers yielded amplified product of the predicted size: 163 bp (outer set) and 107 bp (inner set). The PCR-amplified inner set product were sequenced. The sequence analysis revealed that the MxA fragment had randomly inserted into introns on chromosome 16 (, NW_003612429:30482-30588). Southern blotting targeting clone piglets tails' DNA and Western blotting targeting porcine kidney cells were also performed to demonstrate the authenticity of the MxA expression in these transgenic piglets (Fig. 2c and d).

To detect CSFV replication, adherent cells from tails, kidneys and umbilical cords were isolated and cultured. The cells were infected with 100 $TCID_{50}$ of CSFV for 72 h, and the infected cells were detected using IFA. Only a few MxA-expressing cells exhibited green fluorescence, indicating that most of the cells had been effectively protected by MxA and had resisted viral infection (Figs. 3a-c). To quantify the effect of MxA on viral replication, viral genome copy numbers from porcine tail cells were determined using real-time PCR at 96 hpi. The viral genome copy number per nanogram of total RNA was measured to be 1.05×10^5 copies/ng of total viral RNA from control cells, whereas the MxA-positive cells contained 1.89×10^3, 2.31×10^3, and 2.34×10^3 copies/ng, corresponding to 55-, 143- and 23-fold reductions, respectively (Fig. 4a). Moreover, the tail cells were infected with 100 $TCID_{50}$ of CSFV for 60 h, and the virus-containing supernatant was diluted and used to inoculate PK-15 cells to determine the $TCID_{50}$ values at 60, 72, 84, 96 and 120 h. As shown in Fig. 4b, the MxA protein markedly inhibited infectious virus production at the early time points(60-96hpi) comparing to normal porcine tail cells, however, at later times post-infection (120hpi), the degree of inhibition was reduced (Fig. 4b).

Discussion

Transgenic pigs are of great value for commercial applications and could serve as models for human disease [19, 20]. Pigs are closer to humans in complexity,

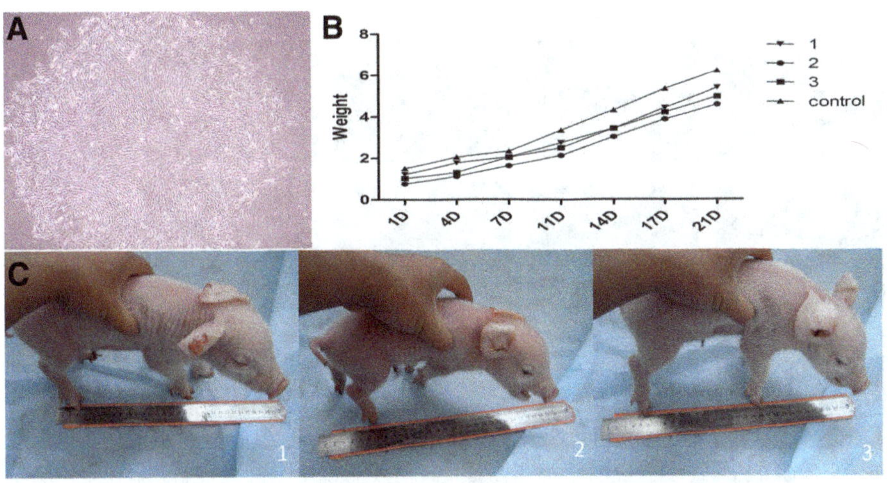

Fig. 1 **a**. The number 34 clone was chosen for NT. Because porcine fetal fibroblasts are capable of a limited number of passages, the cells have a larger and longer shape in this picture. **b**. Three male transgenic piglets were obtained by natural delivery. **c**. The average birth weight was 1.01 kg, and the pigs displayed normal growth rates comparing a non-transgenic piglet born at the same day

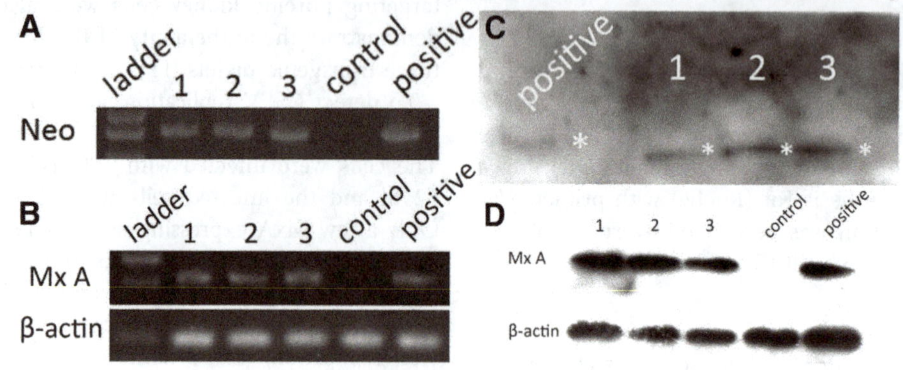

Fig. 2 a-b. PCR data for the neomycin resistance gene (Neo), and RT-PCR data for MxA were performed to confirm the presence of the transgene; the No. 34 clone cells were chosen for the positive control, and normal porcine tails gDNA and blood RNA were chosen as negative control.
c. Southern blotting was performed to detect the vector fragment in the genome; pGKneotAloxp2MxA was chosen as the positive control.
d: Western blotting showed the expression of MxA in all three piglets; a cell strain stably expressing MxA was chosen for the positive control, and tissue from non-transgenic piglets was chosen as a negative control

physiological function and genetics [15, 21]; therefore, we aimed to express human MxA, but not mouse Mx1, in pigs. Somatic cell nuclear transfer is a promising method of producing transgenic animals; however, this cloning strategy has a low success rate (<2 %) for bringing transferred pig embryos to term [22]. It has been well established that unknown mechanisms can affect the development, growth and survival of cloned animals [23]. Despite these potential constraints, we obtained three piglets (one additional piglet died before birth). These piglets did not display abnormal phenotypes in newborn bodyweight and auxodrome before weaning.

In this short report, the transgenes were characterized by PCR, integration site analysis, Southern blotting and Western blotting. To determine the antiviral capacity of MxA against CSFV, some basic in vitro experiments were performed. We used adherent cells from tails, kidneys and umbilical cords to evaluate the antiviral activities of the MxA transgene in the pigs. The results showed that CSFV replicated poorly in the cells of all three transgenic pigs, suggesting that MxA expression markedly inhibited viral growth, but at later time points post-infection(120hpi), the level of inhibition decreased.

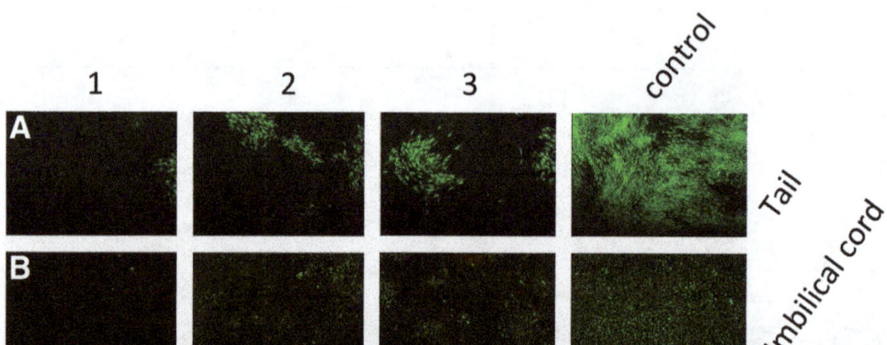

Fig. 3 a-c. IFA demonstrated that the proliferation of CSFV was obviously inhibited in piglet cells, including tail, kidney and umbilical cord cells. Compared with the counterparts from non-transgenic piglet, only a few MxA clone pigs' cells displayed green fluorescence. Moreover, we found that the kidney cells were more sensitive to CSFV than the other two cell types. Our results indicate that the transgenic piglets were effectively protected by MxA

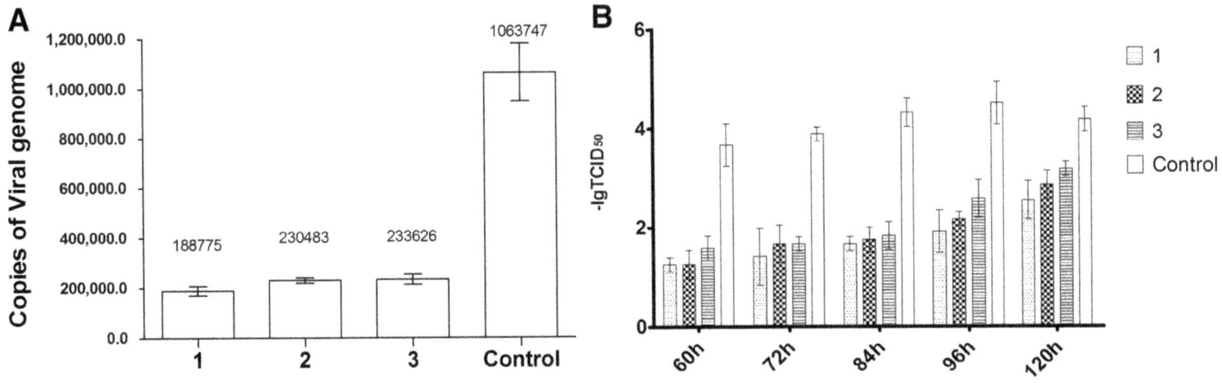

Fig. 4 a. A reduction in the CSFV genome copy number at 96 h post-infection is shown; the copy numbers of CSFV are the means of three repeat experiments. The copy number (viral genomes per nanogram of total RNA) was 1.05×10^5 copies/ng in the control cells, whereas there were 1.89×10^3, 2.31×10^3 and 2.34×10^3 copies/ng in the MxA-positive cells. This result indicates the suppression of CSFV replication in MxA-positive groups. **b**. Inhibition of virus production in piglet cells. Cells were infected with 100 $TCID_{50}$ of CSFV for 60 h, and the viral supernatant was diluted and inoculated onto PK-15 cells to assess the $TCID_{50}$ values from 60 to 120 h. The -log$TCID_{50}$ values represent the means of three repeat titrations after one time infection at each time point. The data indicate that MxA markedly inhibited infectious virus production for the first 3 days, but thereafter, the extent of the inhibition decreased

Conclusions

A conclusion from our study is that high levels of ectopic MxA expression in transgenic swine cells do inhibit CSFV in vitro at early time points post-infection, the inhibitory effects lasted for 96 h post the infection. We expect that this new transgenic model could facilitate animal production for antiviral research targeting RNA viruses.

Acknowledgements

We would like to thank Prof. CC.Tu.(Institute of Veterinary Sciences, Academy of Military Medical Sciences) for kindly providing positive anti-CSFV serum.

Funding

This work was supported by the Fundamental Research Funds for the Heilongjiang Postdoctoral Grant (No. LBH-Z14018), National Nature Science Foundation of China (No. 31502030) and Major Projects of New Varieties of Genetically Modified Organisms (No. 2011ZX08006-001).
Availability of data and materials.

Authors' contributions

Y.C.Z. participated in conceiving the study, participated its design and coordination, helped perform the experiments, helped interpret the results. T.D.W. participated its design and coordination, helped perform the experiments, helped interpret the results. L.Y. and B.L. helped interpret the esults. H.S.O.Y. and C.B.T. participated its design and coordination. Y.C.Z and T.D.W wrote the main manuscript, all authors read and approved the final manuscript.

Competing interests

None of the authors have any competing interests.

Consent for publication

Not applicable.

Author details

[1]College of Life Science, Northeast Forestry University, Harbin, China. [2]College of Animal Sciences, Jilin University, Changchun, China. [3]College of Veterinary Medicine, Inner Mongolia Agricultural University, Hohhot, China.

References

1. Haller O, Staeheli P, Kochs G. Interferon-induced Mx proteins in antiviral host defense. Biochimie. 2007;89(6-7):812–8.
2. Landis H, Simon-Jodicke A, Kloti A, Di Paolo C, Schnorr JJ, Schneider-Schaulies S, Hefti HP, Pavlovic J. Human MxA protein confers resistance to Semliki Forest virus and inhibits the amplification of a Semliki Forest virus-based replicon in the absence of viral structural proteins. J Virol. 1998;72(2):1516–22.
3. Haller O, Frese M, Kochs G. Mx proteins: mediators of innate resistance to RNA viruses. Rev Sci Tech. 1998;17(1):220–30.
4. Chieux V, Chehadeh W, Harvey J, Haller O, Wattre P, Hober D. Inhibition of coxsackievirus B4 replication in stably transfected cells expressing human MxA protein. Virology. 2001;283(1):84–92.
5. Gordien E, Rosmorduc O, Peltekian C, Garreau F, Brechot C, Kremsdorf D. Inhibition of hepatitis B virus replication by the interferon-inducible MxA protein. J Virol. 2001;75(6):2684–91.
6. Netherton CL, Simpson J, Haller O, Wileman TE, Takamatsu HH, Monaghan P, Taylor G. Inhibition of a large double-stranded DNA virus by MxA protein. J Virol. 2009;83(5):2310–20.
7. He DN, Zhang XM, Liu K, Pang R, Zhao J, Zhou B, Chen PY. In vitro inhibition of the replication of classical swine fever virus by porcine Mx1 protein. Antiviral Res. 2014;104:128–35.
8. Kleiboeker SB. Swine fever: classical swine fever and African swine fever. Vet Clin North Am Food Anim Pract. 2002;18(3):431–51.
9. Paton DJ, McGoldrick A, Greiser-Wilke I, Parchariyanon S, Song JY, Liou PP, Stadejek T, Lowings JP, Bjorklund H, Belak S. Genetic typing of classical swine fever virus. Vet Microbiol. 2000;73(2-3):137–57.
10. Summerfield A, Hofmann MA, McCullough KC. Low density blood granulocytic cells induced during classical swine fever are targets for virus infection. Vet Immunol Immunopathol. 1998;63(3):289–301.
11. Summerfield A, Zingle K, Inumaru S, McCullough KC. Induction of apoptosis in bone marrow neutrophil-lineage cells by classical swine fever virus. J Gen Virol. 2001;82(Pt 6):1309–18.
12. Daviet S, Van Borm S, Habyarimana A, Ahanda ML, Morin V, Oudin A, Van Den Berg T, Zoorob R. Induction of Mx and PKR failed to protect chickens from H5N1 infection. Viral Immunol. 2009;22(6):467–72.
13. Seago J, Hilton L, Reid E, Doceul V, Jeyatheesan J, Moganeradj K, McCauley J, Charleston B, Goodbourn S. The Npro product of classical swine fever virus and bovine viral diarrhea virus uses a conserved mechanism to target interferon regulatory factor-3. J Gen Virol. 2007;88(Pt 11):3002–6.
14. Zhao Y, Pang D, Wang T, Yang X, Wu R, Ren L, Yuan T, Huang Y, Ouyang H. Human MxA protein inhibits the replication of classical swine fever virus. Virus Res. 2011;156(1-2):151–5.

15. Yan Q, Yang H, Yang D, Zhao B, Ouyang Z, Liu Z, Fan N, Ouyang H, Gu W, Lai L. Production of transgenic pigs over-expressing the antiviral gene Mx1. Cell Regeneration. 2014;3(1):11.
16. Liu YG, Chen Y. High-efficiency thermal asymmetric interlaced PCR for amplification of unknown flanking sequences. Biotechniques. 2007;43(5): 649–50. 652, 654 passim.
17. Li L, Pang D, Wang T, Li Z, Chen L, Zhang M, Song N, Nie D, Chen Z, Lai L, et al. Production of a reporter transgenic pig for monitoring Cre recombinase activity. Biochem Biophys Res Commun. 2009;382(2):232–5.
18. Xu X, Guo H, Xiao C, Zha Y, Shi Z, Xia X, Tu C. In vitro inhibition of classical swine fever virus replication by siRNAs targeting Npro and NS5B genes. Antiviral Res. 2008;78(3):188–93.
19. Russell SH, Hoopes JL, Odell JT. Directed excision of a transgene from the plant genome. Mol Gen Genet. 1992;234(1):49–59.
20. Yang D, Wang CE, Zhao B, Li W, Ouyang Z, Liu Z, Yang H, Fan P, O'Neill A, Gu W, et al. Expression of Huntington's disease protein results in apoptotic neurons in the brains of cloned transgenic pigs. Hum Mol Genet. 2010; 19(20):3983-94.
21. Rogers CS, Stoltz DA, Meyerholz DK, Ostedgaard LS, Rokhlina T, Taft PJ, Rogan MP, Pezzulo AA, Karp PH, Itani OA, et al. Disruption of the CFTR gene produces a model of cystic fibrosis in newborn pigs. Science. 2008; 321(5897):1837–41.
22. Lai L, Prather RS. Production of cloned pigs by using somatic cells as donors. Cloning Stem Cells. 2003;5(4):233–41.
23. Dean W, Santos F, Stojkovic M, Zakhartchenko V, Walter J, Wolf E, Reik W. Conservation of methylation reprogramming in mammalian development: aberrant reprogramming in cloned embryos. Proc Natl Acad Sci USA. 2001; 98(24):13734–8.

The role of transportation in the spread of *Brachyspira hyodysenteriae* in fattening farms

Enrico Giacomini[1*], Sara Gasparrini[1], Massimiliano Lazzaro[1], Federico Scali[1], Maria Beatrice Boniotti[1], Attilio Corradi[2], Paolo Pasquali[3,4] and Giovanni Loris Alborali[1]

Abstract

Background: Direct and indirect contact among animals and holdings are important in the spread of *Brachyspira hyodysenteriae*. The objective of this study was to investigate the role of slaughterhouse vehicles in spreading *B. hyodysenteriae* between unconnected farms.

Results: Multilocus sequence typing (MLST) and Multiple Locus Variable number tandem repeat Analysis (MLVA) were used to characterize *B. hyodysenteriae* strains isolated from trucks. Before cleaning, 976 batches of finishing pigs transported by 174 trucks from 540 herds were sampled. After cleaning, 763 of the 976 batches were also sampled. Sixty-one of 976 and 4 of 763 environmental swabs collected from trucks before and after cleaning and disinfection operations, respectively, were positive for *B. hyodysenteriae*. The 65 isolates in this study originated from 48 farms. Trucks were classified into five categories based on the number of visited farms as follows: category 1: 1–5 farms, category 2: 6–10 farms, category 3: 11–15 farms, category 4: 16–20 farms, category 5: >21 farms. Although the largest number of vehicles examined belonged to category 1, the highest percentage of vehicles positive for *B. hyodysenteriae* was observed in categories 3, 4 and 5. Specifically, 90.9% of trucks belonging to category 5 were positive for *B. hyodysenteriae*, followed by categories 4 and 3 with 85.7% and 83.3%, respectively. The results of MLST and MLVA suggest that trucks transporting pigs from a high number of farms also play a critical role in spreading different *B. hyodysenteriae* genetic profiles. STVT 83–3, which seems to be the current dominant type in Italy, was identified in 56.25% of genotyped isolates. The genetic diversity of isolated strains from trucks was high, particularly, in truck categories 3, 4 and 5. This result confirmed that MLST and MLVA can support the study of epidemiological links between different *B. hyodysenteriae* farm strains.

Conclusions: This study highlights the potential role of shipments in *B. hyodysenteriae* spread. Moreover, it emphasizes the importance of strict vehicle hygiene practices for biosecurity programmes.

Keywords: Swine dysentery, *Brachyspira hyodysenteriae*, MLST, MLVA, Transportation, Biosecurity

Background

Swine dysentery (SD) is a widely distributed disease that affects pigs in the growing and finishing periods. It can induce high levels of mortality and reduce feed conversion, substantially affecting pig production. The disease's aetiological agent is *Brachyspira hyodysenteriae*, a gram-negative anaerobic bacterium capable of damaging the enterocytes of the large intestine and causing severe muco-haemorragic enteric disease. Furthermore, *Brachyspira hampsonii*, a strongly hemolytic *Brachyspira* species, was also identified as agent of SD [1, 2]. Nevertheless, *B. hampsonii* was never detected in Italy. The transmission of microorganisms occurs mainly by direct contact with infected pigs and the ingestion of contaminated faeces [1]. Moreover, transmission can follow the introduction of contaminated clothing and footwear of animal caretakers or visitors who have had contact with infected pigs, or it can

* Correspondence: Giacominienrico81@gmail.com
[1]Istituto Zooprofilattico Sperimentale della Lombardia e dell'Emilia Romagna [Experimental Zooprophylactic Institute of Lombardy and Emilia Romagna] "Bruno Ubertini", Via Bianchi 7/9, 25124 Brescia, Italy
Full list of author information is available at the end of the article

be conveyed by feral and other animals [1]. Furthermore, motor vehicles used for animal transport seem to be an important potential risk for disease propagation among unconnected farms and slaughterhouses [3]. In fact, vehicles used in animal transportation can be involved in the indirect spread of infectious agents that may cause disease, such as foot and mouth disease (FMD) [4], porcine reproductive respiratory syndrome (PRRS) [5, 6] and porcine epidemic diarrhoea (PED) [7]. It was observed that when animals from different farms are transported separately but in successive shipments, the risk of transmission of infectious agents potentially increases [8, 9]. Therefore, appropriate cleaning and the application of a disinfection protocol for shipment vehicles, as well as biosecurity measures at the farm gate, may be crucial for limiting the spread of disease via shared trucks [10].

In this study, we aimed to investigate the role of trucks in spreading *B. hyodysenteriae* between unconnected farms. To better understand the route of transmission and the source of SD outbreaks, we sampled slaughterhouse vehicle protocols and characterized *B. hyodysenteriae* strains isolated from trucks by combining multilocus sequence typing (MLST) and multiple locus variable number tandem repeat analysis (MLVA).

Methods

Sample collection

A batch of finishing pigs, sent to slaughter by truck, was considered a single epidemiological unit. Between 2012 and 2015, environmental swabs were sampled from trucks for 976 selected epidemiological units. A total of 174 trucks were used to transport those units, which were from 540 different herds. Environmental swabs were collected on trucks at the staging place of the slaughterhouse. Each sample was collected by swabbing the four corners and the perimeter of the low floor of the trucks. One swab per truck was collected before sanitizing procedures and, when possible, one swab was taken after such procedures. Each sample was placed in a single sterile bag, stored in a refrigerated container, and processed within 5 h. Before the cleaning and disinfection operations, 976 samples from 174 trucks were collected. After routine cleaning and disinfection, 763 environmental swabs were taken from 147 of the 174 trucks examined. The procedures applied at the slaughterhouses required that after unloading the animals, the trucks were washed with high-pressure washing systems and disinfected with products based on glutaraldehyde, quaternary ammonium salts, chloramine T and Virkon®.

B. hyodysenteriae isolates

Swab samples kept in sterile bags were washed with 50 ml of saline solution. The liquid was then transferred to a sterile tube and clarified by centrifugation for 5 min at 1500×g. DNA extraction was then performed with 1 ml of the supernatant of each environmental sample using a DNeasy Blood & Tissue Kit (Qiagen GmbH, Germany). The bacterial DNA was eluted into 100 µl of elution buffer. A species-specific real-time PCR assay was performed to detect the presence of *B. hyodysenteriae, B. pilosicoli* and *Lawsonia intracellularis* DNA [11].

Using a pad saturated with washing liquid, each PCR-positive sample was seeded on blood agar culture plates supplemented with rifampicin, vancomycin HCl and colistin and incubated at 37 °C in an anaerobic atmosphere for 5 days. The evaluation of their haemolytic characteristics (strong beta haemolysis) allowed for the identification of samples positive for *B. hyodysenteriae.* Bacterial cells with strong haemolysis were then harvested and resuspended in TE buffer (300 µl). DNA was obtained by boiling the samples at 98 °C for 10 min, and the DNA was stored at 4 °C. A species-specific PCR assay was performed to confirm the classification of *B. hyodysenteriae* or *B. pilosicoli* [11].

Genotyping

The obtained *B. hyodysenteriae* pure isolates were then characterized using MLST and MLVA. MLST was performed on seven loci coding for housekeeping genes [12, 13]. We used the same PCR conditions and purification and PCR sequencing methods as previously described [14]. The sequences obtained were then analysed and codified to obtain a sequence type (ST) [13]. MLVA was conducted by analysing seven multiple variable number tandem repeats (VNTR) loci within the genome using the primers described by Hidalgo and colleagues [15] and the PCR conditions described by Gasparrini and colleagues [14]. The amplicons were analysed on a 2% agarose gel to estimate the locus size and calculate the number of repeats. Hence, the MLVA profiles (VT) were codified [15].

To better characterize the isolates collected, MLST and MLVA profiles were combined (STVT profiles) as previously illustrated [14].

Truck categorisation

The trucks transporting the finishing pig batches were identified and associated with the farms from which the animals originated. The trucks were classified into different categories based on the number of farms visited as follows: category 1: 1–5 farms visited, category 2: 6–10 farms visited, category 3: 11–15 farms visited, category 4: 16–20 farms visited, category 5: >21 farms visited. The percentage of vehicles positive for *B. hyodysenteriae* and the MLST and MLVA profiles of *B. hyodysenteriae* isolates were evaluated according to truck categories.

Statistical analysis

The statistical analysis was conducted by considering two groups of trucks: vehicles transporting pigs from up to five different farms and trucks visiting more than five farms. Differences in the prevalence of positive samples between the two groups were estimated with a chi-square test and odds ratio (OR) with a 95% confidence interval (CI). All statistical computations were performed with GraphPad Prism 6 (GraphPad Software, San Diego, CA, USA). The significance level was set at $P < 0.05$.

Results

Samples

Before cleaning and disinfection operations, 976 environmental samples, one for each batch of pigs, were collected. After the sanitisation routine, 763 of the 976 sampled batches (78.18%) were also sampled.

The real-time PCR analysis performed on the environmental samples collected from trucks before the cleaning and disinfection operations showed that 61 of 976 environmental swabs were positive for *B. hyodysenteriae* (6.25%, Table 1). Four of the 763 environmental swabs collected after routine cleaning and disinfection operations were positive for *B. hyodysenteriae* (0.52%). All four positive samples were collected from trucks where swabs were also positive before cleaning. Two trucks each from categories 4 and 5 had positive samples. Moreover, two of the four positive samples were collected the same day at the same slaughterhouse. Overall, the 65 *B. hyodysenteriae* isolates detected originated from 48 (8.89%) of the 540 tested farms (Table 1).

Truck categories

The finishing pig batches were transported using 174 trucks classified into 5 categories based on the number of farms visited, as described in the Methods section.

In particular, the largest number of vehicles examined belonged to category 1 ($n = 134$). Sixteen trucks were in category 2, 6 trucks were in category 3, 7 trucks were in category 4, and 11 trucks were in category 5 (Fig. 1a). Overall, 22.99% of the trucks were positive for *B. hyodysenteriae* with at least 1 swab.

As shown in Fig. 1b, 90.9% of trucks belonging to category 5 were positive for *B. hyodysenteriae*, followed by truck categories 4 and 3 with 85.7% and 83.3%, respectively. *B. hyodysenteriae* was detected in 7 of the 16 trucks (43.5%) belonging to category 2, and only 13 trucks belonging to category 1 were positive (9.7%).

Genotyping

Sixteen pure isolates of *B. hyodysenteriae* were obtained from the 65 *B. hyodysenteriae* PCR-positive samples collected from different trucks. It was not possible to isolate any strains from 33 *B. hyodysenteriae* PCR-positive swabs, and 16 PCR-positive samples presented a *Brachyspira* spp. mixed culture. The 16 pure isolates, which originated from swab collected before sanitation procedures, were analysed using MLST and MLVA, and the genetic profiles obtained were combined. Eight MLST-MLVA profiles were identified. Table 2 shows the MLST and MLVA profiles of *B. hyodysenteriae* strains isolated from vehicles at slaughterhouses in relation to the 5 truck categories. Thirteen of the 16 isolates were detected in truck categories 3–5, with a high number of farms involved for each vehicle. The most frequent profile was 83–3, found in trucks belonging to all the categories, while several other profiles were isolated in only a single sample (Table 2).

MLST and MLVA strain profiles isolated from trucks are reported in Fig. 2.

Discussion

The results of the investigation of the environmental samples collected from trucks before cleaning and disinfection operations showed that 6.25% of environmental swabs and 8.89% of farms were *B. hyodysenteriae* positive. These data suggest that transportation can play a potential important role in *B. hyodysenteriae* spreading between otherwise unconnected farms and that it can be a critical point for SD control.

Very limited information is available on the role of trucks in spreading SD. It is known that new outbreaks of SD usually occur following introduction of asymptomatic carrier pigs into uninfected herds, by contaminated feed or animal trucks, or by rodents or visitors who have come into contact with infected pigs [4, 16]. The role of the transportation equipment used to move

Table 1 Yearly distribution of total and real-time PCR-positive environmental swabs collected from trucks before and after cleaning and disinfection operations

Year	Before cleaning			After cleaning			Farms[a]		
	Total	Positive	%	Total	Positive	%	Total	Positive	%
2012	247	6	2.43%	174	0	0.00%	134	6	4.48%
2013	110	1	0.91%	86	0	0.00%	72	1	1.39%
2014	89	4	4.49%	76	2	2.63%	70	4	5.71%
2015	530	50	9.43%	427	2	0.47%	264	37	14.02%
TOT	976	61	6.25%	763	4	0.52%	540	48	8.89%

[a]Number of farms from which the pigs transported by trucks originated

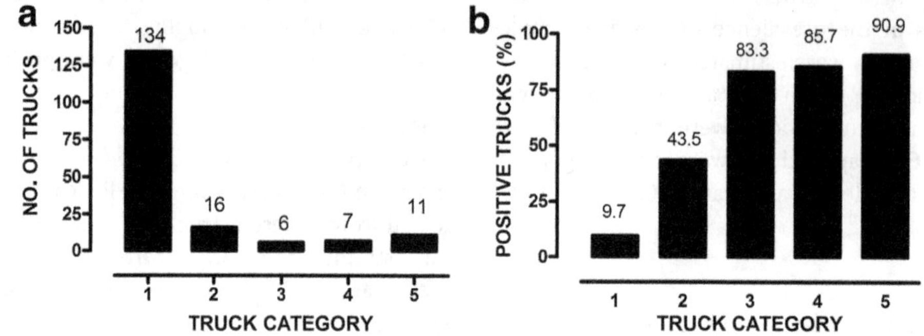

Fig. 1 Distribution of vehicles transporting pigs (**a**) and *B. hyodysenteriae* positive vehicles (**b**) separated by truck categories. Most of the vehicles belonged to category 1, but most of the positive samples were detected in categories 3–5

pigs is well known to spread other diseases, such as porcine epidemic diarrhoea virus (PEDV), transmissible gastroenteritis virus (TGEV) [7] and porcine reproductive respiratory syndrome virus (PRRSV) [6].

The results of our investigations suggest that trucks are involved in *B. hyodysenteriae* spread and that trucks that visit a higher number of farms will have a greater potential of testing positive for *B. hyodysenteriae*. Overall, the percentage of positive samples was significantly higher ($P < 0.0001$) in trucks that visited more than five farms than in trucks that visited fewer than 5 farms (OR = 21.72, 95% CI 8.95–52.67).

The sharing of trucks between farms for the shipment of pigs may increase the risk of disease propagation [8] due to poor cleaning and disinfection of these trucks [17, 18].

The low number of *B. hyodysenteriae*-positive samples (0.52%) after cleaning and disinfecting procedures should not be neglected. The frequency of positive samples after cleaning and disinfecting procedures may be underestimated. Indeed, because of truckers' tight schedules, it was not possible to sample 213 of the 976 shipments (21.82%) after the cleaning routine. It is possible that a transporter who is in a hurry has a higher risk of overlooking some parts of the cleaning and disinfecting routines. All positive samples came from trucks in category 4 or 5, which visited a high number of farms ($n = 47$). Furthermore, two of the four positive samples were collected the same day at the same slaughterhouse, suggesting at least a partial failure of the sanitisation process. *B. hyodysenteriae* is relatively resistant in moist faeces, and it survived for 48 days at 0–10 °C, 7 days at 25 °C, and less than 24 h at 37 °C [19]. It survived at 10 °C for 78 days in soil with 10% pig faeces and for 112 days in pure pig faeces [20]. Moreover, Lambert and colleagues reported that less than one-third of the trucks used for the shipment of pigs in Canada are cleaned and disinfected between successive shipments [18]. Percentage of trucks with inadequate sanitation may differ in the working conditions in which the current study was performed. However, considering that 22.9% of trucks sampled in this study transported at least one *B. hyodysenteriae*-positive batch, shipments may still play an important role in spreading the pathogen among unconnected herds, particularly when farms do not follow strict external biosecurity measures. On the other hand, 33 out of 65 PCR-positive samples were impossible to isolate suggesting that either a low bacterial load was collected or bacteria viability was already reduced before swabbing. Particularly, in the latter case, viability of bacteria to infect animals could be reduced or absent.

MLST and MLVA profile results suggest that trucks transporting pigs from a high number of farms may also play a potential role in spreading different *B. hyodysenteriae* genetic profiles. In general, the same strains isolated in trucks were found in high production areas, as previously reported by Gasparrini and colleagues [14]. Nevertheless, the role of these trucks in spreading different *B. hyodysenteriae* strains should be further investigated because one of the limitations of this study is that only one isolate per batch was identified.

The STVT 83–3 profile, present in 9 of 16 samples, should be the current dominant type in Italy. In two recent studies, STVT 83–3 represented more than 45% of

Table 2 MLST and MLVA profiles of the 16 isolates from vehicle swabs in relation to truck category. All 16 isolates were obtained from swabs collected before cleaning and disinfection operations. The second row displays the sequence type (ST) of each isolate, and the third row displays the variable number tandem repeats type (VT)

Isolate number	1	2	3	4	5	6	7	8	9	10	11	12	13	14	15	16
ST	75	83	83	206	83	83	83	83	76	209	205	83	83	74	83	79
VT	11	3	3	18	3	3	3	3	6	22	2	3	3	2	3	9
Truck category	4	5	4	5	1	3	1	1	3	3	3	4	2	5	5	5

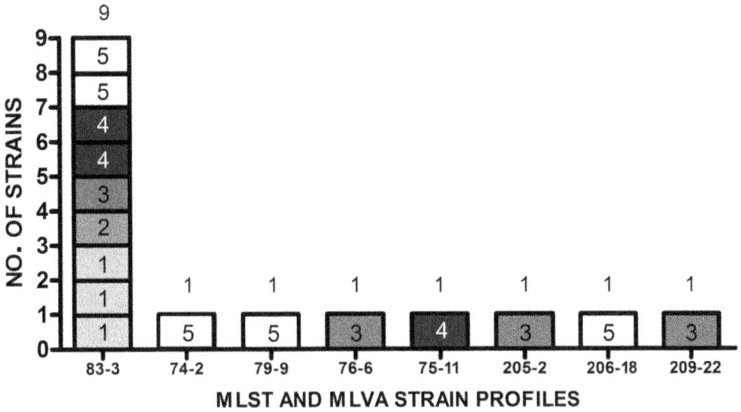

Fig. 2 Number of MLST and MLVA strain profiles isolated from different truck categories. Nine of 16 isolates belonged to the STVT 83–3 profile, while the remaining isolates had different profiles. Each box represents one isolate, and the number within a box represents the category of the source truck

the *B. hyodysenteriae* isolates from 2012 to 2015 [14, 21]. Notwithstanding the low number of isolated strains from trucks, the strain genetic diversity is high. In fact, 8 genetic profiles in 16 isolates were found in the trucks (ratio = 0.5), while 33 of 152 MLST and MLVA profiles were found in the farms (ratio = 0.21) [14], highlighting the role of transportation in collecting and spreading many different *B. hyodysenteriae* strains. The genetic profiles isolated from trucks, but not from outbreaks, belonged to truck categories 3, 4 and 5. This result confirmed that MLST and MLVA can support the study of epidemiological links between different *B. hyodysenteriae* farm strains [22].

Conclusions

Despite its limitations, this study suggests that *B. hyodysenteriae* control measures should include a more stringent application of standardized procedures for hygiene practices to improve the sanitation of vehicles at slaughterhouses. These control measures may be implemented at collection points and slaughterhouses to prevent contaminated vehicles from returning to pig farms and most likely play a role in spreading *B. hyodysenteriae* across vast geographic areas. However, other measures at the farm level, such as loading pigs outside the premises and limiting contact between farmers and trucks during the unloading process, should have a positive effect in reducing the transmission of *B. hyodysenteriae.* Biosecurity measures, at truck and farm levels, are pivotal and require a coordinated effort between producers, transporters and slaughter facility owners to achieve effective implementation. This study on *B. hyodysenteriae* transmission should provide more information regarding the role of shipments, and it highlights the risks that may occur if coordinated biosecurity programmes, which involve finisher transportation, are not properly implemented.

Abbreviations

CI: Confidence interval; FMD: Foot and mouth disease; MLST: Multilocus sequence typing; MLVA: Multilocus variable-number tandem-repeat analysis; OR: Odds ratio; PCR: Polymerase chain reaction; PED: Porcine epidemic diarrhoea; PEDV: Porcine epidemic diarrhoea virus; PRRSV: Porcine reproductive and respiratory syndrome; PRRSV: Porcine reproductive and respiratory syndrome virus; SD: Swine dysentery; ST: Sequence type; STVT: Sequence type and variable number tandem repeats type; TGEV: Transmissible gastroenteritis virus; VNTR: Variable number tandem repeats; VT: Multiple variable number tandem repeats type

Acknowledgements

Not applicable

Funding

The study was fully funded by the Italian Ministry of Health.

Authors' contributions

EG conducted the field research, assisted in data interpretation and wrote the drafts. SG performed MLST and MLVA and assisted in data interpretation. ML conducted the field research and prepared the raw data. FS conducted statistical analyses, interpreted the data, and edited the manuscript. MBB performed MLST and MLVA and assisted in interpretation of MLST and MLVA results. AC, PP and GLA designed and supervised the study. All authors contributed to the final editing and approval of the manuscript.

Consent for publication

Not applicable.

Competing interests

The authors declare that they have no competing interests.

Author details

[1]Istituto Zooprofilattico Sperimentale della Lombardia e dell'Emilia Romagna [Experimental Zooprophylactic Institute of Lombardy and Emilia Romagna] "Bruno Ubertini", Via Bianchi 7/9, 25124 Brescia, Italy. [2]Department of Veterinary Sciences, University of Parma, Parma, Italy. [3]Istituto Superiore di Sanità, Rome, Italy. [4]FAO Reference Center for Veterinary Public Health, Rome, Italy.

References

1. Alvarez-Ordonez A, Martinez-Lobo FJ, Arguello H, Carvajal A, Rubio P. Swine dysentery: aetiology, pathogenicity, determinants of transmission and the fight against the disease. Int J Env Res Public Health. 2013;10(5):1927–47.

2. Mirajkar NS, Phillips ND, La T, Hampson DJ, Gebhart CJ. Characterization and recognition of *Brachyspira hampsonii* sp. nov., a novel intestinal spirochete that is pathogenic to pigs. J Clin Microbiol. 2016;54(12):2942–9.
3. Thakur KK, Revie CW, Hurnik D, Poljak Z, Sanchez J. Analysis of swine movement in four canadian regions: network structure and implications for disease spread. Transbound Emerg Dis. 2016;63(1):e14–26.
4. Alexandersen S, Zhang Z, Donaldson AI, Garland AJM. The pathogenesis and diagnosis of foot-and-mouth disease. J Comp Pathol. 2003;129(1):1–36.
5. Dee S, Deen J, Rossow K, Wiese C, Otake S, Joo HS, Pijoan C. Mechanical transmission of porcine reproductive and respiratory syndrome virus throughout a coordinated sequence of events during cold weather. Can J Vet Res. 2002;66(4):232–9.
6. Dee SA, Deen J, Otake S, Pijoan C. An experimental model to evaluate the role of transport vehicles as a source of transmission of porcine reproductive and respiratory syndrome virus to susceptible pigs. Can J Vet Res. 2004;68(2):128–33.
7. Lowe J, Gauger P, Harmon K, Zhang JQ, Connor J, Yeske P, Loula T, Levis I, Dufresne L, Main R. Role of transportation in spread of porcine epidemic diarrhea virus infection, United States. *Emerging*. Infect Dis. 2014;20(5):872–4.
8. Bigras-Poulin M, Barfod K, Mortensen S, Greiner M. Relationship of trade patterns of the Danish swine industry animal movements network to potential disease spread. Prev Vet Med. 2007;80(2–3):143–65.
9. Smith RP, Cook AJC, Christley RM. Descriptive and social network analysis of pig transport data recorded by quality assured pig farms in the UK. Prev Vet Med. 2013;108(2–3):167–77.
10. Dee S, Deen J, Burns D, Douthit G, Pijoan C. An assessment of sanitation protocols for commercial transport vehicles contaminated with porcine reproductive and respiratory syndrome virus. Can J Vet Res. 2004;68(3):208–14.
11. Willems H, Reiner GA. Multiplex real-time PCR for the simultaneous detection and quantitation of *Brachyspira hyodysenteriae*, *Brachyspira pilosicoli* and *Lawsonia intracellularis* in pig faeces. Berl Munch Tierarztl Wochenschr. 2010;123(5–6):205–9.
12. Mirajkar NS, Gebhart CJ. Understanding the molecular epidemiology and global relationships of *Brachyspira hyodysenteriae* from swine herds in the United States: a multi-locus sequence typing approach. PLoS One. 2014;9(9):e107176.
13. La T, Phillips ND, Harland BL, Wanchanthuek P, Bellgard MI, Hampson DJ. Multilocus sequence typing as a tool for studying the molecular epidemiology and population structure of *Brachyspira hyodysenteriae*. Vet Microbiol. 2009;138(3–4):330–8.
14. Gasparrini S, Alborali GL, Pitozzi A, Guarneri F, Giacomini E, Baldo V, Scali F, Lazzaro M, Beatrice BM. Characterization of *Brachyspira hyodysenteriae* isolates from Italy by multilocus sequence typing and multiple locus variable number tandem repeat analysis. J Appl Microbiol. 2017;123(2):340–451.
15. Hidalgo A, Carvajal A, La T, Naharro G, Rubio P, Phillips ND, Hampson DJ. Multiple-locus variable-number tandem-repeat analysis of the swine dysentery pathogen, *Brachyspira hyodysenteriae*. J Clin Microbiol. 2010;48(8):2859–65.
16. Robertson ID, Mhoma JR, Hampson DJ. Risk factors associated with the occurrence of swine dysentery in Western Australia: results of a postal survey. Aust Vet J. 1992;69(4):92–1.
17. Bottoms K, Poljak Z, Dewey C, Deardon R, Holtkamp D, Friendship R. Evaluation of external biosecurity practices on southern Ontario sow farms. Prev Vet Med. 2013;109(1–2):58–68.
18. Lambert ME, Poljak Z, Arsenault J, D'Allaire S. Epidemiological investigations in regard to porcine reproductive and respiratory syndrome (PRRS) in Quebec, Canada. Part 1: biosecurity practices and their geographical distribution in two areas of different swine density. Prev Vet Med. 2012;104(1–2):74–83.
19. Chia SP, Taylor DJ. Factors affecting the survival of *Treponema hyodysenteriae* in dysenteric pig faeces. Vet Rec. 1978;103(4):68–70.
20. Boye M, Baloda SB, Leser TD, Moller K. Survival of *Brachyspira hyodysenteriae* and *B. pilosicoli* in terrestrial microcosms. Vet Microbiol. 2001;81(1):33–40.
21. Rugna G, Bonilauri P, Carra E, Bergamini F, Luppi A, Gherpelli Y, Magistrali CF, Nigrelli A, Alborali GL, Martelli P, La T, Hampson DJ, Merialdi G. Sequence types and pleuromutilin susceptibility of *Brachyspira hyodysenteriae* isolates from Italian pigs with swine dysentery: 2003-2012. Vet J. 2015;203(1):115–9.
22. Osorio J, Carvajal A, Naharro G, La T, Phillips ND, Rubio P, Hampson DJ. Dissemination of clonal groups of *Brachyspira hyodysenteriae* amongst pig farms in spain, and their relationships to isolates from other countries. PLoS One. 2012;7(6):e39082.

8

Modeling the spatio-temporal dynamics of porcine reproductive & respiratory syndrome cases at farm level using geographical distance and pig trade network matrices

Sara Amirpour Haredasht[1], Dale Polson[2], Rodger Main[3], Kyuyoung Lee[1], Derald Holtkamp[3] and Beatriz Martínez-López[1*]

Abstract

Background: Porcine reproductive and respiratory syndrome (PRRS) is one of the most economically devastating infectious diseases for the swine industry. A better understanding of the disease dynamics and the transmission pathways under diverse epidemiological scenarios is a key for the successful PRRS control and elimination in endemic settings. In this paper we used a two step parameter-driven (PD) Bayesian approach to model the spatio-temporal dynamics of PRRS and predict the PRRS status on farm in subsequent time periods in an endemic setting in the US. For such purpose we used information from a production system with 124 pig sites that reported 237 PRRS cases from 2012 to 2015 and from which the pig trade network and geographical location of farms (i.e., distance was used as a proxy of airborne transmission) was available. We estimated five PD models with different weights namely: (i) geographical distance weight which contains the inverse distance between each pair of farms in kilometers, (ii) pig trade weight (PT_{ji}) which contains the absolute number of pig movements between each pair of farms, (iii) the product between the distance weight and the standardized relative pig trade weight, (iv) the product between the standardized distance weight and the standardized relative pig trade weight, and (v) the product of the distance weight and the pig trade weight.

Results: The model that included the pig trade weight matrix provided the best fit to model the dynamics of PRRS cases on a 6-month basis from 2012 to 2015 and was able to predict PRRS outbreaks in the subsequent time period with an area under the ROC curve (AUC) of 0.88 and the accuracy of 85% (105/124).

Conclusion: The result of this study reinforces the importance of pig trade in PRRS transmission in the US. Methods and results of this study may be easily adapted to any production system to characterize the PRRS dynamics under diverse epidemic settings to more timely support decision-making.

Keywords: Parameter-driven model, Risk assessment, Bayesian approach, Disease dynamics, Risk-based surveillance, Decision making

* Correspondence: beamartinezlopez@ucdavis.edu
[1]Center for Animal Disease Modeling and Surveillance (CADMS), Department of Medicine & Epidemiology, School Veterinary Medicine, University of California, 2108 Tupper Hall, one Shields Avenue, Davis, California 95616, USA
Full list of author information is available at the end of the article

Background

Porcine reproductive and respiratory syndrome virus (PRRSV) is a RNA virus of the family *Arteriviridae* that causes reproductive failure in breeding stock and respiratory disease in piglets. In the US, it has been estimated that the annual economic impact of PRRSV for the pig industry is US$664 million [11]. Previous studies have described three main routes of PRRSV transmission between farms: (i) close contact between pigs, (ii) airborne transmission, particularly in winter and over distances of less than 3 km and, (iii) semen [1]. Spread via semen is relatively easy to control and has been minimized thanks to the increase of biosecurity at boar studs; however transmission through airborne spread or pig movements is more complicated to control as it requires substantial investments and changes in farm management practices (e.g., air filtration, active surveillance, pre-movement testing, etc.). Although the main pathways of transmission between herds have been described, there are few observational studies characterizing the dynamics of PRRS transmission and quantifying the role and relative importance of each pathway in endemic settings. Moreover, very few studies have used information about pig movements and potential airborne transmission (i.e., distance matrices) to forecast PRRS status on farm in an attempt to support the implementation of cost-effective, risk-based interventions. The prevalence of PRRS infection can be high (>40%) particularly in regions with a high density of pigs, large number and frequent pig movements and a lack of vaccination or control measures [1, 9, 14]. However, a better understanding of transmission patterns under specific endemic settings and the prediction of farms at highest risk of PRRS occurrence in subsequent time periods may help producers to prioritize interventions and minimize farm-to-farm transmission, which will facilitate more cost-effective prevention, control and, ultimately, elimination of PRRSV at the farm or regional level.

Mathematical models that quantify the role of each transmission route between farms can be used to better understand the observed distribution of infection as well as predict future outbreaks [5]. Considering the rapid and continuous changes in pig demographics and trade as well as changes in PRRS status and the potential emergence of new diseases (e.g. porcine epidemic diarrhea) there is a need to use models that are flexible to incorporate those changes based on the availability of the data and that allow real-time prediction and modelling of new outbreaks [12].

In this paper, we have expanded and adapted an innovative two-step parameter-driven (PD) approach described by Schrödle et al. [21] which models the spatio-temporal dynamics of PRRS to predict future disease events. The model was computed using integrated nested Laplace approximation (INLA), a recent method for approximate Bayesian inference using latent Gaussian models [19]. INLA is a promising alternative to Markov chain Monte Carlo (MCMC) methods that provides very accurate results within short computational time [20]. We aimed to assess the role that pig trade and geographical distance (as a proxy of airborne transmission) may have on PRRSV transmission and evaluate the predictive ability of PD models to forecast local PRRS cases in a 6 month time frame.

Methods

Data

Data on PRRS diagnostic cases, pig demographics and pig movements were provided by pig producers in one US state. The PRRS data comprised 237 reported PRRS cases and more than 56,731 pig movements occurring between >500 production sites from 2012 to 2015. The state, name and exact number of production sites are omitted here to preserve confidentiality. More information about the data set used regarding farm demographics and pig trade network can be found in Lee et al. [15]. Information on the exact geographical location (x, y coordinates) and number of pigs on the farm were also obtained. PRRS surveillance is primarily conducted in sow farms, nurseries and gilt development units (GDUs), as well as in other types of production sites (e.g., finishers and wean-to-finish farm; WF) Therefore, after an outbreak investigation, we focused only on modeling PRRS cases in sow farms, nurseries and GDU, and the subpopulation of finishers and wean-to-finisher farms that had reported PRRS outbreaks in the last 4 years. In summary a total of 124 farms were considered for the analyses.

Modelling approach

We used a two step approach. First, we used a parameter driven model to identify if there is a spatio-temporal trend of PRRS reported cases from Jan 2012 to July 2014. Then, if a spatio-temporal trend existed, an autoregressive parameter driven model was used to predict the PRRS cases for the last half of 2014 based on different weight matrices. All the analyses were done by using R-INLA software package for R ([19]; www.r-inla.org).

Parameter driven model

We assumed that the general binary observation of PRRS outbreaks in farm i at time t (Y_{it}) follows a Binomial distribution of the form:

$$Y_{it} \sim \text{Binomial}(m_{it},\ \eta_{it}) \text{ with } t = 1, 2, ..., T; i = 1, 2, ..., I \quad (1)$$

where the number of trials, m_{it}, adjusts for possible numbers of tested individuals on farm. In this study we assumed 10% of the animals (i.e. number of trials) in each farm were being tested in a 6-month period. Therefore the probability that the farm is having a outbreak based on the PRRS test result is following binomial distribution. Here T is equal to six corresponding to the number of 6-month time steps from 2012 to 2015, I is equal to 124 (i.e. number of the farms in this study) and η_{it} is the probability of having at least one positive animal in the farm, which is specified as recommended by Blangiardo and Cameletti, [3]:

$$logit(\eta_{it}) = b_0 + u_i + v_i + (\kappa + \delta_i)t \quad (2)$$

where b_0 is the intercept, which quantifies the average PRRS farm status in the entire study, while u_i and v_i are the area-specific effects. The parameter u_i is assumed to be structured in space, which takes into account the PRRS status in neighboring farms [18]. We defined neighboring farms as one located within 6 km radius.

Conditional autoregressive [2], was specified as the structure for the $\boldsymbol{u} = \{u_1,..., u_n\}$. Considering n areas, each characterized by a set of neighbors $\mathcal{N}_i$ and assuming u_i is the following random variable [3]:

$$u_i \mid \boldsymbol{u}{-i}{\sim}Normal\left(\mu_i + \sum_{j=1}^{n} r_{ij}\left(u_j - \mu_j\right), s_i^2\right) \quad (3)$$

where μ_i is the mean for the farm i and $s_i^2 = \sigma_u^2/\mathcal{N}_i$ is the variance for the same farm, which depends on its number of neighbors (e.g., if an farm has many neighbors then its variance will be smaller). This variance structure recognizes the fact that in the presence of strong spatial correlation, the more neighbors a farm has the more information there is in the data about the value of its random effect. While the variance parameter σ_u^2 controls the amount of variation between the spatially structured random effects. The quantity r_{ij} indicates the spatial proximity and can be calculated as $\phi \times W_{ij}$, where $W_{ij} = a_{ij}/\mathcal{N}_i$, a_{ij} is 1 if farms i and j are neighbors and 0 otherwise (note that a_{ii} is set to 0, thus W_{ii} and r_{ii} are 0 as well); and finally, the parameter ϕ controls the properness of the distribution as it was formulated by Cressie [4].

The parameter v_i is a spatially unstructured component which follows a Normal distribution of the form $N(0, \sigma_v^2)$; where σ_v^2 is the variance of the marginal unstructured component. The main linear trend κ, represents the global time effect. A differential trend δ_i, which identifies the interaction between time and space, represents the difference between the global trend (κ) and the area specific trend. If $\delta_i < 0$ then the area specific trend is less steep than the mean trend, whilst $\delta_i > 0$ implies that the area specific trend is steeper than the mean trend.

Autoregressive parameter driven model

For this step we used a hierarchical Bayesian model similar to the one described by Schrödle et al. [21]. Equation 2 can be re-written using two stages.

$$\begin{aligned} &\text{Stage 1}: \text{logit}(\eta_{it}) = b_0 + u_i + v_i + (\kappa + \delta_i)t + \zeta_{it} \\ &\text{Stage 2}: \zeta_{it} = \lambda.\zeta_{i,t-1} + \rho\textstyle\sum_{j\neq i}\omega_{ji}.\zeta_{j,t-1} + \epsilon_{it} \end{aligned} \quad (4)$$

Because PRRS spread follows more an endemic than epidemic pattern in our particular study area u_i and v_i are included in stage one as suggested by [21].

Equation 3 includes an autoregressive process $\zeta_i = (\zeta_{i1}, \ldots, \zeta_{iT})^T$ for each farm i to model the latent spatial spread of the disease based on the georeferenced location of the farms (e.g. [3]). In the second stage, λ and ρ are the autoregressive parameters. We used N(0, 0.25) distributions as priors for λ and ρ in all the models. The term $\sum_{j\neq i} \omega_{ji}.\zeta_{j,t-1}$ is a weighted sum of the past states on other farms j different than the farm of interest (i). Different choices for the weights ω_{ij} are possible (e.g., [16]). Here we used five different weights namely: (i) geographical distance weight which contains only the inverse distance ($1/i \sim j$) between each pair of farms in kilometers, (ii) pig trade (PT_{ji}) weight which contains the number of pig shipments between each pair of farms and, (iii) the product between the distance weight and the standardize relative pig trade weight (PT_{ji}/number of animals in sender farm), (iv) the product between the standardized distance weight (standardized distance ($i \sim j$) between each pair of farms in kilometers) and the standardized relative pig trade weight (standardize pig trade (PT_{ji}) weight/ number of animals in sender farm), and (v) the product of the distance weight and the pig trade weight. For the geographical distance weight the matrix is symmetric. Other combinations using pig trade weight and distance weight in the denominator were tried with but no convergence was obtained. However, the pig trade weight is not symmetric for each pair of farms, because the number of pig traded from farm j to farm i in our study was different from the number of pig traded from farm i to farm j. The errors $\epsilon_i = (\epsilon_{i1}, \ldots, \epsilon_{iT})^T$ were assumed to be independent and normally distributed with variance σ_{ϵ^2}.

We calculated the mean of the first (finite) moment of the predictive probability distribution ($\mu P = E(y_{iT} \mid y - T$) as defined by Schrödle et al. [21]. Here, the vector $y - T$ contains all the observations in all regions i up to time T-1.We used μP to categorize the PRRS status of farms into two groups namely negative and positive (i.e., farm predicted as negative or positive by the model). The optimal threshold based on the μP was calculated using the true positive rate (sensitivity) and true negative rate (specificity). The optimal threshold is the threshold that maximizes the distance to the identity line in the ROC curve [24].

Model selection criteria and prediction ability

We used the deviance information criteria (DIC), which can be easily calculated in INLA, as the selection criterion for the best final Bayesian model [22]. Smaller DIC values indicate a better trade-off between complexity and fit.

In order to determine the discriminating power for distinguishing between PRRS negative and positive farms we calculated the area under the Receiver Operating Characteristic (ROC) curve (AUC) based on the calculated the mean of the first (finite) moment of the predictive probability distribution (μP) of each model [8]. The higher the AUC, the better the model performed in predicting the infected and not infected farms in the last half of 2014. We also computed the simulation error and the model prediction error. The simulation error is the number of times in which the PRRS farm status is incorrectly classified based on the calculated μP from 2012- first half of 2014 (5 time steps). The model prediction error is the sum of the false positive farms and the false negative farms based on the calculated μP of the second half of 2014.

Results

A summary of the distance and number of pig shipments between different types of farms is shown in Fig. 1. The average distance between the farms was 135.4 km. There were 88 pairs of farms out of 7564 pairs of farms that were located in less than 6 km from each other. Most of the shipments (81%) originated from GDUs.

Results of the spatio-temporal parameter driven model of the PRRS status on farm are shown in Figs. 2 and 3. A downward sloping trend in the risk of PRRS cases over time is apparent when plotting the μP of the main time effect (κ_t) together with its 95% credibility interval (Fig. 2). By plotting the μP of the differential time effect (δ_i) we observed that the differential temporal trend is below the average mostly in the GDU and nursery, while the differential temporal trend for the other site types were higher than the average (Fig. 3).

The fit and predictive performance of the different autoregressive PD models (equation 3) are indicated by DIC and AUC (Table 1). The AUC value for the model using only the geographical distance weight had a lower AUC (0.83) compared with the other models suggesting a lower predictive ability. The AUC value of the models using relative pig trade rate combined with distance weight was lower (AUC = 0.86 and AUC = 0.78) than the model using only the pig trade weight matrix (AUC = 0.88). The model using pig trade weight matrix was also the best fit according to the DIC.

The calculated threshold to categorize the farms into two groups based on the μP has the value of 0.1988682.

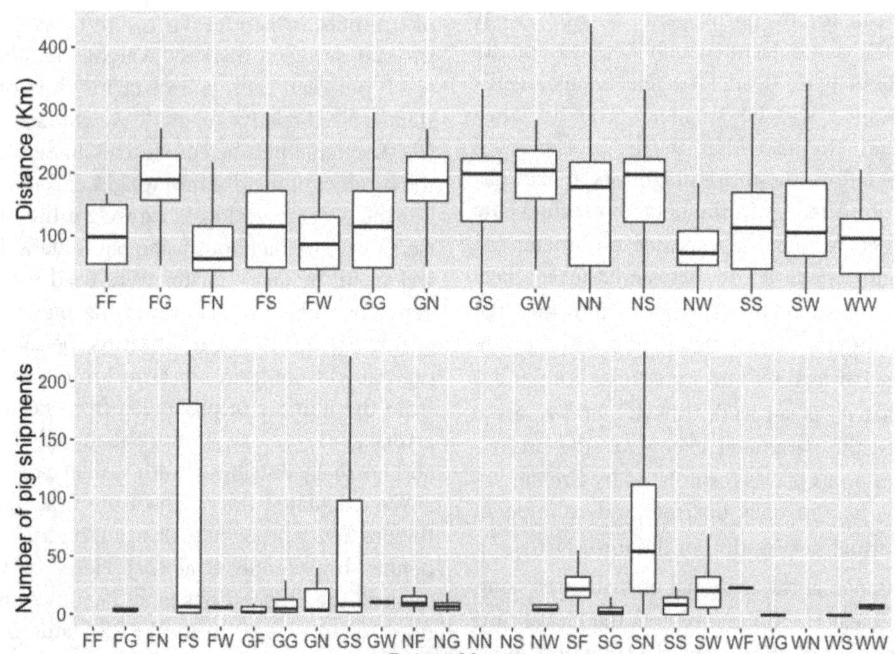

Fig. 1 Boxplots illustrating the distance (*above*) and number of pig shipments (*below*) between pairs of farm types (where F, G, N, S and W stands for finisher, gilt development units, nursery, sow farm and wean-to-finish, respectively). The first letter indicates the origin of the pigs. Notice that only a small fraction of finishers and wean-to-finish were included in the analyses (i.e., only the ones with PRRS outbreaks) therefore movements from and to those farms are not representative of the total volume of movements in the entire population. The horizontal axis (i.e., pairs of farm types) differs in both charts as the pairwise comparison in distance is symmetric but it is asymmetric in movements (i.e., pig movements FG ≠ GF)

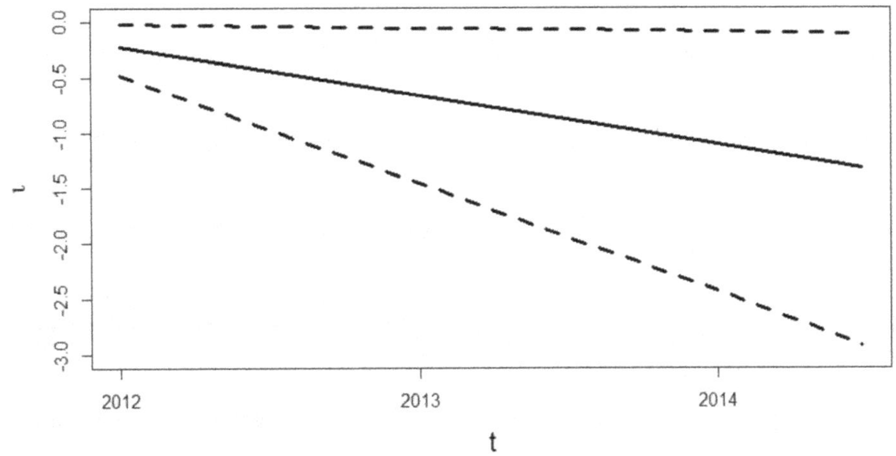

Fig. 2 Global linear temporal trend for PRRS cases from January 2012 to July 2014 using a time step of 6 months. The solid line identifies the posterior mean for ι_t while the dashed lines are 95% credibility interval

The prediction accuracy of the model based on the defined threshold was 85% (105/124) (Fig. 4).

Figure 5 shows how the model performs to simulate the PRRS cases in 124 farms from 2012- first half of 2014 (5 time steps). The model correctly simulated the PRRS status in most of the farms in each of the five time steps except in 27 of the sow farms and three GDU farms.

Discussion

In this paper, we used an advanced two-step parameter-driven approach to evaluate the spatio-temporal dynamics of PRRS from 2012 to July 2014 and predict the subsequent farm status (second half of 2014) in 124 swine production sites of US. The model using the number of pig moved between the farms as a weight matrix

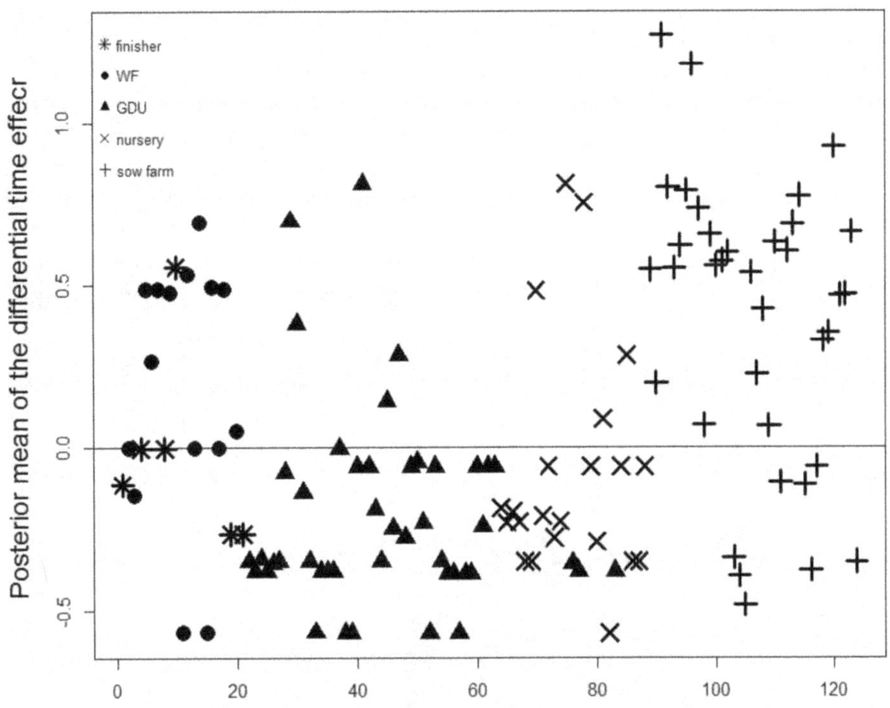

Fig. 3 Posterior mean of the differential time effect (δ_i) for reported PRRS cases of 124 farms from 2012 to 2015. If $\delta_i < 0$ then the farm specific trend is less steep than the mean trend, whilst $\delta_i > 0$ implies that the farm specific trend is steeper than the mean trend. Star, Circle, triangle, multiply and plus represent finisher, WF, GDU, nursery and sow farm, respectively

Table 1 The area under the ROC curve (AUC) based on the calculated posterior mean for the PRRS outbreaks in the farms of second half of 2014 for autoregressive parameter driven model and calculated deviance information criteria (DIC). "std" is the abbreviation for standardize matrix

W_{ji}	AUC	DIC
$1/i \sim j$	0.83	−5540.065
PT_{ji}	0.88	−5382.211
$(PT_{ji}/m_i) . i \sim j$	0.86	NA[a]
$(stdPT_{ji}/m_i) . stdi \sim j$	0.78	−5540.059
$PT_{ji} . i \sim j$	Not converged	Not converged

[a]R-Inla was not able to calculate the DIC for this model

exhibit a better predictive performance than the model just assuming the airborne spread from nearby farms. This suggests that pig trade may have a more important role in PRRS transmission dynamics than airborne transmission, at least in the endemic setting evaluated here. This model was also able to provide a temporal trend for the system (Fig. 2), which may be used to visualize if a system is improving over time and individual farm "scores" (Fig. 3) that could be used for benchmarking and prioritization of risk-reduction measures.

Throughout the global swine industry, extensive efforts have been made to protect commercial swine farms from infection with PRRSV. Extensive efforts are directed to prevent the entry of virus via indirect routes of transmission such as contaminated transport vehicles and insects or aerosols [6, 7]. [6] evaluate the potential of PRRSV-contaminated transport vehicles to infect naïve pigs and assess four sanitation programs for the prevention of virus spread. However, their results support the claim that the movements of animals between farms may play a more important role in the transmission of PRRSV between farms than the nearby airborne transmission of virus.

Previous studies have demonstrated the value of using spatio-temporal models to unravel disease dynamics and identify high risk areas for disease occurrence. To the best of our knowledge very few models have been published to predict PRRS status in the US swine industry. A study conducted by [17] in Ontario, Canada investigated evidence of spread of PRRSV genotypes and determined if spread could be attributed to supplier or ownership connections between herds. The spatial and temporal distributions of six PRRSV genotypes were investigated from 2004 to 2007. Their investigation found no strong evidence of PRRSV spread via aerosol between pig herds in Ontario. They conclude that cluster analysis might not be sensitive for real-time surveillance of PRRSV outbreaks and pig movement network information was more important in the spatial spread of the PRRSV. Kwong et al. [13] examined spatial and temporal spread of PRRSV using individual-level models (ILMs) for infectious diseases, fitted in a Bayesian MCMC framework. Their results showed that the three most important factors for the spread of PRRSV in Ontario (Canada) swine herds were sharing the same herd ownership, gilt source and market trucks. Kwong also suggested that spatial proximity could not be identified as important contributor to PRRSV spread. The results presented in our study provides further evidence that animal movements may be playing a more important role in PRRSV transmission than previously thought in PRRSV endemic settings. Moreover, we have demonstrated the value of using this information to predict, with relatively high accuracy (i.e., 87%) the PRRSV status on farm in subsequent time periods. The model presented here provides a simple, convenient framework and can be employed in real-time using data on the underlying population at risk (i.e., herd size), the PRRS status of farms, the geographical location of farms and, the pig trade network. All this data is usually available for most commercial US pig production systems. Hence our

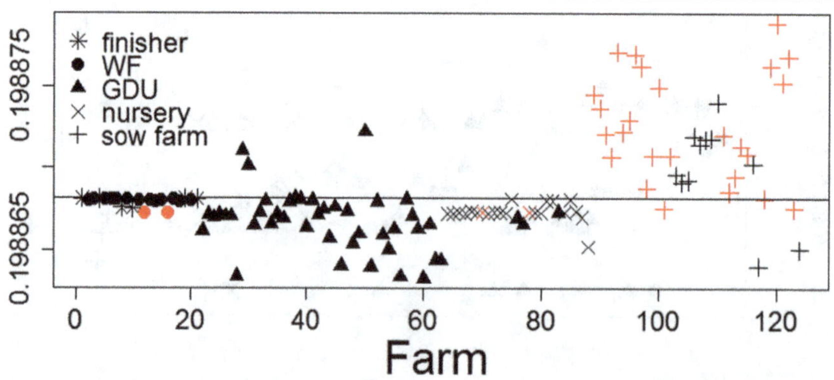

Fig. 4 Posterior mean (μP) for reported PRRS cases of 124 farms for the last half of 2014. The farms below the horizontal line (threshold) are predicted negative and the one above the horizontal line are predicted positive. The reported positive farms in the second half of 2014 are *red* whilst the reported negative farms are *black*. The model prediction accuracy is the sum of the black farms below the threshold and the red farms above the threshold divided by total number of farms (105/124)

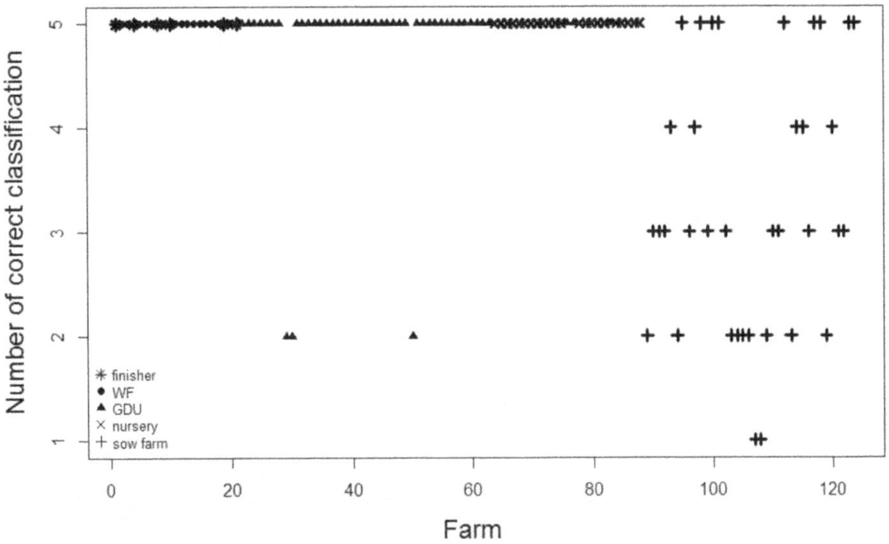

Fig. 5 The number of simulations in which the status of the farm was correctly classified as positive or negative based on the calculated posterior mean from 2012- first half of 2014 (5 time steps)

approach could easily be implemented in operational, real-time surveillance, risk assessment and modeling systems such as Disease BioPortal™ (http://bioportal.ucdavis.edu) to support daily decision making for producers and associated stakeholders.

Most of the prediction errors (11 out of 17 errors in Fig. 4) and all the simulation errors (Fig. 5) occurred in sow farms. The majority of the prediction errors in the sow farms are false positive (seven false positive and four false negative). This result may be associated to some underreporting of PRRS cases in sow farms or to the epidemiological impact and changes in surveillance associated to the introduction and the massive spread of porcine epidemic diarrhea virus (PEDV) during 2013 in the US. PEDV caused significant production losses in the swine industry [23]. The PEDV epidemic also led to an increase of biosecurity measures, disruption of pig trade and reduced sampling and diagnosis of PRRSV [10], which may explain the significant reduction of PRRS reported cases in 2013. Unfortunately, information about biosecurity measures or PED reported cases on farm were not available at the time of this study. The consideration of such information may help to explain some of the simulation and prediction error and potentially increase the predictive accuracy of the model if biosecurity is included as part of the weight matrix.

Another limitation of this study is that PD model does not allow formulating the probability of having at least one positive animal in the farm (i.e., probability that a farm is positive) using multiple weight matrices. However, the weight matrix can be formulated to incorporate different covariates or as a function of different weight matrices to remedy this problem, as it is suggested by Schrödle et al., [21] and as we did in this study (although some of those combinations unfortunately did not converge (Table 1). However, the use of combined weighted matrices limit us in understanding the impact of the each weight matrices and their impact on the probability that a farm is PRRS positive. In this paper we combined the distance weight matrix with the pig trade weight matrix in three different formulations based on the suggestions from Schrödle et al. [21] (Table 1). But none of them had better predictive ability than the model considering only the number of pig movements between farms. One of the reasons why the model using the distance matrix combined with the pig trade weight does not have a better predictive ability than the model using the pig trade weight alone may be that only 1.1% (88/7564*100) of the pair of farms in this study is located less than 6 km from each other. Moreover, farms belonging to other systems that could be near our study farms were excluded from the analyses. Further studies are needed to evaluate if similar results are obtained in higher density areas with more farms within the 6 km range and including other pig production systems.

Conclusion

This study provides a convenient data-driven modelling approach easy to implement and update to characterize PRRS spatio-temporal transmission dynamics and to accurately model PRRS status on farm for subsequent time periods. Model results reveal that pig trade is the most important pathway contributing to PRRSV transmission between farms in the endemic setting under study. A better understanding of pig trade networks and the use of models like the one presented here can help to better predict and control future PRRS outbreaks in US and other endemic settings. These methods will be integrated within the Disease BioPortal™ (http://bioportal.ucdavis.edu) to facilitate the daily use and operational long-term availability of these tools.

Abbreviations

AUC: Area Under the ROC Curve; DIC: Deviance Information Criteria; INLA: Integrated Nested Laplace Approximation; PD : Parameter-Driven; PED: Porcine Epidemic Diarrhea; PEDV: Porcine Epidemic Diarrhea Virus; PRRS: Porcine Reproductive and Respiratory Syndrome; PRRSV: Porcine Reproductive and Respiratory Syndrome Virus; ROC: Receiver Operating Characteristic

Acknowledgment

This study was conducted thanks to the Boehringer Ingelheim gift support and PRRS research award 2015 and the Collaborative Research Agreement between Iowa State University and UC Davis entitled "Epidemiological and information management development and support services through use of the Disease BioPortal™". Authors would like to acknowledge the swine producers for providing data to conduct this study.

Authors' contributions

SAH and BML conceived and designed the study. SAH performed the analysis with the assistance and supervision of BML and drafted the manuscript. DP and KL contributed to data collection, verification and cleaning. DP, RM and DH contributed to the interpretation of the results. All authors read, critically edited and approved the final manuscript.

Competing interests

The authors declare that they have no competing interests.

Consent for publication

Not Applicable.

Author details

[1]Center for Animal Disease Modeling and Surveillance (CADMS), Department of Medicine & Epidemiology, School Veterinary Medicine, University of California, 2108 Tupper Hall, one Shields Avenue, Davis, California 95616, USA. [2]Boehringer-Ingelheim Vetmedica Inc, Saint Joseph, Missouri, USA. [3]Department of Veterinary Diagnostic and Production Animal Medicine, College of Veterinary Medicine, Iowa State University, Ames, USA.

References

1. Albina E. Epidemiology of porcine reproductive and respiratory syndrome (PRRS): an overview. Vet Microbiol. 1997;55(1):309–16.
2. Besag J. Spatial interaction and the statistical analysis of lattice systems. J R Stat soc Series B (Methodological). 1974:192–236.
3. Blangiardo M, Cameletti M. Spatial and spatio-temporal Bayesian models with R-INLA. New York: Wiley; 2015.
4. Cressie N. Statistics for spatial data. New York: Wiley; 1993.
5. Danon L, Ford AP, House T, Jewell CP, Keeling MJ, Roberts GO, et al. Networks and the epidemiology of infectious disease. Interdiscip Perspect Infect Dis. 2011;2011
6. Dee SA, Deen J, Otake S, Pijoan C. An experimental model to evaluate the role of transport vehicles as a source of transmission of porcine reproductive and respiratory syndrome virus to susceptible pigs. Can J Vet Res. 2004a;68(2):128.
7. Dee SA, Schurrer JA, Moon RD, Fano E, Trincado C, Pijoan C. Transmission of porcine reproductive and respiratory syndrome virus under field conditions during a putative increase in the fly population. J Swine Health Prod. 2004b;12:242–5.
8. DeLong ER, DeLong DM, Clarke-Pearson DL. Comparing the areas under two or more correlated receiver operating characteristic curves: a nonparametric approach. Biometrics. 1988:837–45.
9. Evans CM, Medley GF, Green LE. Porcine reproductive and respiratory syndrome virus (PRRSV) in GB pig herds: farm characteristics associated with heterogeneity in seroprevalence. BMC Vet Res. 2008;4(1):1.
10. Geiger J, Connor J. Porcine epidemic diarrhea, diagnosis, and elimination. American Association of Swine Practitioners. 2013;2013:1–4.
11. Holtkamp DJ, Kliebenstein JB, Neumann EJ, Zimmerman JJ, Rotto HF, Yoder TK, et al. Assessment of the economic impact of porcine reproductive and respiratory syndrome virus on United States pork producers. J Swine Health Prod. 2013;21(2):72–84.
12. Jones KE, Patel NG, Levy MA, Storeygard A, Balk D, Gittleman JL, et al. Global trends in emerging infectious diseases. Nature. 2008;451(7181):990–3.
13. Kwong GP, Poljak Z, Deardon R, Dewey CE. Bayesian analysis of risk factors for infection with a genotype of porcine reproductive and respiratory syndrome virus in Ontario swine herds using monitoring data. Prev Vet Med. 2013;110(3):405–17.
14. Lambert M-È, Poljak Z, Arsenault J, D'Allaire S. Epidemiological investigations in regard to porcine reproductive and respiratory syndrome (PRRS) in Quebec, Canada. Part 1: biosecurity practices and their geographical distribution in two areas of different swine density. Prev Vet Med. 2012;104(1):74–83.
15. Lee K, Polson D, Lowe E, Main R, Holtkamp D, Martínez-López B. Unraveling the contact patterns and network structure of pig shipments in the United States and its association with porcine reproductive and respiratory syndrome virus (PRRSV) outbreaks. Prev Vet Med. 2017;138:113–23.
16. Mugglin AS, Cressie N, Gemmell I. Hierarchical statistical modelling of influenza epidemic dynamics in space and time. Stat med. 2002;21(18):2703–21.
17. Rosendal T, Dewey C, Friendship R, Wootton S, Young B, Poljak Z. Spatial and temporal patterns of porcine reproductive and respiratory syndrome virus (PRRSV) genotypes in Ontario, Canada, 2004–2007. BMC vet res. 2014;10(1):1.
18. Rue H, Held L. Gaussian Markov random fields: theory and applications: CRC Press; 2005.
19. Rue H, Martino S, Chopin N. Approximate Bayesian inference for latent Gaussian models by using integrated nested Laplace approximations. J R Stat soc Series B (Statistical Methodology). 2009;71(2):319–92.
20. Schrödle B, Held L. Spatio-temporal disease mapping using INLA. Environmetrics. 2011;22(6):725–34.
21. Schrödle B, Held L, Rue H. Assessing the impact of a movement network on the spatiotemporal spread of infectious diseases. Biometrics. 2012;68(3):736–44.
22. Spiegelhalter DJ, Best NG, Carlin BP, Van Der Linde A. Bayesian measures of model complexity and fit. J R Stat Soc Series B (Statistical Methodology). 2002;64(4):583–639.
23. Stevenson GW, Hoang H, Schwartz KJ, Burrough EB, Sun D, Madson D, et al. Emergence of porcine epidemic diarrhea virus in the United States: clinical signs, lesions, and viral genomic sequences. J Vet Diagn Investig. 2013; 1040638713501675
24. Youden WJ. Index for rating diagnostic tests. Cancer. 1950;3(1):32–5.

9

Development and test of a visual-only meat inspection system for heavy pigs in Northern Italy

Sergio Ghidini[1*], Emanuela Zanardi[1], Pierluigi Aldo Di Ciccio[1], Silvio Borrello[2], Giancarlo Belluzi[3], Sarah Guizzardi[2] and Adriana Ianieri[1]

Abstract

Background: There is a general consensus in recognizing that traditional meat inspection is no longer able to address the hazards related to meat consumption. Moreover, it has been shown that invasive procedures, such as palpation and incision, can increase microbial contamination in carcasses. For these reasons, legislations all over the world are changing meat inspection techniques, moving towards visual-only techniques. Hence, there was also the need to test visual-only inspection in pigs in Italy.

Results: A protocol for visual-only post-mortem inspection was produced together with a 24-class scheme used to record pathological lesions. A list of guidelines needed for univocal interpretation and classification of lesions was developed. To record lesions at the slaughtering line, a light instrument that is resistant to the slaughter environment was designed and then produced in collaboration with an electro-medical company. Six contracted veterinarians were chosen and trained. They performed visual-only post-mortem inspections on 231.673 heavy pigs in three different slaughterhouses of Northern Italy. Visual-only inspection was compared to traditional inspection on 38.819 pig carcasses. No relevant differences were found between the two systems.

Conclusions: The comparison between traditional and visual-only inspection showed that visual-only inspection can be adopted in pig slaughterhouse. The analysis of the performance of the veterinarians stressed the importance of standardization and continuous education for veterinarians working in this field.

Background

Veterinary inspection has been performed for more than a century in slaughterhouses, and it has been effective in protecting consumers against classical hazards such as *Mycobacterium bovis* and parasites. However, there is a consensus around the idea that traditional inspection methods in slaughterhouses no longer cope with the hazards that pose the highest foodborne risks today, such as Salmonella and Yesinia. In industrialised countries, classical diseases are now more effectively controlled with eradication plans [1]. Back in 2011, EFSA [2] stated that the traditional inspection system in swine is not targeted to the main hazards deriving from meat consumption. These hazards are no longer detectable by classical meat inspection because they are no longer caused by pathogens associated with specific lesions and are sometimes related to chemicals. Moreover, procedures such as palpation and incision of the viscera by veterinarians can lead to cross contamination of the carcasses [3].

Considering this evidence, in 2014, the European Commission amended EU Regulation 854/2004 via EU Regulation 219 [4], which laid down specific rules for the organisation of official controls on products of animal origin intended for human consumption [5]. In particular, the regulation stated that starting in June 2014, post-mortem inspection in domestic swine should only be visual and that the official veterinarians shall proceed with additional post-mortem inspection procedures using incision and palpation of the carcass and offal when, in his or her opinion, clinical signs and

* Correspondence: sergio.ghidini@unipr.it
[1]Department of Food and Drug, Parma University, Via Del Taglio, 10, 43126 Parma, Italy
Full list of author information is available at the end of the article

lesions may indicate a possible risk to public health, animal health or animal welfare.

A classification of pig producers as a function of their risk level could help the official veterinarian choose the inspection method [6]. Such a classification should be possible using the food chain information (FCI) module. However, FCI proved to be inefficient in providing such information [7]. In fully integrated chains, it is certainly easier to get more information regarding the farm of origin. Such additional information can be useful for a classification of the farms based on risk.

In Italy, pork production shows a variety of organisational structures and farm size patterns. In 2012, the national pig population was approximately 8.600.000 animals (Eurostat). Southern Italy is characterized by a large number of small-scale farms and many low productivity slaughterhouses, producing a total of 5.700.000 carcasses per year (2012). The North of Italy, where approximately 9.300.000 carcasses are produced per year, is characterized by large-scale indoor intensive farms and high production slaughterhouses (up to 500 carcasses/h). A peculiar feature of swine production in the North of Italy is that there is a very high degree of integration between farmers and meat producers because the majority of swine production in this area processes Protected Designation of Origin products (PDOs). The animals, therefore, share the same genetics, breeding techniques, and feeding schemes, and they have to be born in the North of Italy. In addition, the weight and age of the animals are quite constant since they have to fulfil the requirements of the Parma Ham disciplinary of production. In fact, the animals have to be slaughtered at a minimum age of 9 months and usually weigh approximately 160 kg at the time of slaughtering, with a very small dispersion around the mean because there are economic penalties for lighter and heavier animals [8].

Given this scenario, pig production in the North of Italy can be considered almost fully integrated. Therefore, the holdings in which pigs are raised in this area are fully controlled. When categorizing the holdings according to the risks they pose to public health, they fall into a low-risk class. For this reason, it was considered feasible to test visual-only inspection in this area.

In Italy, there are no data on possible applications of a visual-only inspection system in pigs. In addition, consistent data on post-mortem lesions for pigs at the slaughterhouse are lacking. There have been some local projects in Northern Italy, but the obtained data are not homogenous and comparable. Moreover, in their review, Stark el al. [9] highlighted "a substantial lack of suitable and accessible published data on the frequency of occurrence of many diseases and conditions affecting food animals in Europe." In this context, the Italian Ministry of Health, on behalf of the National Committee for Food Safety, financed a project to study new inspection systems for both the South and the North of Italy.

To fulfil the needs of the high productivity slaughterhouses of the North of Italy, which are characterized by a high working speed, a visual-only inspection system was designed. The system was then tested in three slaughterhouses in the North of Italy to obtain data on the prevalence of post-mortem lesions in pigs dedicated to the production of PDO products. The visual system was then compared to the "traditional" inspection using invasive procedures.

Methods

Study area and population

The Parma Ham Consortium of production limits the area of origin of the animals dedicated to Parma Ham production (and other PDO products) to the following regions: Emilia-Romagna, Veneto, Lombardy, Piedmont, Molise, Umbria, Tuscany, Marche, Abruzzo and Lazio [8]. These regions represent the whole north and a large part of the centre of Italy. The pigs belong to the Large White, Landrace, Duroc breeds and their hybrids. They must be slaughtered at a minimum age of 9 months. At this age, they reach an average weight of 160 kg.

In 2013, 4199 farms in this area produced and then sent to slaughter 8.071.726 animals for transformation into PDO products. Pigs are usually sent to the slaughterhouses in batches of approximately 120 animals. The whole animals are slaughtered in 65 slaughterhouses. All the slaughterhouses have the possibility to buy animals from all the PDO regions mentioned above. Eighteen of these slaughterhouses, which are in only two regions (Emilia-Romagna and Lombardy), process 93% of all the animals [10]. For logistical convenience, the present study was performed in 3 of the 18 slaughterhouses (2 in Lombardy and one in Emilia-Romagna) that share the same layout and slaughtering technique and that are very similar in size and processing speed.

Animal selection

Only heavy pigs following the Parma Ham disciplinary (therefore of national origin) were considered in this study. In the slaughterhouses, no further selection of the animals was performed so that all the animals of the Parma Ham area could have the same probability of being chosen for the study. To minimise the influence of the distance between the farm and the slaughterhouse, the sampling times were homogeneously distributed between the different working days of the week and the working hours of the day.

The study was designed to achieve relative standard errors of the prevalence of lesions lower than 1% for lesions with a prevalence higher than 5% and lower than 10% for lesions with a prevalence as low as 0.1%. Using

FAO [11] formulae, we aimed to inspect 200.000 pig carcasses. The study lasted from January to August 2013.

Visual inspection protocol

A new protocol of visual-only inspection for pigs was developed based on EU Regulation 854/2004 because there were no visual-only inspection protocols at the time of this study. To give an operative tool to veterinarians, the anatomical structures to be inspected were re-arranged into three main groups (carcass, red offal, green offal), which resembles the way organs are found at the end of a slaughtering line.

Together with the veterinary service in the Emilia-Romagna and Lombardy regions and the Italian Ministry of Health, a 24-class scheme (Table 1) was developed. The scheme was designed to be easily adopted in high production slaughterhouses, shared at national level and comparable with schemes adopted by the Food Safety and Inspection Service in the USA [12] and the Food Standard Agency in the UK [13]. A list of guidelines needed for univocal interpretation and classification of lesions was developed (Table 1).

Recording system

An electro-medical company (Omicron T S.R.L., Napoli, Italy) was commissioned to design a light tablet (Fig. 1). The tablet had to record lesions on the slaughtering line and be resistant to the slaughterhouse environment.

The instrument weights 420 g, and it is 24 cm wide, 25 cm height and 1 cm thick. It can be connected to a computer via a mini USB port, which is used for both data downloading and charging. On the front panel, it has 24 square buttons (2 cm on each side), representing the lesions in Table 1. Two larger buttons (2 cm high and 4 cm wide) are used for normal animals and to record a change of batch. A vibration is emitted when a button is pushed. In case of a mistake or a change in diagnosis, the operator can change his decision within 2 s, after which the decision is automatically confirmed by a flashing LED light. The data of each working day are then saved in a file and transferred to the central unit, which handles the database.

Software and data analysis

Software was developed with the help of Omicron T S.R.L., (Napoli, Italy). The software had to build a database, starting from the data recorded on the tablets, and then handle a database of at least 400.000 inspected carcasses. The database system used by this software is MySql Server (Oracle, CA). At present, this software is able to extract the data from the database by using five filters: date, type of farm, distance from slaughterhouse, breeding farm code and veterinarian. In the future, the software could be implemented with other filters if necessary. The results of the queries were exported to MS Excel-compatible datasheets, and MS Excel was used for data elaboration. The mean data were compared using Student's t-test.

Personnel

Six veterinarians experienced in meat inspection of pigs were contracted to perform visual-only post-mortem inspection in the slaughterhouses. First, they were trained to use the recording system and then to handle it in operating conditions. Before collecting the data, each veterinarian was trained in the slaughterhouse for a period of about one month (approximately 5000 carcasses). After this period, their results were analysed and they were given further training on the classification of lesions, following the previously developed guidelines. The veterinarians then inspected approximately 40,000 carcasses each to achieve the target of 200,000 carcasses that was previously set. The contracted veterinarians were regularly rotated between the three slaughterhouses.

Place of work

The three slaughterhouses had a capacity varying from 380 to 450 carcasses per hour. In these slaughterhouses, the contracted veterinarians were placed before the official colleagues performing traditional inspections to prevent the contracted veterinarians from diagnosing lesions by relying on cuts made by the official colleagues. To minimise mutual influence, the contracted and official veterinarians were always the maximum possible distance apart in the slaughtering environment (never <5 m) .

Visual-only vs. traditional inspection comparison

In the last period of the study, the developed recording system was also given to official veterinarians, and the data from visual-only (performed by the contracted veterinarians) and traditional inspections (performed by the official veterinarians) of the same pigs were compared on 38.919 pig carcasses. In this period, the work was conducted only in one slaughterhouse to minimise environmental effects. Furthermore, because a different tool to record lesions was already in use in the chosen slaughterhouse, the official veterinarians working there were already trained to perform post-mortem inspections while recording data on an electronic device.

The study was submitted to the Institutional Review Board of The University of Parma that gave a favourable opinion since compliant with ethical principles.

Results

Overall, 231.673 carcasses were inspected by means of a visual-only post-mortem inspection. The carcasses composed 1.832 batches (mean of 126 animals/batch) and came from 323 different farms. A batch is defined as a

Table 1 Lesion classification and the guidelines adopted to record the data

Apparatus	Lesion	Guideline
Respiratory	Pneumonia	Detect both pneumonia and outcomes of pneumonia. Detect pneumonia when an entire lobe is interested, or when not involving the entire lobe, it involves two contralateral lobes. Always consider specific pneumonia. Consider lung abscesses (even one) as pneumonia.
	Pleuropneumonia	Is recognized when adhesions are present on the carcass. Is recognised when fibrin is present on the visceral layer of the pleura.
Digestive	Hepatitis	Hepatitis and outcomes of hepatitis. The presence of fibrin on the capsule should not be classified as hepatitis (classified as peritonitis).
	Hepatosis/hepatic dystrophies	Steatosis and necrosis are to be classified only in cases involving at least an entire lobe or parts of several lobes.
	Peritonitis/perihepatitis	
	Enteritis	Haemorrhagic or necrotic. Thickening of the small intestine.
Reproductive-Urinary	Nephritis	Nephritis and glomerulonephritis.
	Nephrosis	Cystitis and hydronephrosis.
	Cryptorchidism	
Cardio Circulatory	Myocarditis	Involvement of pericarditis. Do not classify degenerative processes in the absence of inflammation as myocarditis.
	Pericarditis	
Integumentary	Dermatitis	Recognized when there is a thickening of the skin. Detect when lesions exceed 50% of the body surface and not when confined to the abdominal region and chest. Detect carcasses massively affected by bites of ectoparasites as dermatitis.
	Erysipelas	Detect whenever the typical skin lesions are encountered.
Locomotor	Arthritis	
	Muscle colour alteration (PSE/DFD)	PSE / DFD
	Oedema/emaciation	
Other (carcass)	Jaundice	
	Abscesses	Detect all abscesses that are not located in the lung or in the liver. Also detect phlegmons as abscesses.
	Neoplasms / tumours	
	Biliary or faecal contamination	Both faecal and bile contamination. In addition, the residual presence of parts of the rectal mucosa is considered contamination.
	Trauma	Skin
		Bruises and injuries due to mismanagement during loading / unloading (bruises and haematomas). Wounds from intraspecific fights and numerous injuries that get to in the derma, possibly infected.
		Skeletal muscle
		Splay-leg animals (open). Do not report results of old injuries.
	Lymphadenopathy	Mesenteric lymph nodes, lung, and generally an increase in the volume of lymph nodes in the carcass.
	Splenomegaly	Detect when affecting more than 50% of the organ.
	Petechial haemorrhages	

group of animals from one farm delivered on one day, usually transported by a single truck. In Table 2, the number and percentage of each lesion detected in each slaughterhouse and an estimate of the prevalence for each lesion. Table 3 presents the results of the comparison between traditional and visual-only inspections. Table 4 shows the total variability achieved and the variability within each lesion (standard deviation and variation coefficient).

Discussion

The majority of lesions were at the respiratory level (Table 2). In fact, more than 20% of the animals had pneumonia or pleuropneumonia. This result is not surprising because intensively bred, fat animals nine months in age were inspected. Furthermore, these data are consistent with those coming from international literature. For instance, in a review of post-mortem data in pig slaughterhouses of New Zealand from 2000 to 2010,

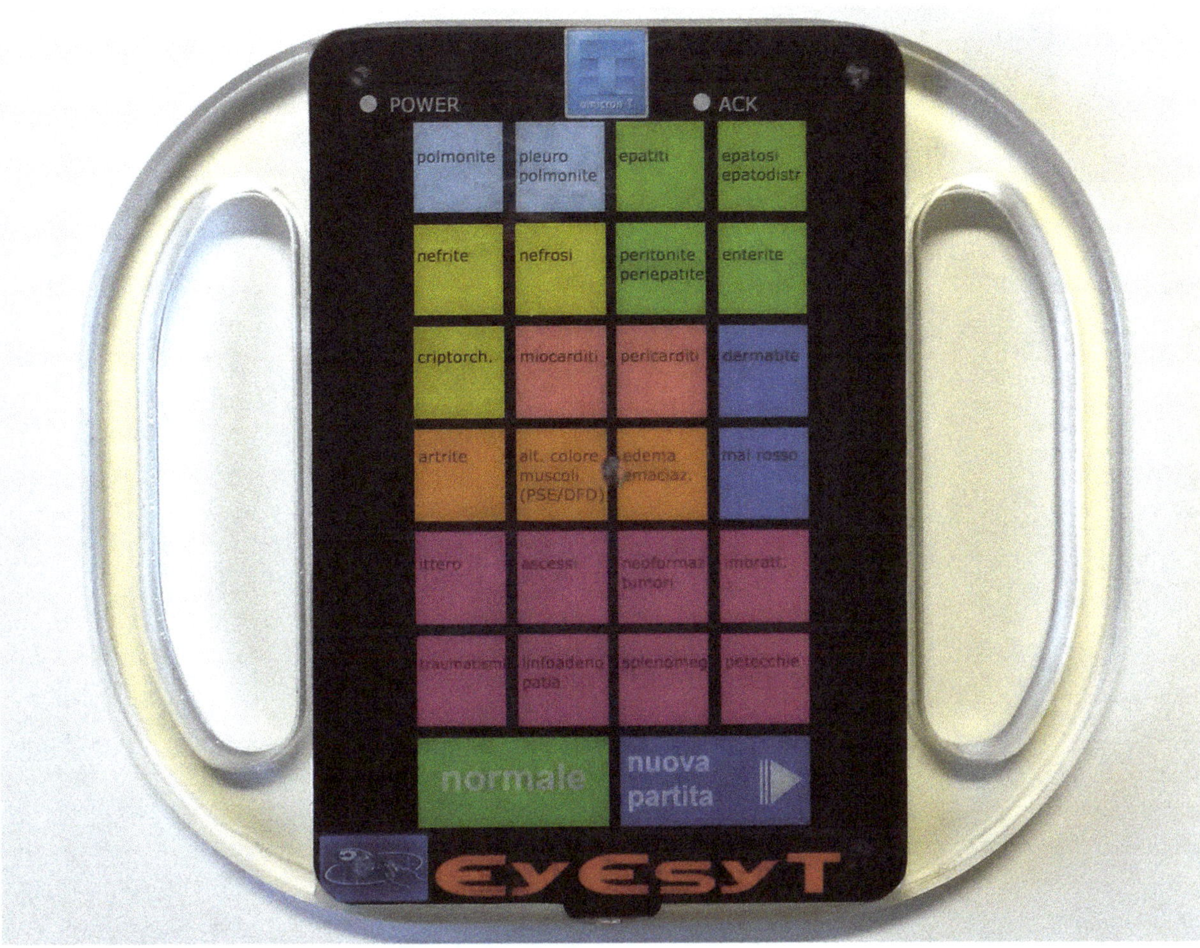

Fig. 1 The recording system developed in cooperation with Omicron T

Neumann et al. [14] found a prevalence of pleurisy, pneumonia and pleuropneumonia of approximately 16%. This prevalence is slightly lower than the one found in the present study, which can be explained by the lower age and weight of their animals at the time of slaughter.

For heavy pigs from Northern Italy, Merialdi et al. [15], found a prevalence of respiratory lesions of up to 40%, which is even higher than the prevalence in the present study. However, the focus of this previous study was different, and the researchers probably included all minimal lung lesions. In the present study, pneumonia was considered only if the lesion (Table 1) intersected a whole lobe. They found a prevalence of milk spot lesions near 10%, while in the present study, the prevalence of hepatic lesions was 16%. Milk spot lesions composed the majority of hepatic lesions in the present study, but the fact that all hepatic lesions were not classified in more detail can explain the difference in results.

According to European Union Regulation (EC) No. 854/2004, erysipelas should be detected ante-mortem, and the slaughtering must be deferred. Nevertheless, erysipelas can be undiagnosed ante-mortem because the typical lesions become evident only after scalding and bristle removal. In this case, swine carcasses affected by erysipelas must either undergo skin removal or be destroyed depending on the disease stage. Occasional cases of erysipelas were recorded during post-mortem inspection, but the number was very low. In all of these cases, the carcasses were destroyed.

No large differences were detected between the three slaughterhouses. In particular, as could be expected due to the homogeneity of the animals, no relevant differences in lesions related to animal health were found. Only a relevant difference in biliary or faecal contamination was found. In particular, one slaughterhouse showed an prevalence of carcass contamination (3.6%) that was much higher than that of the other two slaughterhouses (2.2% and 2.5%). The slaughtering lines of the three plants did not have relevant technological differences. The two slaughterhouses with lower incidences had a visual inspection of carcasses for faecal or biliary contamination, defined as a critical control point in their

Table 2 Number and percentage of each lesion detected during the work in the three slaughterhouses and an estimate of the prevalence of each lesion

	Slaughterhouse 1		Slaughterhouse 2		Slaughterhouse 3		Tot.		
	number	%	number	%	number	%	number	Prevalence %	standard error
Pneumonia	5100	5.40	8840	8.99	1911	4.91	15,851	6.43	0.050
Pleuropneumonia	15,242	16.14	12,654	12.87	6756	17.35	34,652	15.46	0.074
Hepatitis	21,972	23.27	10,535	10.71	5594	14.37	38,101	16.12	0.075
Hepatosis/hepato-dystrophies	625	0.66	3537	3.60	618	1.59	4780	1.95	0.028
Peritonitis/perihepatitis	355	0.38	730	0.74	71	0.18	1156	0.43	0.013
Enteritis	206	0.22	514	0.52	137	0.35	857	0.36	0.012
Nephritis	234	0.25	261	0.27	113	0.29	608	0.27	0.011
Nephrosis	134	0.14	137	0.14	224	0.58	495	0.29	0.011
Cryptorchidism	139	0.15	140	0.14	115	0.30	394	0.20	0.009
Myocarditis	11	0.01	3	0.00	4	0.01	18	0.01	0.002
Pericarditis	3341	3.54	3345	3.40	1059	2.72	7745	3.22	0.036
Dermatitis	832	0.88	1120	1.14	858	2.20	2810	1.41	0.024
Erysipelas	29	0.03	115	0.12	291	0.75	435	0.30	0.011
Arthritis	0	0.00	8	0.01	0	0.00	8	0.00	0.000
Muscle colour alteration (PSE/DFD)	7	0.01	2	0.00	4	0.01	13	0.01	0.002
Oedema/emaciation	22	0.02	12	0.01	4	0.01	38	0.02	0.003
Jaundice	79	0.08	11	0.01	9	0.02	99	0.04	0.004
Abscesses	571	0.60	865	0.88	422	1.08	1858	0.86	0.019
Neoplasms / tumours	25	0.03	7	0.01	9	0.02	41	0.02	0.003
Biliary or faecal contamination	2126	2.25	3582	3.64	956	2.46	6664	2.78	0.034
Trauma	405	0.43	1316	1.34	674	1.73	2395	1.17	0.022
Lymphadenopathy	138	0.15	47	0.05	25	0.06	210	0.09	0.006
Splenomegaly	254	0.27	173	0.18	176	0.45	603	0.30	0.011
Petechial haemorrhages	24	0.03	1	0.00	0	0.00	25	0.01	0.002
Tot.	51,871	54.94	47,955	48.77	20,235	51.45	119,965	51.72	0.102
Animals	94,411		98,333		38,929		231,590		

self-control plan, while the third slaughterhouse did not. This difference probably resulted in the operators paying greater attention during the evisceration phases.

No differences in trauma lesions were found between the slaughterhouses. The relatively low number of cases (2395, 1.03%) shows that the operators pay attention to animal welfare and handling during transportation and ante-mortem care.

Overall, the kidney conditions of the animals were good, and nephritis or nephrosis lesions were detected in less than 0.3% of the cases.

Dermatitis lesions were found in approximately 1.4% of cases. This figure is much lower than the data recorded by Neuman et al. [14], who found mange lesions in 3.6% of the animals. Still, the data can be considered comparable because dermatitis in the present study was recorded only when the lesion involved more than 50% of the whole skin surface (Table 1).

Regarding peritonitis/perihepatitis, enteritis, cryptorchidism, pericarditis, abscesses and splenomegaly, it is almost impossible to compare these data with international literature since these data are scarce.

Myocarditis, arthritis, muscle colour alteration, oedema/emaciation, jaundice, neoplasms/tumours, lymphadenopathy and petechial haemorrhages cannot be considered since their prevalence was lower than 0.1%, and at this level, the relative standard error of the estimate is too high to make reliable conclusions.

Visual vs. traditional inspections

As a whole, the visual-only inspection showed greater efficiency than the traditional inspection in detecting lesions (Table 3). In fact, the visual-only inspection detected lesions in 52% of the animals, while the traditional inspection detected lesions in only 42% of the animals. There was a large difference in the sensitivity in

Table 3 Results of the comparison between traditional and visual-only inspections

	Traditional	%	Visual-only	%	δ % over traditional	Relative δ % over traditional
Pneumonia	2709	6.96	1911	4.91	−2.05	−29.5
Pleuropneumonia	4150	10.66	6756	17.35	6.69	62.8
Total respiratory	6859	17.62	8667	22.26	4.64	
Hepatitis	6566	16.87	5594	14.37	−2.50	−14.8
Hepatosis/hepato-dystrophies	1	0.00	618	1.59	1.58	61,700
Peritonitis/perihepatitis	66	0.17	71	0.18	0.01	7.58
Enteritis	38	0.10	137	0.35	0.25	261
Total digestive	6671	17.14	6420	16.49	−0.65	
Nephritis	35	0.09	113	0.29	0.20	223
Nephrosis	163	0.42	224	0.58	0.16	37.4
Cryptorchidism	40	0.10	115	0.30	0.19	188
Total reproductive-urinary	238	0.61	452	1.16	0.55	
Myocarditis	1	0.00	4	0.01	0.01	300
Pericarditis	575	1.48	1059	2.72	1.24	84.2
Total cardio-circulatory	576	1.48	1063	2.73	1.25	
Dermatitis	520	1.34	858	2.20	0.87	65.0
Erysipelas	148	0.38	291	0.75	0.37	96.6
Total tegumentary	668	1.72	1149	2.95	1.24	
Arthritis	0	0.00	0	0.00	0.00	
Muscle colour alteration (PSE/DFD)	0	0.00	4	0.01	0.01	
Oedema/emaciation	3	0.01	4	0.01	0.00	33.3
Total locomotor	3	0.01	8	0.02	0.01	
Jaundice	4	0.01	9	0.02	0.01	125
Abscesses	454	1.17	422	1.08	−0.08	−7.05
Neoplasms / tumours	3	0.01	9	0.02	0.02	200
Biliary or faecal contamination	685	1.76	1161	2.98	1.22	69.5
Trauma	103	0.26	674	1.73	1.47	554
Lymphadenopathy	6	0.02	25	0.06	0.05	317
Splenomegaly	111	0.29	176	0.45	0.17	58.6
Petechial haemorrhages	1	0.00	0	0.00	0.00	−100
Total other	1367	3.51	2476	6.36	2.85	
Tot lesions	16,382		20,235			
Tot Animals	38,929		38,929			
% lesions	42.09		51.98			

pneumonia and pleuropneumonia detection probably because official veterinarians performing traditional inspections did not undergo training for lesion classification before the trial. As a matter of fact, if we consider respiratory lesions (pneumonia and pleuropneumonia) together, the difference is much lower and not statistically relevant. In synthesis, comparable numbers of respiratory diseases were detected by both systems, but the lesion classifications were different.

In addition, the difference in hepatitis detection ability was not statistically relevant, but it is not surprising that traditional liver palpation leads to more sensitivity in this area.

As a whole, almost the same sensitivity was noticed in detecting lesions in red and green offal, while visual-only inspection showed greater sensitivity in detecting lesions on the carcass. The slaughtering line was working at 380 pigs per hour, meaning that there was less than 10 s to perform a whole post-mortem inspection. If the veterinarian had to perform invasive actions, the time available for looking at the whole carcass was probably too short.

Table 4 Means, standard deviations and percent variation coefficients of lesion detection achieved by contracted veterinarians in the preliminary phase, when they inspected 5000 carcass each (not included in the global database), and the comparison period at the end of the study, after the guidelines were applied

	Preliminary period			Final period			
	mean	st. dev.	v. c.	mean	st. dev.	v. c.	Δ v.c. after training
Pneumonia	8.58	8.88	103.52	4.69	3.83	81.66	−21.85
Pleuropneumonia	10.86	7.21	66.39	17.29	1.78	10.31	−56.08
Hepatitis	17.00	9.10	53.54	14.56	2.81	19.26	−34.28
Hepatosis/hepato-dystrophies	1.72	2.61	151.90	1.36	2.17	159.73	7.83
Peritonitis/perihepatitis	0.55	0.54	97.81	0.20	0.17	83.45	−14.36
Enteritis	0.30	0.27	90.53	0.38	0.22	59.68	−30.84
Nephritis	0.18	0.07	40.29	0.26	0.15	59.44	19.14
Nephrosis	0.16	0.16	97.47	0.55	0.25	45.50	−51.98
Cryptorchidism	0.14	0.03	24.34	0.30	0.06	20.80	−3.55
Myocarditis	0.02	0.02	150.55	0.01	0.02	113.93	−36.62
Pericarditis	2.96	1.02	34.43	2.71	0.50	18.61	−15.82
Dermatitis	0.96	0.67	69.44	1.97	1.11	56.40	−13.04
Erysipelas	0.06	0.09	154.20	0.71	0.68	96.10	−58.10
Arthritis	0.01	0.01	167.33	0.00	0.00	0.00	−167.33
Muscle colour alteration (PSE/DFD)	0.00	0.01	154.92	0.01	0.01	115.72	−39.20
Oedema/emaciation	0.02	0.02	89.57	0.01	0.01	120.94	31.36
Jaundice	0.04	0.03	88.06	0.03	0.03	96.50	8.44
Abscesses	0.74	0.28	38.07	1.09	0.35	31.87	−6.20
Neoplasms / tumours	0.01	0.01	77.46	0.04	0.08	200.00	122.54
Biliary or faecal contamination	2.44	0.90	36.85	3.10	0.88	28.44	−8.41
Trauma	0.56	0.71	125.58	1.58	1.13	71.25	−54.33
Lymphadenopathy	0.14	0.19	143.46	0.06	0.04	62.70	−80.77
Splenomegaly	0.24	0.19	82.18	0.46	0.24	50.97	−31.21
Petechial haemorrhages	0.02	0.02	150.55	0.00	0.00	0.00	−150.55
Total	47.66	19.02	39.91	51.37	5.51	10.73	−29.19

The analytical results agree with an assessment of risk associated with changes in meat inspections conducted by the Danish Agriculture and Food Council in 2014 [16], which found higher sensitivity for visual inspections than traditional inspections. Hill in 2013 [17], Mousing in 1997 [18] and Blagojevich in 2015 [19] also stressed that switching to visual inspection in pigs does not imply an increase in risk, even if the pigs are raised outdoors. Figure 2 graphically represents the differences between the two inspection systems.

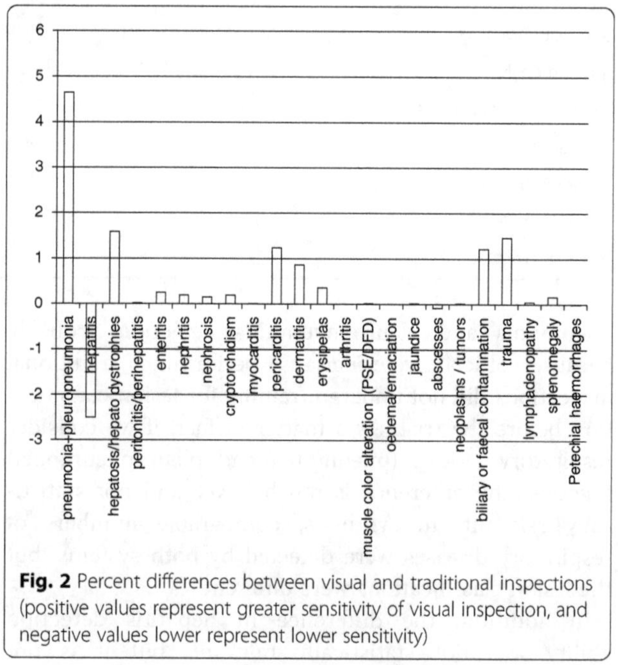

Fig. 2 Percent differences between visual and traditional inspections (positive values represent greater sensitivity of visual inspection, and negative values lower represent lower sensitivity)

Pre- and post-training evaluation of veterinarians

To conduct this analysis, it was postulated that on a very large number of inspected animals, each operator should obtain the same mean data. This approach was only possible in field conditions. In such a scenario, the deviation from the median is a good parameter to define how good the inspector is compared to other colleagues. Obviously, such a system is most reliable and meaningful for the most common lesions, and it is not reliable for more "exotic" lesions.

After setting guidelines and training, a generally low variation was achieved at the end of the study period, as shown by a decrease in the variation coefficient of almost every lesion category (Table 4). The decrease was present in common lesions and in the total number of lesions, showing that training is crucial to obtain homogenous judgements by veterinarians. This approach was not successful for detecting and classifying every lesion (e.g., hepatosis and nephritis), but one of the functions of such an instrument is the ability to address future training actions.

Official vs. contracted veterinarians

The same principle used for evaluating pre- and post-training performance was adopted to compare the performance of official and contracted veterinarians. Following this principle, the official veterinarians that inspected a low number of animals were excluded from this analysis. The classification and recording of lesions can be extremely useful because these data can be used for epidemiological purposes, for farming suggestions and even for farm classification. However, such a system can be effective only if the inspector's judgements are repeatable and reliable. As much as possible, the inspections have to be independent of the individuals conducting the inspections. Moreover, these judgements have extremely important economic relevance since different condemnation rates of single organs or whole carcasses imply different costs both for slaughterers and for famers.

From the data in Table 5, it is clear that the trained contracted veterinarians achieved a globally lower variability than the official colleagues. The fact that the official veterinarians were not trained to apply the guidelines can easily explain the difference. The data

Table 5 Means, standard deviations and percent variation coefficients of lesion detection achieved by the official veterinarians performing traditional inspection and by the contracted veterinaries performing visual-only inspection in the comparison period

	Official veterinarians			Contracted veterinarians			
	mean	st. dev.	v. c.	mean	st. dev.	v. c.	δ over official
Pneumonia	5.82	4.39	75.57	4.69	3.83	81.66	6.09
Pleuropneumonia	10.70	2.86	26.76	17.29	1.78	10.31	−16.45
Hepatitis	14.96	8.80	58.83	14.56	2.81	19.26	−39.56
Hepatosis/hepato-dystrophies	0.00	0.00	300.00	1.36	2.17	159.73	−140.27
Peritonitis/perihepatitis	0.11	0.26	239.75	0.20	0.17	83.45	−156.30
Enteritis	0.04	0.07	181.11	0.38	0.22	59.68	−121.43
Nephritis	0.05	0.06	123.58	0.26	0.15	59.44	−64.15
Nephrosis	0.21	0.32	152.40	0.55	0.25	45.50	−106.91
Cryptorchidism	0.06	0.09	161.92	0.30	0.06	20.80	−141.13
Myocarditis	0.00	0.00	300.00	0.01	0.02	113.93	−186.07
Pericarditis	1.81	1.20	66.13	2.71	0.50	18.61	−47.52
Dermatitis	0.80	1.65	205.77	1.97	1.11	56.40	−149.37
Erysipelas	0.39	0.32	82.58	0.71	0.68	96.10	13.52
Arthritis	0.00	0.00	0.00	0.00	0.00	0.00	0.00
Muscle colour alteration (PSE/DFD)	0.00	0.00	0.00	0.01	0.01	115.72	115.72
Oedema/emaciation	0.01	0.01	217.58	0.01	0.01	120.94	−96.64
Jaundice	0.01	0.01	198.29	0.03	0.03	96.50	−101.79
Abscesses	0.97	0.55	56.44	1.09	0.35	31.87	−24.57
Neoplasms / tumours	0.02	0.05	254.11	0.04	0.08	200.00	−54.11
Biliary or faecal contamination	1.96	0.64	32.94	3.10	0.88	28.44	−4.50
Trauma	0.10	0.21	205.51	1.58	1.13	71.25	−134.26
Lymphadenopathy	0.01	0.02	198.62	0.06	0.04	62.70	−135.92
Splenomegaly	0.14	0.19	135.20	0.46	0.24	50.97	−84.24
Petechial haemorrhages	0.00	0.00	300.00	0.00	0.00	0.00	−300.00
Total	38.15	16.30	42.71	51.37	5.51	10.73	−31.98

Nine official veterinarians conducted inspections during the study, but two of these veterinarians were excluded in this evaluation since they inspected less than 1000 carcasses

demonstrate that it is essential to reach a high level of standardisation, which can be achieved only through the adoption of strict operative guidelines and training veterinarians to adopt and follow these guidelines. The training should be aimed towards reaching a lower variability in judgement by understanding and following the guidelines.

Conclusions

The data derived from local projects on post-mortem lesions in slaughterhouses in Northern Italy were not homogenous and comparable.

For the first time, a classification of lesions was developed and shared with the Ministry of Health and the two most productive regions in the swine sector. Moreover, a relevant dataset of these lesions and instruments able to further expand this database were built.

In industrial high-speed slaughtering lines of pigs, visual inspection was shown to be comparable to traditional inspection and was even more sensitive for some lesions.

Post-mortem inspection is a human judgement and is therefore prone to large error. To minimize error and to achieve a high level of standardization, it is necessary to develop operative guidelines. In addition, training the operators involved is crucial for obtaining consistent data. Only with reliable data can post-mortem inspection reports be used for several purposes, such as epidemiological studies or the classification of farms based on risk. It is therefore important to have the same classification and guidelines, and the veterinarians involved in meat inspection should undergo continuous education.

Acknowledgements
The authors want to acknowledge the veterinary services of the Emilia Romagna and Lombardy regions and all the slaughterhouse personnel who were involved in the project.

Funding
The project was financed by the Italian Ministry of Health.

Authors' contributions
SG, EZ, PADC and AI designed the study, followed the work and analysed the data. SB, GB and SG contributed to the study design and its implementation in the field scenario. All authors read and approved the final manuscript.

Consent for publication
Not applicable

Competing interests
The authors declare that they have no competing interests.

Author details
[1]Department of Food and Drug, Parma University, Via Del Taglio, 10, 43126 Parma, Italy. [2]Italian Ministry of Health, Via Giorgio Ribotta, 5, 00144 Rome, Italy. [3]Italian Ministry of Health, Viale Tanara 31/A, 43100 Parma (PR), Italy.

References

1. Huey R. Toroughly modern meat inspection. Vet Rec. 2014;170(3):68–70.
2. EFSA. Scientific opinion on the public health hazards to be covered by inspection of meat (swine). EFSA J. 2011;9(10):2351. [198 pp.]
3. Buncic S, Nychas GJ, Lee Michael RF, Koutsoumanis K, Hebraud M, Desvaux M, Chorianopoulos N, Bolton D, Blagojevic B, Antic D. Microbial pathogen control in the beef chain: recent research advances. Meat Sci. 2014;97(3):288–97.
4. Commission Regulation (EU) No 219/2014 amending Annex I to Regulation (EC) No 854/2004 of the European Parliament and of the Council as regards the specific requirements for post-mortem inspection of domestic swine. Official Journal of the European Union. L 69/99. 206. 08 March 2014;
5. Regulation (EC) No. 854/2004. Official Journal of the European Union. L155. 206. 29 April 2004;
6. Heinonen M, Grohn YT, Saloniemi H, Eskola E, Tuovinen V. K. The effects of health classification and housing and management of feeder pigs on performance and meat inspection findings of all-in-all-out swine-finishing herds. Prev Vet Med. 2001;49(1–2):41–54.
7. Felin E, Jukola E, Raulo S, Heinonen J, Fredriksson-Ahomaa M. Current food chain information provides insufficient information for modern meat inspection of pigs. Prev Vet Med. 2016;127:113–20.
8. Prosciutto di Parma. Disciplinary of Production. 2015. Available at http://www.prosciuttodiparma.com/pdf/it_IT/disciplinare.28.11.2013.it.pdf. Accessed 7 June 2015.
9. Stärk KDC, Alonso S, Dadios N, Dupuy C, Ellerbroek L, Georgiev M, Hardstaff J, Huneau-Salaün A, Laugier C, Mateus A, Nigsch A, Afonso A, Lindberg A. Strengths and weaknesses of meat inspection as a contribution to animal health and welfare surveillance. Food Control. 2014;39:154–62.
10. Istituto Parma Qualità. Rapporto sull'attività dei servizi coordinati di controllonell'anno 2013. 2014. Available at http://www.google.it/url?sa=t&rct=j&q=&esrc=s&source=web&cd=8&ved=0CEYQFjAHahUKEwjjnq_nj5bGAhUKXBQKHX0IAHg&url=http%3A%2F%2Fineqweb.it%2Findex.php%2Ffiles%2F7dcee9883e139530df552ecdb3da8e948927fc1b.pdf%3Faction%3Ddownload&ei=uBaBVePiCoq4Uf2QgMAH&usg=AFQjCNFOijufCr_9C9ZZ1-3zfONrRpOFwg&sig2=lRajHTlzllxPfzi5yrPPVQ&bvm=bv.96041959.d.d24&cad=rja. Accessed 5 June 2015.
11. FAO. The Epidemiological Approach to Investigate Disease Problems. 2013. Available at http://www.fao.org/wairdocs/ilri/x5436e/x5436e06.htm#4.4%20sample%20sizes. Accessed on November 2012;
12. Food Safety and Inspection Service. FSIS Directive 6100.2 17/09/2007. 2007. Available at http://www.fsis.usda.gov/OPPDE/rdad/FSISDirectives/6100.2.pdf;
13. Food Standard Agency. Trial of visual inspection of fattening pigs from non-controlled housing conditions. 2013. Available at https://www.food.gov.uk/science/research/choiceandstandardsresearch/meatcontrolsprojects/fs145003/#.UqhAieKmYxA
14. Neumann EJ, Hall WF, Stevenson MA, Morris RS, Ling Min Than J. Descriptive and temporal analysis of post-mortem lesions recorded in slaughtered pigs in New Zealand from 2000 to 2010. N Z Vet J. 2014; 62(3):110–6.
15. Merialdi G, Dottori M, Bonilauri P, Luppi A, Gozio S, Pozzi P, Spaggiari B, Martelli P. Survey of pleuritis and pulmonary lesions in pigs at abattoir with a focus on the extent of the condition and herd risk factors. Vet J. 2012;193:234–9.
16. Danish Agriculture and Food Council. Assessment of risk associated with a change in meat inspection, 2014. Available at http://lf.dk/Aktuelt/Publikationer/Svinekod.aspx#. Accessed on November 2015;
17. Hill A, Adam Brouwer A, Donaldson N, Lambton S, Buncic S, Griffiths I. A risk and benefit assessment for visual-only meat inspection of indoor and outdoor pigs in the United Kingdom. Food Control. 2013;30:255–64.
18. Mousing J, Kyrval J, Jensen T. K, Aalbaek B, Buttensch J, Svensmark B, Willeberg P. Meat safety consequences of implementing visualpostmortem meat inspection procedures in Danish slaughter pigs. Vet Rec. 1997;140(8):472–77.
19. Blagojevic B, Dadios N, Reinmann K, Guitian J, Stärk KDC. Green offal inspection of cattle, small ruminants and pigs in the United Kingdom: impact assessment of changes in the inspection protocol on likelihood of detection of selected hazards. Res Vet Sci. 2015;100:31–8.

10

An indirect enzyme-linked immunosorbent assay for the identification of antibodies to Senecavirus A in swine

Cheryl M. T. Dvorak[1*], Zeynep Akkutay-Yoldar[1,2], Suzanne R. Stone[1], Steven J.P. Tousignant[3], Fabio A. Vannucci[4] and Michael P. Murtaugh[1]

Abstract

Background: *Senecavirus A (SVA)*, a member of the family *Picornaviridae*, genus *Senecavirus*, is a recently identified single-stranded RNA virus closely related to members of the *Cardiovirus* genus. SVA was originally identified as a cell culture contaminant and was not associated with disease until 2007 when it was first observed in pigs with Idiopathic Vesicular Disease (IVD). Vesicular disease is sporadically observed in swine, is not debilitating, but is significant due to its resemblance to foreign animal diseases, such as foot-and-mouth disease (FMD), whose presence would be economically devastating to the United States. IVD disrupts swine production until foreign animal diseases can be ruled out. Identification and characterization of SVA as a cause of IVD will help to quickly rule out infection by foreign animal diseases.

Methods: We have developed and characterized an indirect ELISA assay to specifically identify serum antibodies to SVA. Viral protein 1, 2 and 3 (VP1, VP2, VP3) were expressed, isolated, and purified from *E. coli* and used to coat plates for an indirect ELISA. Sera from pigs with and without IVD symptoms as well as a time course following animals from an infected farm, were analyzed to determine the antibody responses to VP1, VP2, and VP3.

Results: Antibody responses to VP2 were higher than VP1 and VP3 and showed high affinity binding on an avidity ELISA. ROC analysis of the SVA VP2 ELISA showed a sensitivity of 94.2% and a specificity of 89.7%. Compared to IFA, the quantitative ELISA showed an 89% agreement in negative samples and positive samples from 4–60 days after appearance of clinical signs. Immune sera positive for FMDV, encephalomyocarditis virus, and porcine epidemic diarrhea virus antibodies did not cross-react.

Conclusions: A simple ELISA based on detection of antibodies to SVA VP2 will help to differentially diagnose IVD due to SVA and rule out the presence of economically devastating foreign animal diseases.

Keywords: Seneca valley virus, SVV, Senecavirus A, SVA, Swine, ELISA, Veterinary diagnostics, Immunology

Background

Senecavirus A (SVA), a member of the family *Picornaviridae*, genus *Senecavirus*, is a recently identified single-stranded RNA virus closely related to members of the *Cardiovirus* genus [1, 2]. SVA was originally identified as a cell culture contaminant and was not associated with disease until 2007 when it was first observed in pigs with Idiopathic Vesicular Disease (IVD) [2, 3]. Vesicular disease is sporadically observed in swine, is not debilitating, but is significant due to its resemblance to foreign animal diseases, such as foot-and-mouth disease (FMD), whose presence would be economically devastating to the United States [3, 4]. IVD disrupts swine production until foreign animal diseases can be ruled out. Identification and characterization of SVA as a cause of IVD will help to quickly rule out infection by foreign animal vesicular disease pathogens.

IVD in association with SVA has been observed recently in Canada, the United States, and Brazil, in the absence of other vesicular foreign animal diseases [3, 5, 6]. A quick

* Correspondence: dvora013@umn.edu
[1]Department of Veterinary and Biomedical Sciences, University of Minnesota, 1971 Commonwealth Ave, St. Paul, MN 55108, USA
Full list of author information is available at the end of the article

test to diagnose SVA infection is necessary to help rule out infection by foreign animal diseases without prolonged disruption of animal movement. As of now, SVA infection is diagnosed by RT-PCR, a serum neutralizing assay, indirect fluorescent antibody test (IFA), or competitive enzyme-linked immunosorbent assay (cELISA) [6–9]. RT-PCR is a rapid method to determine if animals are acutely infected with virus or if vesicles contain virus, but a negative result cannot be used to rule out previous herd exposure since clinical signs of infection are usually resolved within 1–2 weeks [6, 10]. Presence of antibodies to SVA may indicate previous infection and possible presence of the virus in a herd. Although serum neutralization and IFA test for the presence of serum antibodies, ELISA is more rapid and convenient. A rapid, specific and sensitive assay for the detection of SVA-specific antibodies is needed. A cELISA for the detection of SVA antibodies is available, but requires an antibody competition between well characterized monoclonal antibodies and serum antibodies for binding to inactivated viral antigen [7]. An indirect ELISA only requires a purified antigen and so is not susceptible to mutations that change reactivity of the monoclonal antibody-binding epitope. An SVA VP1 ELISA has recently been used to examine antibody presence in sows and piglets naturally infected with SVA, however a comprehensive validation of this assay was not shown [11]. Although numerous ELISA kits used for the detection of viral antibodies are commercially available, an indirect ELISA kit is not yet commercially available for the detection of anti-SVA antibodies in pigs.

An optimized, well characterized, quick and inexpensive indirect ELISA for the detection of SVA antibodies as well as a thorough examination of antibodies and their levels over a time course following infection is needed. The aim of this study was to develop and characterize an indirect ELISA assay to identify serum antibodies to SVA as well as examine the kinetics of the presence and levels of SVA antibodies over a time course following infection. The SVA VP2 ELISA developed in this study can now be used to help differentially diagnose IVD due to SVA, helping to quickly rule out the presence of an economically devastating foreign animal disease.

Methods

Cloning, expression and purification of SVA VP1, VP2, and VP3 protein

The full length gene sequences for SVA VP1, VP2, and VP3 from strain 11-55910-3 (Genbank ID AGM16001) was optimized for expression in *E. coli*, synthesized (Integrated DNA Technologies, Inc., Coralville, IA), and cloned into a modified pET24b vector (Novagen, Madison, WI) [12] using the In-Fusion cloning kit (Clontech, Mountain View, CA) following the manufacturer's directions. Gene sequences for VP1, VP2, and VP3 antigens were confirmed by sequencing. Protein expression and purification was performed as previously described [13]. Purity was analyzed by SDS-PAGE, stained using Imperial™ protein stain (ThermoFisher Scientific, Waltham, MA). Protein concentrations used to establish plate coating conditions were determined using the Quick-start Bradford protein assay following manufacturer's instructions (Bio-Rad Laboratories, Inc., Hercules, CA) using a Bio-tek Epoch plate reader (BioTek Instruments, Inc., Winooski, VT).

Serum samples

Recent and archived porcine serum samples that had been previously submitted to the University of Minnesota Veterinary Diagnostic Laboratory (UMN-VDL) for routine diagnostics or specific viral pathogen evaluation were obtained. The samples were provided for diagnostic purposes, not specifically for use in this study. In addition, positive serum samples were obtained from 34 sows clinically diagnosed with vesicular lesions and bled periodically over a 60-day period starting at the first observation of clinical signs (sampling at day 0, 4, 11,18, 25, 39, and 60) ($n = 205$). Serum samples that tested negative for SVA by PCR ($n = 116$) were obtained from sows and finishing pigs from various farms with no prior evidence of vesicular disease. These animals were assumed to be SVA antibody-negative and were treated as such in this study. Porcine epidemic diarrhea virus (PEDV) seropositive samples ($n = 40$) were archived samples from our laboratory and encephalomyocarditis virus (EMCV) seropositive samples were obtained from the UMN-VDL ($n = 8$). FMD seropositive samples ($n = 21$) were archived samples from Plum Island Animal Disease Center representing 8 different serotypes, 2 field samples, and ranged from 0 to 36 days post-infection/post-challenge. The FMDV samples were examined for cross-reactivity against the SVA VP1, VP2, and VP3 ELISA at Plum Island Animal Disease Center (PIADC) facilities following the ELISA protocol described here.

Antibody detection by ELISA and IFA

Detection of antibodies to SVA VP1, VP2, and VP3 protein was performed by indirect ELISA as previously described [12, 13] on microtiter plates coated with either 500 ng or 200 ng of antigen per well or a combination of all 3 proteins at 100 ng each (300 ng total protein per well). Positive and negative control serum samples were run on each plate.

An avidity ELISA was performed following the ELISA protocol above, coating with 200 ng of VP2 antigen per well, and with the addition of a guanidine HCl wash step. Before secondary antibody was added, 1 M guanidine HCl in phosphate buffered saline (PBS) + 0.05% Tween-20, pH 7.4, was added to each well and incubated for 10 min. Plates were then washed as usual, secondary antibody was added, and the remainder of the ELISA protocol was performed as above. The avidity index was determined by dividing the optical density (OD) of the sample treated with guanidine by the OD of the sample without guanidine treatment (OD_{Gn+}/OD_{Gn-}).

The UMN-VDL performed a diagnostic IFA test to detect anti-SVA antibodies present in serum. Briefly, human lung cancer NCI-H1299 cells were inoculated with an SVA strain isolated in 2015 from an outbreak in the U.S. Infected cells were washed with PBS, fixed with acetone and incubated using two-fold dilutions of serum from 1:20 to 1:320 at 37 °C for 1 h. After fluorescein labeled goat anti-pig IgG diluted 1:50 in PBS was added into the wells and incubated at 37 °C for 1 h, the cells were observed under fluorescence microscopy. A positive signal at a sample dilution of 1:20 was considered suspect and a 1:40 or higher dilution was considered to be positive.

Statistical methods

ELISA analysis, receiver-operator characteristics (ROC) analysis, and comparison to the IFA results were performed using GraphPad Prism software (Version 5.0a, GraphPad Software, Inc., La Jolla, CA).

Results

SVA protein expression and ELISA development

The SVA VP1, VP2, and VP3 proteins were cloned, expressed, and purified. Protein preparations were observed to be >90% pure (Fig. 1). ELISA plates were coated with 500 ng/well of VP1, VP2 or VP3 protein and samples were examined for anti-SVA antibody reactivity. SVA-negative samples from a neighboring farm ($n = 28$) were used to determine the cut-off values for negative ($<OD_{avg} + 1SD$) and positive ($>OD_{avg} + 2SD$) samples. Suspect positive samples occurred if the OD value fell between the negative and positive sample cut-off values.

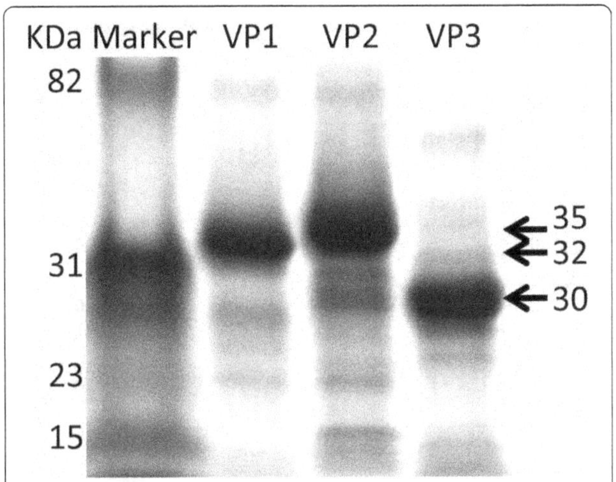

Fig. 1 SVA VP1, VP2, and VP3 purified proteins. Purity of the proteins eluted from cobalt affinity columns were visualized by SDS-PAGE. Molecular weights are determined by comparison to kaleidoscope pre-stained standards (Bio-rad, Hercules, CA) run on the same gel

The SVA ELISA was first evaluated using samples from a farm showing clinical signs, starting at the day clinical signs were first observed (Day 0) and sampled up to 60 days post-break (Days 4, 11, 18, 25, 39, 60). Comparison of antibody reactivity to VP1, VP2, or VP3 showed that VP2 was significantly different than VP1 and VP3 ($p < 0.0001$) giving the largest range of OD values and the biggest difference between positive and negative sample values (Fig. 2). VP1 showed some negative values at all time points and lower values overall, while VP3 showed limited immunoreactivity and discriminated poorly between positive and negative. A coating combination of 100 ng each of VP1, VP2, and VP3 together on the same samples shown in Fig. 2 gave results that were correlated with VP2 antigen alone ($r^2 = 0.927$, $p < 0.0001$).

SVA VP2 ELISA optimization and validation

Further optimization of VP2 ELISA sensitivity and specificity led to coating plates with 200 ng VP2 protein per well. ROC analysis was performed using 116 negative samples and 205 positive samples. At a positive/negative sample cut-off value of OD = 0.6, the area under the curve to differentiate positive from negative was 0.9622 with a p value <0.0001. Test sensitivity was 94.2% and specificity was 89.7%.

Cross-reactivity of the SVA VP2 ELISA was evaluated by testing samples that were seropositive for PEDV, a coronavirus, EMCV, a closely related picornavirus, and FMDV, a high-consequence animal picornavirus pathogen that causes vesicular lesions. We observed that 3% of PEDV-positive serum samples in a herd with no history of SVA exposure tested positive (ODavg = 0.081, SD = 0.119) (Fig. 3). All EMCV seropositive samples were negative for SVA antibodies ($OD_{avg} = 0.085$, SD = 0.040) (Fig. 3). FMD seropositive samples were examined for cross-reactivity on the VP1, VP2, and VP3 ELISAs. The FMDV ELISA was run at PIADC and the absorbance values (including positives and negatives) were lower than when the ELISA tests were run in our laboratory. Thus the cut-off values were adjusted based on the OD values of the positive and negative controls (Fig. 3). In the VP1 ELISA, 1 of the positive control samples was identified as suspect instead of positive and the VP3 ELISA identified 2 positive control samples as negative and 1 as suspect. For the FMDV-seropositive samples, 2 were identified as SVA VP1 positive and 4 as suspect, and no samples were positive for the VP3 ELISA. On the VP2 ELISA, 20 of the 21 (95.3%) samples tested negative and one (4.7%) sample tested positive. The FMDV positive sample that

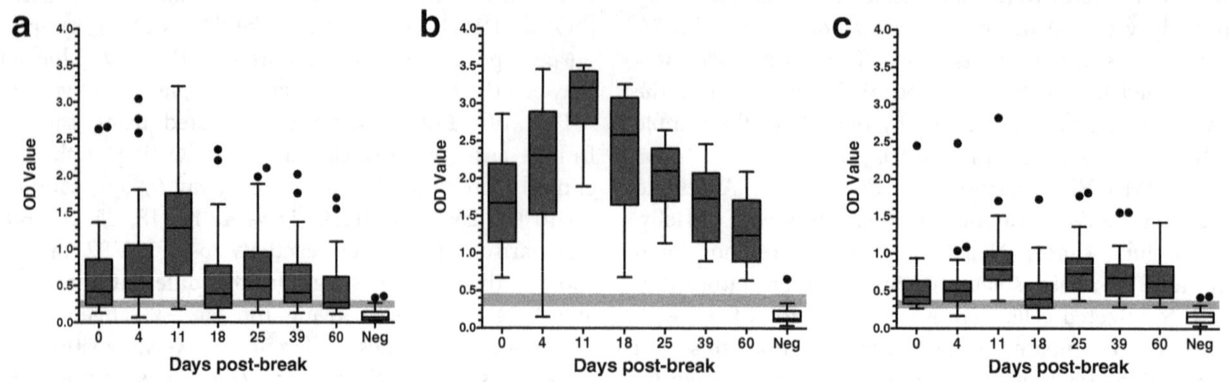

Fig. 2 Time course of antibody responses to SVA VP1, VP2, and VP3. Serum samples collected from sows at the onset of clinical signs until 60 days later were tested in duplicate wells coated with 500 ng of each antigen. Negative control serum (Neg) was from a matched SVA-negative farm. Results are shown as a box whisker plot using the Tukey method for outliers for (**a**) VP1, (**b**) VP2, and (**c**) VP3 proteins. The suspect positive OD range is shown as a grey bar with negatives below and positives above the bar

cross-reacted on the SVA VP2 ELISA was serotype A24. Notably, this sample also reacted with SVA VP1, suggesting that it was a true positive reaction and not cross-reactivity, since antibodies reacted against 2 SVA antigens.

Avidity ELISA confirmation of reactivity

Avidity, or functional affinity, measures the strength of a polyclonal antibody interaction with antigen, based on reduction in ELISA reactivity caused by incubation of the antigen-antibody complex with a denaturing agent. Figure 4 shows that the avidity index increased until 25 days after clinical signs were first observed. In addition, the proportion of samples with an avidity index >0.5 was greater than 80% at all times after 25 days (Fig. 4).

The avidity ELISA was also used to evaluate non-specific antibody reactivity against SVA VP2 protein that would give rise to false positive interpretations. The PEDV seropositive samples that cross-reacted with the SVA VP2 ELISA were evaluated by the avidity ELISA. These samples were clearly negative using the avidity ELISA (avidity index = 0.04). By contrast, the lowest avidity index in SVA seropositive samples from infected herds was 0.12 on the day clinical signs were first observed and the average avidity index of SVA seropositive samples was 0.52.

Comparison of ELISA to IFA

Comparison of negative samples and positive samples from the infection time course showed that ELISA and IFA were correlated ($n = 231$, $p < 0.0001$) (Fig. 5). The IFA has a specificity of 100% and a sensitivity of 90.3%. Agreement on negative samples was 89% and agreement from 4 to 60 days after appearance of clinical signs varied from 73 to 100%. However, on the day that clinical signs were first observed (Day 0), test agreement was

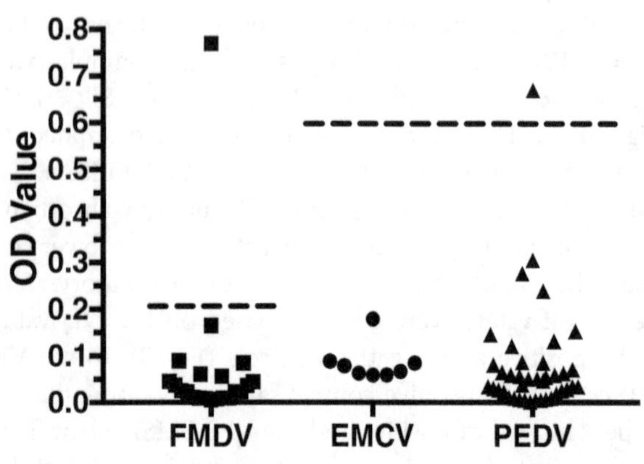

Fig. 3 Cross-reactivity analysis of SVA VP2 ELISA to other virus seropositive samples. The SVA VP2 ELISA was performed on pig samples that were seropositive to other viruses (FMDV, EMCV, or PEDV), but whose SVA antibody status was unknown. The positive/negative cut-off values for EMCV and PEDV tested at the University of Minnesota, and FMDV tested at PIADC are shown by the dashed line

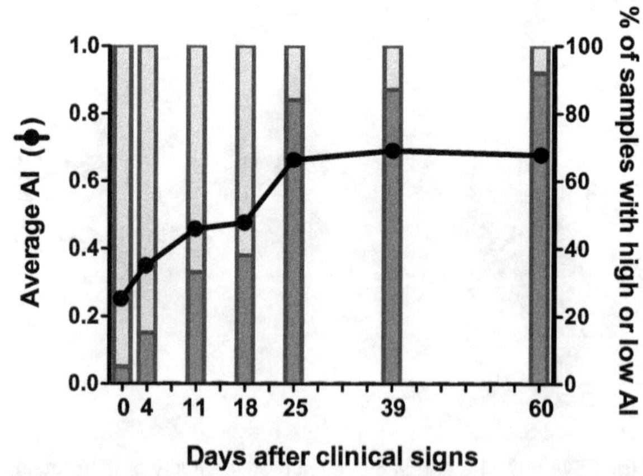

Fig. 4 Avidity analysis on VP2 ELISA positive samples. The average avidity index (AI, *black line*) and percent of samples with low (<0.5, *light grey bar*) or high (>0.5, *dark grey bar*) AI are shown at each time point

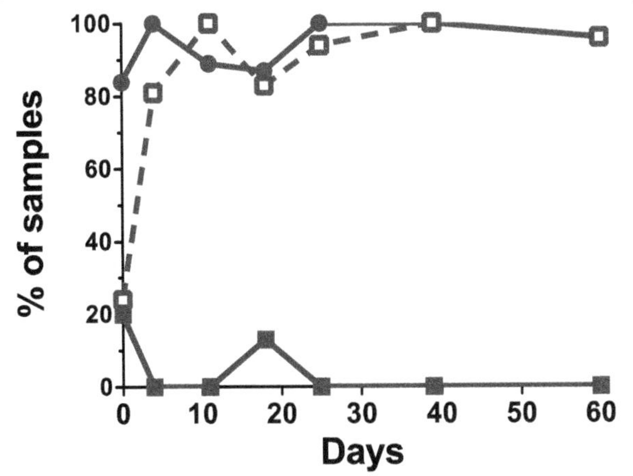

Fig. 5 VP2 ELISA and IFA comparison. The percent of VP2 ELISA positive (*closed circles*) samples and the percent of IFA positive (*open squares*) and IFA suspect (*closed squares*) samples are shown over a 60 day time course

40%, which was due to samples testing ELISA positive, but IFA negative or suspect (Fig. 5). In cases of disagreement, ELISA was usually positive while IFA was negative or suspect. Three percent of total samples were ELISA negative, but IFA positive (days 11, 18, and 60).

Discussion

Rapid diagnostic methods to test for SVA exposure in cases of vesicular disease are critical to the U.S. swine industry since animal movement, an essential aspect of modern swine production, can be halted if foot-and-mouth disease virus (FMDV) infection is suspected. The incidence of SVA has greatly increased since mid-2015, creating a compelling need for a simple, high-throughput test [10]. We have developed a sensitive and specific SVA ELISA for the detection and diagnosis of SVA-specific antibodies.

Surprisingly, VP2 antigen was substantially more immunogenic than VP1 and VP3 in the population as a whole, although occasional pigs were observed with high antibody levels to one or both of VP1 and VP3, as shown in Fig. 2. The sensitivity and specificity of the VP2 ELISA, 94.2 and 89.7%, respectively, indicate that it would be a reliable test to identify infected herds. The VP1 protein in picornaviruses is the most external and immunodominant [14] and has been used for numerous ELISA assays to detect picornavirus antibodies. However, many of the monoclonal antibody epitopes have been identified in VP2 and, because VP2 is more conserved than VP1, VP2 may be better able to detect across serotypes [15, 16]. Even though VP2 is conserved, cross-reactivity of the SVA VP2 ELISA to immune serum of the closely related picornavirus, EMCV, was not observed. Reactivity was observed in one (4.7%) FMDV seropositive sample. Since this serum sample, alone among 21 in total, also reacted with VP1, the most likely explanation is that the source animal was cryptically infected with SVA. The pig had been obtained from a commercial supplier and did not show clinical symptoms of disease, but its prior history was not known.

An avidity ELISA assesses the strength of antibody binding to antigen, thus denaturing weak interactions that are a common source of cross-reactivity and background noise [17]. Its use helps to increase assay specificity and to confirm suspect samples as positive or negative. In addition, an increase in avidity of the time course of an immune response can be used to monitor B lymphocyte maturation and antibody affinity increase that occurs during isotype switching and hypersomatic mutation in light and heavy chains [18]. We observed that the avidity index was low until about 3 weeks post-clinical signs, thus indicating that the humoral response was in an early stage and that infection was recent. It suggests that the avidity ELISA may be a useful indicator of outbreak initiation. Comparison of ELISA and IFA showed that ELISA also was more sensitive in diagnosing early infection. At later times (day 4–11 and later), ELISA and IFA were both able to identify SVA positive animals at similar rates, as shown in Fig. 5. Identification of SVA antibody-positive animals by SVA VP2 ELISA along with either the avidity ELISA or IFA as a confirmatory test in case of suspected false negatives, may be ideal for the immuno-diagnosis of SVA infection.

The kinetics of the antibody response to SVA have been recently examined. In a naturally infected farm ELISA-positive antibodies (anti-SVA VP1) were observed in pig serum at 1 week post-clinical signs in less than 15% of animals [11]. However, at 3 weeks post-clinical signs over 70% of animals were seropositive and by 6 weeks over 90% of animals were seropositive [11]. Experimental SVA infection of 9 week old pigs showed that all animals seroconverted by 15 days post-infection as determined by an indirect fluorescent antibody test [10]. In this study, we observed that SVA VP2 antibodies were present in 84% of animals when clinical signs were first observed and persisted for 60 days after clinical signs were first observed, though they were in decline from peak levels observed on day 11. In experimental infection of 9 week old pigs, vesicular lesions were first observed on the feet at 4 days, and nearly all pigs showed lesions at 5 days [10]. Since antibodies typically are not detected until 7 to 10 days after antigen exposure, it suggests that antibodies would not be present on the day clinical signs were first observed, as was observed by SVA IFA (only 24% of animals are seropositive by IFA on day 0) and by SVA VP1 ELISA, which was even less sensitive [11]. By contrast, the SVA VP2 ELISA is more sensitive, detecting antibodies in 84% of animals on the day of clinical signs.

Conclusions

An indirect ELISA based on SVA VP2 can rapidly and reliably detect SVA antibodies present in swine. Identification of SVA infection as the cause of IVD can help to quickly rule out the presence of economically devastating foreign animal diseases in swine, enable producers to return to normal production after clinical signs have resolved, and make informed management decisions.

Acknowledgements

The authors would like to thank The Foreign Animal Disease Diagnostic Laboratory, National Veterinary Services Laboratories, Veterinary Services, Animal Plant Health Inspection Service, United States Department of Agriculture, Greenport, NY 11944 for providing FMDV seropositive samples and testing them using the SVA ELISA and the University of Minnesota Veterinary Diagnostic Laboratory for providing porcine serum samples for this project.

Funding

Dr. Akkutay-Yoldar was funded by the Scientific and Technological Research Council of Turkey (TUBITAK) Scholarship.

Authors' contributions

CMTD, SJT, FAV, and MPM conceived the study and participated in its design and coordination. CMTD, ZA-Y, and SRS performed experiments and interpreted results. FAV helped interpret results. CMTD wrote the main manuscript. MPM helped interpret results and write the manuscript. All authors read and approved the final manuscript.

Competing interests

CMTD and MPM have applied for a patent pertaining to the results presented in the manuscript. Other authors declare no competing interests.

Author details

[1]Department of Veterinary and Biomedical Sciences, University of Minnesota, 1971 Commonwealth Ave, St. Paul, MN 55108, USA. [2]Department of Virology, Ankara University, Faculty of Veterinary Medicine, Diskapi, 06110 Ankara, Turkey. [3]Swine Vet Center P.A., 1608 S. Minnesota Ave, St. Peter, MN 56082, USA. [4]Department of Veterinary Population Medicine, University of Minnesota, 1365 Gortner Ave, St. Paul, MN 55108, USA.

References

1. Adams MJ, Lefkowitz EJ, King AM, Bamford DH, Breitbart M, Davison AJ, Ghabrial SA, Gorbalenya AE, Knowles NJ, Krell P, et al. Ratification vote on taxonomic proposals to the International Committee on Taxonomy of Viruses (2015). Arch Virol. 2015;160(7):1837–50.
2. Hales LM, Knowles NJ, Reddy PS, Xu L, Hay C, Hallenbeck PL. Complete genome sequence analysis of Seneca Valley virus-001, a novel oncolytic picornavirus. J Gen Virol. 2008;89(Pt 5):1265–75.
3. Pasma T, Davidson S, Shaw SL. Idiopathic vesicular disease in swine in Manitoba. Can Vet J. 2008;49(1):84–5.
4. Resolution Number 14, Research on Seneca Valley Virus. In: 116th Annual Meeting of the United States Animal Health Association. Greensboro, NC: United States Animal Health Association; 2012. This article can be found at: http://www.usaha.org/Committees/TransmissibleDiseasesOfSwine.aspx.
5. Vannucci FA, Linhares DC, Barcellos DE, Lam HC, Collins J, Marthaler D. Identification and complete genome of Seneca Valley virus in vesicular fluid and sera of pigs affected with idiopathic vesicular disease, Brazil. Transbound Emerg Dis. 2015;62(6):589–93.
6. Leme RA, Zotti E, Alcântara BK, Oliveira MV, Freitas LA, Alfieri AF, Alfieri AA. Senecavirus A: an emerging vesicular infection in Brazilian pig herds. Transbound Emerg Dis. 2015;62(6):603–11.
7. Yang M, van Bruggen R, Xu W. Generation and diagnostic application of monoclonal antibodies against Seneca Valley virus. J Vet Diagn Invest. 2012;24(1):42–50.
8. Bracht AJ, O'Hearn ES, Fabian AW, Barrette RW, Sayed A. Real-time reverse transcription PCR assay for detection of Senecavirus A in swine vesicular diagnostic specimens. PLoS One. 2016;11(1):e0146211.
9. Rudin CM, Poirier JT, Senzer NN, Stephenson J, Loesch D, Burroughs KD, Reddy PS, Hann CL, Hallenbeck PL. Phase I clinical study of Seneca Valley virus (SVV-001), a replication-competent picornavirus, in advanced solid tumors with neuroendocrine features. Clin Cancer Res. 2011;17(4):888–95.
10. Montiel N, Buckley A, Guo B, Kulshreshtha V, VanGeelen A, Hoang H, Rademacher C, Yoon KJ, Lager K. Vesicular disease in 9-week-old pigs experimentally infected with Senecavirus A. Emerg Infect Dis. 2016;22(7):1246–8.
11. Gimenez-Lirola LG, Rademacher C, Linhares D, Harmon K, Rotolo M, Sun Y, Baum DH, Zimmerman J, Piñeyro P. Serological and molecular detection of Senecavirus A associated with an outbreak of swine idiopathic vesicular disease and neonatal mortality. J Clin Microbiol. 2016;54(8):2082–9.
12. Puvanendiran S, Stone S, Yu W, Johnson CR, Abrahante J, Jimenez LG, Griggs T, Haley C, Wagner B, Murtaugh MP. Absence of porcine circovirus type 1 (PCV1) and high prevalence of PCV 2 exposure and infection in swine finisher herds. Virus Res. 2011;157(1):92–8.
13. Dvorak CMT, Yang Y, Haley C, Sharma N, Murtaugh MP. National reduction in porcine circovirus type 2 prevalence following introduction of vaccination. Vet Microbiol. 2016;189:86–90.
14. Rossmann MG, Arnold E, Erickson JW, Frankenberger EA, Griffith JP, Hecht HJ, Johnson JE, Kamer G, Luo M, Mosser AG. Structure of a human common cold virus and functional relationship to other picornaviruses. Nature. 1985; 317(6033):145–53.
15. Yang M, Clavijo A, Suarez-Banmann R, Avalo R. Production and characterization of two serotype independent monoclonal antibodies against foot-and-mouth disease virus. Vet Immunol Immunopathol. 2007;115(1–2):126–34.
16. Freiberg B, Höhlich B, Haas B, Saalmüller A, Pfaff E, Marquardt O. Type-independent detection of foot-and-mouth disease virus by monoclonal antibodies that bind to amino-terminal residues of capsid protein VP2. J Virol Methods. 2001;92(2):199–205.
17. Inouye S, Hasegawa A, Matsuno S, Katow S. Changes in antibody avidity after virus infections: detection by an immunosorbent assay in which a mild protein-denaturing agent is employed. J Clin Microbiol. 1984;20(3):525–9.
18. Bannard O, Cyster JG. Germinal centers: programmed for affinity maturation and antibody diversification. Curr Opin Immunol. 2017;45:21–30.

11

Causes, consequences and biomarkers of stress in swine

Silvia Martínez-Miró[1*], Fernando Tecles[2*], Marina Ramón[1], Damián Escribano[2], Fuensanta Hernández[1], Josefa Madrid[1], Juan Orengo[1], Silvia Martínez-Subiela[2], Xavier Manteca[3] and José Joaquín Cerón[2]

Abstract

Background: In recent decades there has been a growing concern about animal stress on intensive pig farms due to the undesirable consequences that stress produces in the normal physiology of pigs and its effects on their welfare and general productive performance. This review analyses the most important types of stress (social, environmental, metabolic, immunological and due to human handling), and their biological consequences for pigs.

The physio-pathological changes associated with stress are described, as well as the negative effects of stress on pig production. In addition an update of the different biomarkers used for the evaluation of stress is provided. These biomarkers can be classified into four groups according to the physiological system or axis evaluated: sympathetic nervous system, hypothalamic-pituitary-adrenal axis, hypothalamic-pituitary-gonadal axis and immune system.

Conclusions: Stress it is a process with multifactorial causes and produces an organic response that generates negative effects on animal health and production. Ideally, a panel of various biomarkers should be used to assess and evaluate the stress resulting from diverse causes and the different physiological systems involved in the stress response. We hope that this review will increase the understanding of the stress process, contribute to a better control and reduction of potential stressful stimuli in pigs and, finally, encourage future studies and developments to better monitor, detect and manage stress on pig farms.

Keywords: Stress, Pigs, Biomarkers

Background

The worldwide increase in the demand for animal products in recent decades has led to the use of intensive systems that have been demonstrated to produce stress in animals [1]. Since Hans Selye first introduced the concept of stress as "the non-specific response of the body to any demand for change" [2], the concept has received several definitions, so that nowadays its meaning can vary depending of the biological field in which it is used. According to Fink [3], stress in behavioral sciences is regarded as the perception of threat, with resulting anxiety, discomfort, emotional tension, and difficulty in adjustment. In terms of pure neuroendocrinology, stress is any stimulus that provokes release of the adrenocorticotropic hormone (ACTH) and adrenal glucocorticoids; and for the sociologists, it is any social disequilibrium that produces disturbances in the social structure within which a population lives [3]. Despite this variability in meaning, one of the most accepted definitions of stress is "the biological response elicited when an individual perceives a threat to its homeostasis" [4] which can apply to both humans and animals. In this review we will study the main types of stress that can affect pigs in intensive farming conditions, its consequences and the main biomarkers that can be used to detect whether the pigs are enduring stressful conditions.

* Correspondence: silviamm@um.es; ftecles@um.es
[1]Department of Animal Production, Campus of Excellence Mare Nostrum, Universidad de Murcia, 30100 Murcia, Spain
[2]Department of Animal Medicine and Surgery, Campus of Excellence Mare Nostrum, Universidad de Murcia, 30100 Murcia, Spain
Full list of author information is available at the end of the article

Various classifications of stress have been described in the literature. From a practical point of view, it is of interest to classify the stress according to its duration and also to its causes. Regarding the duration of the stress, it can be acute (short in duration; lasting minutes or various days) or chronic (lasting weeks, months or even years). In addition, depending of its cause, the stress can be classified as social, environmental, metabolic, immunological or due to human practices and manipulation of animals.

Main causes of stress

In the following lines we will study the main causes of stress, as well the situations in the current intensive production systems where the pigs can be more exposed to these causes. It is important to point out that different external factors can produce a similar stress response, but on the other hand, the same stressful stimulus can produce a different response in the animal depending on its age, genetics, production system or previous exposure to the stimulus.

Social stress

Pigs are regrouped with unfamiliar conspecifics at different times of their productive cycle such as during gestation or after weaning, during the fattening period or before transport to slaughter. In these situations, pigs may fight in order to establish a new dominance hierarchy and this generates stress [5]. Such social stress can be acute, immediately following regrouping, or chronic, when the animals are socially subordinate or isolated [6], or as a result of repeated social regrouping [7].

Social stress can vary depending of the group size, space available and gender and genetic of the pig. Larger groups seem to have less social stress than smaller groups, reflecting a lower probability of monopolizing resources as the group size increases [8]. Intensive housing involves a reduction in the space per animal, which causes stress because of restricted movements and freedom to feed themselves [9]. It has been demonstrated that the frequency of social interactions and aggressive behaviour increases as the space allowance decreases in group-housed sows [10, 11] and the growth rate decreases linearly as the space allowance per pig decreases [12]. Response to social stress is higher in males than in females [13]. Aggressive behavior after regrouping varies between individuals and to some extent such individual differences have a genetic basis. As a result, some lines of pigs seem to fight less than other when unacquainted individuals are mixed [14].

Environmental stress

Intensive pig farming requires control of the temperature, humidity, light, concentration of dust and gases, ammonia levels and sound intensity [15–20]. For example, ambient temperature should be as close as possible to the thermal neutrality for the age of the pig being housed, (i.e. for prenursery pigs between 28 and 32 °C, for nursery pigs between 22 and 28 °C (depending on live weight, with lower live weight requiring higher temperature), for growing animals close to 20 °C, for finishing pigs between 16 and 18 °C, for pregnant sows between 15 and 18 °C, and for lactating sows and boars close to 16 °C) [15]. However, sometimes optimal environmental conditions cannot be maintained in farms producing stress in animals. For example, in areas where there are extreme hot or cold seasons, in farms located in areas of high noise or in the case of equipment failure. It is important to bear in mind that the effects of the thermal environment on pigs do not depend solely on ambient temperature, but on the so-called effective temperature, which depends on ambient temperature, ventilation and flooring, among other factors.

It should also be pointed out that the barren environments of modern production systems have a negative effect on animal welfare due to the lack of bedding material and/or slatted pen floors. They create a poor environment where pigs cannot develop their natural behaviour [21]. Inability to perform highly motivated behaviors may lead to a stress response. This is the case, for example, when sows are prevented from showing nest-building behavior before farrowing [22].

Metabolic stress

This stress results from food and/or water restriction or deprivation [23–25]. Although most studies in the literature induce metabolic stress by means of experimental models, metabolic stress can also appear in intensive farming conditions when pregnant sows are subjected to restrict feeding, which has been shown to result in chronic hunger [26]. Likewise, in the process of mixing pregnant sows, it is usual for the more submissive animals to have less or no access to food [27].

In any case, the negative effects of food deprivation will depend on the length of the fasting period. When an animal is food-deprived, its glucose levels in blood drop and enters in a catabolic state that requires the use and production of alternative fuels such as non-esterified fatty acids (NEFA), beta-hydroxybutyrate and glycerol for energetic needs [28, 29]. These analytes could be used as indicators of metabolic stress [29].

Immunological stress

Immunological stress is produced when an animal is challenged by infectious agents [30], which may occur due to the presence of disease or after vaccination. Stress can be considered as a possible cause but also a consequence of infectious disseases. A situation of stress produces changes in numbers and proportions of blood leukocytes [31], mitogen-induced cell proliferation, natural killer cell cytotoxicity and circulating inflammatory factors [32], which can result in increased susceptibility to any infectious disease [33]. And in the case of an existing disease, the stress associated may predispose pigs to the emergence of a different disease that complicates the process [13, 34].

Stress by animal handling

On commercial farms, pigs are subjected to handling practices which can cause acute stress. Some of these practices such as snaring or vena cava blood sampling produce a high stress, whereas others such as tattoing or electric shocks induced a more moderate stress in a previous study [35]. Similarly, castration, a common operation on some farms, has been shown to cause stress when carried out without anesthetics or analgesics [36].

Situations in intensive production systems where pigs are more exposed to stressors

There are two particular situations in the productive system, namely weaning and transport, when animals are more exposed to the causes of stress described above, and which generate a high degree of stress in the animals. Weaning is a period full of challenges to the piglet such as abrupt separation from the sow, transportation to a new physical environment, a different food source, commingling with pigs from other litters, greater exposition to pathogens and dietary or environmental antigens and handling practices such as vaccination and drug administration [37].

Transport either to another holding or slaughterhouse also includes exposure to different stressful events such as departure from the usual room, truck loading and unloading, fasting, different temperature and humidity, noise, vibration of the vehicle or inappropriate stocking densities [16, 38].

Therefore, special care should be taken in weaning, providing high-quality diets to minimize the risk of diarrhoea and reinforce immune system. Highly digestible animal proteins and feed additives such as enzymes and dietary acids may be used to improve the digestibility of the diet. Another option would be to offer low-protein and amino acid-fortified diets to limit the amount of fermentable protein presented to the gut and the use of pre- and probiotics, n-3 long chain polyunsaturated fatty acids and n-6 linoleic acid. Moreover, special attention should be paid to environmental and sanitary conditions in the post weaning stage, and an all-in, all-out management system should be used to minimize disease exposure [37, 39].

In addition, there are published reports and official documents with guidelines to improve the welfare and production of pigs during transport [16, 40]. These guidelines include avoiding extreme temperatures and the overloading of trucks, minimizing the time the pigs are on the truck, using non-slip flooring on loading ramps and providing an adequate handling to the pigs by well-trained people [16, 40].

Consequences of stress in pigs

Biological response

The stressors mentioned above are perceived by pigs as a threat to their homeostasis, which trigger a variety of biological responses (behavioural, neuroendocrine and immunological).

Behavioural responses

Avoiding a threat, facing up to it or hiding from it can be described as normal behaviour, whereas stereotypes (a repetitive, invariant behaviour pattern with no obvious goal or function) are considered as abnormal behaviours that can appear after a stress [41]. In addition, frequent defecation can be an indicator of fear and stress, and excessive aggressive behaviour as well as tail and ear biting are considered abnormal behaviours [42, 43]. A behavioural ethogram to evaluate the external response of pigs to stress has been proposed by Ruis et al. [44], which covers exploring, defecation/urination, inactive (sleeping, lying, sitting and standing), ingestive (feeding and drinking), vocalizing and walking behaviours.

Sympathetic-adrenal-medullary axis response (SAM)

Catecholamines (epinephrine and norepinephrine) are released by the chromaffin cells of the adrenal medulla when the sympathetic nervous system is activated by a stress stimulus. An increase in heart rate and blood pressure is one of the consequences of this activation. Other changes, such as constriction of the intestine and skin vessels, dilatation of skeletal muscle vessels, dilatation of the pupils, or release of glucose and lipids from the liver are also observed. All these short-term changes prepare the animal to face the stressful stimulus or to escape from it [45].

Hypothalamic-pituitary-adrenal axis response (HPA)

Corticotropin-releasing factor is released by the hypothalamus once the stressful stimulus is detected. As a consequence of this, the adrenocorticotropic hormone (ACTH) is released by the anterior pituitary gland. Finally, glucocorticoids are produced and released by the adrenal cortex to increase the catabolism of tissues rich in protein and fat to produce glucose [45].

Hypothalamic-pituitary-gonadal axis response (HPG)

Stress is generally accompanied by both an increase in the HPA activity and a decrease in HPG [46]. Glucocorticoids inhibit the release of luteizing hormone (LH) from the pituitary and estradiol and progesterone secretion by the ovary [47], as well testosterone from the testes [48], decreasing blood concentrations of these hormones. Prolonged or chronic stress usually results in inhibition of reproduction, while the effect of transient or acute stress in certain cases may be stimulatory [49].

Immune system response

This response depends on the mediator released in the process of stress: catecholamines or glucocorticoids [50]. Catecholamines, which are usually produced at the beginning of stress or during a short-term stressful stimulus, produce an increase in leukocytes (mainly granulocytes and lymphocytes), which are released into the systemic circulation. On the other hand, cortisol which predominates when stressful stimuli are prolonged, mainly decreases the number of lymphocytes in blood. Glucocorticoids can also suppress the production of cytokines and immunoglobulins [50–52].

Consequences for pig production

Pigs in intensive systems have to cope with long-term and intense short-term stressful stimuli that affect their welfare. High levels of stress and poor welfare have negative effects on five main factors related with pig production: pig performance, reproduction, behaviour, immunity and meat quality [53]. The magnitude of these effects will vary depending on stress duration and intensity, and on the early experience, age and genetics of the animal [4]. Some representative examples of these negative effects are provided below.

Any stressful condition can produce a decrease in performance parameters of pigs such as feed intake, daily gain or body weight (Table 1). For example, pigs housed at 32.2 °C had a 32.3 % decrease in average daily feed intake, 39.3 % lower average daily gain, 9.8 % lower final body weight and a 16.3 % lower gain:feed ratio compared with pigs housed at 23.9 °C [17]. Indeed, feed intake can decrease by up to 47 % in pigs housed at temperatures above the thermoneutral zone [19]. Similarly, Hyung et al. [54] found that growth rates were reduced by 15.7 and 7.1 % as a result of crowding and mixing, respectively, and showed a decrease in daily gain and gain:feed ratio of about 15 and 10 %, respectively, when the space available per pig was reduced from 0.56 to 0.25 m^2/pig. Similarly, Lee et al. [55] showed that weaner pigs housed in a clean environment consumed about 8 % more feed and grew faster (about 10 %) than those housed in a dirty environment, and Hicks et al. [56] described that shipping by 4 h in weaner pigs produced a loss of 2.9 % body weight.

Table 1 Summary of stressful stimuli that produce a decreased in pig performance

Parameter affected	Stressful stimuli	Decrease, %	Reference
ADFI	Heat stress	32.3	White et al. [17]
		47.0	Pearce et al. [19]
	Dirty environment	8.0	Lee et al. [55]
ADG	Heat stress	39.3	White et al. [17]
	Crowding	15.7	Hyung et al. [54]
	Mixing	7.1	Hyung et al. [54]
	Decreasing space availability	15.0	Hyung et al. [54]
	Dirty environment	10.0	Lee et al. [55]
BW	Heat stress	9.8	White et al. [17]
	Shipping (4 h)	2.9	Hicks et al. [56]
G:F	Heat stress	16.3	White et al. [17]
	Decreasing space availability	10.0	Hyung et al. [54]

ADFI average daily feed intake, *ADG* average daily gain, *BW* body weight, *G:F* Gain:Feed ratio

A negative effect on the reproductive system has been described in boars in situations of stress, with a reduction in both ejaculate volume and semen quality, while gilts and sows may show fewer born piglets per litter and reduced rebreeding rate, as well as irregular rebreeding, higher weaning-to-oestrus interval [49], leading to a fall in farm production parameters.

In stressful situations there may be a reduction in the normal function of the immune system [31, 34], which may even suppress the response after vaccination [13]. This will result in an increase in the presence of diseases [57], with a subsequent increase in costs and decrease in production.

In addition, stress affects meat quality and an increase in incidence of pale, soft and exudative (PSE) and dark, firm and dry (DFD) meats, and reduced meat quality was found when stressful handling systems were used [16].

Biomarkers of stress studied in pigs

There is no a "gold standard" procedure to determine with accuracy the degree of animal welfare and the level of stress of an animal. Methodologies frequently used to quantify stress in animals include: (1) direct behavioural observations using behaviour scoring systems [44, 53, 58] or automated behaviour recognition video analysis [59, 60], and (2) biomarkers that can reflect the pathophysiological responses to stress [61–63]. There is a tendency to evaluate a panel of various biomarkers representing the different body systems involved: SAM, HPA axis, HPG axis and immune system.

Sympathetic Nervous System: alpha-amylase and chromogranin A

Alpha-amylase

This enzyme is used in humans as a stress biomarker because it increases after both physical and psychological stress [64]. It is measured in saliva and its activity is correlated with plasma catecholamine concentrations, being a marker of SAM activation [64–66]. In pigs alpha-amylase activity increases after 1 min of immobilization with nasal snares, however, high inter-individual variability in the responses was observed and some pigs did not present evident changes after this stressful stimulus [67]. Further studies would be necessary to clarify the role of this enzyme in porcine stress.

Chromogranin A

Chromogranin A (CgA) is an acidic soluble protein belonging to the granins family [68]. It was initially detected in chromaffin granules of the adrenal medulla, [69]. Later, CgA was found in secretory vesicles of endocrine, neuroendocrine and neuronal cells [70, 71]. During stress CgA is secreted into the blood by the adrenal medulla and anterior pituitary gland, with a smaller amount also released from sympathetic nerve endings [68]. In addition, CgA has been detected in salivary glands of humans and various animal species [72–74]. The release of CgA in saliva is mediated by the secretion of catecholamines [75], and has been related to the activation of SAM [76]. In humans, the measurement of CgA in saliva has been used as a reliable marker of SAM activation as an alternative to adrenaline and noradrenaline [77], which have high variability in results and low stability in saliva [78–80].

In pig, CgA has been used as a marker of SAM activation in different situations such as immobilization with a nasal snare [80], after refeeding following a period of food deprivation [25] and after isolation or regrouping [63]. CgA is not affected by age, gender or circadian rhythms [81]. This could be considered as an advantage compared with other stress biomarkers such as cortisol [82, 83], or Ig A [84] which are both influenced by these factors.

Hypothalamic-Pituitary-Adrenal Axis: Glucocorticoids

Cortisol is one of the most widely used biomarkers to detect stress in pigs, and is the main glucocorticoid in this species [85]. Its increase is related with HPA axis activation [86–88].

Despite its wide use, cortisol is influenced by factors such as circadian rhythm and genetics that could limit its use as a stress biomarker [89, 90]. Cortisol concentrations follow a circadian rhythm, with morning levels being up to 40 % higher than afternoon levels [91, 92], although a peak during the afternoon has been observed by several authors [83, 93, 94]. Furthermore, the average concentration of cortisol in pigs decrease with age, reaching a stable profile around 20 weeks of age, when levels were about 37 % lower than at 12 weeks of age [91, 95]. In addition, gender is another source of variation, with concentration in barrows being about 15 % higher than in gilts [91].

Plasma or serum has been the most widely used samples to measure cortisol in pigs and they reflect both the fraction of protein-bound cortisol and the free cortisol [91, 96]. However, there is a growing tendency to use saliva for cortisol measurements because it can be obtained by non-invasive techniques and reflects only the free cortisol which is the active fraction [43, 83, 97].

Although most stress stimuli tend to increase cortisol, in some situations cortisol such levels remain unchanged and show a large variability between individuals. For example, after 24 and 48 h transport, cortisol concentrations were not modified [98], and similarly, cortisol concentrations were not affected by feed deprivation or isolation, with a large variability between individual pigs [25, 63]. Likewise, McGlone et al. [99] found no significant change in plasma cortisol levels after shipping.

Hypothalamic-pituitary-gonadal axis: testosterone

Testosterone is a circulating androgen produced by the testes in males and by the ovaries in females, with a small amount being produced by the adrenal gland. The production of testosterone depends on the secretion of gonadotropin releasing hormone (GnRH) by the hypothalamus. GnRH binds to the gonadotrophs of the anterior pituitary to stimulate the secretion of luteinizing hormone (LH) and follicle stimulating hormone (FSH). FSH acts on Sertoli cells to aid spermatogenesis while LH induces the secretion of testosterone by Leydig cells in testes and by Theca cells in ovaries [100].

Although chronic stress has an inhibitory effect testosterone secretion [101], acute stress has been seen to increase testosterone levels in blood [102] and saliva [103]. For example, in pigs, an increase in salivary testosterone was detected after immobilization with a nose-snare or after short road transport [103]. The cause of this increase of testosterone in stress conditions is unclear, but could be due to increased sensitivity of the testes to LH, as a result of the activation of the SAM axis [102]. In addition, the administration of ACTH to boars induced a rapid increase in testosterone levels and adrenals could be a source of testosterone in stress situations [104].

Immune System: acute phase proteins, immunoglobulin A and interleukin-18

Acute phase proteins

Acute phase proteins (APPs) are blood proteins whose concentration is modified in response to inflammation, infection, and physical or psychological stress [105]. They are primarily synthesized by the liver [106] and released into the systemic circulation to restore the homeostasis of the organism [107]. They serve as a tool for disease diagnosis in pigs, especially to detect acute inflammation, but they have also been studied as stress biomarkers in plasma [105, 108, 109] and saliva [110].

A hypothesis was developed by Murata [111] to explain the link between APP and stress. This hypothesis starts with the SAM and HPA axis activation. The release of catecholamines by the SAM leads to the induction of pro-inflammatory cytokines such as interleukin-6 [112], which is known to be a strong inducer of hepatic APP production in pigs [113]. In swine, numerous studies have measured APP in stressful conditions; however, there is no clear pattern of APP response in stress situations and in some cases contradictory results were obtained. For example, while haptoglobin levels increased after 20 min of transport and 3 h lairage [114], 45 min transport or social isolation produced no significant changes in this APP [110]. Another example is the case of serum amyloid A, which increased in isolated animals [110] but did not change after stress induced by changes in the pattern of food administration [115]. So, further studies would be needed to clarify to the link between stress and the acute phase response.

Immunoglobulin A

Immunoglobulin A (IgA) is the most abundant antibody in mucous membranes, where it has a protective role against infectious agents, allergens and foreign proteins [116]. IgA has been described as a stress biomarker in rats [117], dogs [118] and humans [119]. In pigs, an increase in saliva IgA has been reported after immobilization [84, 120], in endotoxemia [121], and after isolation [63]. In the case of isolation, IgA was more strongly affected than other markers such as cortisol and testosterone [63].

Interleukin-18

Interleukin-18 (IL-18) is a proinflammatory cytokine initially detected in Kupffer cells in mice, although it has been located in other sites such as adrenal cortex, astrocytes, microglia or keratinocytes [122, 123]. It is as an interferon-gamma inducing factor [122], and also has anti-tumor and antimicrobial activity [124, 125].

Based on its increase in rats after ACTH administration [126], IL-18 has been proposed as a stress biomarker. Although studies in domestic animals are very scarce, an increase in IL-18 concentration in saliva has been described in pigs after 1 h of immobilization [120].

Conclusions

In this paper the main causes and consequences of stress in pigs, as well as the biomarkers that can be used for its evaluation are reviewed. Stress is a process with multifactorial causes, producing an organic response that generates negative effects in the health and production of the animals affected. Due to the diverse causes that can produce stress and the various physiological systems involved in the stress response, ideally a panel of various biomarkers should be used to assess the stress response in animals. We hope that this review can increase the understanding of the stress process, contribute to a better control and reduction of potential stressful stimuli in pigs, and encourage further studies and developments to better monitor, detect and manage stress on pig farms.

Abbreviations

ACTH, adrenocorticotropic hormone; ADFI, average daily feed intake; ADG, average daily gain; APPs, acute phase proteins; BW, Body weight; CgA, chromogranin A; DFD, dark, firm, dry; FSH, follicle stimulating hormone; G:F, gain:feed ratio; GnRH, gonadotropin-releasing hormone; HPA, hypothalamic-pituitary-adrenal axis; HPG, hypothalamic-pituitary-gonadal axis; IgA, immunoglobulin A; IL-18, interleukin-18; LH, luteinizing hormone; PSE, pale, soft, exudative; SAM, Sympathetic-adrenal-medullary axis

Acknowledgements

This study was funded by the Spanish Ministry of Economy and Competitiveness (AGL 2012–33612) and by the Seneca Foundation of Murcia Region (project 19894/GERM/15).

Authors' contributions

All authors participated in the design and helped to draft the manuscript and to include updated information in it. Once completed, all authors read and approved the final manuscript. SMM, FT and JJC conceptualized the review. JJC coordinated the process of writing the manuscript.

Competing interests

The authors declare that they have no competing interests.

Consent for publication

Not applicable.

Author details

[1]Department of Animal Production, Campus of Excellence Mare Nostrum, Universidad de Murcia, 30100 Murcia, Spain. [2]Department of Animal Medicine and Surgery, Campus of Excellence Mare Nostrum, Universidad de Murcia, 30100 Murcia, Spain. [3]Department of Animal and Food Science, Universitat Autònoma de Barcelona, 08193 Bellaterra, Barcelona, Spain.

References

1. Barnett JL, Hemsworth PH, Cronin GM, Jongman E, Hutson GD. A review of the welfare issues for sows and piglets in relation to housing. Aust J Agric Res. 2001;52:1–28.
2. Selye H. A syndrome produced by diverse nocuous agents. Nature. 1936;138:32.
3. Fink G. Stress: definition and history. In: Squire LR, editor. Encyclopaedia of Neuroscience. London: Elsevier; 2009. p. 549–55.
4. Moberg GP. Biological response to stress: implications for animal welfare. In: Moberg GP, Mench JA, editors. The biology of animal stress: Basic Principles and Implications for Animal Welfare. USA: CABI Publishing; 2000. p. 1–22.
5. Pitts AD, Weary DM, Pajor EA, Fraser D. Mixing at young ages reduces fighting in unacquainted domestic pigs. Appl Anim Behav Sci. 2000;68:191–7.
6. Arnone M, Dantzer R. Does frustration induce aggression in pig? Appl Anim Ethol. 1980;6:351–62.
7. Coutellier L, Arnould C, Boissy A, Orgeur P, Prunier A, Veissier I, Meunier-Salaün MC. Pig's responses to repeated social regrouping and relocation during the growing-finishing period. Appl Anim Behav Sci. 2007;105:102–15.
8. Andersen IL, Naevdal E, Bakken M, Boe KE. Aggression and group size in domesticated pigs, Sus scrofa: 'When the winner takes it all and the loser is standing small'. Anim Behav. 2004;68:965–75.
9. Verdon M, Hansen CF, Rault JL, Jongman E, Hansen LU, Plush K, Hemsworth PH. Effects of group housing on sow welfare: a review. J Anim Sci. 2015;93:1999–2017.

10. Weng RC, Edwards SA, English PR. Behaviour, social interactions and lesion scores of group-housed sows in relation to floor space allowance. Appl Anim Behav Sci. 1998;59:307–16.
11. Remience V, Wavreille J, Canart B, Meunier-Salau MC, Prunier A, Bartiaux-Thill N, Nicks B, Vandenheede M. Effects of space allowance on the welfare of dry sows kept in dynamic groups and fed with an electronic sow feeder. Appl Anim Behav Sci. 2008;112:284–96.
12. Randolph JH, Cromwell GL, Stahly TS, Kratzer DD. Effects of group size and space allowance on performance and behaviour of swine. J Anim Sci. 1981; 53(4):922–7.
13. de Groot J, Ruis MAW, Scholten JW, Koolhaas JM, Boersma WJA. Long-term effects of social stress on antiviral immunity in pigs. Physiol Behav. 2001;73: 145–58.
14. Muráni E, Ponsuksii S, D'Eath RB, Turner SP, Kurt E, Evans G, Thölking L, Klont R, Foury A, Mormède P, Wimmers K. Association of HPA axis related genetic variation with stress reactivity and aggressive behaviour in pigs. BMC Genet. 2010;11:74.
15. Wathes C, Whittemore C. Environmental management of pigs. In: Kyriazakis I, Whittemore C, Whittemore CT, editors. Whitemore's science and practice of pig production. Oxford: Blackwell Publishing; 2006. p. 533–90.
16. Warriss PD. The welfare of slaughter pigs during transport. Anim Welfare. 1998;7:365–81.
17. White HM, Richert BT, Schinckel AP, Burgess JR, Donkin SS, Latour MA. Effects of temperature stress on growth performance and bacon quality in grow-finish pigs housed at two densities. J Anim Sci. 2008;86:1789–98.
18. O'Connor EA, Parker MO, McLeman MA, Demmers TG, Lowe JC, Cui L, Davey EL, Owen RC, Wather CM, Abeyesinghe SM. The impact of chronic environmental stressors on growing pigs, sus scrofa (Part 1): Stress physiology, production and play behaviour. Animal. 2010;4:1899–909.
19. Pearce SC, Gabler NK, Ross JW, Escobar J, Patience JF, Rhoads RP, Baumgard LH. The effects of heat stress and plane of nutrition on metabolism in growing pigs. J Anim Sci. 2013;91:2108–18.
20. Sanz MV, Johnson JS, Abuajamieh M, Stoakes SK, Seibert JT, Cox L, Kahl S, Elsasser TH, Ross JV, Isom SC. Effects of heat stress on carbohydrate and lipid metabolism in growing pigs. Physiol Rep. 2015;3(2):e12315.
21. Beattie VE, O'Connell NE, Kilpatrick DJ, Moss BW. Influence of environmental enrichment on welfare-related behavioural and physiological parameters in growing pigs. J Anim Sci. 2000;70(3):443–50.
22. Oczak M, Maschat K, Berckmans D, Vranken E, Baumgartner J. Classification of nest-building behaviour in non-crated farrowing sows on the basis of accelerometer data. Biosyst Eng. 2015;140:48–58.
23. Toscano MJ, Lay DC, Craig BA, Pajor EA. Assessing the adaptation of swine to fifty-seven hours of feed deprivation in terms of behavioural and physiological responses. J Anim Sci. 2007;85:441–51.
24. Lallès JP, David JC. Fasting and refeeding modulate the expression of stress proteins along the gastrointestinal tract of weaned pigs. J Anim Physiol Anim Nutr. 2011;95:478–88.
25. Ott O, Soler L, Moons CPH, Kashiha MA, Bahr C, Vandermeulen J, Janssens S, Gutiérrez AM, Escribano D, Cerón JJ, Berckmans D, Tuyttens FAM. Different stressors elicit different responses in the salivary biomarkers cortisol, haptoglobin, and chromogranin A in pigs. Res Vet Sci. 2014;97:124–8.
26. Arellano PE, Pijoan C, Jacobson ID, Algers B. Stereotyped behaviour, social interactions and suckling pattern of pigs housed in groups or in single crates. Appl Anim Behav Sci. 1992;2:157–66.
27. Brouns F, Edwards SA. Social rank and feeding behaviour of group-housed sows fed competitively or ad libitum. Appl Anim Behav Sci. 1994;39:225–35.
28. Razdan P, Mwanza AM, Kindahl H, Hultén F, Einarsson S. Impact of postovulatory food deprivation on the ova transport, hormonal profiles and metabolic changes in sows. Acta Vet Scand. 2001;42:45–55.
29. Tucker AL, Atkinson JL, Millman ST, Widowski TM. Metabolic indicators of nutritional stress are not predictive of abnormal oral behavior in piglets. Physiol Behav. 2010;100(4):277–83.
30. Song C, Jiang J, Han X, Yu G, Pang Y. Effect of immunological stress to neuroendocrine and gene expression in different swine breeds. Mol Biol Rep. 2014;41:3569–76.
31. Tuchscherer A, Kanitz E, Puppe B, Tuchscherer A, Viergutz T. Changes in endocrine and immune responses of neonatal pigs exposed to a psychosocial stressor. Res Vet Sci. 2009;87:380–8.
32. Wrona D, Trojniar W, Borman A, Ciepielewski Z, Tokarski J. Stress induced changes in peripheral natural killer cell cytotoxicity in pigs may not depend on plasma cortisol. Brain Behav Immun. 2001;15:54–64.
33. Wirtz PH, von Känel R, Emini L, Suter T, Fontana A, Ehlert U. Variations in anticipatory cognitives stress appraisal and differential proinflammatory cytokine expression in response to acute stress. Brain Behav Immun. 2007;21:851–9.
34. Morrow-Tesch JL, McGlone JJ, Salak-Johnson JL. Heat and social stress effects on pig immune measures. J Anim Sci. 1994;72(10):2599–609.
35. Merlot E, Mounier AM, Prunier A. Endocrine response of gilts to various common stressors: A comparison of indicators and methods of analysis. Physiol Behav. 2011;102:259–65.
36. Prunier A, Mounier AM, Hay M. Effects of castration, tooth resection, or tail docking on plasma metabolites and stress hormones in young pigs. J Anim Sci. 2005;83:216–22.
37. Campbell JM, Crenshaw JD, Polo J. The biological stress of early weaned piglets. J Anim Sci Biotechnol. 2013;4:19–23.
38. Brown SN, Knowles TG, Wilkins LJ, Chadd SA, Warriss PD. The response of pigs to being loaded or unloaded onto commercial animal transporters using three systems. Vet J. 2005;170:91–100.
39. Goodband B, Tokach M, Dritz S, de Rouchey J, Woodworth J. Practical starter pig amino acid requirements in relation to immunity, gut health and growth performance. J Anim Biotechnol. 2014;5:12–23.
40. Council Regulation (EC) No 1/2005 of 22 December 2004. on the protection of animals during transport and related operations and amending Directives 64/432/EEC and 93/119/EC and Regulation (EC) No 1255/97. Official Journal of European Union. 5.1.2005.
41. Squires EJ. Effects on Animal Behaviour. Health and Welfare. In: Squires EJ, editor. Applied Animal Endocrinology. Cambridge: CABI Publishing; 2003. p. 192–225.
42. Sonoda LT, Fels M, Oczak M, Vranken E, Ismayilova G, Guarino M, Viazzi S, Bahr C, Berckmans D, Hartung J. Tail biting in pigs-causes and management intervention strategies to reduce the behavioural disorder. A review. Berl Munch Tierarztl Wochenschr. 2013;126:104–12.
43. Valros A, Munsterhjelm C, Puolanne E, Ruusunen M, Heinonen M, Peltoniemi OAT, Pösö AR. Physiological indicators of stress and meat and carcass characteristics in tail bitten slaughter pigs. Acta Vet Scand. 2013;55:75.
44. Ruis MA, Brake JH, Engel B, Buist WG, Blokhuis HJ, Koolhaas JM. Adaptation to social isolation. Acute and long-term stress responses of growing gilts with different coping characteristics. Physiol Behav. 2001;73:541–51.
45. Dallman MF, Hellhammer D. Regulation of the hypothalamo-pituitary-adrenal axis, chronic stress, and energy: The role of the brain and networks. In: Contrada RJ, Baum A, editors. The Handbook of Stress Science: Biology, Psychology, and Health. New York: Springer Publishing Company; 2011. p. 11–36.
46. Rivier C, Rivest S. Effect of stress on the activity of the hypothalamic-pituitary-gondal axis: Peripheral and central mechanisms. Biol Reprod. 1991;45:523–32.
47. Chrousos GP, Torpy DJ, Gold PW. Interactions between the hypothalamic-pituitary-adrenal axis and the female reproductive system: clinical implications. Ann Intern Med. 1998;129:229–40.
48. Norman RL, Smith CJ. Restraint inhibits luteinizing hormone and testosterone secretion in intact male rhesus macaques: effects of concurrent naloxone administration. Neuroendocrinol. 1992;55:405–15.
49. Einarsson S, Brandt Y, Lundeheim N, Madej A. Stress and its influence on reproduction in pigs: a review. Acta Vet Scand. 2008;50:48.
50. Dhabhar FS. Enhancing versus suppressive effects of stress on immune function: Implications for immunoprotection and immunopathology. Neuroimmunomodulat. 2009;16:300–17.
51. Dhabhar FS, Miller AH, McEwen BS, Spencer RL. Effects of stress on inmune cell distribution-dynamics and hormonal mechanisms. J Immunol. 1995;154:5511–27.
52. Dhabhar FS, McEwen BS. Bidirectional effects of stress and glucocorticoid hormones on immune function: possible explanations for paradoxical observartions. In: Ader R, Felten DL, Cohen N, editors. Psychoneuroimmunology. San Diego: Elsevier Academic Press; 2001. p. 301–38.
53. Smulders D, Verbeke G, Mormède P, Geers R. Validation of a behavioural observation tool to assess pig welfare. Physiol Behav. 2006; 89:438–47.
54. Hyung Y, Ellis M, Johnson RW. Effects of feeder type, space allowance, and mixing on the growth performance and feed intake pattern of growing pigs. J Anim Sci. 1998;76(11):2771–8.
55. Lee C, Gilesc LR, Brydena WL, Downing JL, Owense PC, Kirby AC, Wynn PC. Performance and endocrine responses of group housed weaner pigs

exposed to the air quality of a commercial environment. Livest Prod Sci. 2005;93:255–62.
56. Hicks TA, McGlone JJ, Whisnant CS, Kattesh HG, Norman RL. Behavioural, endocrine, immune and performance measures for pigs exposed to acute stress. J Anim Sci. 1998;76:474–83.
57. Proudfoot K, Habing G. Social stress as a cause of diseases in farm animals: current knowledge and future directions. Vet J. 2015;206:15–21.
58. O'Driscoll K, Teixeirab DL, O'Gormana D, Taylora S, Boyle LA. The influence of a magnesium rich marine supplement on behaviour, salivary cortisol levels, and skin lesions in growing pigs exposed to acute stressors. Appl Anim Behav Sci. 2013;145:92–101.
59. Ott S, Moons CPH, Kashiha MA, Bahr C, Tuyttens FAM, Berckmans D, Niewold TA. Automated video analysis of pig activity at pen level highly correlates to human observations of behavioural activities. Livest Sci. 2014;160:132–7.
60. Nilsson M, Herlin AH, Ardö H, Guzhva O, Åström K, Bergsten C. Development of automatic surveillance of animal behaviour and welfare using image analysis and machine learned segmentation technique. Animal. 2015;9(11):1859–65.
61. Ayala I, Martos N, Silvan G, Gutierrez-Panizo C, Clavel J, Illera J. Cortisol, adrenocorticotropic hormone, serotonin, adrenaline, and noradrenaline serum concentrations in relation to disease and stress in the horse. Res Vet Sci. 2012;93:103–7.
62. Hart KA. The use of cortisol for the objective assessment of stress in animals: pros and cons. Vet J. 2012;192(2):137–9.
63. Escribano D, Tvarijonaviciute A, Tecles F, Cerón JJ. Serum paraoxonase type-1 activity in pigs: Assay validation and evolution after an induced experimental inflammation. Vet Immunol Immunop. 2015;163(3–4):210–5.
64. Nater UM, Rohleder N. Salivary alpha-amylase as a non-invasive biomarker for the sympathetic nervous system: Current state of research. Psychoneuroendocrino. 2009;34:486–96.
65. Granger DA, Kivlighan KT, El-Sheikh M, Gordis EB, Stroud LR. Salivary alpha-amylase in biobehavioural research: recent developments and applications. Ann NY Acad Sci. 2007;1098:122–44.
66. DeCaro JA. Methodological considerations in the use of salivary a-amylase as a stress marker in field research. Am J Hum Biol. 2008;20:617–9.
67. Fuentes M, Tecles F, Gutiérrez A, Otal J, Martínez-Subiela S, Cerón JJ. Validation of an automated method for salivary alpha-amylase measurements in pigs (Sus Scrofa Domesticus) and its application as a stress biomarker. J Vet Diagn Invest. 2011;23:282–7.
68. Taupenot L, Harper KL, O'Connor DT. Mechanisms of disease: The chromogranin-secretogranin family. N Engl J Med. 2003;348:1134–49.
69. Takiyyuddin MA, Cervenka JH, Sullivan PA, Pandian MR, Parmer RJ, Barbosa JA, O'Connor DT. Is physiologic sympathoadrenal catecholamine release exocytotic in human? Circulation. 1990;81(1):185–95.
70. Winkler H, Fischer-Colbrie R. The chromogranins A and B: The first 25 years and future perspectives. Neuroscience. 1992;49:497–528.
71. Hendy GN, Bevan S, Mattei MG, Mouland AJ. Chromogranin A. Clinical and investigative. Medicine. 1995;18(1):47–65.
72. Sato F, Kanno T, Nagasawa S, Yanaihara N, Ishida N, Hasegawa T, Iwanaga T. Immunohistochemical localization of chromogranin A in the acinar cells of equine salivary glands contrasts with rodent glands. Cells Tissues Organs. 2002;172:29–36.
73. Saruta J, Tsukinoki K, Sasaguri K, Ishii H, Yasuda M, Osamura YR, Watanabe Y, Sato S. Expression and localization of chromogranin A gene and protein in human submandibular gland. Cells Tissues Organs. 2005;180:237–44.
74. Huang Y, Liu W, Yin C, Zhao R, Yang X. Response to lipopolysaccharide in salivary components and the submandibular gland of pigs. Livest Sci. 2014; 167:323–30.
75. Kanno T, Asada N, Yanase H, Iwanaga T, Nishikawa Y, Hoshino M, Yanaihara N. Autonomic control of submandibular chromogranin A secretion in the anaesthetized rat. Biomed Res. 1998;19:411–4.
76. Akiyoshi H, Aoki M, Shimada T, Noda K, Kumagai D, Saleh N, Sugii S, Ohashi F. Measurement of plasma chromogranin A concentrations for assessment of stress responses in dogs with insulin-induced hypoglycemia. Am J Vet Res. 2005;66:1830–5.
77. Dimsdale JE, O'Connor DT, Ziegler M, Mills P. Chromogranin A correlates with norepinephrine release rate. Life Sci. 1992;51:519–25.
78. Gallina S, Di Mauro M, D'Amico MA, D'Angelo E, Sablone A, Di Fonso A, Bascelli A, Izzicupo P, Di Baldassarre A. Salivary chromogranin A, but not a-amylase, correlates with cardiovascular parameters during high-intensity exercise. Clin Endocrinol. 2011;75:747–52.
79. Kennedy B, Dillon E, Mills PJ, Ziegler MG. Catecholamines in human saliva. Life Sci. 2001;69:87–99.
80. Escribano D, Soler L, Gutiérrez AM, Martínez-Subiela S, Cerón JJ. Measurement of chromogranin A in porcine saliva: Validation of a time-resolved immunofluorometric assay and evaluation of its application as a marker of acute stress. Animal. 2013;7:640–7.
81. Escribano D, Gutiérrez AM, Fuentes-Rubio M, Cerón JJ. Saliva chromogranin A in growing pigs: A study of circadian patterns during daytime and stability under different storage conditions. Vet J. 2014;199(3):355–9.
82. Gallangher NL, Giles LR, Wynn PC. The development of a circadian pattern of salivary cortisol secretion in the neonatal piglet. Biol Neonate. 2002;81: 113–8.
83. Hillmann E, Schrader L, Mayer C, Gygax L. Effects of weight, temperature and behaviour on the circadian rhythm of salivary cortisol in growing pigs. Animal. 2008;2:405–9.
84. Muneta Y, Yoshikawa T, Minagawa Y, Shibahara T, Maeda R, Omata Y. Salivary IgA as a useful non-invasive marker for restraint stress in pigs. J Vet Med Sci. 2010;72:1295–300.
85. Bottoms GD, Roesel OF, Rausch FD, Akins EL. Circadian variation in plasma cortisol and corticosterone in pigs and mares. Am J Vet Res. 1972;33(4): 785–90.
86. Lawrence AB, Petherick JC, McLean KA, Dean LA, Chirnside J, Vaughan A, Clutton E, Terlouw EMC. The effects of environment on behaviour, plasma cortisol and prolactin in parturient sows. Appl Anim Behav Sci. 1994;39:313–30.
87. Barnett JL, Cronin GM, McCallum TH. Effects of grouping unfamiliar adults pigs after dark, after treatment with amperozide and by using pens with stalls, on aggression, skin lesions and plasma cortisol concentrations. Appl Anim Behav Sci. 1996;50:121–33.
88. Pol F, Courboulay V, Cotte J, Martrenchar A, Hay M, Mormède P. Urinary cortisol as an additional tool to assess the welfare of pregnant sows kept in two types of housing. Vet Res. 2002;33:13–22.
89. Mormède P, Andanson S, Aupérin B, Beerda B, Guémené D, Malmkvist J, Manteca X, Manteuffel G, Prunet P, Van Reenen CG, Richard S, Veissier I. Exploration of the hypothalamic-pituitary-adrenal function as a tool to evaluate animal welfare. Physiol Behav. 2007;92:317–39.
90. Désautés C, Bidanel JP, Mormède P. Genetic study of behavioural and pituitary-adrenocortical reactivity in response to an environmental challenge in pigs. Physiol Behav. 1997;62:337–45.
91. Ruis MAW, Brake JHA, Engel B, Ekkel ED, Buist WG, Blokhuis HJ, Koolhaas JM. The circadian rhythm of salivary cortisol in growing pigs: effects of age, gender, and stress. Physiol Behav. 1997;62:623–30.
92. Möstl E, Palme R. Hormones as indicators of stress. Domest Anim Endocrin. 2002;23:67–74.
93. de Jong IC, Prelle TI, van De Burgwal JA, Lambooij E, Korte SM, Blokhuis HJ, Koolhaas JM. Effects of environmental enrichment on behavioural responses to novelty, learning, and memory, and the circadian rhythm in cortisol in growing pigs. Physiol Behav. 2000;68:571–8.
94. de Leeuw JA, Ekkel ED. Effects of feeding level and the presence of a foraging substrate on the behaviour and stress physiological response of individually housed gilts. Appl Anim Behav Sci. 2004;86:15–25.
95. Ekkel ED, Dieleman SJ, Schouten WGP, Portela A, Corni-Lissen G, Tielen MJM, Halberg F. The circadian rhythm of cortisol in the saliva of young pigs. Physiol Behav. 1996;60:985–9.
96. Evans FD, Christopherson RJ, Aherne FX. Development of the cyrcadian rhythm of cortisol in the gilt from weaning until puberty. Can J Anim Sci. 1988;68:1105–11.
97. Escribano D, Fuentes-Rubio M, Cerón JJ. Validation of an automated chemiluminescent immunoassay for salivary cortisol measurements in pigs. J Vet Diagn Invest. 2012;24:918–23.
98. Piñeiro M, Piñeiro C, Carpintero R, Morales J, Campbell FM, Eckersall PD, Toussaint MJM, Lampreave F. Characterisation of the pig acute phase protein response to road transport. Vet J. 2007;173:669–74.
99. McGlone JJ, Salak JL, Lumpkin EA, Nicholson RI, Gibson M, Norman RL. Shipping stress and social status effects on pig performance, plasma cortisol, natural killer cell activity, and leukocyte numbers. J Anim Sci. 1993;71(4):888–96.
100. Nargund VH. Effects of psychological stress on male fertility. Nat Rev Urol. 2015;12:373–82.
101. Toufexis D, Rivarola MA, Lara H, Viau V. Stress and the reproductive axis. J Neuroendocrinol. 2014;26(9):573–86.

102. Chichinadze K, Chichinadze N. Stress-induced increase of testosterone: Contributions of social status and sympathetic reactivity. Physiol Behav. 2008;94:595–603.
103. Escribano D, Fuentes-Rubio M, Cerón JJ. Salivary testosterone measurements in growing pigs: validation of an automated chemiluminescent immunoassay and its possible use as an acute stress marker. Res Vet Sci. 2014;97(1):20–5.
104. Bilandzic N, Simic B, Kmetic I. Effect of three-day ACTH administration on concentrations of cholesterol, cortisol, progesterone, testosterone and LH in the boars. Slov Vet Res. 2012;49(3):123–32.
105. Murata H, Shimada N, Yoshioka M. Current research on acute phase proteins in veterinary diagnosis: an overview. Vet J. 2004;168:28–40.
106. Baumann H, Gauldie J. The acute phase response. Immunol Today. 1994;15:74–80.
107. Cray C, Zaias J, Altman NH. Acute phase response in animals: a review. Comparative Med. 2009;59(6):517–26.
108. Eckersall PD. Recent advances and future prospects for the use of acute phase proteins as markers of disease in animals. Rev Med Vet-Toulouse. 2000;151(7):577–84.
109. Piñeiro C, Piñeiro M, Morales J, Andrés M, Lorenzo E, Pozo MD, Álava MA, Lampreave F. Pig-MAP and haptoglobin concentration reference values in swine from commercial farms. Vet J. 2009;179:78–84.
110. Soler L, Gutiérrez A, Escribano D, Fuentes M, Cerón JJ. Response of salivary haptoglobin and serum amyloid A to social isolation and short road transport stress in pigs. Res Vet Sci. 2013;95:298–302.
111. Murata H. Stress and acute phase protein response: An inconspicuous but essential linkage. Vet J. 2007;173:473–4.
112. Johnson JD, Campisi J, Sharkey CM, Kennedy SL, Nickerson BN, Greenwood BN, Fleshner M. Catecholamines mediate stress-induced increases in peripheral and central inflammatory cytokines. Neuroscience. 2005;135:1295–307.
113. González-Ramón N, Hoebe K, Álava MA, Van Leengoed L, Piñeiro M, Carmona S, Iturralde M, Lampreave F, Piñeiro A. Pig MAP/ITIH4 and haptoglobin are interleukin-6-dependent acute phase serum proteins in porcine primary cultured hepatocytes. Eur J Biochem. 2000;267:1878–85.
114. García-Celdrán M, Ramis G, Quereda JJ, Armedo E. Reduction of transport-induced stress on finishing pigs by increasing lairage time at the slaughter house. J Swine Health Prod. 2012;20(3):118–22.
115. Piñeiro C, Piñeiro M, Morales J, Carpintero R, Campbell FM, Eckersall PD, Toussaint MJM, Álava MA, Lampreave F. Pig acute-phase protein levels after stress induced by changes in the pattern of food administration. Animal. 2007;1:133–9.
116. Zaine L, Ferreira C, Gomes Mde O, Monti M, Tortola L, Vasconcellos RS, Carciofi AC. Faecal IgA concentration is influenced by age in dogs. Brit J Nutr. 2011;106:183–6.
117. Guhad FA, Hau J. Salivary IgA as a marker of social stress in rats. Neurosci Lett. 1996;216:137–40.
118. Kikkawa A, Uchida Y, Nakade T, Taguchi K. Salivary secretory IgA concentrations in beagle dogs. J Vet Med Sci. 2003;65(6):689–93.
119. Wetherell MA, Hyland ME, Harris JE. Secretory immunoglobulin A reactivity to acute and cumulative acute multi-tasking stress: relationships between reactivity and perceived workload. Biol Psychol. 2004;66:257–70.
120. Muneta Y, Minagawa Y, Nakane T, Shibahara T, Yoshikawa T, Omata Y. Interleukin-18 expression in pig salivary glands and salivary content changes during acute immobilization stress. Stress. 2011;14:549–56.
121. Escribano D, Campos PHRF, Gutiérrez AM, Le Floc N, Cerón JJ, Merlot E. Effect of repeated administration of lipopolysaccharide on inflammatory and stress markers in saliva of growing pigs. Vet J. 2014;200(3):393–7.
122. Conti B, Jahng JW, Tinti C, Son JH, Joh TH. Induction of interferon-γ inducing factor in the adrenal cortex. J Biol Chem. 1997;272:2035–7.
123. Stoll S, Müller G, Kurimoto M, Saloga J, Tanimoto T, Yamauchi H, Okamura H, Knop J, Enk AH. Production of IL-18 (IFN-gamma-inducing factor) messenger RNA and functional protein by murine keratinocytes. J Immunol. 1997;159(1):298–302.
124. Kawakami K, Qureshi MH, Zhang T, Okamura H, Kurimoto M, Saito A. IL-18 protects mice against pulmonary and disseminated infection with Cryptococcus neoformans by inducing IFN-gamma production. J Immunol. 1997;159(11):5528–34.
125. Micallef MJ, Yoshida K, Kawai S, Hanaya T, Kohno K, Arai S, Tanimoto T, Torigoe K, Fuji M, Ikeda M, Kurimoto M. In vivo antitumor effects of murine interferon-gamma-inducing factor/interleukin-18 in mice bearing syngeneic Meth A sarcoma malignant ascites. Cancer Immunol Immun. 1997;43:361–7.
126. Conti B, Sugama S, Kim Y, Tinti C, Kim H, Baker H, Volpe B, Attardi B, Joh T. Modulation of IL-18 production in the adrenal cortex following acute ACTH or chronic corticosterone treatment. Neuroimmunomodulation. 2000;8(1):1–7.

12

Modeling livestock population structure: a geospatial database for Ontario swine farms

Salah Uddin Khan[1*], Terri L. O'Sullivan[1], Zvonimir Poljak[1], Janet Alsop[2] and Amy L. Greer[1*]

Abstract

Background: Infectious diseases in farmed animals have economic, social, and health consequences. Foreign animal diseases (FAD) of swine are of significant concern. Mathematical and simulation models are often used to simulate FAD outbreaks and best practices for control. However, simulation outcomes are sensitive to the population structure used. Within Canada, access to individual swine farm population data with which to parameterize models is a challenge because of privacy concerns. Our objective was to develop a methodology to model the farmed swine population in Ontario, Canada that could represent the existing population structure and improve the efficacy of simulation models.

Results: We developed a swine population model based on the factors such as facilities supporting farm infrastructure, land availability, zoning and local regulations, and natural geographic barriers that could affect swine farming in Ontario. Assigned farm locations were equal to the swine farm density described in the 2011 Canadian Census of Agriculture. Farms were then randomly assigned to farm types proportional to the existing swine herd types. We compared the swine population models with a known database of swine farm locations in Ontario and found that the modeled population was representative of farm locations with a high accuracy (AUC: 0.91, Standard deviation: 0.02) suggesting that our algorithm generated a reasonable approximation of farm locations in Ontario.

Conclusion: In the absence of a readily accessible dataset providing details of the relative locations of swine farms in Ontario, development of a model livestock population that captures key characteristics of the true population structure while protecting privacy concerns is an important methodological advancement. This methodology will be useful for individuals interested in modeling the spread of pathogens between farms across a landscape and using these models to evaluate disease control strategies.

Keywords: Synthetic population, Swine, Pigs, Farms, Ontario, Infectious disease transmission model

Background

The Canadian swine industry has gone through a major transformation in the last century. The number of pig farms has decreased from 8.1 in 1921 to 0.6 per 100 inhabitants in 2011 [1], but the average number of pigs raised per farm has continued to grow in Canada. In 2011, the swine industry was the fourth largest agricultural industry (CAD 3.9 billion value) in Canada after canola, dairy products and beef cattle [1]. During the same year, Canada exported more than one million tons of pork valued at $2.9 billion to more than 80 countries and was ranked as the fifth largest pork exporter in the world [2]. Ontario is considered to be the second largest swine producing province in Canada with 24.4% of all pigs and the majority are in southern Ontario [3]. It is hypothesized that areas with a high density of farms are at greater risk for infectious disease introduction and spread [4, 5].

Infectious diseases in farmed animals have economic, social, and animal health consequences as well a possible human health consequences [6]. Foreign animal diseases (FAD) of swine are of significant concern in terms of animal health and welfare and also due to the anticipated economic losses that would arise as a result of a FAD incursion in Ontario [2]. Because FAD introductions are rare events especially in more developed countries with rigorous importation regulations on animals and animal products, mathematical and epidemiological

* Correspondence: sukhanbd@uoguelph.ca; agreer@uoguelph.ca
[1]Department of Population Medicine, Ontario Veterinary College, University of Guelph, Guelph, ON, Canada
Full list of author information is available at the end of the article

modeling are often used to simulate the extent of such outbreaks and best practices for control using what are considered to be the "most likely" scenarios [7].

Disease modeling provides a cost-effective approach for researchers to develop an understanding of the determinants of disease spread within a population and factors contributing to effective disease control [8]. Host-pathogen relationships frequently demonstrate non-linear trends. Such complex relationships are often best described by computer simulation models [8]. This methodology has contributed to our understanding of disease dynamics and how best to intervene in order to prevent the spread of an infectious disease [8, 9]. However, simulation outcomes are sensitive to the geographic location of livestock enterprises, the number of animals present at each location, and the frequency of both direct and indirect movement events between livestock enterprise locations [10, 11]. In Canada, access to individual swine farm population data with which to parameterize models is limited because of privacy concerns. Authorities responsible for disease outbreak response such as Canadian Food Inspection Agency (CFIA) and Ontario Ministry of Agriculture, Food and Rural Affairs (OMAFRA) do not maintain a livestock population database of animals susceptible to FAD or other reportable diseases. Rather, they rely on premise and animal identification databases maintained by the provincial or territorial governments and/or by livestock traceability administrators, such as Pig Trace Canada (*Personal communication: Pascale Aubry, CFIA and Tim Pasma, OMAFRA*). Although CFIA and OMAFRA have a data sharing agreement in the event of an outbreak, access to the livestock location database is restricted to use during an animal disease emergency. Therefore, our objective was to develop a methodology to model farmed swine population in Ontario, Canada that captured the most important aspects of the existing swine farm population structure in Ontario in order to improve the realism of computer simulation models.

Methods

Swine farming in Ontario and 2011 census database structure

Statistics Canada conducts an agricultural census once every five years and detailed data for the most recent agricultural census (2011) was publicly available from the Statistics Canada website [3]. The Canadian census data on swine farming consisted of the number and types of farms, and the aggregated number of animals (Additional file 1: Table S1, Figure S1, S2). The smallest unit of the aggregated farming data was Census Consolidated Subdivisions (CCS). Formation of a CCS depended on multiple factors that included a census subdivision consisting of a land area greater than 25 km^2 or having a human population size greater than 100,000 [12].

Swine farm data were extracted from the 2011 Agricultural Census by CCS, the smallest aggregated geographical unit. However, there were two limitations related to the spatial resolution of the data available for analysis. First, a large proportion of data on the total number of animals in a farm were missing. Based on production type, the missing data ranged from 33% to 48% (Additional file 1: Table S1). And second, the format of the census data did not distinguish mixed farm types (e.g. farms having multiple swine production types), which is a feature of the swine population commonly observed in Southern Ontario [13]. These limitations made the dataset less useful for assessing the overall number of pigs and types of swine farms in each CCS. Therefore, we only utilized the total number of pig farms as reported in the 2011 census for our model. We performed additional data processing to match geographic boundary files of Ontario CCS with the 2011 Census swine population data to develop a geospatial database that matched the swine farm density reported in the 2011 Census data (Additional file 1: Figure S1, S2).

Data processing and evaluation

We have described the estimation and validation of the spatial locations of swine farms in Ontario, Canada as a six-step process: This included 1) identifying ecological and anthropogenic factors that may affect swine farming; 2) defining the relative importance of the factors affecting swine farming, 3) generating an algorithm to achieve a likelihood score for swine farming in a particular location; 4) estimating the suitability of a location for swine farming; 5) generating random farm locations equal to the swine farm density reported in the 2011 Census of Agriculture, and 6) validate the methods for estimating swine farming likelihood.

Understanding the factors influencing the locations of swine farms in Ontario

We consulted with swine experts in Ontario (Drs. Zvonimir Poljak and Terri L. O'Sullivan, Ontario Veterinary College, University of Guelph, and Dr. Tim Pasma, Lead Veterinarian and Epidemiologist, Animal Health and Welfare Branch of the Ontario Ministry of Agriculture, Food and Rural Affairs, Guelph, Ontario, Canada) through multiple face-to-face meetings, and email communications, reviewed available farm data, and performed literature searches to determine the factors influencing swine farming in Ontario (Table 1) [14, 15]. Like any other commercial operation, we assumed that access to transportation was one of the key drivers for the establishment of a swine farm. Additionally, we assumed that the local regulations for agricultural land use, land availability and facilities supporting farm infrastructure also played key roles in determining suitable swine farm locations [14, 15]. Key drivers for zoning regulations by the local and provincial authorities included

Table 1 Factors influencing the locations of swine farms in Ontario, scoring guidelines, and geographic information system data used to assign scores

Attributes	Scoring guideline	GIS Data
Zoning and Local Regulations		
Population centers	Farms are not allowed to be established within a municipality or a population center	Ontario Population Centers /Residential Land Use
Agricultural zone	Swine farms are encouraged to be established within the area zoned for agricultural use	Agricultural ecumene
Roads within population center	Although farms are almost always near a road network, the roads passing within a population center or residential area should be away from a swine farm	Road Network Passing through a population Center/ Residential Location
Land Availability		
Crown Land	Crown Land - MNR Unpatented Land Public are not supposed to have any private establishment. However, since the most recent update in the database (2010), a proportion of the land may have been given access to public. Therefore, we assigned a suitability score of 5% within the Crown Land, and 100% for the remainder	Crown Land - MNR Unpatented Land Public
Crown Game Preserves	Farms are not allowed to be established on land designated for Crown game preserves	Crown Game Preserves
Government Institutional Land Use	Farms are not allowed to be established on land designated for government institutions	Government Institutional Land Use
Industrial Land Use	Farms are not generally allowed to be established on land designated for industrial establishments	Resources and Industrial Land Use
Camp, Recreation	Farms should be located a certain distance from camp and recreational establishments	Camp, Recreation
Facilities Supporting Farm Infrastructure		
Road Network	Roads that do not got through population centers have a higher likelihood of being near swine farms	Road Network
	Swine farms could be located near highways, but their access to transportation will depend on the local road network connecting the farms, thus we only kept the local road network attribute.	
Geographic Barriers		
Waterbodies	Swine farms are generally not located near shorelines of the large waterbodies (e.g. Great Lakes). Therefore, we considered that it would be unlikely that farms would be within 1 km of the shorelines of the Great Lakes.	Great Lakes
Large Inland Waterbodies	We consider it highly unlikely that a swine farm would be located within the boundaries of large inland waterbodies (e.g. rivers and lakes).	Inland lakes and rivers

concerns related to water and air pollution and odour control [15]. Production waste (i.e. manure) resulting from intense swine farming was identified as a key environmental concern [15]. Because swine farm waste materials contain a high concentrations of nitrate, phosphate, salts, and bacteria, they may pollute nearby open water sources [15], triggering risks for the health of human, animal, and aquatic ecosystems. As a result, many of the regulations and guidelines focus on containing swine farms within specific agricultural zones in order to have sufficient space to store, handle, and process farm waste materials. Since southern Ontario mostly consists of gently rolling plains, larger waterbodies were the only noticeable natural barriers for the establishment of swine farms [16]. However, because of the current regulations for environmental safety, we assumed that swine farms needed to be situated a reasonable distance from large open waterbodies to prevent contaminants from farm waste materials. Other factors, such as the land designated for population and urban centers, government institutional uses, industrial zones, Crown game preserves, camps and recreational uses, and Crown lands added additional restrictions for areas that could support swine farming in Ontario (Table 1).

Developing geospatial data layers and assigning suitability scores

To assess the factors influencing swine farming in Ontario (Additional file 1: Figure S3), we identified the geospatial databases that could capture zoning and local regulations, farm land availability, facilities supporting farm infrastructure, and geographic barriers (Table 2). Multiple data processing steps were necessary to assign and combine the suitability scores into a single geospatial dataset. We re-projected all of our geographical data layers to The Lambert Conformal Conic map projection, a map projection system frequently used in Ontario [17].

We divided the province of Ontario into 1 km^2 geospatial grids as data units and calculated the distance between each unit and the nearest factors influencing swine farming (Table 2). The next step included assigning suitability scores based on the distance between the outer boundary of a geospatial grid and a factor influencing swine farming (Table 2). For example, the likelihood of a farm being within 300 m of a road that does not intersect a residential location is very high because of the ease of transporting animals and goods. However, as a farm location unit moves further away from road networks, transportation logistics become more difficult. With a conservative approach, we assumed that it would not be logistically feasible to establish a farm five kilometers away from the nearest road network. Similarly, because of the local regulations [15], pig farms could not be established within a population center or residential zone, thus we assigned a likelihood score of zero to these area of the geospatial grid. Initially, we assumed that pig farms would need to maintain a sufficient distance from provincial population centers. However, when we assessed publicly available pig farm location data from Ontario (n = 45, data not shown), there were a small proportion of farms within the two kilometer buffer outside the population centers. Therefore, we assigned a lower likelihood score to the geospatial units within the two kilometer buffer outside the population centers than the geospatial units more than two

Table 2 Geospatial data layers and the associated suitability scores for the prospect of having a swine farm in a particular geographical location

GIS data layers	Data source	Categories	Suitability scores
Road Network (excluding highways)	StatCan	Roads passing through population centers	0
		Roads that don't pass through population centers.	
		- Within 300 m	100
		- Between 301 and 500 m	50
		- Between 501 and 5000 m	25
		- More than 5 KM	0
Agricultural Ecumene[a]	StatCan	- Intersect	100
		- Do not intersect	10
Population Centers/ Residential Zones	StatCan and DMTI Spatial Inc.	- Within a population center/residential zone	0
		- Within a 2 KM buffer around the outer perimeter of a population center	25
		- Between 2.001 and 15 KM buffer around a population center	95
		- More than 15 KM away from the outer perimeter of a population center	50
Crown Land - MNR Unpatented Land Public	Ontario Land use information, Ministry of Natural resources	- Intersect	5
		- Do not intersect	100
Camp and Recreation spots	Ontario Land use information, Ministry of Natural resources	- Intersect within 1KM buffer of the outer perimeter	0
		- Outside 1KM buffer of the outer perimeter	100
Government Institutional Land Use	DMTI Spatial Inc.	- Intersect	0
		- Do not intersect	100
Resource and Industrial Land Use	DMTI Spatial Inc.	- Intersect	0
		- Do not intersect	100
Waterbodies – Great Lakes	NOAA	- Intersect within 1KM buffer of the outer perimeter	0
		- Outside 1KM buffer of the outer perimeter	100
Large Inland Waterbodies	StatCan	Larger waterbodies (e.g. ranking 1, 2 and 3). A geographical reference location:	
		- Intersect within 1KM buffer of the outer perimeter	0
		- Outside 1KM buffer of the outer perimeter	100

[a]Agricultural Ecumene refers to the occupied land surface used for agricultural or any other economic purposes

kilometers outside the population centers. We also assumed that the likelihood of a farm being more than 15 km away from the nearest population center is lower because of the logistics and costs associated with animal, animal product, and farm supplies and consumables transportation. Agricultural zones were of specific focus for assigning probability scores because the majority of the surface within the zone consisted of the loam soil types. This particular soil type supports the storage and draining of organic waste materials produced on a farm [14] and for this reason we assigned a high likelihood score for geospatial units within a defined agricultural zone. Because of the current local regulations relating to open water pollution, farms should maintain sufficient distance from open-water sources. Hence, we created a 1-km buffer around the larger waterbodies and calculated the distance between a geospatial unit and the nearest water source. The geospatial units that intersected a water body, received a likelihood score of zero. However, assigning probability scores to the geospatial units near waterbodies presented a challenge because a single geospatial unit may intersect with the 1 km buffer zone, but a large proportion of the surface of the unit might have sufficient space to accommodate a farm (Additional file 1: Figure S4). For this reason, we subtracted the land surface covered by the polygons generated from the '1-km buffer to the waterbodies' from the dataset. Performing this action allowed us to retain portions of a geospatial unit with space that could accommodate a swine farm.

Combined suitability score for pig farming operations and random farm placement

To develop a combined pig farm suitability surface, we developed an algorithm consistent with the suitability scores calculated for each of the individual level factors that were identified as influencing pig farming in Ontario. Figure 1 is an example of calculating a combined suitability surface: step 1 consisted of the process of multiplying the input parameters with scores assigned for each of the geospatial units and step 2 consisted of regressing the combined suitability scores to a scale ranging from zero to one. With zero being completely unsuitable and one being completely suitable based on the defined algorithm.

Once we calculated the combined pig farm placement suitability scores, we generated random farm locations within the geospatial units that exceeded a defined threshold (methods described in the model accuracy assessment section). The random points generated within a CCS were equal to the number of farms reported in the 2011 agricultural census [18]. Additionally, random points were not permitted within 300 m of each other. The minimum distance of 300 m were selected based on the observed distance characteristics of the publicly available pig farm data in Ontario (data not shown).

Validate the methods for estimating swine farming likelihood

To assess the accuracy of the models, we followed standard approaches to generate agreement matrices [19–21] in order to compare the level of agreement between the predicted combined suitability score of the models and the "reference" presence or absence data. The presence/absence pig farm data for a geographical unit served as a reference dataset for evaluating the classification accuracy of the predictive models.

The reference data on pig farm premises for validation of the model-generated swine population was derived from the Ontario Provincial Premises Registry collected by the Ontario Ministry of Agriculture, Food, and Rural Affairs [22]. The Provincial Premises Registry provides a premises identification number for those who voluntarily registered their agri-food businesses, which includes livestock farms. Although premises registration was voluntary, the compliance rate was very close to 100% because the farms were required to have a premises identification number to report pig movements to meet federal reporting regulation (Personal communication, Ontario Ministry of Agriculture, Food, and Rural Affairs). Most importantly, for the purpose of validating the modeled swine population

Step 1

Road Network				Population Centers				Crown Land				Combined Score		
0	100	75	X	0	50	95	X	100	100	100	=	0	500000	712500
5	50	50		50	95	30		100	100	5		25000	475000	7500

Step 2

Combined Score				Combined Suitability Surface		
0	500000	712500	$/100^3$ =	0.00	0.50	0.71
25000	475000	7500		0.03	0.48	0.01

Fig. 1 An example of calculating a combined suitability surface: step 1 of the process required multiplying the input parameters with the scores assigned for each of the geospatial units, and step 2, consisted of regressing the combined suitability scores to a scale ranging from 0 to 1

algorithm, premise registration records included information regarding the geographic location of the centroid of a parcel of land where the farm is located or individual barns of the swine farms. The total number of registered premises within the province of Ontario was approximately double the number of farms listed in the 2011 agricultural census likely because many of the farms registered multiple premises or there was an underreporting of swine farms in the 2011 census or both.

To assess model validity, we compared the algorithm-generated swine farm locations for the modeled swine datasets that received no score (i.e. zero, not suitable for pig farm) with those that received a positive score (i.e. non-zero, could support a pig farm) to the geographical location units that had presence or absence information on pig farm operations from the Provincial Premises Registry. The Provincial Premises Registry served as the reference dataset for model validation.

We developed multiple models by varying the combinations of explanatory variables. To begin with, we identified a minimal required set of explanatory variables that could explain probable pig farming locations and assess the accuracy. Considering the logistical challenges with assigning suitability scores to the surfaces intersecting with waterbodies (Additional file 1: Figure S4) and the probability that farms could have been placed near waterbodies before regulations were in place (e.g. previously described publicly available swine farm location data identified 4.4% of the farms were within one kilometer near a waterbody), we removed the variables explaining different types of waterbodies (from small to large) from models 2 through 5 to assess the changes in model accuracy (Table 3). We initially assumed that the explanatory variables included in model 1 were sufficient to assign a probability score for swine farm locations. However, since the Crown land database (Crown Land - MNR Unpatented Land) was somewhat dated (last update in 2010), we included this variable in model 4 to assess the difference in model accuracy. We also hypothesized that the explanatory variables in model 1 would be sufficient to represent agricultural zones because they excluded the population centers and other non-agricultural related land uses. To explore this, we included the agricultural ecumene to model 6 to assess the changes in model efficacy.

Since we developed multiple models based on a range of different assumptions, we followed a two-step approach for model selection and assessment of validity. First, for each of the population models (Table 3), we calculated the area under the receiver operating characteristic (ROC) curve using the Mann-Whitney U statistic [23]. The hypothesis was that that a randomly chosen 1-km^2 surface with a pig farm present (from the Provincial Premises Registry) would receive a higher likelihood score compared to the randomly chosen geographical unit without any pig farms. In the second step, True Skill Statistics (measured as: sensitivity + specificity - 1) [24] and Kappa values were calculated to identify an optimal threshold cut-off for the model's combined suitability score that demonstrated maximum sensitivity and specificity [21, 25].

Once we identified an optimal threshold for the model with the highest area under the ROC curve (AUC), we generated random spatial points from a uniform distribution [18] to represent farm locations for the population model within the geographical surface that scored equal to or above the threshold likelihood score. The

Table 3 Accuracy statistics of the model swine populations: area under the receiver operating characteristics curve (AUC) and standard deviations (Sd)

Models	AUC (Sd.)
Model1	0.74 (0.004)
Road network + population centers and residential zones + camp and recreational spots + government institutional land use + resources and industrial land use + great lakes + large inland waterbodies + small inland waterbodies	
Model2	0.75 (0.004)
Removed[a] small inland waterbodies from *Model1*	
Model3	0.76 (0.004)
Removed large inland waterbodies with 1 KM buffer from *Model2* surface	
Model4	0.76 (0.003)
Included Crown Land - MNR Unpatented public land to *Model3*	
Model5	0.89 (0.003)
Removed great lakes with 1 KM buffer from *Model4* surface	
Model6	0.90 (0.003)
Included agricultural ecumene to *Model5*	

[a]Removed was defined as the section(s) of a surface unit intersecting with a predictor which was not included in the computation

number of random modeled farm location points within a Census Consolidated Subdivision (CCS) was equal to the number of pig farms described in the 2011 Agricultural Census. Once the farm locations were assigned, we randomly assigned the type of swine operation (e.g. farrow to finish, finisher farm types) proportional to the recently surveyed operation types [13]. The farm types were also randomly assigned a size (number of pigs per farm) based on the farm-level population distribution from the 2011 census information.

Results

Attributes that received a suitability score to support swine farming had varying degrees of land surface coverage: highest land surface (31%) was covered by the proximity to the road network and the least (0.6%) was by government and institutional land use (Additional file 1: Table S2). Models to generate a combined likelihood scores to identify pig farming locations in Ontario demonstrated relatively high accuracy (Table 3). A suitable model (Model 6, Fig. 2) was achieved by incorporating distance information on road networks, population centers and residential zones, camps and recreational centers, land used by government, resources, and industrial purposes, and agricultural zoning and subtracting the landscape areas that had larger waterbodies or were within a 1 km buffer zone of a larger waterbody. Model 6 demonstrated a very high predictive accuracy (AUC: 0.90, Standard deviation (SD): 0.003) (Fig. 3) when compared to the premises registry information describing pig farming in Ontario (Table 3). The model predicted 9.6% of the Ontario's land surfaces, mostly in southern Ontario suitable for supporting pig farms. When comparing model algorithms to the true pig farming locations (premises registry), we used the higher threshold cut-off identified between two distinct approaches: True Skill Statistics and Kappa Statistics. A likelihood threshold of 0.82 was identified as an optimal cut-off (Sensitivity: 72%, Specificity: 96%) (Figs. 3 and 4). The land surfaces that scored on and above this threshold cut-off were selected to generate random farm locations (n = 2485) equal to the number of swine farms documented in the 2011 Canadian agricultural census. When compared to the known pig farming locations (census consolidated subdivisions) described in the 2011 census, the randomly generated farm location points (Fig. 5) demonstrated very high accuracy (AUC: 0.93, SD: 0.01).

Discussion

We developed a model to generate a swine population to represent the farm population structure for commercially raised pigs in Ontario. Publicly available data from the 2011 Canadian agricultural census and geospatial information were used to generate a swine population

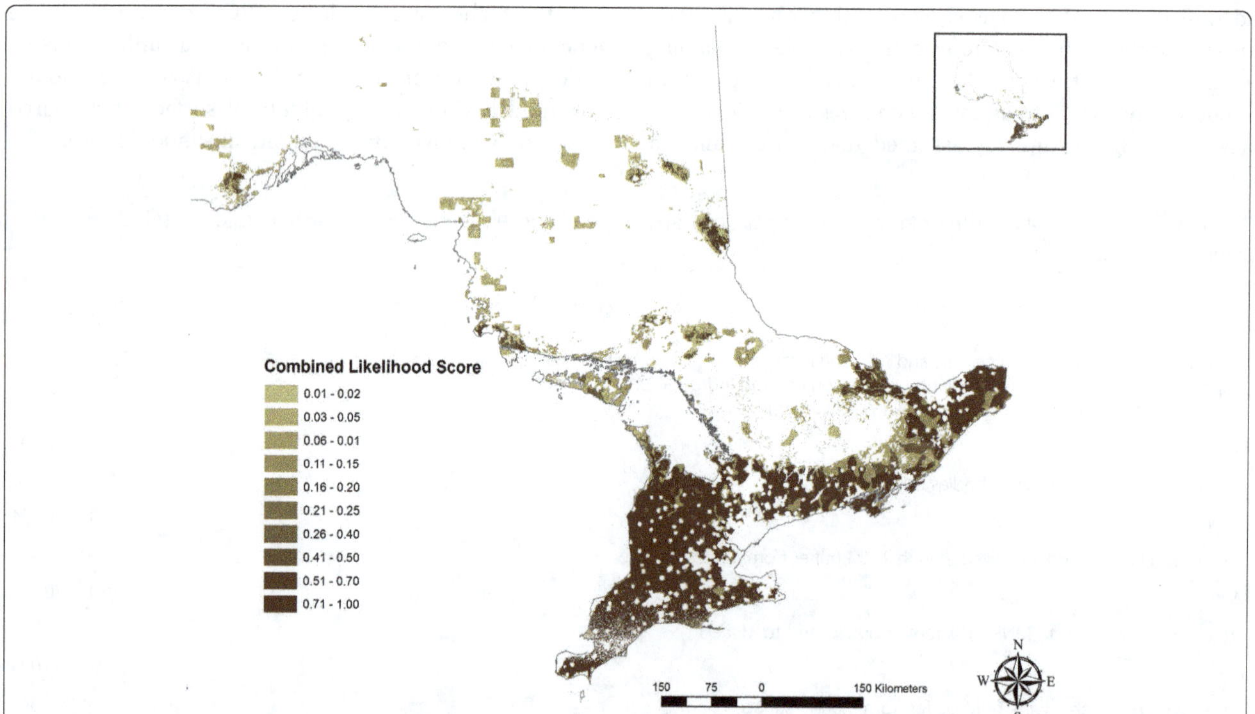

Fig. 2 A map of Ontario showing the combined pig farming likelihood scores generated through model 6. The intensity of the color represents the combined likelihood score (range 0–1): the areas with a higher likelihood score (darker color) represent a greater probability of having a pig farm and the surfaces in white represent areas with no probability of having a pig farm

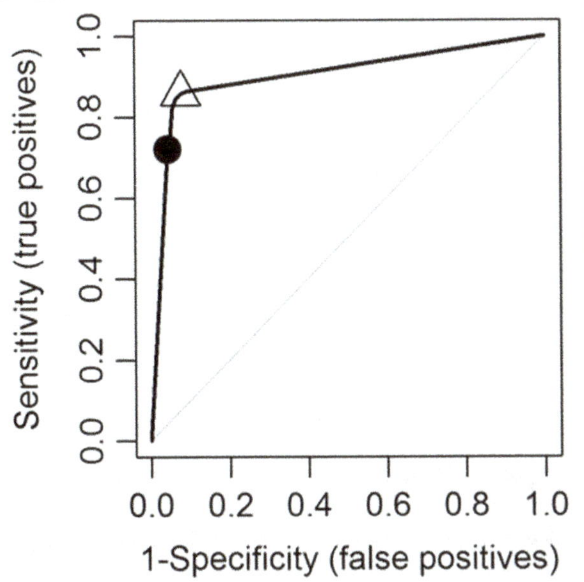

Fig. 3 A receiver operating characteristic (ROC) plot for the combined likelihood score's predictability of model 6, with the optimal threshold marked along the ROC curve. The hollow triangle shape and the black circle indicate the sensitivity and specificity associated with True Skill Statistics (0.04) and the maximum Kappa value (0.82) respectively

structure that represents an improvement over alternative methods, such as the random placement of farm locations across the landscape [26]. When compared with the actual geospatial location information for pig farms in Ontario, the model demonstrated high accuracy.

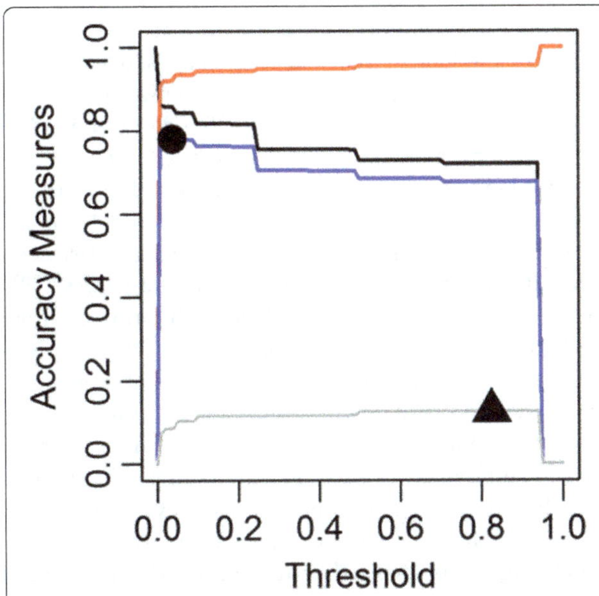

Fig. 4 A graph of error measures (sensitivity, specificity, True Skill Statistics and Kappa) as a function of the threshold for model 6. The colored lines representing sensitivity (black), specificity (red), True Skill Statistics (blue), and Kappa (gray). The black circle indicates the threshold cut-off (0.04) where True Skill Statistics was highest and the triangle shape indicates the threshold cut-off (0.82) where maximum Kappa value was achieved

Generating a well validated model population of swine farms means that this model population could be used as an input into disease simulation models. This will enable researchers to examine questions related to the prevention and control of pathogens within the swine industry including FAD, while at the same time protecting the privacy of individual pork producers. This approach could be replicated for other agricultural commodity groups (e.g. poultry, beef cattle etc.) for which limited individual level data exist.

Our approach was to identify a minimum set of predictors required to assign each cell of a regular grid applied across the geographical extent of Ontario a score reflecting the probability that a pig farm would be present. We hypothesized that regional, cultural, regulation, and landscape factors would be major drivers of the establishment of swine farms. We assigned suitability scores based on a combination of expert opinion, literature reviews, and logic. The models developed based on different combinations of predictors have demonstrated moderate to high accuracy (Table 3). The combination of predictors to create multiple models further helped to assess the predictor selection procedure, particularly the importance of incorporating 'logic' (step 6) to improve model accuracy. In addition, we matched the production types and number of animals on each farm based on the known distribution from recent surveys [13] and the 2011 census [3] to develop a realistic population structure for the province of Ontario. Our findings provide a methodology to estimate the likely geographic location of swine enterprises in a given area. This approach can be used to simulate a population of farms that provides a reasonable estimate of both the number of farms and the location of farms in a study area. A similar approach has been used to model commercial poultry farm locations in the United States [26]. The modeled poultry population was later used to generate parameter estimates for highly pathogenic avian influenza transmission models [26, 27].

There has been tremendous growth in the Canadian swine industry over the past few decades. However, profits have varied dramatically for several reasons, including the increased input costs (e.g. feed), disease outbreaks, changes in the value of the Canadian dollar, and changes in North American pork prices [28]. FAD outbreaks are particularly important not only because of the direct impact on production, but also because of the destruction of healthy animals due to welfare slaughter, import bans by Canadian trading partners, and the risk of a long-term import ban by some countries [2, 3]. Between 1921 and 2011, agricultural intensification in commercial swine production has decreased the number of Canadian swine farms from 711,090 to 7371, but in the same time period, the number of pigs raised has increased from 9

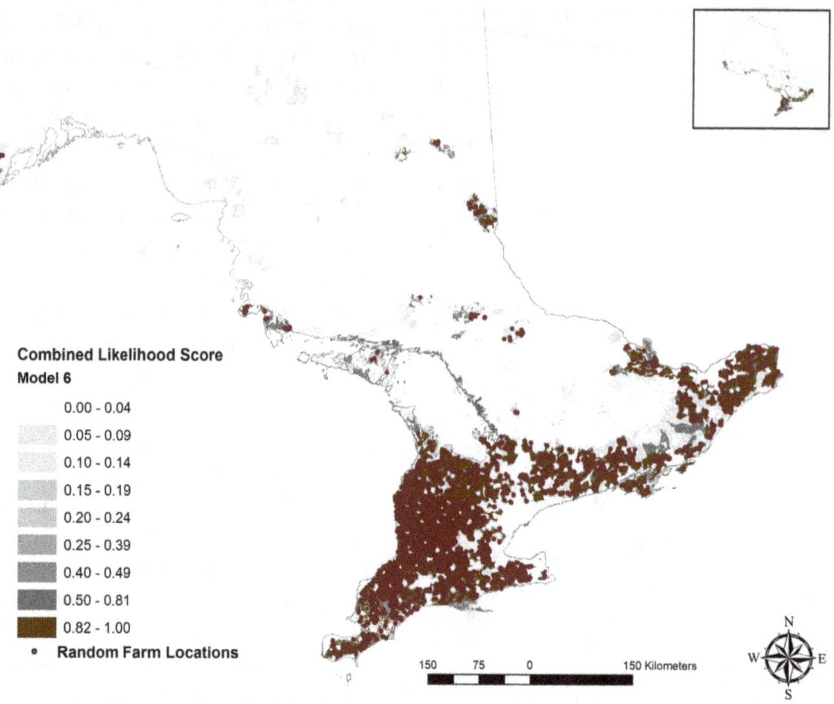

Fig. 5 Random pig farm locations generated using model 6 and based on a combined likelihood threshold cut-off value of 0.82.The red dots ($n = 2485$) represent the locations of model pig farms generated on the surfaces that fall above the likelihood threshold cut-off value. The color intensity on the background represents the combined likelihood threshold

million to 33 million pigs [29]. Although the transformation from backyard swine farms to commercial farming operations increases the likelihood that good biosecurity practices will be carried out, the potential introduction of a FAD remains a major concern for the Canadian swine industry. One recent example was in 2009, when countries such as China and Russia placed a ban on Canadian pork imports because of pandemic influenza A (H1N1). This forced some producers to downsize or exit the industry through government assistance programs [1, 30].

The introduction of a FAD into the Canadian swine industry would have an enormous economic impact. In order to mitigate this risk, preparedness planning is required to estimate the possible extent of an FAD outbreak, the expected efficacy of the control and eradication measures that would be applied in the event of an outbreak, and the human resource and infrastructure requirements (e.g. the number of veterinarians, technicians, disposal services etc.) necessary to effectively carry out control and eradication measures. One of the key requirements for preparedness planning requires the development and parameterization of disease transmission models that incorporate accurate farm population structure that would serve as the base for the disease transmission model [10, 11]. The methodology described here, provides one such example of how this population structure can be derived. The spread of a livestock pathogen is primarily influenced by three factors: first, the variability of disease susceptibility in different production types, second, the geographical proximity and clustering of farms, and third, the direct and indirect movement of animals, people, feed, fomites, vehicles and animal products between different production types [31–34]. Estimating the direct and indirect movements between farms was out of the scope of this research however, to capture the static swine farm characteristics, we developed a spatially explicit population of swine farm locations in Ontario, classified the farms to different production types based on a recent survey [13], and assigned numbers of animals in each farm based on the farm-level population distribution from 2011 agricultural census. The farm locations were randomly generated across the land surface with a likelihood of supporting a swine farm and farm density matched with the census units. The production types and the numbers of animals in each farm were assigned based on surveys, reports, and census data in order to best replicate the existing swine population in the modeled population [3, 13]. The accuracy statistics demonstrated the geographical locations generated for random farm placement using our model algorithm had a very high agreement with the actual observed swine farm locations and therefore, the model swine population generated is a suitable surrogate for incorporation into disease transmission models.

Although the modeled population was a suitable representation of the actual swine farm locations in Ontario, this is not without limitations. First, the number of farms generated in the models were based on the 2011 agricultural census. Underreporting of swine farms, particularly small and backyard farms in the census could have resulted in generating fewer farms in our model. Moreover, a farm with modest number of pigs (e.g. ~700 heads) could have multiple barns located in geographically dispersed location and it was unclear if the census recorded them as a single farm or counted them separately (Personal communication: Dr. Zvonimir Poljak, Department of Population Medicine, Ontario Veterinary College, University of Guelph, Guelph, ON, Canada). On the other hand, the premises registry listed almost twice the number of farm premises. This is likely because individual farm owners had the option to register multiple barns of a single "farm" separately. However, because of the restricted nature of premise registry data, we were unable to verify the proportion of farms that may have registered multiple barns. One way to overcome this issue would be to include a 'correction factor' to adjust the estimated number of farms so it better matches the number of farms derived from a different farmed animal data source(s). However, introducing a 'correction factor' would require a thorough understanding of the proportion of missing data from the primary data source, in our case the 2011 agricultural census. Since we were unable to identify a credible data source for the proportion of farms missing in the census data, we did not include a 'correction factor' with an assumption that the proportional density of the swine farms in the model would be about the same as the actual population. Second, we defined a threshold cut-off using Kappa statistics. This measure is dependent on the prevalence of an outcome [24] and could result in poor agreement when the prevalence is low. In our case, the number of 1-km^2 grid cells having swine farms was very low compared to the total land surface of the province (0.028 vs. 1). A way to overcome this low-prevalence issue would be to calculate True Skill Statistics. However, the threshold defined by True Skill Statistics was extremely low (Fig. 4). Therefore, we took a conservative approach and selected the threshold cut-off where the Kappa value minimized commission error (higher specificity). Third, we did not incorporate the waterbodies that had extremely small surface areas. The reason for such consideration was because our measurement units were 1 km^2 geographic blocks. Even if a unit contained a small waterbody, it would have had an adequate amount of surface areas remaining to also accommodate a swine farm (Additional file 1: Figure S4). Finally, we did not incorporate a separate geospatial data layer on soil types in the models. Although loam type soil facilitates farm waste storage, the incorporation of an agricultural ecumene data layer that included much of the land surface with supported soil types as well as easy access to local grain production for swine feeding management was considered to be a reasonable substitute.

Conclusions

In the absence of a full, identifiable population structure dataset for swine farms in Ontario, developing a model swine population that captures the key characteristics of the observed population structure while protecting producer privacy is an important methodological advancement. Such a population structure will be useful for individuals interested in modeling the spread of pathogens between farms across a landscape and using models to evaluate disease control and eradication measures.

Additional file

Additional file 1: Modeling Livestock Population Structure: A Geospatial Database for Ontario Swine Farms. Description of data: **Table S1.** Data structure and missing data in 2011 agriculture census: pig farm types and number of heads. **Figure S1.** Frequency of pig farms in Ontario's census consolidated subdivisions: Canadian Agricultural Census 2011. **Figure S2.** Frequency of pigs in Ontario's census consolidated subdivisions: Canadian Agricultural Census 2011. **Figure S3.** A map of Canada showing the administrative boundaries of the provinces. **Figure S4.** An example of relative occupancies of small waterbodies in the 1-km^2 spatial grids. **Table S2.** Land surface covered by the attributes with a suitability score (above zero) supporting swine farms in Ontario. (PDF 336 kb)

Abbreviations

AUC: Area Under the Receiver Operating Characteristics Curve; CCS: Census Consolidated Subdivisions; CIFA: Canadian Food Inspection Agency; FAD: Foreign animal diseases; GIS: Geographical Information System; OMAFRA: Ontario Ministry of Agriculture, Food and Rural Affairs; ROC: Receiver Operating Characteristics; SD: Standard deviation

Acknowledgements

We acknowledge the funding support of the Natural Sciences and Engineering Research Council (NSERC) and the Canada Research Chairs (CRC) Program. We also acknowledge data support from the Provincial Premises Registry, Ontario Ministry of Agriculture, Food and Rural Affairs, particularly Dr. Tim Pasma, Lead Veterinarian, Epidemiology, Animal Health and Welfare Branch and Alexander Heim, Coordinator, Premises Information Management for sharing the anonymized swine premises information for the model validation step and Pascale Aubry, Canadian Food Inspection Agency (CFIA) for providing information on livestock farm identification process during the event of an outbreak.

Funding

This research is funded by the Natural Sciences and Engineering Research Council (NSERC) and the Canada Research Chairs (CRC) Program.

Authors' contributions

ALG, SUK, TLS, ZP, JA conceived the study design, SUK extracted and organized the data, performed analysis, and drafted the manuscript. All co-authors reviewed the draft and consented for submission to a journal. All authors read and approved the final manuscript.

Consent for publication
Not applicable

Competing interests
The authors declare that they have no competing interests

Author details
[1]Department of Population Medicine, Ontario Veterinary College, University of Guelph, Guelph, ON, Canada. [2]Ontario Ministry of Agriculture, Food and Rural Affairs, Guelph, ON, Canada.

References

1. Brisson Y: The changing face of the Canadian hog industry: Canadian Agriculture at a Glance. Statistics Canada, Agriculture Division. Available at: http://www.statcan.gc.ca/pub/96-325-x/2014001/article/14027-eng.htm. Accessed on: 18 Oct 2016. In.; 2014.
2. Whiting TL. Foreign animal disease outbreaks, the animal welfare implications for Canada: risks apparent from international experience. Can Vet J. 2003; 44(10):805–15.
3. Statistics-Canada: Census of Population and Agriculture, 2011. In.; 2011.
4. Drew T. The emergence and evolution of swine viral diseases: to what extent have husbandry systems and global trade contributed to their distribution and diversity? Revue Scientifique et Technique-OIE. 2011;30(1):95.
5. Jones BA, Grace D, Kock R, Alonso S, Rushton J, Said MY, McKeever D, Mutua F, Young J, McDermott J. Zoonosis emergence linked to agricultural intensification and environmental change. Proc Natl Acad Sci. 2013;110(21):8399–404.
6. Gibbs EP. The evolution of one health: a decade of progress and challenges for the future. Vet Rec. 2014;174(4):85–91.
7. Harvey N, Reeves A, Schoenbaum MA, Zagmutt-Vergara FJ, Dube C, Hill AE, Corso BA, McNab WB, Cartwright CI, Salman MD. The north American animal disease spread model: a simulation model to assist decision making in evaluating animal disease incursions. Prev Vet Med. 2007;82(3–4):176–97.
8. Anderson RM, RM. M: infectious diseases of humans: dynamics and control. Oxford: Oxford University Press; 1991.
9. Hethcote HW. Qualitative analyses of communicable disease models. Math Biosci. 1976;28(3):335–56.
10. Sattenspiel L. Population structure and the spread of disease. Hum Biol. 1987;59(3):411–38.
11. Miller JC, Volz EM. Incorporating disease and population structure into models of SIR disease in contact networks. PLoS One. 2013;8(8):e69162.
12. Census of Population, Available at: http://www.statcan.gc.ca/pub/92-195-x/2011001/geo/ccs-sru/ccs-sru-eng.htm, accessed on: 31 Jan 2017.
13. Ken McEwan, Marchand L: Benchmarking the Ontario Swine Industry 2011: A Report to Ontario Pork. Available at: http://www.ridgetownc.uoguelph.ca/research/documents/mcewan_Benchmarking_Project_Final_Report.pdf. Accessed on: 6 Feb 2017. In.; 2012.
14. Anonymous: Canadian Code of Practice for Environmentally Sound Hog Production. Canadian Pork Council. Available at: http://manitobapork.com/wp-content/uploads/Canadian_Code_of_Practice_for_Environmentally_Sound_Hog_Production.pdf. Accessed on: 8 Feb 2017. In.; 1996.
15. Lynn Marchand, McEwan K: The Impact of Township Zoning By-Laws on Ontario Swine Farms: A report to Ontario Pork. Ridgetown College, University of Guelph. Available at: http://agrienvarchive.ca/bioenergy/download/sec1_3.pdf. Accessed on: 8 Feb 2017. In.; 1997.
16. Resources MoN: Ontario Radar DSM, Metadata record, Geographic Information Branch, Science and Information Resources Division, Ministry of Natural Resources. Available at: https://www.javacoeapp.lrc.gov.on.ca/geonetwork/srv/en/main.home. Accessed on: 7 Feb 2017. 2012.
17. Statistics-Canada: The Lambert conformal conic map projection. Available at: http://www.statcan.gc.ca/pub/92-195-x/2011001/other-autre/mapproj-projcarte/m-c-eng.htm. Accessed on: 09 Feb 2017. 2015.
18. Generate Random Points. Available at: www.ianbroad.com. Accessed on 22 Feb 2017.
19. Stehman SV, Czaplewski RL. Design and analysis for thematic map accuracy assessment: fundamental principles. Remote Sens Environ. 1998;64(3):331–44.
20. Watson PF, Petrie A. Method agreement analysis: a review of correct methodology. Theriogenology. 2010;73(9):1167–79.
21. Fielding AH, Bell JF. A review of methods for the assessment of prediction errors in conservation presence/absence models. Environ Conserv. 1997;24(01):38–49.
22. OMAFRA: Provincial Premises Registry: Ontario Ministry of Agriculture, Food, and Rural Affairs. Available at: https://www.ontarioppr.com/home_en.html?font=M. Accessed on: 4th Mar 2017. 2012.
23. DeLong ER, DeLong DM, Clarke-Pearson DL. Comparing the areas under two or more correlated receiver operating characteristic curves: a nonparametric approach. Biometrics. 1988:837–45.
24. Allouche O, Tsoar A, Kadmon R. Assessing the accuracy of species distribution models: prevalence, kappa and the true skill statistic (TSS). J Appl Ecol. 2006; 43(6):1223–32.
25. Manel S, Williams HC, Ormerod SJ. Evaluating presence–absence models in ecology: the need to account for prevalence. J Appl Ecol. 2001;38(5):921–31.
26. Bruhn MC, Munoz B, Cajka J, Smith G, Curry RJ, Wagener DK, Wheaton WD: Synthesized population databases: A geospatial database of US poultry farms. RTI Press publication No. MR-0023-1201. Research Triangle Park, NC: RTI Press. Retrieved from https://www.rti.org/sites/default/files/resources/13649076_mr-0023-1201-bruhn.pdf. Accessed on: 3rd Oct 2016. In.; 2012.
27. Rorres C, Pelletier ST, Bruhn MC, Smith G. Ongoing estimation of the epidemic parameters of a stochastic, spatial, discrete-time model for a 1983-84 avian influenza epidemic. Avian Dis. 2011;55(1):35–42.
28. Fabiosa JF: Assessing the impact of the exchange rate and its volatility on Canadian pork and live swine exports to the United States and Japan. 2002.
29. Statistics-Canada: Census of Population and Agriculture, 1921 and 2011. In.
30. Council CP: Cull Breeding Swine Program: Annual Report For the Fiscal Year Ending March 31, 2010. Available from: http://www.cpc-ccp.com. Accessed on: 24 Oct 2016 2010.
31. Boklund A, Goldbach SG, Uttenthal A, Alban L. Simulating the spread of classical swine fever virus between a hypothetical wild-boar population and domestic pig herds in Denmark. Prev Vet Med. 2008;85(3–4):187–206.
32. Martínez-López B, Ivorra B, Ramos A, Sánchez-Vizcaíno JM. A novel spatial and stochastic model to evaluate the within-and between-farm transmission of classical swine fever virus. I. General concepts and description of the model. Vet Microbiol. 2011;147(3):300–9.
33. Kitching RP, Thrusfield MV, Taylor NM. Use and abuse of mathematical models: an illustration from the 2001 foot and mouth disease epidemic in the United Kingdom. Revue Scientifique et Technique-Office International des Epizooties. 2006;25(1):293.
34. Morris R, Wilesmith J, Stern M, Sanson R, Stevenson M. Predictive spatial modelling of alternative control strategies for the foot-and-mouth disease epidemic in great Britain, 2001. In: II international symposium on application of modelling as an innovative Technology in the Agri-Food Chain; MODEL-IT 566: 2001; 2001. p. 337–47.

13

Characterization and virulence clustering analysis of extraintestinal pathogenic *Escherichia coli* isolated from swine in China

Yinchu Zhu[1,2†], Wenyang Dong[1,2†], Jiale Ma[1,2], Lvfeng Yuan[1], Hassan M.A. Hejair[1,2], Zihao Pan[1,2], Guangjin Liu[1,2] and Huochun Yao[1,2*]

Abstract

Background: Swine extraintestinal pathogenic *Escherichia coli* (ExPEC) is an important pathogen that leads to economic and welfare costs in the swine industry worldwide, and is occurring with increasing frequency in China. By far, various virulence factors have been recognized in ExPEC. Here, we investigated the virulence genotypes and clonal structure of collected strains to improve the knowledge of phylogenetic traits of porcine ExPECs in China.

Results: We isolated 64 Chinese porcine ExPEC strains from 2013 to 14 in China. By multiplex PCR, the distribution of isolates belonging to phylogenetic groups B1, B2, A and D was 9.4%, 10.9%, 57.8% and 21.9%, respectively. Nineteen virulence-related genes were detected by PCR assay; *ompA*, *fimH*, *vat*, *traT* and *iutA* were highly prevalent. Virulence-related genes were remarkably more prevalent in group B2 than in groups A, B1 and D; notably, *usp*, *cnf1*, *hlyD*, *papA* and *ibeA* were only found in group B2 strains. Genotyping analysis was performed and four clusters of strains (named I to IV) were identified. Cluster IV contained all isolates from group B2 and Cluster IV isolates had the strongest pathogenicity in a mouse infection model. As phylogenetic group B2 and D ExPEC isolates are generally considered virulent, multilocus sequence typing (MLST) analysis was performed for these isolates to further investigate genetic relationships. Two novel sequence types, ST5170 and ST5171, were discovered. Among the nine clonal complexes identified among our group B2 and D isolates, CC12 and CC95 have been indicated to have high zoonotic pathogenicity. The distinction between group B2 and non-B2 isolates in virulence and genotype accorded with MLST analysis.

Conclusion: This study reveals significant genetic diversity among ExPEC isolates and helps us to better understand their pathogenesis. Importantly, our data suggest group B2 (Cluster IV) strains have the highest risk of causing animal disease and illustrate the correlation between genotype and virulence.

Keywords: Porcine extraintestinal pathogenic *Escherichia coli*, Genotype, Virulence, Multilocus sequence typing

Background

Extraintestinal pathogenic *Escherichia coli* (ExPEC) is a major pathogenic agent causing disease worldwide. It can lead to many kinds of extraintestinal diseases, including newborn meningitis, sepsis, and urinary tract disease [1]. It has been reported to cause death in animals and humans in Europe and North America [2, 3]. ExPEC can be distinguished from intestinal pathogenic *E. coli* and commensal *E. coli* by isolation site and genetic patterns [4]. Based on the isolation site, ExPEC can be classified as uropathogenic *E. coli* (UPEC), avian pathogenic *E. coli* (APEC), newborn meningitis *E. coli* (NMEC) or sepsis *E. coli* (SEPEC). The infectivity of ExPEC involves various extraintestinal virulence-associated factors in microbe-host interactions, rather than a simple mechanism [5]. Genome plasticity of ExPEC is the basis for rapid adaptation to the changing environment, which in turn increases the diversity of *E. coli* populations.

* Correspondence: yaohch@njau.edu.cn
†Equal contributors
1College of Veterinary Medicine, Nanjing Agricultural University, Nanjing 210095, China
2Key Lab of Animal Bacteriology, Ministry of Agriculture, Nanjing Agricultural University, Nanjing 210095, China

ExPEC is a major pathogen in the swine industry, responsible for considerable economic losses [6]. Alongside rapid development of industrial swine husbandry in China, an increasing trend of porcine ExPEC outbreaks has become an urgent problem [7]. Furthermore, the similarities in ExPEC isolates from human and animal infection cases suggest that there is cross-infection potential between different hosts, including humans, companion animals, pigs and birds [8]. I.e., ExPEC has high zoonotic potential, which makes porcine ExPEC a significant danger to public health.

E. coli consists of phylogenetic groups, namely A, B1, B2 and D. Most virulent ExPEC strains belong to group B2, followed by Group D. Generally, isolates assigned to groups A or B1 are less likely to cause disease in healthy animals [9]. The presence of virulence-related (VR) genes has a close connection with the virulence phenotype. Many genes have been identified as VR in ExPEC, and are involved in adhesion (P, S fimbriae, F1C fimbriae, Dr-binding adhesin and type I fimbriae), invasion (*ibeA*, invasive of brain endothelium), iron acquisition (siderophores), toxicity (hemolysin, vacuolating toxin, cytotoxic necrotizing factor) and surface protection (capsule) [10]. To identify combinations of VR genes associated with disease, the virulence genotyping method has previously been used in studies of UPEC [11]. However, such data is still limited for porcine ExPEC. In this study, we performed virulence genotyping, animal infection experiments and multilocus sequence typing (MLST) analysis, to provide insight into the associations between genotypes, phylogenetic groups and virulence phenotypes of ExPEC.

Results

Hemolytic activity tests

Of 64 tested ExPEC isolates, five produced β-hemolysin in 7% sheep blood agar, namely strains DCE-1, DCE-2, DCE-5, DCE-6, DCE-9.

Prevalence of VFs

The prevalence of VR genes was diverse (Additional file 1). *iutA, vat, fimH, traT* and *ompA* appeared in >60% of strains (*ompA* was observed in all isolates). Among adhesion factors, *fimH* was the most prevalent (81.2%). Among siderophore factors, *iutA* (60.9%) was more frequently detected than *fyuA, ireA* and *iroN*. The prevalence of *cnf1, focG, ibeA, kpsMIII, afa, hlyD, sfaA, papA* was <10%, and *focG* was not detected in any isolate. Table 1 shows these results in detail.

Phylogenetic group classification revealed that 9.4% (6/64) of the porcine ExPEC isolates belonged to group B1, 10.9% (7/64) to group B2, 57.8% (37/64) to group A and 21.9% (14/64) to group D. The phylogenetic group classification was associated with genetic patterns. The average number of VR genes in phylogenetic group B2 (12.1) was significantly higher than that in groups A (4.4), B1 (3.8), and D (4.3) (Fisher test, $P < 0.05$). *hlyD, ibeA, usp, cnf1, papA* were only observed in group B2 and *sfaA, afa* were only detected in group A. *ireA, papA, sfaA, afa, kpsMIII, ibeA* were rarely detected in any of the phylogenetic groups. Additional file 2: Table S1 shows statistical analysis of associations between virulence-associated factors.

Cluster structure analysis

Based on virulence gene profiles, four virulence clusters (I, II, III, IV) were identified using BioNumerics software according to a previous method (Fig. 1). Seven strains belonged to Cluster I, with an average of 2.43 virulence-associated genes per strain. Four stains belonged to Cluster II, with average of 2.7 virulence-associated genes. Cluster III contained 46 isolates, with an average of 4.92 virulence–associated genes. Cluster IV contained seven isolates with an average 12 virulence–associated genes. In general, the virulence of phylogenetic group B2 *E. coli* isolates is considered to be highest, followed by group D, which is in turn higher than that of phylogenetic groups A or B1 [12]. In this study, all phylogenetic group B2 isolates were found in Cluster IV. The dependency between Cluster IV and phylogenetic group B2 was significant (χ^2 test, $P < 0.05$), but no significance was found between other clusters and phylogenetic groups. In addition, it was always observed the number of virulence-associated genes in an isolate was significantly correlated with its phylogenetic group, thus B2 isolates contained more virulence-associated genes than non-B2 isolates (χ^2 test, $P < 0.05$). The prevalence of virulence-associated genes between clusters was also compared (Table 2), but no characteristic pattern was found for ExPEC. However, the presence of *hlyD, ibeA, usp, cnf1, papA* in Cluster IV is a difference from the other three clusters, indicating that those five genes are possible markers for the prediction of highly virulent ExPEC.

MLST analysis

Among 21 isolates belonging to phylogenetic groups D and B2, 13 different STs were identified, including 11 known STs (ST1011, ST354, ST788, ST405, ST117, ST12, ST95, ST961, ST141, ST648 and ST457) (Additional file 1). Two novel STs were identified in this study, namely, ST5170 and ST5171. Four STs included all seven B2 group isolates, namely ST12, ST961, ST141, and ST95. Other STs were found for group D

Table 1 Distribution of virulence factors classified according to phylogenetic group

Virulence factors	NO. of ExPEC isolates(%)				
	Total ($n = 64$;%)	Group A ($n = 37$;57.8%)	GroupB1 ($n = 6$;9.4%)	GroupB2 ($n = 7$;10.9%)	Group D ($n = 14$;21.9%)
Siderophores					
iutA	39(60.1)	24(64.9)[a]	1(16.7)[b]	7(100)[b]	7(50)[b]
iroN	17(26.6)	4(10.9)[a]	3(50)[b]	6(85.7)[b]	4(28.6)[b]
fyuA	15(23.4)	5(13.5)[a]	0(0)[a]	7(100)[b]	3(21.4)[c]
ireA	7(10.9)	3(8.1)	0(0)	1(14.3)	3(21.4)
Adhesins					
fimH	52(81.3)	23(62.2)	6(100)	7(103)	11(78.6)
papC	14(21.9)	5(13.5)[a]	1(16.7)[ab]	5(71.4)[b]	3(21.4)[b]
papA	3(4.7)	0(0)[a]	0(0)[ab]	3(42.9)[b]	0(0)[b]
sfaA	1(1.6)	1(2.7)	0(0)	0(0)	0(0)
hraA	13(20.3)	4(10.9)[a]	0(0)[a]	5(71.4)[b]	4(28.6)[b]
afa	3(4.7)	3(8.1)	0(0)	0(0)	0(0)
Toxin					
cnf1	5(7.8)	0(0)[a]	0(0)[a]	5(71.4)[b]	0(0)[c]
hlyD	5(7.8)	0(0)[a]	0(0)[a]	5(71.4)[b]	0(0)[c]
vat	42(65.6)	23(62.2)	4(66.7)	7(100)	8(57.1)
Miscellaneous					
ompA	64(100)	37(100)	6(100)	7(100)	14(100)
ups	7(10.9)	0(0)[a]	0(0)[a]	7(100)[b]	0(0)[c]
traT	40(62.5)	30(81.1)[a]	4(66.7)[ab]	3(42.9)[b]	3(21.4)[b]
Invasion					
ibeA	2(3.1)	0(0)[a]	0(0)[ab]	2(28.6)[b]	0(0)[b]
Capsule					
kpsMII	10(15.7)	0(0)[a]	0(0)[a]	7(100)[b]	3(21.4)[c]
kpsMIII	1(1.6)	0(0)	0(0)	0(0)	1(7.1)

a,b,c $P < 0.05$

isolates. To further analyze the phylogenetic relationships of these 21 ExPEC isolates, a phylogenetic tree were generated (Fig. 2). The phylogenetic analysis showed that the group B2 and group D isolates could each be grouped (Fig. 2). All isolates in the group B2 section of the tree were classified into Cluster IV in the virulence genotyping analysis; the isolates in the group D part of the tree were from Clusters I, II and III (Fig. 2).

eBURST analysis of these 21 isolates identified nine clonal complex (CCs), namely, CC1011, CC457, CC117, CC141, CC405, CC354, CC648, CC12 and CC95 (Fig. 3). ST774 is a single locus variant (SLV) of ST648, which is the primary founder of CC648. ST961 was connected to ST12 as a member of CC12. Three STs were not classified into any CCs, i.e., they were singletons (ST5170, ST788, and ST5171). Strains from CC12 and CC95 have been indicated to have strong pathogenicity and zoonotic potential (Table 3).

Virulence evaluation of representative ExPEC isolates

Seven group B2 strains selected from Cluster IV showed high virulence in a mouse infection model (Table 4): the mortalities varied from 60% (3/5) to 100% (5/5) at a challenge dose of 4×10^7 CFU; the mortalities were more diverse at a challenge dose of 4×10^6 CFU, but of particular note, isolate JX131101 caused 100% mortality (5/5), indicating high virulence. The 14 group D strains showed obvious diversity in virulence: PxECZ01C and PxECZF4d did not cause any mortality at a dose of 4×10^7 CFU, while strains SXE-20 and SXE-14 presented high virulence; all of group D strains have no pathogenicity at a challenge dose of 4×10^6 CFU. No abnormality was found in mice in the control group injected with PBS.

Discussion

The importance of ExPEC has been recognized, and many ExPEC related diseases in cows, humans and food have been reported in the North America and

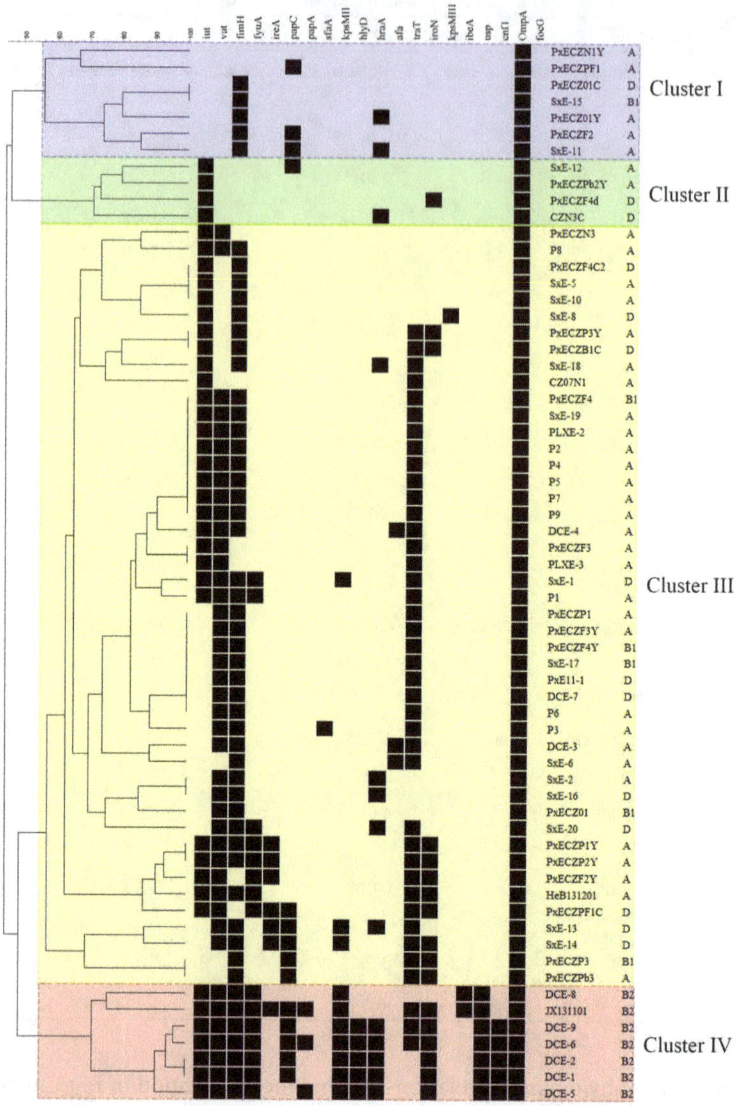

Fig. 1 Clustering of the 64 ExPEC isolates based on the presence or absence of virulence-associated factors. Each column shows the results for a single gene. *Black*: gene present; *blank*: gene absent

Europe. In China, ExPEC has become a frequent pathogen in the swine industry [13, 14]. However, understanding of the pathogenesis and epidemiology of porcine ExPEC is still limited. Some reports showed that >50% of ExPEC isolates from swine belong to phylogenetic groups A and B1 [15], which is consistent with our results. In this study, only a few isolates were classified as phylogenetic group B2, which is an obvious contrast with the fact that most ExPECs isolated from humans or companion animals belong to groups B2 and D [3]. In this study, the isolates were considered as ExPEC based organ origin. Johnson et al [16] proposed a molecular approach to delimit ExPEC, by considering the presence of 2 of the 5 virulence markers (*papA/papC, sfa/foc, afa/dra, iutA* and *kpsMTII*) in an *E. coli* strain as ExPEC. According to this criterion, 13 of 69 strains in this study were identified as ExPEC, which contained all 7 B2 strains (Additional file 3: Table S3). Notably, the prevalence of ExPEC that qualified to criterion was larger within high virulence strains (9/12, 75%; mortality ≥ 3) than within low virulence strains (2/9, 22.2%; mortality ≤ 2) in the mouse infection model. This indicated that Johnson's criterion is more strict and selective compared to the robust standard we used in this study, and is able to identify strains with a higher potential to cause diseases.

A single virulence factor does not determine bacterial pathogenicity. Thus, in this study, 19 major virulence-associated genes of ExPEC were selected

Table 2 Distribution of virulence factors classified according to clusters

Virulence factors	NO. of ExPEC isolates(%)				
	Total ($n = 64$;%)	Cluster I ($n = 7$;10.9%)	Cluster II ($n = 4$;6.25%)	Cluster III ($n = 46$;71.9%)	Cluster IV ($n = 7$;10.9%)
Siderophores					
iutA	39(60.1)	$0(0)^{a}$	$4(100)^{b}$	$28(60.1)^{b}$	$7(100)^{b}$
iroN	17(26.6)	$0(0)^{a}$	$1(25)^{ab}$	$10(21.7)^{a}$	$6(85.7)^{b}$
fyuA	15(23.4)	$0(0)^{a}$	$0(0)^{a}$	$8(17.4)^{a}$	$7(100)^{b}$
ireA	7(10.9)	0(0)	0(0)	6(13)	1(14.3)
Adhesins					
fimH	52(81.3)	$5(71.4)^{ac}$	$0(0)^{b}$	$40(86.9)^{c}$	$7(100)^{c}$
papC	14(21.9)	3(42.9)	1(25)	5(10.9)	5(71,4)
papA	3(4.7)	0(0)	0(0)	0(0)	3(42.9)
sfaA	1(1.6)	0(0)	0(0)	1(2.2)	0(0)
hraA	13(20.3)	2(28.6)	1(25)	5(10.9)	5(71.4)
afa	3(4.7)	0(0)	0(0)	3(6.5)	0(0)
Toxin					
cnf1	5(7.8)	$0(0)^{a}$	$0(0)^{a}$	$0(0)^{a}$	$5(71.4)^{b}$
hlyD	5(7.8)	$0(0)^{a}$	$0(0)^{a}$	$0(0)^{a}$	$5(71.4)^{b}$
vat	42(65.6)	$0(0)^{a}$	$0(0)^{a}$	$35(76.1)^{b}$	$7(100)^{b}$
Miscellaneous					
ompA	64(100)	7(100)	4(100)	46(100)	7(100)
ups	7(10.9)	$0(0)^{a}$	$0(0)^{a}$	$0(0)^{a}$	$7(100)^{b}$
traT	40(62.5)	$0(0)^{a}$	$0(0)^{a}$	$37(80.4)^{b}$	$3(42.9)^{b}$
Invasion					
ibeA	2(3.1)	0(0)	0(0)	0(0)	2(28.6)
Capsule					
kpsMIII	1(1.6)	0(0)	0(0)	1(2.2)	0(0)
kpsMII	10(15.7)	$0(0)^{a}$	$0(0)^{a}$	$3(6.5)^{a}$	$7(100)^{b}$

a,b,c $P < 0.05$

for a comprehensive analysis with phylogenetic investigation, aiming to reveal genotypic traits related to virulence. These 19 virulence-associated genes contribute to the fitness of ExPEC and increase its adaptability and competitiveness in colonizing host animals. Four clusters were identified in the genotyping analysis. Cluster IV included only B2 group isolates and showed a higher prevalence of virulence-associated genes than the other three clusters. Animal infection experiments confirmed higher virulence of isolates from Cluster IV, which is consistent with B2 group strains leading to serious diseases [17]. The distinction between B2 and non-B2 ExPEC is clear, shown by MLST, virulence genotyping and virulence assessment. In addition, group D ExPEC isolates are considered to be more pathogenic than groups A and B1, although in this study some group D strains presented similar virulence to group A or B1 isolates. Furthermore, group D isolates were mixed with group A and B1 isolates in Clusters I, II and III in the genotyping analysis. In MLST analysis, no obvious correlations were observed with genotypic cluster virulence in group D strains. Group D isolates thus present high diversity in genotype and phenotype.

MLST analysis can provide other information besides phylogenetic relationships [18]. After comparing our results with the MLST database (http://pubmlst.org/), we found STs in this study that have been reported to be present in diseases of birds, dogs and humans. For example, strain JX131101 belonged to ST95 in CC95; ST95 is the most important pathogenic sequence type in human-associated cases [19]. ST95 isolates are frequently reported to be related to newborn meningitis (NM) and uropathogenic infection (UTI) in Europe and the North America [20, 21]. Group D isolate CZN3C is assigned to ST354, which

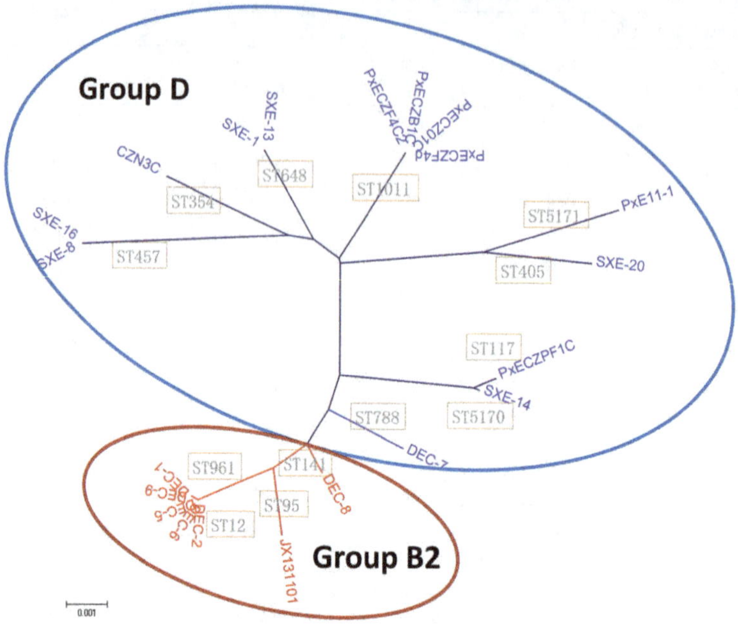

Fig. 2 Phylogenetic organization of group B2 and D isolates of different multi locus sequence types based on the neighbor-joining method. Numbers at the nodes are bootstrap values and the *bar* represents 0.001 nucleotide changes. Group B2 strains gather together (*red circle*), as do group D strains (*blue circle*)

is a common ST type in isolates causing UTI and NM in humans, companion animals and swine [22, 23]. Some ST1011 isolates lead to UTI in avians and companion animals [24], but several group D ST1011 isolates showed low virulence in this study. Our data suggest that isolates from the same ST can have different pathogenic phenotypes, and indicate the diversity and complexity of pathogenic *E. coli*.

A study by Tan *et al.* showed that *fimH, traT* and *iutA* were highly prevalent in porcine ExPEC isolates, which is in consistent with our results, but the prevalence of *fyuA*, *cnf1*, *kpsMTII,* and *iroN* differ between our study and theirs; the *focG* gene was not detected in any isolates in this study, which is similar to Tan's research [25]. Interestingly, the results of VR gene detection in ExPEC isolates from retail pork is quite different from that from pigs on farms [26]. This suggests that *E. coli* strains isolated from pork may originate from processes such as meat production or transportation.

We found five VR genes to be highly prevalent specifically in Cluster IV (which contained only group B2 isolates), namely *papA, hlyD, usp, ibeA* and *cnf1*, suggesting that these five genes may be closely related to strong pathogenicity. This result contains a risk factor that similar geographical of B2 isolated in this study might lead to a prevalence bias of virulence factors. Both *hlyD* and *cnf1* are well-known toxin genes in ExPEC. *ibeA* is associated with neonatal meningitis [27] and is an important virulence-associated factor widely distributed among APEC and NMEC [28]. *usp*, the uropathogenic-specific gene, was reported in a large number of strains from patients and animals with pyelonephritis or prostatitis [29]. Both our results and a previous study of virulence genotypes of canine ExPEC [11] indicate that *cnf1, hlyD, ups* and *kpsMII* could be possible marker genes for high virulence in ExPEC, although this point still needs to be verified in further study or using a larger collection of ExPEC isolates.

Conclusions

In this study, a total of 19 VR genes in 64 Chinese porcine ExPEC strains were detected by PCR. Based on VR gene profiles, those isolates were divided into four clusters (named I to IV). Notably, all Cluster IV isolates were from group B2, and VR genes were remarkably more prevalent in group B2 than in groups A, B1 and D. The distinction between group B2 and non-B2 isolates in virulence and genotype accorded with MLST analysis. Considering Cluster IV isolates had the strongest pathogenicity in a mouse infection model, genes that were only found in group B2 strains (that *cnf1, hlyD, ups* and *kpsMII*) could be possible marker genes for high virulence in ExPEC. This study revealed the genetic differences between

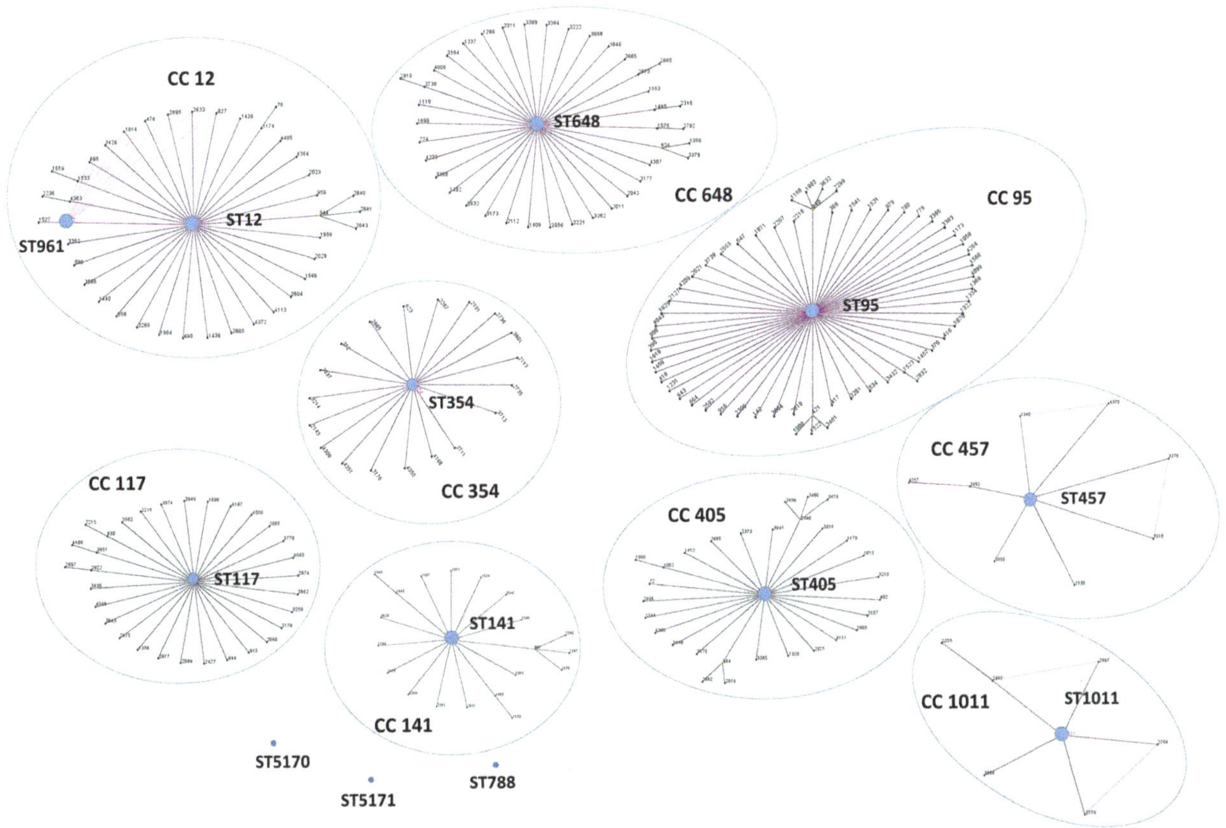

Fig. 3 eBURST analysis of 13 STs of porcine extraintestinal *Escherichia coli*. The clonal structure of ExPEC is demonstrated by eBURST plots based on the profile of seven allelic housekeeping genes. Two STs differing in one locus but sharing the other six loci constitute a single locus variant (SLV); a double locus variant (DLV) means the STs contain two different loci. STs that did not include any SLVs with others are termed singletons. We observed nine main clonal complexes (CCs; CC12, CC648, CC354, CC141, CC405, CC457, CC1011, CC117 and CC95), and three singletons (ST788, ST5170 and ST5171). Strains from the same ancestor are grouped together in *blue circles*

porcine ExPEC strains from China and enlarges the knowledge of the porcine ExPEC virulence.

Methods

Bacterial isolation and culture conditions

From April 2013 to August 2014, a total of 64 ExPEC strains were isolated from clinically diseased pigs in five provinces (Jiangsu, Zhejiang, Shandong, Hebei, Shanxi and Jiangxi) of China (Additional file 4: Table S2). All the isolates were recovered from extraintestinal organs, including spleen, lung, liver, kidney and brain, and MacConkey agar was used for initial purification. Isolates were grown in Luria-Bertani broth for 6 h and then stored in 50% glycerol at −70 °C until further characterization.

Hemolytic activity tests

The hemolytic activities of clinical ExPEC isolates were determined by culture on 7% sheep blood agar. The formation of beta-hemolysin was observed.

PCR detection of virulence-related genes and phylogenetic group identification

The genomic DNA of bacteria was extracted using an E.Z.N.A. bacterial DNA kit (Omega, Beijing, China) following the manufacturer's instructions. Individual PCR assays were performed for 19 ExPEC VR genes, including *kpsMII, kpsMIII, iroN, fyuA, ireA, iutA, papC, hra, sfaS, papA, fimH, afa, hlyD, vat, cnf1, ompA, traT, usp* and *ibeA*. The phylogenetic group was determined by multiplex PCR with three pairs of primers, *chuA, yjaA* and *TspE4.C2* [30]. All PCR primers used in this study are listed in Table 5.

Cluster analysis of virulence genotype

The presence or absence of putative virulence-associated genes among isolates was visualized using BioNumerics (version 6.6, Applied Maths, Kortrijk, Belgium) to study similarity among isolates, according to the method applied in a previous report [11]. These data were analyzed using a simple matching coefficient. Cluster analysis was performed by the

Table 3 Sequence types and clonal complex of group D and B2 isolates

Sequence type (ST)	Strains	Clusters	Clonal complex
ST1011	PxECZ01C	Cluster I	CC1011
ST1011	PxECZF4d	Cluster II	CC1011
ST354	CZN3C	Cluster II	CC354
ST1011	PxECZB1C	Cluster III	CC1011
ST1011	PxECZF4C2	Cluster III	CC1011
ST457	SXE-8	Cluster III	CC457
ST648	SXE-1	Cluster III	CC648
ST648	SXE-13	Cluster III	CC648
ST5171	PxE11-1	Cluster III	None
ST788	DCE-7	Cluster III	None
ST457	SXE-16	Cluster III	CC457
ST405	SXE-20	Cluster III	CC405
ST117	PxECZPF1C	Cluster III	CC117
ST5170	SXE-14	Cluster III	None
ST961	DCE-9	Cluster IV	CC12
ST961	DCE-1	Cluster IV	CC12
ST12	DCE-6	Cluster IV	CC12
ST12	DCE-2	Cluster IV	CC12
ST12	DCE-5	Cluster IV	CC12
ST141	DCE-8	Cluster IV	CC141
ST95	JX131101	Cluster IV	CC95

Table 4 Experimental virulence of representative isolates in BALB/c mice

Clusters	Strains	Mortality		Phylogenetic groups	Virulence
		4×10^7	4×10^6		
Cluster I	PxECZ01C	0/5	0/5	D	None virulence
Cluster II	PxECZF4d	0/5	0/5	D	None virulence
Cluster II	CZN3C	2/5	0/5	D	Less virulence
Cluster III	PxECZF4C2	1/5	0/5	D	Less virulence
Cluster III	SXE-8	3/5	0/5	D	Less virulence
Cluster III	PxECZB1C	2/5	0/5	D	Less virulence
Cluster III	SXE-1	2/5	0/5	D	Less virulence
Cluster III	PxE11-1	2/5	0/5	D	Less virulence
Cluster III	DCE-7	1/5	0/5	D	Less virulence
Cluster III	SXE-16	3/5	0/5	D	Less virulence
Cluster III	SXE-20	4/5	0/5	D	Less virulence
Cluster III	PxECZPF1C	3/5	0/5	D	Less virulence
Cluster III	SXE-13	1/5	0/5	D	Less virulence
Cluster III	SXE-14	5/5	1/5	D	Virulence
Cluster IV	DCE-9	3/5	0/5	B2	Less virulence
Cluster IV	DCE-6	4/5	1/5	B2	Virulence
Cluster IV	DCE-2	3/5	0/5	B2	Less virulence
Cluster IV	DCE-5	4/5	3/5	B2	Virulence
Cluster IV	DCE-1	4/5	2/5	B2	Virulence
Cluster IV	DCE-8	4/5	2/5	B2	Virulence
Cluster IV	JX131101	5/5	5/5	B2	Virulence
	PBS	No mortality			

All these strains were able to kill BALB/c mice in doses of 10^8 cfu, including PxECZ01C and PxECZF4d

unweighted pair group method using arithmetic averages (UPGMA).

Multilocus sequence typing

MLST is a useful method to track genetic variation of microbes and survey epidemics. It provides an accurate and highly discriminatory genotyping system for bacteria. In this study, group D and group B2 ExPEC isolates were used to perform MLST tests. The DNA fragments of seven housekeeping genes (*purA, fumC, icd, mdh, recA, gyrB* and *adk*) were amplified by PCR and the products were sequenced. Allele sequence determination was performed using the *E. coli* MLST database (http://mlst.ucc.ie/mlst/dbs/E. coli). Any new alleles (i.e. those not recognized by the *E. coli* MLST system) were submitted to the database curator to be assigned new allele numbers. Sequence types (STs) were identified based on the allele profiles.

Phylogenetic analyses were conducted on the basis of the concatenation of seven MLST loci (*purA, fumC, icd, mdh, recA, gyrB* and *adk*) using the MEGA v4.1 software as previously described [31]. The result is presented as a neighbour-joining tree; the robustness of the groupings was assessed by bootstrap resampling of 1,000 replicates. eBURST (http://eburst.mlst.net) analysis was also performed to identify potential clonal complexes (CCs) and founders [18], and the overall population structures were determined.

Statistical analysis

The prevalence of VR genes in ExPEC isolates in different clusters was compared using Fisher's exact test (Statistica 5.0, StatSoft Inc., Tulsa, OK, USA). A chi-square test (χ^2 test) was used to calculate the correlation between clusters, phylogenetic groups and the quantity of virulence-associated genes. Results were considered significant if $P < 0.05$.

Animal infection experiments

E. coli strains belonging to groups D and B2 have a higher risk of causing severe disease. Using the results of genotype clustering, 21 group D and B2 ExPEC strains were tested in a mouse infection model. All

Table 5 Virulence genes primers for PCR in this study

PCR assay	Gene	Primer sequence	PCR product size/bp
Virulence-associated genes	*papA*	ATGGCAGTGGTGTCTTTTGGTG	717
		CGTCCCACCATACGTGCTCTTC	
	papC	GTGGCAGTATGAGTAATGACCGTTA	203
		ATATCCTTTCTGCAGGGATGCAATA	
	iutA	ATCGGCTGGACATCATGGGAAC	314
		CGCATTTACCGTCGGGAACGG	
	vat	CTTACCTCTCTGGCACTATCTG	1021
		GTCAGTGAACCGGCACC	
	fimH	TGCAGAACGGATAAGCCGTGG	508
		GCAGTCACCTGCCCTCCGGTA	
	fyuA	TGATTAACCCCGCGACGGGAA	787
		CGCAGTAGGCACGATGTTGTA	
	ireA	GATGACTCAGCCACGGGTAA	254
		CCAGGACTCACCTCACGAAT	
	kpsMTII	GCGCATTTGCTGATACTGTTG	272
		CATCCAGACGATAAGCATGAGCA	
	hlyD	CTCCGGTACGTGAAAAGGAC	904
		GCCCTGATTACTGAAGCCTG	
	sfaS	GTCTCTCACCGGATGCCAGAATAT	240
		GCATTACTTCCATCCCTGTCCTG	
	hra	GTAACTCACACTGCTGTCACCT	139
		CGAATCGTTGTCACGTTCAG	
	cnf1	CTTTACAATATTGACATGCTG	446
		TCGTTATAAAATCAAACAGTG	
	afa	TAAGGAAGTGAAGGAGCGTG	210
		CCGCCCTGAAGAAGTATCAC	
	kpsMTIII	TCCTCTTGCTACTATTCCCCCT	392
		AGGCGTATCCATCCCTCCTAAC	
	ibeA	AATGAGTGCCGCTCGTGAAGG	548
		CCCCCCAGTCTCCATATTTAG	
	iroN	CTCCGACGATGATAATGACGA	440
		TGGGACGTTTGGTAATGATGT	
	ompA	GATCAGTGCAGCACGCTGTTT	385
		GGGCGAAGCAGCTCCAGTAG	
	traT	CGATGAGCACAGCAATCAAGA	486
		CATTATCCGTTGTCACCGTTG	
	usp	GAGCGGTTATTTATTGAAATC	448
		CACAGCAGTCATCAACCACTG	

isolates tested were grown in LB medium with shaking at 37 °C for about 4–5 h to reach a concentration of 10^9 CFU/ml.

A total of 215 female BALB/c mice (5-weeks-old) were purchased from the Comparative Medicine Center of Yangzhou University. Mice were housed in the Animal Experimental Center of Nanjing Agricultural University, by a full-time staff. Temperature and humidity are controlled, food and water are accessible. The mice were divided into 43 groups, five mice per group. Mice in groups 1 to 42 were inoculated with the 21 selected strains by intraperitoneal injection (0.2 mL) at doses of 4×10^6 or 4×10^7 CFU per mouse. Group 43 was the uninoculated control and received phosphate buffered saline (PBS). The mice were monitored for survival twice a day for 1 week.

Additional files

Additional file 1: MLST and VR genes profiles. (XLSX 16 kb)

Additional file 2: Table S1. Statistical analysis of associations between virulence-associated factores(VFs). *P* values by Fisher's exact test, shown only where < .10. *P* < .10 reflects statistical significance ;*P* values between .01 and .05 reflect possible statistical significance. (DOCX 19 kb)

Additional file 3: Table S2. The isolation sources of strains in this study. (DOCX 18 kb)

Additional file 4: Table S3. The information of isolates identified as ExPEC with Johnson et al's criterion (DOCX 15 kb)

Abbreviations

ExPEC: Extraintestinal pathogenic *Escherichia coli*; MLST: Multilocus sequence typing; VR: Virulence-related

Acknowledgements

We would like to thank Dr. Xian Qi and Dr. Chen Dong (Jiangsu Provincial Center for Disease Control and Prevention) for their help in using BioNumerics software.

Funding

This work was supported by grants from the National Nature Science Foundation of China (No. 31372455) and the project funded by the Priority Academic Program Development of Jiangsu Higher Education Institutions (PAPD).

Authors' contributions

HY conceived and designed the experiments. YZ, WD, LY, JM and MA performed the experiments. GL contributed materials and analysis tools. YZ, JM, and ZP analyzed the data. YZ and WD drafted the manuscript. ZP and HY revised the manuscript. HY coordinated the study. All authors have read and approved the final manuscript version.

Competing interests

The authors declare that they have no competing interests.

References

1. Johnson JR, Johnston B, Clabots CR, Kuskowski MA, Roberts E, DebRoy C. Virulence genotypes and phylogenetic background of Escherichia coli serogroup O6 isolates from humans, dogs, and cats. J Clin Microbiol. 2008;46(2):417–22.
2. Dezfulian H, Batisson I, Fairbrother JM, Lau PCK, Nassar A, Szatmari G, Harel J. Presence and characterization of extraintestinal pathogenic Escherichia coli virulence genes in F165-positive E-coli strains isolated from diseased calves and pigs. J Clin Microbiol. 2003;41(4):1375–85.

3. Maynard C, Bekal S, Sanschagrin F, Levesque RC, Brousseau R, Masson L, Lariviere S, Harel J. Heterogeneity among virulence and antimicrobial resistance gene profiles of extraintestinal Escherichia coli isolates of animal and human origin. J Clin Microbiol. 2004;42(12):5444–52.
4. Kohler CD, Dobrindt U. What defines extraintestinal pathogenic Escherichia coli? Int J Med Microbiol. 2011;301(8):642–7.
5. Picard B, Garcia JS, Gouriou S, Duriez P, Brahimi N, Bingen E, Elion J, Denamur E. The link between phylogeny and virulence in Escherichia coli extraintestinal infection. Infect Immun. 1999;67(2):546–53.
6. Russo TA, Johnson JR. Medical and economic impact of extraintestinal infections due to Escherichia coli: focus on an increasingly important endemic problem. Microbes Infect. 2003;5(5):449–56.
7. Normile D. Infectious diseases - WHO probes deadliness of China's pig-borne disease. Science. 2005;309(5739):1308–9.
8. Moulin-Schouleur M, Schouler C, Tailliez P, Kao MR, Bree A, Germon P, Oswald E, Mainil J, Blanco M, Blanco J. Common virulence factors and genetic relationships between O18: K1: H7 Escherichia coli isolates of human and avian origin. J Clin Microbiol. 2006;44(10):3484–92.
9. Boerlin P, Travis R, Gyles CL, Reid-Smith R, Janecko N, Lim H, Nicholson V, McEwen SA, Friendship R, Archambault M. Antimicrobial resistance and virulence genes of Escherichia coli isolates from swine in Ontario. Appl Environ Microbiol. 2005;71(11):6753–61.
10. Johnson JR, Delavari P, Kuskowski M, Stell AL. Phylogenetic distribution of extraintestinal virulence-associated traits in Escherichia coli. J Infect Dis. 2001;183(1):78–88.
11. Mateus L, Henriques S, Merino C, Pomba C, da Costa LL, Silva E. Virulence genotypes of Escherichia coli canine isolates from pyometra, cystitis and fecal origin. Vet Microbiol. 2013;166(3-4):590–4.
12. Moreno E, Prats G, Planells I, Planes AM, Perez T, Andreu A. Characterization of Escherichia coli isolates derived from phylogenetic groups A and B1 causing extraintestinal infection. Enferm Infecc Microbiol Clin. 2006;24(8):483–9.
13. Tang X, Tan C, Zhang X, Zhao Z, Xia X, Wu B, Guo A, Zhou R, Chen H. Antimicrobial resistances of extraintestinal pathogenic Escherichia coli isolates from swine in China. Microb Pathog. 2011;50(5):207–12.
14. Liu C, Chen Z, Tan C, Liu W, Xu Z, Zhou R, Chen H. Immunogenic characterization of outer membrane porins OmpC and OmpF of porcine extraintestinal pathogenic Escherichia coli. FEMS Microbiol Lett. 2012;337(2):104–11.
15. Ding Y, Tang X, Lu P, Wu B, Xu Z, Liu W, et al. Clonal analysis and virulent traits of pathogenic extraintestinal Escherichia coli isolates from swine in China. BMC veterinary research. 2012;8:140.
16. Johnson JR, Murray AC, Gajewski A, Sullivan M, Snippes P, Kuskowski MA, Smith KE. Isolation and molecular characterization of nalidixic acid-resistant extraintestinal pathogenic Escherichia coli from retail chicken products. Antimicrob Agents Chemother. 2003;47(7):2161–8.
17. Vangchhia B, Abraham S, Bell JM, Collignon P, Gibson JS, Ingram PR, et al. Phylogenetic diversity, antimicrobial susceptibility and virulence characteristics of phylogroup F Escherichia coli in Australia. Microbiol. 2016;162(11):1904–12.
18. Feil EJ, Li BC, Aanensen DM, Hanage WP, Spratt BG. eBURST: Inferring patterns of evolutionary descent among clusters of related bacterial genotypes from multilocus sequence typing data. J Bacteriol. 2004; 186(5):1518–30.
19. Tivendale KA, Logue CM, Kariyawasam S, Jordan D, Hussein A, Li G, Wannemuehler Y, Nolan LK. Avian-pathogenic Escherichia coli strains are similar to neonatal meningitis E. coli strains and are able to cause meningitis in the rat model of human disease. Infect Immun. 2010; 78(8):3412–9.
20. Moriel DG, Bertoldi I, Spagnuolo A, Marchi S, Rosini R, Nesta B, Pastorello I, Corea VA, Torricelli G, Cartocci E, et al. Identification of protective and broadly conserved vaccine antigens from the genome of extraintestinal pathogenic Escherichia coli. Proc Natl Acad Sci U S A. 2010;107(20):9072–7.
21. Bauchart P, Germon P, Bree A, Oswald E, Hacker J, Dobrindt U. Pathogenomic comparison of human extraintestinal and avian pathogenic Escherichia coli–search for factors involved in host specificity or zoonotic potential. Microb Pathog. 2010;49(3):105–15.
22. Guo S, Wakeham D, Brouwers HJ, Cobbold RN, Abraham S, Mollinger JL, Johnson JR, Chapman TA, Gordon DM, Barrs VR, et al. Human-associated fluoroquinolone-resistant Escherichia coli clonal lineages, including ST354, isolated from canine feces and extraintestinal infections in Australia. Microbes Infect / Institut Pasteur. 2015;17(4):266–74.
23. Mora A, Blanco M, Lopez C, Mamani R, Blanco JE, Alonso MP, Garcia-Garrote F, Dahbi G, Herrera A, Fernandez A, et al. Emergence of clonal groups O1: HNM-D-ST59, O15:H1-D-ST393, O20:H34/HNM-D-ST354, O25b:H4-B2-ST131 and ONT:H21,42-B1-ST101 among CTX-M-14-producing Escherichia coli clinical isolates in Galicia, northwest Spain. Int J Antimicrob Agents. 2011;37(1):16–21.
24. Maluta RP, Logue CM, Casas MR, Meng T, Guastalli EA, Rojas TC, et al. Overlapped sequence types (STs) and serogroups of avian pathogenic (APEC) and human extra-intestinal pathogenic (ExPEC) Escherichia coli isolated in Brazil. Plos One. 2014;9(8):e105016.
25. Tan C, Tang X, Zhang X, Ding Y, Zhao Z, Wu B, Cai X, Liu Z, He Q, Chen H. Serotypes and virulence genes of extraintestinal pathogenic Escherichia coli isolates from diseased pigs in China. Vet J. 2012;192(3):483–8.
26. Xia X, Meng J, Zhao S, Bodeis-Jones S, Gaines SA, Ayers SL, McDermott PF. Identification and antimicrobial resistance of extraintestinal pathogenic Escherichia coli from retail meats. J Food Prot. 2011;74(1):38–44.
27. Bingen E, Picard B, Brahimi N, Mathy S, Desjardins P, Elion J, Denamur E. Phylogenetic analysis of Escherichia coli strains causing neonatal meningitis suggests horizontal gene transfer from a predominant pool of highly virulent B2 group strains. J Infect Dis. 1998;177(3):642–50.
28. Germon P, Chen YH, He L, Blanco JE, Bree A, Schouler C, Huang SH, Moulin-Schouleur M. ibeA, a virulence factor of avian pathogenic Escherichia coli. Microbiol-Sgm. 2005;151:1179–86.
29. Rijavec M, Muller-Premru M, Zakotnik B, Zgur-Bertok D. Virulence factors and biofilm production among Escherichia coli strains causing bacteraemia of urinary tract origin. J Med Microbiol. 2008;57(11):1329–34.
30. Clermont O, Bonacorsi S, Bingen E. Rapid and simple determination of the Escherichia coli phylogenetic group. Appl Environ Microbiol. 2000; 66(10):4555–8.
31. Wang Y, Zhu J, Lu C, Wu B, Liu D, Hang W, Liu H, Liu X. Evidence of circulation of an epidemic strain of Pasteurella multocida in Jiangsu, China by multi-locus sequence typing (MLST). Infect Genet Evol. 2013;20:34–8.

14

Pigs immunized with a novel E2 subunit vaccine are protected from subgenotype heterologous classical swine fever virus challenge

Rachel Madera[1†], Wenjie Gong[1,5†], Lihua Wang[1], Yulia Burakova[1,4], Karen Lleellish[1], Amy Galliher-Beckley[1], Jerome Nietfeld[2], Jamie Henningson[2], Kaimin Jia[3], Ping Li[3], Jianfa Bai[2], John Schlup[4], Scott McVey[6], Changchun Tu[5*] and Jishu Shi[1*]

Abstract

Background: Classical swine fever (CSF) or hog cholera is a highly contagious swine viral disease. CSF endemic countries have to use routine vaccination with modified live virus (MLV) vaccines to prevent and control CSF. However, it is impossible to serologically differentiate MLV vaccinated pigs from those infected with CSF virus (CSFV). The aim of this study is to develop a one-dose E2-subunit vaccine that can provide protection against CSFV challenge. We hypothesize that a vaccine consisting of a suitable adjuvant and recombinant E2 with natural conformation may induce a similar level of protection as the MLV vaccine.

Results: Our experimental vaccine KNB-E2 was formulated with the recombinant E2 protein (Genotype 1.1) expressed by insect cells and an oil-in-water emulsion based adjuvant. 10 pigs (3 weeks old, 5 pigs/group) were immunized intramuscularly with one dose or two doses (3 weeks apart) KNB-E2, and 10 more control pigs were administered normal saline solution only. Two weeks after the second vaccination, all KNB-E2 vaccinated pigs and 5 control pigs were challenged with 5×10^5 $TCID_{50}$ CSFV Honduras/1997 (Genotype 1.3, 1 ml intramuscular, 1 ml intranasal). It was found that while control pigs infected with CSFV stopped growing and developed high fever (>40 °C), high level CSFV load in blood and nasal fluid, and severe leukopenia 3–14 days post challenge, all KNB-E2 vaccinated pigs continued to grow as control pigs without CSFV exposure, did not show any fever, had low or undetectable level of CSFV in blood and nasal fluid. At the time of CSFV challenge, only pigs immunized with KNB-E2 developed high levels of E2-specific antibodies and anti-CSFV neutralizing antibodies.

Conclusions: Our studies provide direct evidence that pigs immunized with one dose KNB-E2 can be protected clinically from CSFV challenge. This protection is likely mediated by high levels of E2-specific and anti-CSFV neutralizing antibodies.

Keywords: Classical swine fever, Vaccine, E2, Adjuvant, CSF, CSFV, KNB-E2

Abbreviations: CSF, Classical swine fever; MLV, Modified live virus; CSFV, Classical swine fever virus; $TCID_{50}$, 50 % tissue culture infective dose; DIVA, Differentiation of infected from vaccinated animals; HCLV, Hog cholera lapinised virus; WBC, White blood cells; PBS, Phosphate-buffered saline; DPV, Days post vaccination; DPC, Days post challenge; ELISA, Enzyme-linked immunosorbent assay; VNA, Virus neutralizing antibody; β-ME, β-mercaptoethanol

* Correspondence: changchun_tu@hotmail.com; jshi@vet.k-state.edu
[†]Equal contributors
[5]Institute of Military Veterinary Medicine, Academy of Military Medical Sciences, Changchun, China
[1]Department of Anatomy and Physiology, Kansas State University, Manhattan, KS 66506, USA
Full list of author information is available at the end of the article

Background

Classical swine fever (CSF) or hog cholera, causes severe economic losses to the swine industry worldwide and presents a significant agro-security threat to CSF free countries such as the U.S. CSF is a highly contagious viral disease of swine, including wild (feral) pigs. CSF is caused by an enveloped Pestivirus named classical swine fever virus (CSFV) [1]. The CSFV genome consists of a single, positive-stranded RNA of approximately 12.3 kb encoding a polyprotein of 3898 amino acids. The translated polyprotein is processed by viral as well as cellular proteases to the mature forms of four structural (C, E^{rns}, E1, and E2) and eight nonstructural viral proteins (N^{pro}, p7, NS2, NS3, NS4A, NS4B, NS5A, and NS5B) [2].

The genotypes of CSF viruses can be classified into three major groups with eleven subgroups [3–5]. Group 1 (1.1, 1.2, 1.3, & 1.4) contains primarily historical strains isolated from many regions of the world and includes all live-attenuated vaccine strains. Group 2 (2.1, 2.2, & 2.3) contains most of the currently circulating strains, whose prevalence has increased and caused epidemic infection since the 1980s. Group 3 (3.1, 3.2, 3.3, & 3.4) contains most of the strains distributed in separated geographic regions such as Taiwan, Korea, Japan, Thailand and the United Kingdom. Recent phylogenetic analyses have indicated a "switch" of field CSFV from the historical group 1 or 3 to the more recently prevalent group 2 in Europe and Asia [6, 7].

In contrast to the non-vaccination and stamping-out policy in CSF-free zones, CSF endemic countries have to use routine vaccination to prevent and control CSF. When used properly, vaccination can be an effective approach to limit transmission of the CSFV, prevent disease outbreaks, and establish protective immunity in naïve pig populations. To date, three types of CSF vaccines have been developed commercially: 1) modified live virus (MLV) vaccines which are manufactured and widely used in CSF endemic countries [8, 9]; 2) subunit vaccines based on CSF viral envelope protein E2 [10–13] , and 3) a chimeric live recombinant viral vector vaccine [14–17]. Although they are important tools for CSF outbreak control, better CSF vaccines are needed for the U.S. to maintain the CSF-free status because of the intrinsic limitations of the current commercial vaccines.

MLV CSF vaccines are generally safe and effective. However, it is impossible to serologically differentiate MLV vaccinated pigs from those infected with CSFV. Thus, a long and costly non-vaccination and stamping-out eradication process would have to be followed if MLV are the only vaccines available. In addition, it would be unsafe and costly to manufacture MLV vaccines in CSF-free countries such as the U.S. In 2015, Suvaxyn CSF Marker, a chimeric CSF vaccine that contains live bovine viral diarrhea virus (BVDV) which has been modified to express CSF E2 gene was approved by the European Union. However, Suvaxyn CSF Marker is approved only for emergency vaccination (page 6 in SUMMARY OF PRODUCT CHARACTERISTICS, http://ec.europa.eu/health/documents/community-register/2016/20160704135310/anx_135310_en.pdf).

Compared to MLV vaccines, subunit vaccines are designed to meet the DIVA (differentiation of infected from vaccinated animals) requirement for vaccination. Two CSFV envelope glycoproteins E^{rns} and E2 have been targeted for vaccine development. Although the effectiveness of E^{rns} as a vaccine target has been controversial [18, 19], two vaccines (*BAYOVAC CSF E2* from Bayer and *Porcilis Pesti* from MSD) based on baculovirus-expressed E2 were marketed commercially in Europe. Vaccinated pigs develop antibodies exclusively to the E2 protein; whereas, naturally infected animals may also develop antibodies to E^{rns}, thus permitting detection of vaccinated animals via this negative marker [20].

However, these subunit vaccines are no longer commercially available because of two significant weaknesses compared with conventional MLV CSF vaccines: they need two vaccinations and offer incomplete protection. In addition to insect cells, yeast and mammalian cells are also used to produce E2 antigens for vaccine development [18, 21]. However, two vaccinations are also required for these yeast- or mammalian cell-based E2 subunit vaccines to achieve homologous protection in pigs. Despite the limitations of E2-subunit vaccines, E2 protein is well recognized as the protective antigen that is essential and may be sufficient for vaccine-mediated protection against CSFV.

One major objective of our CSF research is to develop a DIVA CSF vaccine that can be safely manufactured and used in the U.S. We have recently found that the monoclonal anti-E2 antibody WH211 has much stronger affinity to the dimeric E2 than the monomer. Others have recently shown that antibodies specific to one genotype E2 might not have strong affinity to other genotype E2 proteins on CSFV [22], and this may partially explain why limited protection against heterologous CSFV occurred in pigs vaccinated with E2-subunit vaccines in which E2-specific antibodies play an important role in protective immunity. In addition, we have recently demonstrated that adjuvants can enhance vaccine-mediated cross-protection against porcine reproductive and respiratory syndrome virus (PRRSV) [23] and swine influenza virus [24]. Thus, we hypothesize that a vaccine consisting of a suitable adjuvant and recombinant E2 with natural conformation from the C-strain may induce similar levels of protection as MLV CSF vaccines. Here we provide the first evidence that pigs immunized with a novel one-dose E2-subunit vaccine (KNB-E2) are protected clinically from CSFV challenge. This protection is likely mediated by high levels of E2-specific anti-CSFV neutralizing antibodies.

Methods

Virus and cells

Classical swine fever virus isolate Honduras/1997 (a field isolate from Honduras) was kindly provided by Dr. Sabrina Swenson from the Animal and Plant Health Inspection Service (APHIS), United States Department of Agriculture (USDA). This CSFV isolate was passaged four times in swine testicle cells (ST; ATCC) cultured in DMEM (Gibco) supplemented with 10 % fetal bovine serum (FBS; Atlanta Biologicals) and 1 % Penicillin-streptomycin solution (Gibco). For recombinant E2 production in insect cells, *Spodoptera frugiperda* insect cells (Sf9; ATCC) were grown in Grace's insect medium (Gibco) supplemented with 10 % FBS and 1 % antibiotic-antimycotic solution (Gibco), and High Five insect cells (Invitrogen) were grown in Express Five SFM medium (Gibco).

Expression and purification of recombinant CSFV E2 and E^{rns} protein

PCR-amplified CSFV E2 and E^{rns} genes from hog cholera lapinised virus C-strain (HCLV, Genotype 1.1) was cloned into pFastBacTMI Baculovirus Expression System plasmid vector using the following primers: HCLV-E2-F: 5′-CGCGGATCCACCATAACCATTGCATTCCTCATC-3′, HCLV-E2-R: 5′-CCGGAATTCTTAAT-GATGGTGATG ATGCGCATCCAGGTCAAACCAG-3′; HCLV-E^{rns}-F: 5′-CGCGGATCCACCATGGAAAAAGCCCTATT-GGC ATG-3′, and HCLV-E^{rns}-R: 5′-CCGGAATTCTTAATG GTGATGGTGATGATGCACCCTCGCTGCTCCCTGT C-3′. The desired PCR products were then transformed into DH10BacTM *E. coli* host strain that contains a baculovirus shuttle vector (bacmid) and a helper plasmid. Upon screening of colonies, positive *E. coli* transformants with recombinant E2 and E^{rns} bacmid were upscaled by overnight culture in liquid media and the bacmid was isolated using Purelink® HiPure Plasmid Midiprep Kit (Invitrogen). To generate recombinant baculovirus stock for E2 and E^{rns} expression, Sf9 insect cells were transfected using Cellfectin II Reagent (Invitrogen) and passaged three times to amplify the E2- or E^{rns} bearing recombinant baculovirus. At passage 3, Sf9 cell culture supernatant was collected and clarified by centrifugation at $500 \times g$ for 5 min to obtain the baculovirus stock that was used to infect High Five™ Cells for E2 or E^{rns} expression. E2 and E^{rns} protein was purified using Ni-NTA Agarose (Novex™) as described by the manufacturer. CSFV E2 protein expression and purification was verified by SDS-PAGE and subsequently by western blot using E2 monoclonal antibody WH211 (APHA Scientific) as we described previously [25].

Pigs, E2-subunit vaccine, vaccination, and challenge

Conventional Large White-Duroc crossbred weaned specific-pathogen free male piglets (3 weeks of age) were purchased from a commercial vendor. The pigs were fed with standard commercial diet and kept under laboratory biosafety level III Agriculture (BSL3-Ag) conditions at the Biosecurity Research Institute (BRI), Kansas State University.

The CSFV E2 subunit vaccine KNB-E2 was prepared by simple hand mixing of purified CSFV E2 with an oil-in-water emulsion adjuvant [24]. One dose (2 ml) KNB-E2 contains 75 μg of purified E2 protein. The pigs were randomly allotted into 4 groups ($n = 5$ for each group) with two control groups and two vaccinated groups. The control groups including non-vaccinated, non-challenged (−/−) and non-vaccinated, CSFV challenged (−/+) pigs were given intramuscularly 2 ml Phosphate-buffered saline (PBS). All vaccinated pigs were immunized intramuscularly with 2 ml of KNB-E2. One vaccinated group received only one dose of the KNB-E2 (One-dose group) and the second vaccinated group received two doses of KNB-E2 with the second dose given 21 days later (Two-dose group). Two weeks after the second vaccination, pigs were challenged with 5×10^5 $TCID_{50}$ CSFV isolate Honduras/1997 (1 ml intramuscular, 1 ml intranasal). Honduras/1997 was evaluated as a moderate virulent strain in our previous study. E2 sequencing and nucleotide BLAST analysis indicate that this isolate belongs to CSFV subgenotype 1.3 (GenBank Accession#: KU716076) and has 97 % nucleotide sequence identity to a CSFV isolated in nearby Guatemala (Accession # JX028200).

Pigs were monitored daily for clinical signs and rectal temperatures. Sera were collected on study day 0 (Dose 1) and 21 days post first vaccination (21 DPV; Dose 2). Whole blood, serum and nasal swabs were collected on 35 DPV (also as 0 DPC) and every 3 days after challenge until the end of this study, at 15 days post challenge (15 DPC). All pigs that survived were humanely euthanized at 15 DPC. Total white blood cell (WBC) and leukocyte differentiation counts were performed with VetScan HM5 Analyzer (Abaxis). Tonsil, lymph node, kidney, and lung were collected for virus identification by immunohistochemical staining with anti-E2 antibody WH303 as described earlier with some modification [26].

Measurement of anti-E2 and anti-E^{rns} antibodies in pigs

Anti-E2 and anti-E^{rns} antibodies were determined in E2-vaccinated and CSFV-infected pig sera by enzyme-linked immunosorbent assay (ELISA). Briefly, 62.5 ng/ml of purified E2 or E^{rns} was used as coating antigen on 96-well flat-bottomed microtiter plates (Corning®). Diluted sera (each sample in duplicate) were added to plates and incubated for 1 h at room temperature. Then, horseradishperoxidase (HRP)-conjugated goat anti-porcine IgG was used as secondary antibody (Southern Biotech). The ELISA plates were developed using 3,3,5,5 tetramethylbenzidine (TMB) stabilized chromogen (Novex™), and the reactions were stopped with 2 N sulfuric acid. Relative antibody concentrations were determined using optical spectrophotometer readings at 450 nm using a SpectraMAX microplate reader and analyzed with Softmax® Pro 6.4 Software (Molecular Devices).

RNA isolation and real-time RT-PCR for virus quantification in sera and nasal swabs

Viral RNA from sera and nasal swabs were isolated using IBI Viral Nucleic Acid Extraction Kit II (IBI Scientific) as prescribed by the manufacturer. Real-time RT-PCR was performed using CSFV-specific primers and PCR cycling parameters as previously described [27]. For quantification, passage 4 CSFV stock (10^7 $TCID_{50}$) was serially diluted (10^7 to 10^2) before viral RNA isolation and used for standard curve. Viremia was calculated and determined using StepOne™ Software v2.3 (Applied Biosystems).

Serum anti-CSFV neutralization assay

The anti-CSFV neutralizing antibody titers in the serum were determined using indirect fluorescent antibody assay (IFA). Briefly, serum samples collected at 35 DPV (0 DPC) and 15 DPC were first diluted five-fold and then serially diluted two-fold, the diluted serum samples (in duplicate) were incubated with 100 $TCID_{50}$ of CSFV Honduras/1997 in DMEM with 10 % FBS for 1 h at 37 °C. Residual virus infectivity was determined by adding 1.0×10^4 ST cells to each well with serum-virus mixture in 96-well plate and incubated at 37 °C for 3 days. The cells were subjected to

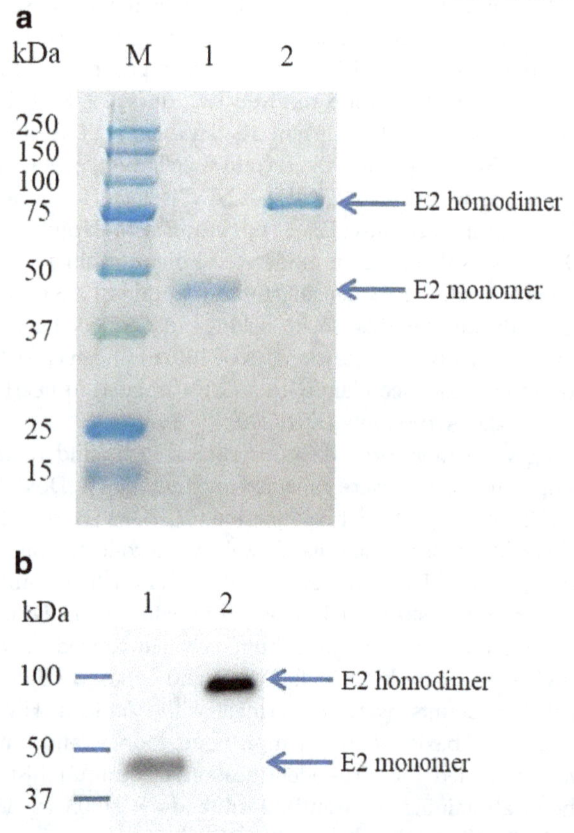

Fig. 1 Production and characterization of recombinant CSFV E2 protein. **a** SDS-PAGE analysis. Lane 1, E2 protein (1 µg) treated with Laemmli sample buffer with addition of reducing reagent β-mercaptoethanol (β-ME); Lane 2, E2 protein (1 µg) treated with Laemmli sample buffer without β-ME. **b** Western blot of purified E2 protein. Lane 1, E2 protein (1 µg) treated with β-ME; Lane 2, E2 protein (50 ng) purified and stored under non-reducing conditions. E2-specific Mab WH211 was used for the western blot

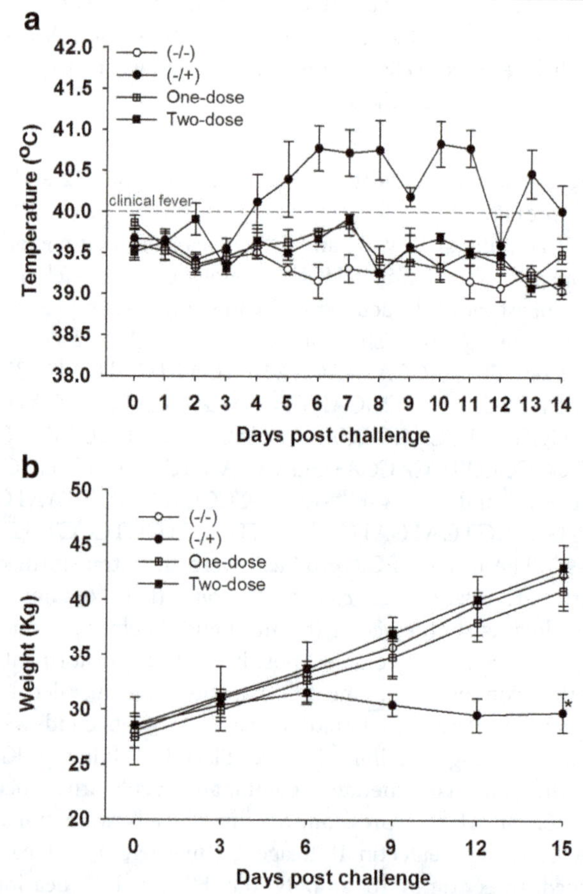

Fig. 2 Pigs immunized with E2 subunit vaccine KNB-E2 were protected clinically from CSFV challenge. Pigs were immunized with KNB-E2 on Day 0 for the One-dose group and a second dose on 21 DPV for the Two-dose group. Two weeks after the second vaccination (35 DPV), pigs were challenged with 5×10^5 $TCID_{50}$ CSFV strain Honduras/1997. **a** Body temperature was monitored daily after CSFV infection. Vaccinated pigs did not have body temperatures higher than 40.5 °C. **b** Shown are body weight measured every 3 days after CSFV challenge. Data are mean ± SEM for five pigs per group. * $p < 0.05$

immunofluorescence staining with E2-specific mAb WH211 and Alexa Fluor 488 goat anti-mouse IgG (H + L) (Life Science). Neutralizing antibody titers in serum samples were expressed as the reciprocal of the highest dilution that caused 50 % neutralization.

Statistical analysis

The variations between groups were analyzed by one-way analysis of variance (ANOVA) followed by post-hoc Dunnett's method using Sigmaplot 11 software (Systat). Differences were considered statistically significant when $p < 0.05$.

Results

Recombinant CSFV E2 proteins produced by insect cells existed as homodimers and had stronger affinity to anti-E2 antibody than that of the monomeric E2 proteins

CSF virus E2 gene from the HCLV was cloned into the recombinant baculovirus and recombinant E2 protein was produced using High Five insect cells. The culture medium was then collected by centrifugation and subjected to protein purification with Ni-NTA agarose beads. As shown in Fig. 1a, pure recombinant E2 protein was obtained from the condition medium. Under reducing conditions, recombinant E2 protein appeared to be 45 kDa, while the native E2 protein mainly existed as homodimer under non-reducing conditions with a molecular weight of ~90 kDa (Fig. 1a). The dimerization of recombinant E2 protein expressed in insect cells was further confirmed by western blot analysis with anti-E2 mAb WH211. It is worth noting that although the amount of E2 dimer protein loaded in lane 2 on Fig. 1b was only 1/20 of the monomeric E2 (50 ng vs. 1 μg), E2 dimers seem to have a higher affinity to WH211 than did the E2 monomer as evidenced by the difference in intensity of the E2 bands on western blot (Fig. 1b).

Pigs immunized with one dose KNB-E2 were protected from heterologous CSFV challenge

To test the efficacy of CSFV E2 subunit vaccine, pigs in both vaccinated groups and the (−/+) group were challenged with CSFV isolate Honduras/1997. After CSFV inoculation, pigs in the (−/+) group displayed clinical signs of CSF, including high fever (Fig. 2a), loss of body weight (Fig. 2b), severe leukopenia (Fig. 3), convulsion, diarrhea, and one of the five pigs, #59, had to be euthanized due to severe clinical symptoms at 9 DPC. In contrast, pigs vaccinated with KNB-E2 - the E2 subunit vaccine (One-dose and Two-dose groups) did not show elevated body temperature after CSFV challenge (Fig. 2a). More importantly, body weight gains in the two vaccinated groups were almost identical to that in healthy

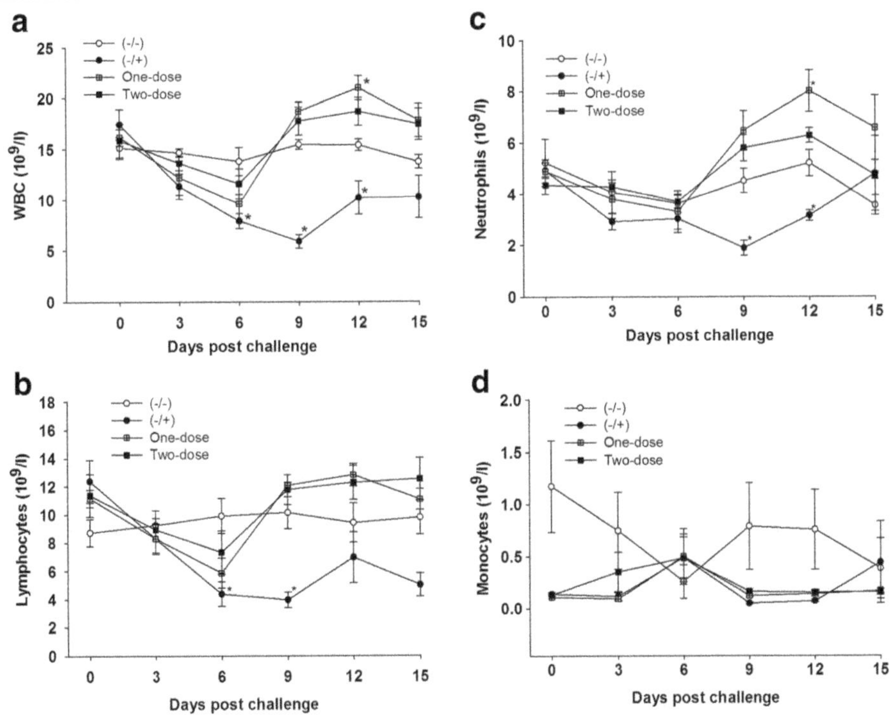

Fig. 3 Pigs vaccinated with KNB-E2 were protected from CSFV-induced leukopenia. Blood cell counts including WBC (**a**), lymphocytes (**b**), neutrophils (**c**), and monocytes (**d**) were monitored on 0, 3, 6, 9, 12, and 15 DPC. A slight decrease but not statistically different in the numbers of WBC, lymphocytes, and neutrophils of all vaccinated pigs were observed at 3 DPC and 6 DPC, these numbers were recovered by 9 DPC. Data are mean ± SEM for five pigs per group. *p < 0.05

control pigs (−/−) before and after CSFV challenge (Fig. 2b).

WBC and lymphocyte counts in (−/+) pigs challenged with CSFV were significantly reduced after CSFV inoculation and reached the lowest levels at 9 DPC (Fig. 3a and b), respectively. In contrast, there was a slight decrease in the numbers of WBC and lymphocytes in pigs vaccinated with KNB-E2 at 3 and 6 DPC; however, the numbers of these cells in vaccinated pigs, especially for pigs in the One-dose group, increased significantly at 9 DPC and then after (Fig. 3a and b, respectively). Similarly, the numbers of neutrophils in the (−/+) group were significantly reduced at 9 and 12 DPC (Fig. 3c), while the numbers of neutrophils in pigs immunized with KNB-E2 were increased significantly at 9 and 12 DPC. The numbers of monocytes in all pig groups seem not to be affected significantly by the CSFV challenge (Fig. 3d).

Vaccination prevents CSF virus replication in blood, nasal cavity, lung, lymph node, tonsil, and kidney in pigs immunized with KNB-E2

CSFV was detected in both serum and nasal swab samples from the (−/+) pigs at 6 DPC. The virus loads in these pigs continued to increase at 9 and 12 DPC and reduced slightly at the time of necropsy on 15 DPC (Tables 1 and 2). In contrast, pigs vaccinated KNB-E2 (One-dose or Two-dose) had undetectable or extremely low levels of CSFV RNA in the blood and nasal fluids by real-time RT-PCR analysis (Tables 1 and 2). CSFV was not detected in any of the serum samples from KNB-E2 vaccinated pigs when they were added to ST cells (10 μl/well in a 96-well plate) for virus isolation (data not shown); and using the same method, CSFV was detected in serum samples from (−/+) pigs collected on 6 and 9 DPC (data not shown). Surprisingly, one of the (−/+) pigs, #56, had significantly less CSFV in the blood and nasal fluid than that of other pigs in the (−/+) group.

Using immunohistochemical staining with E2-specifc antibody WH303, we also determined whether CSFV were present in the lung, lymph nodes, kidney, and tonsil collected from all groups at necropsy (15 DPC). It was found that CSFV were present in the tonsil, lymph node, lung, and kidney in 4/5 of the (−/+) pigs (data not shown). Consistent with the real-time RT-PCR data shown above, CSFV was not detected in any of the tissues from pig #56. CSFV was not

Table 1 Pigs vaccinated with E2 subunit vaccine did not develop viremia after CSFV challenge

Serum		3 DPC		6 DPC		9 DPC		12 DPC		15 DPC	
Treatment	Pig #	Ct value	$TCID_{50}$	Ct value	$TCID_{50}$	Ct value	$TCID_{50}$	Ct value	$TCID_{50}$	Ct value	$TCID_{50}$
(−/−)	51	(−)	(−)	ND	ND	ND	ND	ND	ND	ND	ND
(−/−)	52	37	98	ND	ND	ND	ND	(−)	(−)	(−)	(−)
(−/−)	53	(−)	(−)	(−)	(−)	ND	ND	(−)	(−)	36	112
(−/−)	54	(−)	(−)	(−)	(−)	(−)	(−)	(−)	(−)	(−)	(−)
(−/−)	55	(−)	(−)	(−)	(−)	(−)	(−)	(−)	(−)	(−)	(−)
(−/+)	56	(−)	(−)	29	4330	30	2774	28	17,617	35	163
(−/+)	57	36	78	25	47,547	20	1,460,325	19	4,993,009	21	1,036,940
(−/+)	58	(−)	(−)	28	7090	23	222,328	20	2,587,042	21	1,095,457
(−/+)	59	(−)	(−)	26	28,553	22	480,384	pig died			
(−/+)	60	(−)	(−)	29	5169	22	507,102	21	1,019,529	21	1,003,013
One-dose	61	37	42	28	7192	35	160	38	29	38	58
One-dose	62	(−)	(−)	34	170	(−)	(−)	39	21	(−)	(−)
One-dose	63	34	179	35	160	36	68	(−)	(−)	(−)	(−)
One-dose	64	36	56	33	330	34	169	36	131	(−)	(−)
One-dose	65	(−)	(−)	35	100	(−)	(−)	(−)	(−)	(−)	(−)
Two-dose	66	(−)	(−)	36	56	35	106	(−)	(−)	(−)	(−)
Two-dose	67	(−)	(−)	34	279	(−)	(−)	(−)	(−)	(−)	(−)
Two-dose	68	(−)	(−)	36	85	(−)	(−)	(−)	(−)	(−)	(−)
Two-dose	69	(−)	(−)	(−)	(−)	(−)	(−)	(−)	(−)	(−)	(−)
Two-dose	70	(−)	(−)	35	97	(−)	(−)	(−)	(−)	(−)	(−)

ND not done; (−): Undetectable; Pigs were challenged with CSFV 35 days post first vaccination. CSFV RNA in the blood was measured by real-time RT-PCR as described in Methods section

(−/−): Control pigs without CSFV challenge; (−/+): Control pigs challenged with CSFV

One-dose: Pigs vaccinated with one dose KNB-E2 and then challenged with CSFV

Two-dose: Pigs vaccinated with KNB-E2 twice and then challenged with CSFV

Table 2 CSFV were cleared from the nasal cavity in pigs vaccinated with E2 subunit vaccine 15 days post challenge

Nasal swab		3 DPC		6 DPC		9 DPC		12 DPC		15 DPC	
Treatment	Pig #	Ct value	$TCID_{50}$	Ct value	$TCID_{50}$	Ct value	$TCID_{50}$	Ct value	$TCID_{50}$	Ct value	$TCID_{50}$
(–/–)	51	ND	ND	ND	ND	ND	ND	ND	ND	(–)	(–)
(–/–)	52	ND	ND	ND	ND	ND	ND	(–)	(–)	(–)	(–)
(–/–)	53	(–)	(–)	(–)	(–)	(–)	(–)	(–)	(–)	(–)	(–)
(–/–)	54	(–)	(–)	(–)	(–)	39	37	(–)	(–)	(–)	(–)
(–/–)	55	(–)	(–)	34	184	34	560	(–)	(–)	(–)	(–)
(–/+)	56	(–)	(–)	35	95	33	1521	28	19,033	33	2867
(–/+)	57	(–)	(–)	32	876	24	300,220	20	1,882,476	22	904,988
(–/+)	58	37	31	34	293	24	411,326	21	1,438,113	21	1,502,256
(–/+)	59	(–)	(–)	32	1065	21	3,182,081	pig died			
(–/+)	60	38	19	34	261	25	293,326	21	1,451,296	22	745,304
One-dose	61	(–)	(–)	35	124	36	166	36	106	(–)	(–)
One-dose	62	(–)	(–)	(–)	(–)	38	52	37	42	36	109
One-dose	63	(–)	(–)	37	35	37	83	33	495	(–)	(–)
One-dose	64	(–)	(–)	34	224	(–)	(–)	37	68	(–)	(–)
One-dose	65	(–)	(–)	36	68	37	78	34	301	(–)	(–)
Two-dose	66	(–)	(–)	37	38	39	28	35	145	(–)	(–)
Two-dose	67	(–)	(–)	36	60	38	67	35	221	(–)	(–)
Two-dose	68	(–)	(–)	(–)	(–)	34	2398	34	283	(–)	(–)
Two-dose	69	(–)	(–)	36	56	37	79	34	269	37	42
Two-dose	70	(–)	(–)	36	58	(–)	(–)	34	330	(–)	(–)

ND not done; (–): Undetectable; Pigs were challenged with CSFV 35 days post first vaccination. CSFV RNA in the blood was measured by real-time RT-PCR as described in Methods section

(–/–): Control pigs without CSFV challenge; (–/+): Control pigs challenged with CSFV

One-dose: Pigs vaccinated with one dose KNB-E2 and then challenged with CSFV

Two-dose: Pigs vaccinated with KNB-E2 twice and then challenged with CSFV

detected in any tissues from pigs vaccinated with KNB-E2 (One-dose or Two-dose).

Pigs vaccinated with KNB-E2 developed high levels of E2-specific antibodies and anti-CSFV neutralizing antibody (VNA) titers after vaccination and challenge

As shown in Fig. 4a, all vaccinated pigs developed E2-specific antibody after immunization. E2-specific antibody level in the One-dose group increased dramatically after challenge and was even higher than that in the Two-dose group at 9 DPC. The level of E2-specific antibody in the Two-dose group increased dramatically after the boost vaccination, but decreased significantly in the first 9 days post challenge. E2-specific antibody was not detected in control pigs before or after the challenge (Fig. 4a). In contrast to E2-specpific antibody response, E^{rns}-specific antibody was only detected in the (–/+) pigs at 15 DPC (Fig. 4b).

Similar to E2-specific antibody response, all vaccinated pigs developed anti-CSFV neutralizing antibody before challenge at 35 DPV (Table 3). The VNA titers in the One-dose group were lower than that in the Two-dose group at 35 DPV. However, the VNA titers in the One-dose group were higher than that in the Two-dose group at 15 DPC. Pigs in the control groups had no detectable neutralizing antibody at 35 DPV and 15 DPC. Thus, there seems to be close correlation between anti-CSFV neutralizing antibody titers and levels of E2-specific antibodies in pigs after KNB-E2 vaccination and CSFV challenge. Consistent with its viremia status, pig #56 in the (–/+) group had detectable anti-CSFV neutralizing antibody at 15 DPC.

Discussion

Commercial E2 subunit vaccines previously available in Europe were marketed as two-dose vaccines for basic vaccination for homologous protection. Here we present data showing that vaccination with one dose KNB-E2 protects pigs from subgenotype heterologous (1.1 vs. 1.3) CSFV challenge. Pigs vaccinated with KNB-E2 did not have any fever or growth retardation after CSFV challenge. CSFV was not detected in the blood, nasal cavity, lung, kidney, lymph node, and tonsil in vaccinated pigs 15 days post challenge. Our report demonstrates that subunit vaccine KNB-E2 is safe and effective at stimulating immunity against

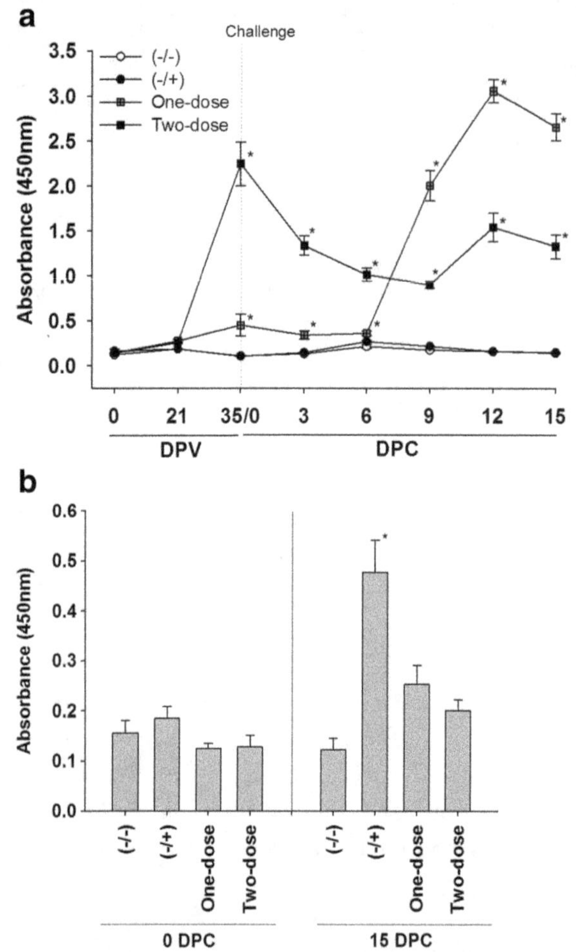

Fig. 4 E2-specific antibodies were detected by ELISA only in pigs vaccinated with KNB-E2 before and after challenge. E2- and E^{rns}-specific antibodies were measured by ELISA as we described in Materials and Methods. **a** E2-specific antibody in serum samples collected after vaccination and challenge. **b** E^{rns}-specific antibody in serum samples collected at 0 DPC and 15 DPC. Data are shown as mean ± SEM for five pigs per group. * $p < 0.05$

heterologous and geographically (Central-South America) relevant CSFV in an experimental setting in the U.S.

It has been well established that CSFV E2 protein is the major protective antigen and can elicit neutralizing antibody, thus it is frequently used as the antigen for subunit vaccine development (see reviews [6, 9, 28]). Because attenuated CSFV vaccine HCLV strain is well-known for its efficacy and safety, the HCLV E2 gene (genotype 1.1) was cloned and expressed with the insect cell/baculovirus system in this study. Purified E2 proteins mainly present as homodimers, which is identical to the native glycosylated E2 protein reported in previous studies [21, 29]. Furthermore, we found that E2 homodimers have higher affinity to E2-specific mAb WH211 than do the monomers, indicating that oligomerization and glycosylation of E2 protein are important for the induction of protective immune response and neutralizing antibodies.

The efficacy of the two commercial E2 subunit vaccines has been extensively evaluated in various vaccination-challenge studies in pigs. The E2 antigen in *BAYOVAC CSF E2* was originated from CSF Brescia [30], a genotype 1.2. Although a single vaccination with this vaccine can significantly reduce mortality of pigs challenged with homologous CSFV up to 13 months after a single vaccination [13], it did not protect pigs from developing fever [11]. Different from *BAYOVAC CSF E2,* the E2 antigen in *Porcilis Pesti* was originated from CSFV Alfort/Tubingen [28], a genotype 2.3. It was reported that single vaccination with *Porcilis Pesti* failed to protect immunized pigs and prevent horizontal transmission of CSFV (Alfort/187, genotype 1.1) to unvaccinated sentinel pigs [31]. Others have shown that *Porcilis Pesti* can totally prevent horizontal transmission 14 DPV and significantly reduce transmission 7 DPV [10].

In contrast, pigs immunized with one dose KNB-E2 are protected from a subgenotype heterologous CSFV challenge without the development of fever and growth retardation, and CSFV was cleared from the pigs by 15 DPC. The differential efficacy between KNB-E2 and the commercial E2 subunit vaccines may be due to the fact that we use E2 protein from genotype 1.1 C-strain CSFV and/or the E2 antigens in KNB-E2 are in the native dimeric conformation. This speculation is consistent with the report from others showing that sows vaccinated with E2 proteins from CSFV genotype 1.2 were better protected against clinical CSF than sows vaccinated with E2 proteins from CSFV genotype 2.3 when these pigs were challenged with CSFV genotype 2.1 [32]. Alternatively, the higher (75 μg/dose for KNB-E2 vs. 32 μg/dose for BAYORVAC CSF E2) amount of E2 protein used in our vaccine may also contribute to the superior efficacy after one dose immunization.

In addition, we have also found that pigs immunized with one dose or two doses of KNB-E2 have different antibody responses to CSFV challenge. Prior to challenge, the VNA titer and E2-specific antibody in pigs from the One-dose group were lower than that from pigs in the Two-dose group (Table 3 and Fig. 4). However, pigs in the One-dose group generated higher anti-CSFV neutralizing antibody and E2-specific antibody after challenge than that of pigs in the Two-dose group. It seems that CSFV challenge with Honduras/1997 may function as a booster vaccination with live viruses, which resulted in the induction of a stronger immunological response and a larger amounts of neutralizing antibody than does a boost vaccination with a subunit vaccine. We speculate that the high levels of VNA and E2-specific antibodies prior to challenge in the Two-dose pigs may accelerate the inactivation and removal of

Table 3 Pigs vaccinated with E2 subunit vaccine developed high titers of anti-CSFV neutralizing antibodies

Treatment	Pig #	35 DPV	15 DPC	Treatment	Pig #	35 DPV	15 DPC
(−/−)	51	0	0	(−/+)	56	0	>160
(−/−)	52	0	0	(−/+)	57	0	0
(−/−)	53	0	0	(−/+)	58	0	0
(−/−)	54	0	0	(−/+)	59	0	0
(−/−)	55	0	0	(−/+)	60	0	0
One-dose	61	15	10,240	Two-dose	66	960	7680
One-dose	62	240	>10,240	Two-dose	67	640	7680
One-dose	63	320	>10,240	Two-dose	68	1920	10,240
One-dose	64	20	>10,240	Two-dose	69	7680	7680
One-dose	65	640	5120	Two-dose	70	480	2560

DPV day post vaccination (first dose), *DPC* day post challenge. Pigs were challenged on 35 DPV
(−/−): Control pigs without challenge; (−/+): Control pigs challenged with CSFV
One-dose: Pigs vaccinated with one dose KNB-E2 and then challenged with CSFV
Two-dose: Pigs vaccinated with KNB-E2 twice and then challenged with CSFV

circulating CSFV post challenge, which may lead to fewer or no live CSFV available for further immunological stimulation.

The dynamics of anti-CSFV neutralizing antibody produced in the vaccinated groups after challenge is consistent with the changes of white blood cells. As shown in Figs. 3 and 4, the trends (decrease or increase) of WBC and lymphocytes parallel the trends of E2-specific antibody levels and VNA titers in vaccinated pigs compared with that in control pigs. Interestingly, the impact of KNB-E2 vaccination on leukocyte homeostasis is different from that of MLV C-strain vaccine, as evidenced by the fact that dramatic increase of leukocyte cells in pigs vaccinated with KNB-E2 was not observed in pigs immunized with the C-strain vaccine [33]. The meaning of this difference has yet to be explored in future studies.

In contrast to all vaccinated pigs, control pigs challenged with CSFV developed significant levels of anti-E^{rns} antibody at 15 days post challenge. This observation indicates that KNB-E2 has the DIVA characteristic as a CSF vaccine. However, we do recognize that although the challenge CSFV strain Honduras/1997 used in our study is from the Americas and heterologous to the origin strain of the E2 gene, it is not a recent outbreak strain. Our study design was limited by the current availably of CSFV in an academic setting in the U.S. – a CSF-free country. Because most of the presently circulating strains in the world belong to genotype 2, future studies are planned to better understand the protective ability of KNB-E2 against the CSFV in the field.

Conclusion

CSFV E2 protein was successfully generated by insect cell/baculovirus expression system and the purified E2 protein was formulated with an oil-in-water emulsion adjuvant as a CSF subunit vaccine (KNB-E2) for pigs. Pigs immunized with one dose KNB-E2 can be clinically protected from CSFV challenge. This novel subunit vaccine has DIVA characteristics, can be manufactured in CSF-free regions, and is suitable for CSF prevention and control in both CSF endemic area and emergency outbreaks.

Acknowledgements

We thank Dr. Brooke Bloomberg and the rest of the Comparative Medicine staff at Kansas State University for their technical help. Thanks to husbandry staff at the Biosecurity Research Institute at K-State for providing high-level quality of animal care. We thank Dr. Paul Hauer, Dr. Sabrina Swenson, and Ms. Melinda Jenkins-Moore for their assistance in obtaining the CSFV isolates from the National Veterinary Services Laboratories (NVSL), USDA APHIS.

Funding

This research was supported by an award from the National Bio and Agro-Defense Facility Transition Fund, a Kansas Bioscience Authority grant KBA-CBRI 611310, and a USDA ARS Specific Cooperative Agreement 59-5430-001-23S, NP-103.

Authors' contributions

RM, WG, LW, YB, KL, AGB, KJ, and PL carried out the animal studies, participated in the production and characterization of recombinant E2, adjuvant production, and helped in drafting the manuscript. JN, JH participated in the animal studies, pathology evaluation, and assisted in drafting the manuscript. RM, JB, JS, SM, and CT participated in formulating the vaccine, study design, statistical analysis. JS conceived and coordinated the study, formulated the vaccine and participated in data analysis, and drafted the manuscript. All authors read and approved the final manuscript.

Competing interests

The authors declare that they have no competing interests.

Consent for publication

Not applicable.

Author details

[1]Department of Anatomy and Physiology, Kansas State University, Manhattan, KS 66506, USA. [2]Department of Diagnostic Medicine and

Pathobiology, Kansas State University, Manhattan, KS 66506, USA. [3]Department of Chemistry, Kansas State University, Manhattan, KS 66506, USA. [4]Department of Chemical Engineering, Kansas State University, Manhattan, KS 66506, USA. [5]Institute of Military Veterinary Medicine, Academy of Military Medical Sciences, Changchun, China. [6]United States Department of Agriculture, Agricultural Research Service, Arthropod Borne Animal Disease Research Unit, Manhattan, KS 66502, USA.

References

1. Moennig V. Introduction to classical swine fever: virus, disease and control policy. Vet Microbiol. 2000;73(2–3):93–102.
2. Meyers G, Thiel HJ, Rumenapf T. Classical swine fever virus: recovery of infectious viruses from cDNA constructs and generation of recombinant cytopathogenic defective interfering particles. J Virol. 1996;70(3):1588–95.
3. Paton DJ, McGoldrick A, Greiser-Wilke I, Parchariyanon S, Song JY, Liou PP, Stadejek T, Lowings JP, Bjorklund H, Belak S. Genetic typing of classical swine fever virus. Vet Microbiol. 2000;73(2–3):137–57.
4. Postel A, Moennig V, Becher P. Classical swine fever in Europe–the current situation. Berl Munch Tierarztl Wochenschr. 2013;126(11–12):468–75.
5. Postel A, Schmeiser S, Perera CL, Rodriguez LJ, Frias-Lepoureau MT, Becher P. Classical swine fever virus isolates from Cuba form a new subgenotype 1. 4. Vet Microbiol. 2013;161(3–4):334–8.
6. Huang YL, Deng MC, Wang FI, Huang CC, Chang CY. The challenges of classical swine fever control: modified live and E2 subunit vaccines. Virus Res. 2014;179:1–11.
7. Everett H, Salguero FJ, Graham SP, Haines F, Johns H, Clifford D, Nunez A, La Rocca SA, Parchariyanon S, Steinbach F, Drew T, Crooke H. Characterisation of experimental infections of domestic pigs with genotype 2.1 and 3.3 isolates of classical swine fever virus. Vet Microbiol. 2010;142(1–2):26–33.
8. Blome S, Meindl-Bohmer A, Loeffen W, Thuer B, Moennig V. Assessment of classical swine fever diagnostics and vaccine performance. Rev Sci Tech. 2006;25(3):1025–38.
9. van Oirschot JT. Vaccinology of classical swine fever: from lab to field. Vet Microbiol. 2003;96(4):367–84.
10. Dewulf J, Laevens H, Koenen F, Mintiens K, de Kruif A. Efficacy of E2-sub-unit marker and C-strain vaccines in reducing horizontal transmission of classical swine fever virus in weaner pigs. Prev Vet Med. 2004;65(3–4):121–33.
11. Bouma A, de Smit AJ, de Kluijver EP, Terpstra C, Moormann RJ. Efficacy and stability of a subunit vaccine based on glycoprotein E2 of classical swine fever virus. Vet Microbiol. 1999;66(2):101–14.
12. van Rijn PA, van Gennip HG, Moormann RJ. An experimental marker vaccine and accompanying serological diagnostic test both based on envelope glycoprotein E2 of classical swine fever virus (CSFV). Vaccine. 1999;17(5):433–40.
13. de Smit AJ, Bouma A, de Kluijver EP, Terpstra C, Moormann RJ. Duration of the protection of an E2 subunit marker vaccine against classical swine fever after a single vaccination. Vet Microbiol. 2001;78(4):307–17.
14. Blome S, Aebischer A, Lange E, Hofmann M, Leifer I, Loeffen W, Koenen F, Beer M. Comparative evaluation of live marker vaccine candidates "CP7_E2alf" and "flc11" along with C-strain "Riems" after oral vaccination. Vet Microbiol. 2012;158(1–2):42–59.
15. Eble PL, Geurts Y, Quak S, Moonen-Leusen HW, Blome S, Hofmann MA, Koenen F, Beer M, Loeffen WL. Efficacy of chimeric Pestivirus vaccine candidates against classical swine fever: protection and DIVA characteristics. Vet Microbiol. 2013;162(2–4):437–46.
16. Renson P, Le Dimna M, Keranflech A, Cariolet R, Koenen F, Le Potier MF. CP7_E2alf oral vaccination confers partial protection against early classical swine fever virus challenge and interferes with pathogeny-related cytokine responses. Vet Res. 2013;44:9.
17. Rangelova D, Nielsen J, Strandbygaard B, Koenen F, Blome S, Uttenthal A. Efficacy of marker vaccine candidate CP7_E2alf in piglets with maternally derived C-strain antibodies. Vaccine. 2012;30(45):6376–81.
18. Lin GJ, Deng MC, Chen ZW, Liu TY, Wu CW, Cheng CY, Chien MS, Huang C. Yeast expressed classical swine fever E2 subunit vaccine candidate provides complete protection against lethal challenge infection and prevents horizontal virus transmission. Vaccine. 2012;30(13):2336–41.
19. Gladue DP, Holinka LG, Largo E, Fernandez Sainz I, Carrillo C, O'Donnell V, Baker-Branstetter R, Lu Z, Ambroggio X, Risatti GR, Nieva JL, Borca MV. Classical swine fever virus p7 protein is a viroporin involved in virulence in swine. J Virol. 2012;86(12):6778–91.
20. de Smit AJ, Bouma A, van Gennip HG, de Kluijver EP, Moormann RJ. Chimeric (marker) C-strain viruses induce clinical protection against virulent classical swine fever virus (CSFV) and reduce transmission of CSFV between vaccinated pigs. Vaccine. 2001;19(11–12):1467–76.
21. Hua RH, Huo H, Li YN, Xue Y, Wang XL, Guo LP, Zhou B, Song Y, Bu ZG. Generation and efficacy evaluation of recombinant classical swine fever virus E2 glycoprotein expressed in stable transgenic mammalian cell line. PLoS One. 2014;9(9):e106891.
22. Luo L, Nishi K, Macleod E, Sabara MI, Lin M, Handel K, Pasick J. Baculovirus expression and antigenic characterization of classical swine fever virus E2 proteins. Transbound Emerg Dis. 2013;60(2):143–51.
23. Li X, Galliher-Beckley A, Huang H, Sun X, Shi J. Peptide nanofiber hydrogel adjuvanted live virus vaccine enhances cross-protective immunity to porcine reproductive and respiratory syndrome virus. Vaccine. 2013;31(41):4508–15.
24. Galliher-Beckley A, Pappan LK, Madera R, Burakova Y, Waters A, Nickles M, Li X, Nietfeld J, Schlup JR, Zhong Q, McVey S, Dritz SS, Shi J. Characterization of a novel oil-in-water emulsion adjuvant for swine influenza virus and Mycoplasma hyopneumoniae vaccines. Vaccine. 2015;33(25):2903–8.
25. Li Y, Wang L, Pappan L, Galliher-Beckley A, Shi J. IL-1β promotes stemness and invasiveness of colon cancer cells through Zeb1 activation. Mol Cancer. 2012;11:87.
26. Belak K, Koenen F, Vanderhallen H, Mittelholzer C, Feliziani F, De Mia GM, Belak S. Comparative studies on the pathogenicity and tissue distribution of three virulence variants of classical swine fever virus, two field isolates and one vaccine strain, with special regard to immunohistochemical investigations. Acta Vet Scand. 2008;50:34.
27. Hoffmann B, Beer M, Schelp C, Schirrmeier H, Depner K. Validation of a real-time RT-PCR assay for sensitive and specific detection of classical swine fever. J Virol Methods. 2005;130(1–2):36–44.
28. Dong XN, Chen YH. Marker vaccine strategies and candidate CSFV marker vaccines. Vaccine. 2007;25(2):205–30.
29. Lin GJ, Liu TY, Tseng YY, Chen ZW, You CC, Hsuan SL, Chien MS, Huang C. Yeast-expressed classical swine fever virus glycoprotein E2 induces a protective immune response. Vet Microbiol. 2009;139(3–4):369–74.
30. Hulst MM, Westra DF, Wensvoort G, Moormann RJ. Glycoprotein E1 of hog cholera virus expressed in insect cells protects swine from hog cholera. J Virol. 1993;67(9):5435–42.
31. Ziegler U, Kaden V. Vaccination of weaner pigs against classical swine fever with the subunit vaccine "Porcilis Pesti": influence of different immunization plans on excretion and transmission of challenge virus. Berl Munch Tierarztl Wochenschr. 2002;115(7–8):267–73.
32. Depner KR, Bouma A, Koenen F, Klinkenberg D, Lange E, de Smit H, Vanderhallen H. Classical swine fever (CSF) marker vaccine. Trial II. Challenge study in pregnant sows. Vet Microbiol. 2001;83(2):107–20.
33. Graham SP, Everett HE, Haines FJ, Johns HL, Sosan OA, Salguero FJ, Clifford DJ, Steinbach F, Drew TW, Crooke HR. Challenge of pigs with classical swine fever viruses after C-strain vaccination reveals remarkably rapid protection and insights into early immunity. PLoS One. 2012;7(1):e29310.

15

Coinfection modulates inflammatory responses, clinical outcome and pathogen load of H1N1 swine influenza virus and *Haemophilus parasuis* infections in pigs

Małgorzata Pomorska-Mól*, Arkadiusz Dors, Krzysztof Kwit, Ewelina Czyżewska-Dors and Zygmunt Pejsak

Abstract

Background: Respiratory co-infections are important factor affecting the profitability of pigs production. Swine influenza virus (SIV) may predispose to secondary infection. *Haemophilus parasuis* (*Hps*) can be a primary pathogen or be associated with other pathogens such as SIV. To date, little is known about the effect of coinfection with SIV and *Hps* on the disease severity and inflammatory response and the role of *Hps* in the induction of pneumonia in the absence of other respiratory pathogens. In the study we investigated the influence of SIV and *Hps* coinfection on clinical course, inflammatory response, pathogens shedding and load at various time points following intranasal inoculation. The correlation between local concentration of cytokines and severity of disease as well as serum acute phase proteins (APP) concentration has been also studied.

Results: All co-infected pigs had fever, while in single inoculated pigs fever was observed only in part of animals. Necropsy revealed lesions in the lungs all SIV-inoculated and co-inoculated pigs, while in *Hps*-single inoculated animals only 1 out of 11 pigs revealed gross lung lesions. The SIV shedding was the highest in co-inoculated pigs. There were no differences between *Hps*-single inoculated and co-inoculated groups with regard to *Hps* shedding. The significant increase in *Hps* titre in the lung has been found only in co-inoculated group. All APP increased after co-infection. In single-inoculated animals various kinetics of APP response has been observed. The lung concentrations of cytokines were induced mostly in SIV + *Hps* pigs in the apical and middle lobe. These results correlated well with localization of gross lung lesions.

Conclusions: The results revealed that SIV increased the severity of lung lesions and facilitated *Hps* (PIWetHps192/2015) replication in the porcine lung. Furthermore, *Hps* influenced the SIV nasal shedding. Enhanced *Hps* and SIV replication, together with stronger systemic and local inflammatory response contributed to a more severe clinical signs and stronger, earlier immune response in co-inoculated animals. We confirmed the previous evidence that single-*Hps* infection does not produce significant pneumonic lesions but it should be in mind that other strains of *Hps* may produce lesions different from that reported in the present study.

Keywords: Pigs, Respiratory co-infections, Disease severity, Immunity, Pathogens shedding

* Correspondence: mpomorska@piwet.pulawy.pl
Department of Swine Diseases, National Veterinary Research Institute, Partyzantów 57, 24-100 Pulawy, Poland

Background

Respiratory infections in pigs are very important factor affecting the profitability of pig production [1, 2]. Although various bacteria or viruses could induce the respiratory infection separately, it has commonly been caused by coinfection with more pathogens under field conditions [1–3]. The most important infectious agents responsible for infection of the respiratory tract in pigs are: swine influenza virus (SIV), porcine reproductive and respiratory syndrome virus (PRRSV), *Pasteurella multocida* (Pm), *Actinobacillus pleuropneumoniae* and *Mycoplasma hyopneumoniae* [2, 4–6]. Besides, the above mentioned pathogens, the *Haemophilus parasuis (Hps)* can also be recovered from the lungs of pigs with pneumonia [1, 7–10]. In these cases *Hps* is often isolated along with other bacterial or viral pathogens and, therefore, the role of *Hps* in producing pneumonia is not clear [8, 11].

Bacterial pneumonia secondary to influenza is often observed in pigs [12]. SIV is a significant contributor to the respiratory diseases and may predispose to secondary bacterial infection. *Hps* is an important and common respiratory pathogen of pigs [13]. It can be a primary pathogen or be associated with other diseases such as SIV [3, 8]. It could be also isolated from nasal cavity, tonsils and trachea of apparently healthy pigs [8, 14]. Under favorable conditions, *Hps* can cause severe systemic infection characterized by fibrinous polyserositis, arthritis and meningitis [8, 11, 14]. Factors leading to systemic infection by *Hps* have not been clarified to date [9, 14].

Although there are previous reports of experimental reproduction of *Hps* or SIV infection in conventional pigs, little is known about the effect of concurrent infection with SIV and *Hps* on the disease severity and inflammatory response in pigs, even if this coinfection is common under field conditions [13, 15–17]. There are also limited data on the role of *Hps* in the production of pneumonia in the absence of other respiratory pathogens. Furthermore, the kinetics of acute phase protein (APP) response in SIV/*Hps* co-infected pigs has not been studied to date. As it has been shown for other pathogens, the exposure to several pathogens can lead to a stronger APP response, as compare to single infection [18–20]. Thus, in order to investigate the influence of SIV and *Hps* coinfection on clinical outcome, both local and systemic inflammatory response as well as pathogen shedding and load at various time points following intranasal inoculation, three experimental infections (*Hps*- and SIV-single infection, SIV/*Hps* co-infection) has been performed in the present study. The correlation between local concentration of cytokines and severity of infection (clinical score, lung score) as well as serum APP concentration has been also studied.

Results

Clinical signs

All pigs from co-infected group had fever for at least one day (rectal temperature ≥40° C). In SIV – inoculated group fever was observed in 7 out of 11 pigs, while in *Hps* - inoculated pigs only in 3 out of 11 pigs (Fig. 1). The mean clinical scores (±SD) in all groups are presented in Fig. 2. In single-inoculated pigs, the individual clinical score ranged from 0 to 1 (*Hps*) or from 0 to 5 (SIV), while in co-inoculated pigs the individual clinical score ranged from 1 to 6. Pigs from the control group did not revealed clinical signs of any disease. Significant differences were observed between mean clinical score in SIV- and *Hps* + SIV – inoculated pigs and the controls ($p \leq 0.05$). There was also significant difference between co-inoculated and *Hps*-inoculated group ($p \leq 0.05$). No differences were observed between mean clinical score in SIV-single inoculated and co-inoculated animals as well as between *Hps*-inoculated and control animals.

Pathological examination

Postmortem examination revealed macroscopic lesions (well-demarcated plum-colored or dark red lesions) in the lungs all SIV-inoculated and co-inoculated pigs, while in *Hps*-single inoculated animals only 1 out of 11 pigs revealed macroscopic changes in the lung. None of the control pigs had visible pneumonia. The mean lung scores (±SD) are presented in Fig. 3. There were no significant differences between lung score observed at different days post inoculation

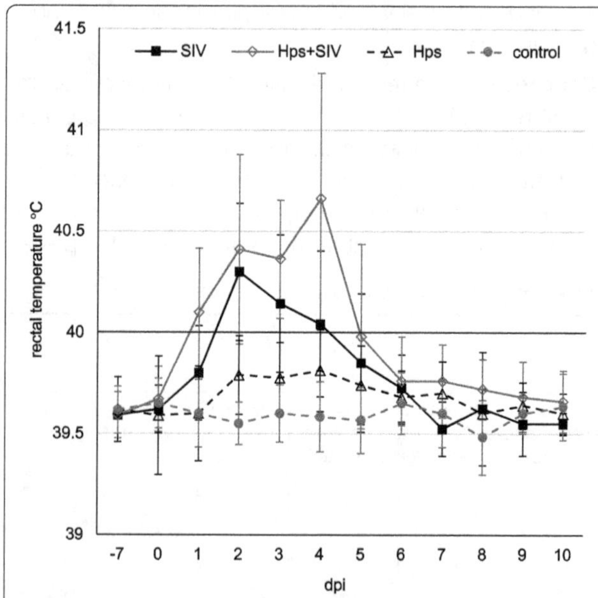

Fig. 1 Rectal temperature (mean ±SD) in pigs single or dual inoculated with swine influenza virus (SIV) and/or *Haemophilus parasius* (Hps). Number of pigs affected: *Hps* + SIV 11/11; SIV 7/11; *Hps* 3/11

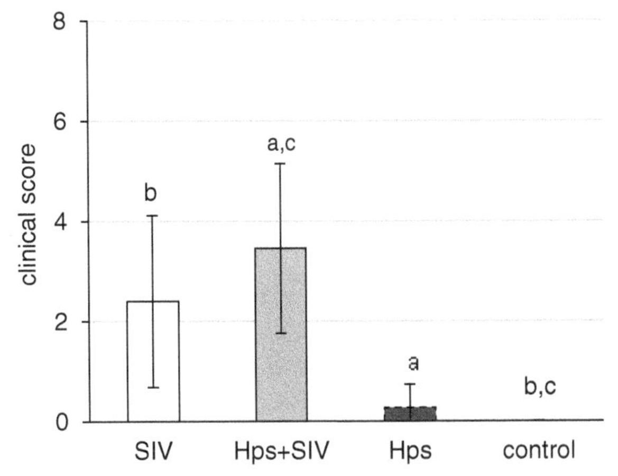

Fig. 2 Clinical score (mean±SD) of pigs single or dual inoculated with swine influenza virus (SIV) and/or *Haemophilus parasius* (Hps). The significant differences between groups are indicated with the same superscripts

within each group ($p > 0.05$). Significant differences were found between mean lung score observed co-inoculated and *Hps*-inoculated groups and control animals ($p < 0.05$). There was no difference between lung score noted in co-inoculated and SIV-only inoculated animal. No differences were also found between mean lung score in *Hps*-inoculated and control pigs.

Pathogens shedding and load

The highest SIV shedding (expressed as mean SIV titre ($\log_{10}$ $TCID_{50}$ titre/100 mg secrete from nasal swabs) was observed in co-inoculated pigs. Significant differences between single-SIV and dual inoculated pigs were found from 3 to 7 DPI ($p < 0.05$). Compared to control pigs, significantly higher ($p < 0.05$) mean SIV titers were observed in both SIV-single inoculated pigs and co-inoculated pigs from 1 to 5 DPI and 1 to 7 DPI, respectively (Fig. 4.). The mean *Hps* titre in the nasal swabs (expressed as $\log_{10}$ CFU titre/100 mg secretion) in piglets from SIV + *Hps* and *Hps* groups increased significantly from day 1 post inoculation and remaining at the significantly higher level to the end of study ($p < 0.05$). There were no differences between *Hps*-single inoculated and co-inoculated groups with regard to *Hps* nasal shedding (Fig. 5.).

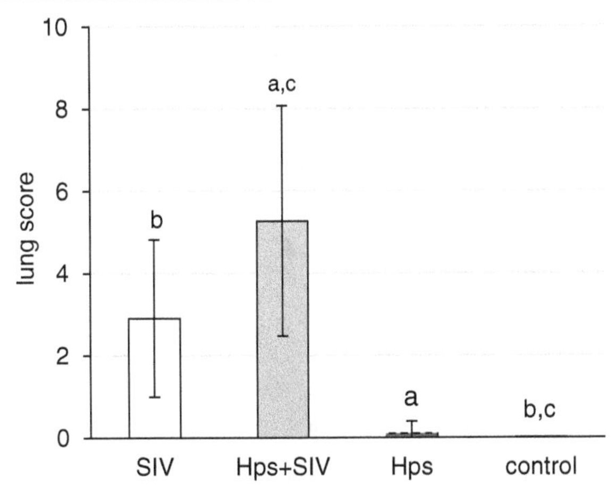

Fig. 3 Lung score (mean±SD) of pigs single or dual inoculated with swine influenza virus (SIV) and/or *Haemophilus parasius* (Hps). The significant differences between groups are indicated with the same superscripts

The SIV and *Hps* titres in the lungs at 2, 4 and 10 dpi are presented in Figs. 6 and 7, respectively. All pigs inoculated with SIV were virus positive in samples taken from right lungs at 2 and 4 DPI. At 10 DPI the virus was detected in 1 out of 5 lungs in SIV-single inoculated animals, while in pigs co-inoculated with *Hps* in 2 out of 5 lungs and no significant differences between virus inoculated groups were found. The mean SIV $TCID_{50}$ titres were highest in co-inoculated pigs at 2 and 4 DPI ($p < 0.05$).

The significant increase in *Hps* titre in the lung were found only in co-inoculated group ($p < 0.05$). The significant differences were detected between the mean titre of *H. parasuis* in the lungs taken from pigs from *Hps* and SIV + *Hps* groups during whole study period (2, 4 and 10 DPI) ($p < 0.05$).

Humoral immune response to SIV and *Hps*

The onset of specific humoral response after inoculations with SIV and/or *Hps* is presented in Figs. 8 and 9, respectively.

A specific humoral response against SIV was observed at 7 DPI in 80% of pigs (4/5) co-inoculated and 40% of pigs (2/5) single inoculated with SIV. All animals inoculated with SIV (single or dual) developed specific antibodies at 10 DPI (the HI titre ranged from 20 to 80 in co-inoculated pigs and from 20 to 40 in SIV-only inoculated group). There were no differences with regard to HI titre at 7 and 10 DPI between groups inoculated with SIV (single or dual) ($p \geq 0.05$). None of pigs not inoculated with SIV had antibodies against this pathogen (<20 HI titre).

Significant differences between co-inoculated and single-inoculated or control pigs with regard to *Hps* specific antibodies was observed at 7 DPI ($p \leq 0.05$). Furthermore, in groups inoculated with *Hps* (single or dual) the mean ELISA ratio at 10 DPI was significantly higher than in SIV – inoculated and control animals ($p \leq 0.05$). The ELISA ratio in control group did not differ significantly from the observed in SIV-inoculated pigs during study period.

Systemic levels of acute phase proteins

All studied APP increased after co-infection, with mean maximum concentrations from 3 to 7 DPI (Fig. 10.) ($p <$ 0.05). In single-inoculated animals different kinetics of acute phase response has been noted. In the control group concentrations of all APP were constant.

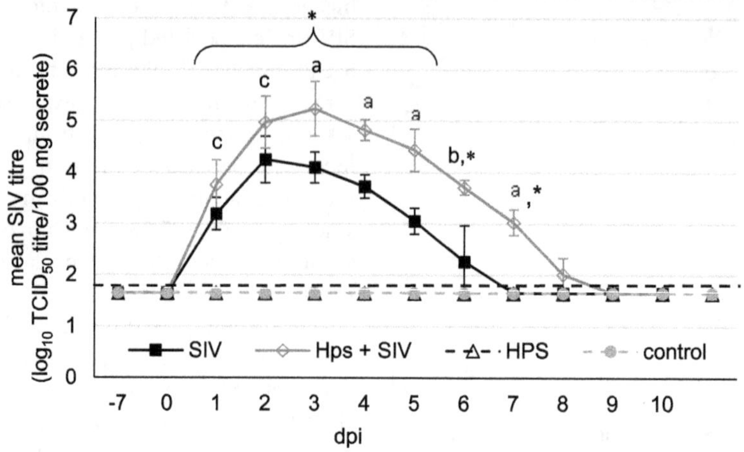

Fig. 4 Nasal virus shedding (mean ±SD) after inoculation of pigs with swine influenza virus (A/Poland/Swine/14131/2014) and or *Haemophilus parasius*. Mean virus titres (determined by cell culture) in nasal swabs collected during study period. The dashed line represents the detection limit. * - the significant differences compared to control group; a - the significant differences between inoculated groups; b - the significant differences between SIV and *Hps* + SIV inoculated groups; c – the significant differences between SIV, *Hps* + SIV and *Hps*

C-reactive protein

Significant increase in the mean concentration of CRP compared to control pigs has been observed in co-inoculated animals from 1 to 7 DPI. At 2 DPI the significant difference compared to control group was noted also for the *Hps*-inoculated pigs ($p < 0.05$). The maximum mean level of CRP in co-inoculated animals was observed at 3 DPI and reached 224.61 ± 96.80 μg/ml (almost 8-fold increase comparing to the day 0 level). In pigs inoculated only with *Hps* the maximum mean concentration of CRP was observed at 2 DPI (2.5 fold increase comparing to day 0 level). In pigs from SIV group the mean levels of CRP did not differ significantly from that determined in the control animals.

Haptoglobin

The concentration of Hp increased significantly in all inoculated groups comparing to control animals. The strongest and the most prolonged Hp response was found in SIV + *Hps* group. The mean concentration of Hp in this group had increased by 48 h after co-inoculation and were notably higher compared to control pigs ($p < 0.05$) to the end of study. Significant differences between single and dual-inoculated groups were observed from 3 to 10 DPI ($p < 0.05$). The highest mean concentrations of Hp in co-inoculated pigs were observed at 5 DPI. The mean maximal concentration was almost 9-fold higher, compared to the mean baseline concentration. The highest concentration of

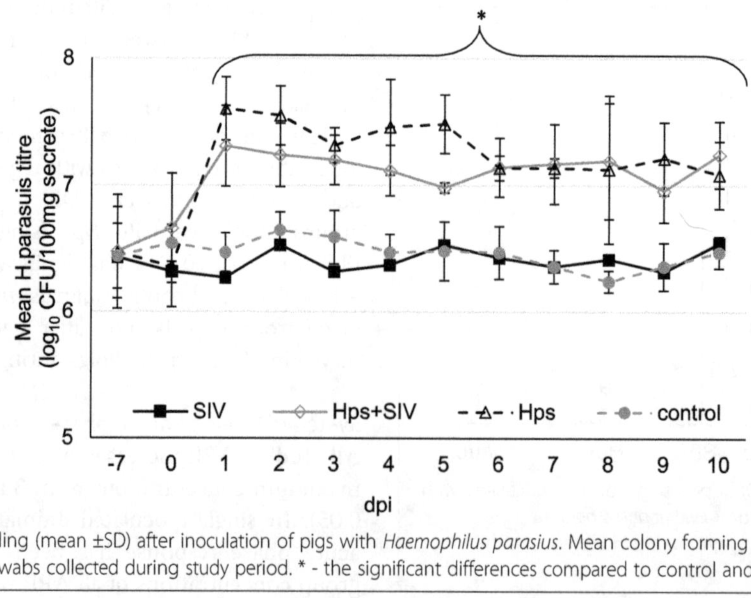

Fig. 5 Nasal bacteria shedding (mean ±SD) after inoculation of pigs with *Haemophilus parasius*. Mean colony forming units (CFU) (determined by quantitative PCR) in nasal swabs collected during study period. * - the significant differences compared to control and SIV group

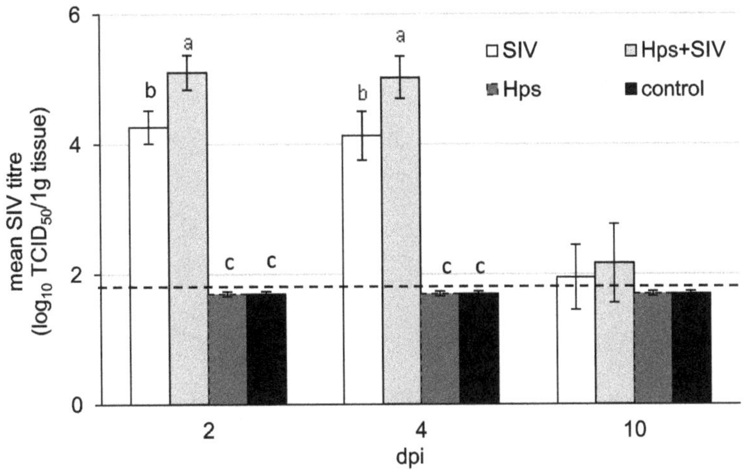

Fig. 6 Swine influenza virus titre (mean ±SD) (determined by cell culture) in the lung at 2, 4 and 10 days after single or dual inoculation of pigs with swine influenza virus and/or *Haemophilus parasius*. The dashed line represents the detection limit. Columns with various superscripts within the same day of study differ significantly

Hp in particular animal after coinfection reached 7.03 mg/ml (at 3 DPI). In pigs single inoculated with SIV or *Hps* only short-term increase in Hp level was recorded (at 2 and 3 DPI in SIV-inoculated and at 3 dpi in *Hps*-inoculated pigs).

Serum amyloid

A. Significant increase of SAA concentration was found in all inoculated groups ($p < 0.05$). No significant changes were found in control pigs ($p \geq 0.05$). The strongest reaction has been noted in co-inoculated animals. The mean peak concnetration in mentioned group was detected at 3 DPI and reached 254.31 ± 181.32 μg/ml (over 100-fold increase comparing to the day 0 level). Significantly higher concentration compared to the controls was observed from 1 to 5 DPI ($p < 0.05$). In the remaining, single-inoculated groups the mean maximum concentrations were observed at 2 DPI (over 15-fold increase) and significant differences compared to controls were noted from 2 to 3 DPI ($p < 0.05$).

Pig major acute phase protein

Baseline levels of Pig-MAP in experimental animals were found to be below 0.92 mg/ml. Concentration of Pig-MAP increased significantly 72 h after co-inoculation and inoculation with *Hps* ($p < 0.05$). In co-inoculated pigs the concentration of Pig-MAP remained significantly elevated till 10 DPI (end of study), while in *Hps*-single inoculated pigs till 5

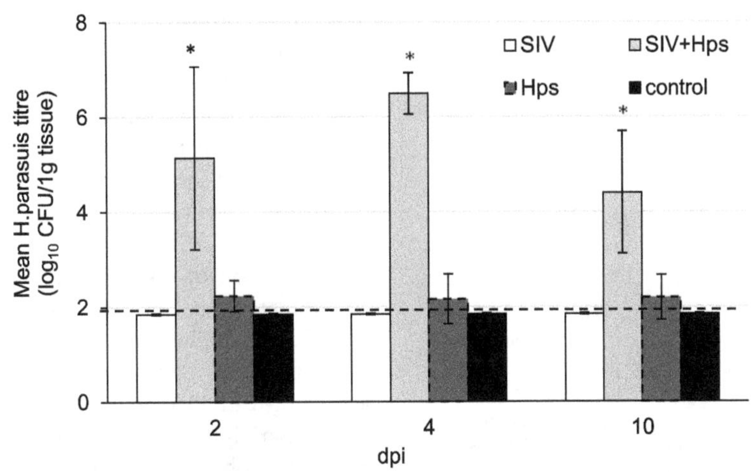

Fig. 7 *H. parasuis* titres (mean ±SD) (determined by quantitative PCR) in the lung at 2, 4 and 10 days after single or dual inoculation of pigs with swine influenza virus and/or *Haemophilus parasius*. The dashed line represents the detection limit. * - significant differences compared to remaining groups

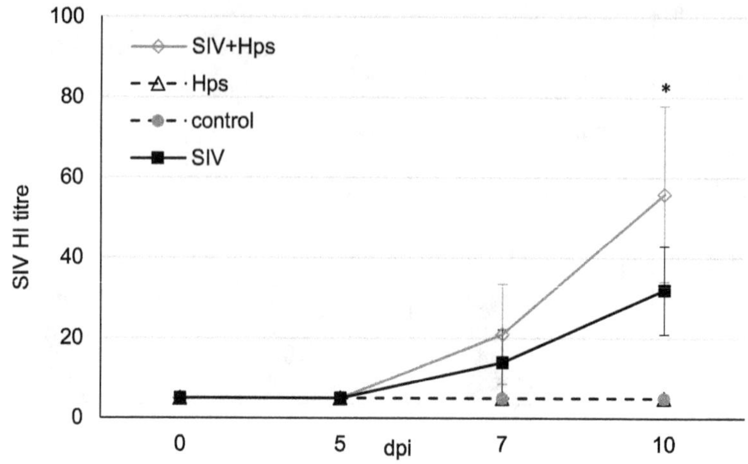

Fig. 8 Mean (±SD) HI antibody titres against A/Poland/Swine/14131/2014 SIV in of pigs single or dual inoculated with swine influenza virus (SIV) and/or *Haemophilus parasius* (Hps). * - significant differences compared to groups not inoculated with SIV

dpi. The highest Pig-MAP mean levels were observed between 5 to 7 DPI. The maximum mean concentration of Pig-MAP, observed at 7 DPI in piglets from SIV + *Hps* group was almost 3 times higher compared to day 0-level (baseline concentration). There were no significant differences in the kinetics of Pig-MAP response between co-inoculated and *Hps*-single inoculated pigs. In pigs single inoculated with SIV as well as in control animals the level of Pig-MAP in serum was constant during study period.

Cytokines – Local lung response

In general the local concentrations of TNF-α, IFN-γ, IL-1β, IL-6 and IL-10 were induced mostly in SIV + *Hps* pigs (Fig. 11). In control pigs the concentrations of all investigated cytokines were relatively constant ($p \geq 0.05$).

At 2 DPI, concentrations of proinflammatory cytokines (IL-1β, IL-6, TNF-α) and IFN-γ were significantly higher in the lungs of co-inoculated pigs compared to controls (with exception of IL-1β and TNF-α in apical lobes). Furthermore significant differences were observed between co-inoculated and single inoculated pigs, with exception of IL-1β and TNF-α in apical lobes, and IFN-γ in middle and accessory lobes. In particular differences were noted between *Hps* and SIV + *Hps* group with regard to IFN-γ (all lobes) and TNF-α, IL-1β and IL-6 (except apical lobes) as well as between co-inoculated and SIV groups with regard to IFN-γ and IL-1β. No significant differences were found between control and single inoculated pigs with regard to IL-1β and IL-10 level in all lobes from the upper part of the right lung at that time. The highest concentrations of cytokines were generally observed in right middle lobes what positively correlated with the lesions detected during necropsy.

At 4 DPI the concentrations of all investigated cytokines were significantly higher in co-inoculated pigs, compared to controls ($p < 0.05$). No significant differences were observed with regard to IL-1β and IL-10 in single-inoculated groups, compared to controls ($p \geq 0.05$). With regard to SIV + *Hps* group the significantly higher concentration of investigated cytokines was observed in all evaluated parts of the lung. In SIV inoculated animals significantly higher concentration of IFN-γ compared to control group was observed in middle and accessory lobes, IL-6 in all lobes and TNF-α in apical and middle lobes. No significant increase in the level of cytokines tested was observed in *Hps* inoculated group ($p \geq 0.05$).

At 10 DPI the lung concentrations of cytokines generally decreased compared to 2 and 4 DPI, but in the case of IL-1β, IL-6 and IL-10 (in co-inoculated animals) were

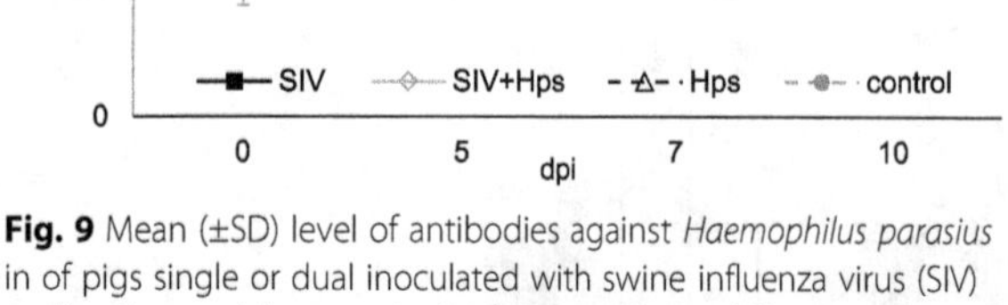

Fig. 9 Mean (±SD) level of antibodies against *Haemophilus parasius* in of pigs single or dual inoculated with swine influenza virus (SIV) and/or *Haemophilus parasius* (*Hps*) * - significant differences compared to control group; a - significant differences between co-inoculated pigs and *Hps* single-inoculated groups. ELISA ratio (ER) was calculated as directed by the manufacturer (Swinecheck®HPS, Biovet, Canada) according to the following formula: Er $= \frac{\text{OD of test serum from wells with Ag-OD of test serum from wells without Ag}}{\text{mean OD (+) from wells with Ag-mean OD (+) from wells without Ag}}$ (+) - positive control, Ag - antigen

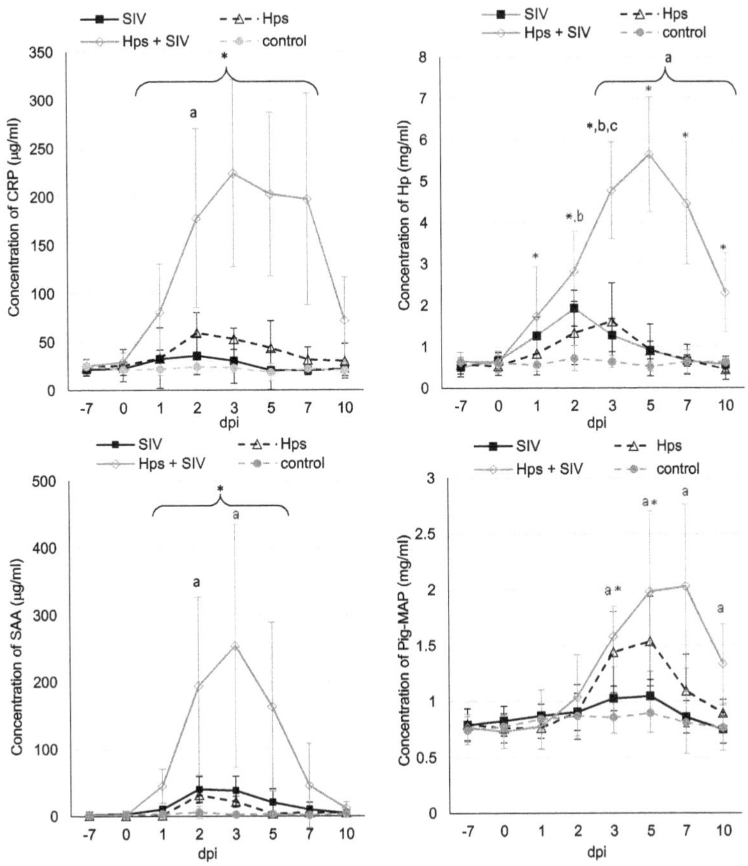

Fig. 10 Concentrations of SAA, Pig-MAP, Hp and CRP (mean ±SD) in serum of pigs before and on various time-point after single or dual inoculation with swine influenza virus (SIV) and/or *Haemophilus parasius* (Hps). CRP: * - significant differences between co-inoculated and control group; a - significant differences between *Hps*-inoculated and control group; Hp: a- significant differences between single and dual-inoculated groups; * - significant differences between co-inoculated and control pigs; b - significant differences between SIV and control groups, c - significant differences between *Hps* and control groups. SAA: * - significantly differences between co-inoculated and control pigs, a – significant differences between single-inoculated and control pigs. Pig-MAP: a – significant differences between co-inoculated and control pigs; * - significant differences between Hps and control group

still significantly higher compared to controls ($p < 0.05$). Significantly greater concentrations were observed for IL-1β with regard to middle and accessory lobes, for IL-6 with regard to apical lobe and for IL-10 with regard to all lobes ($p < 0.05$). No significant differences between local concentrations of all investigated cytokines in single-inoculated and control animals were found for all lung lobes at 10 dpi.

Summarizing, the maximum concentrations of cytokines in general were observed at 4 DPI. The highest concentrations of most cytokines were found in the apical and middle lobe. These results correlated well with localization of gross lung lesions. Significant correlations were found between lung concentration of IL-1β, IL-6, IFN-γ and TNF-α and pathological changes in the lungs (R-Spearman = 0.65; 0.63; 0.71 and 0.62 respectively; $p < 0.05$). A positive correlation was also observed between concentrations of IL-1β and IFN-γ in the lungs and clinical signs (R-Spearman = 0.64 and 0. 67 respectively, p < 0.05). No significant correlation between local cytokine concentration and systemic APP response were found.

Discussion

Swine influenza is commonly characterized by fever, respiratory and systemic nonspecific symptoms (i.e. loss of appetite, apatia) [16]. In the enzootic form, clinical signs may be less obvious. Subclinical infection is also quite common [17, 21, 22]. During uncomplicated infection the morbidity can be as high as 100% but the mortality is relatively low (ranges from less than 1% to 4%). The most common complications of swine influenza are secondary bacterial pneumonia and PRDC [3, 12]. Coinfections often lead to overproduction of cytokines that may be harmful to the host [12]. There are several mechanisms, by which SIV infection predisposes to secondary bacterial infection, including: increased expression of cell receptors leading to increased colonization and modification of host immune responses (i.e. impairing of

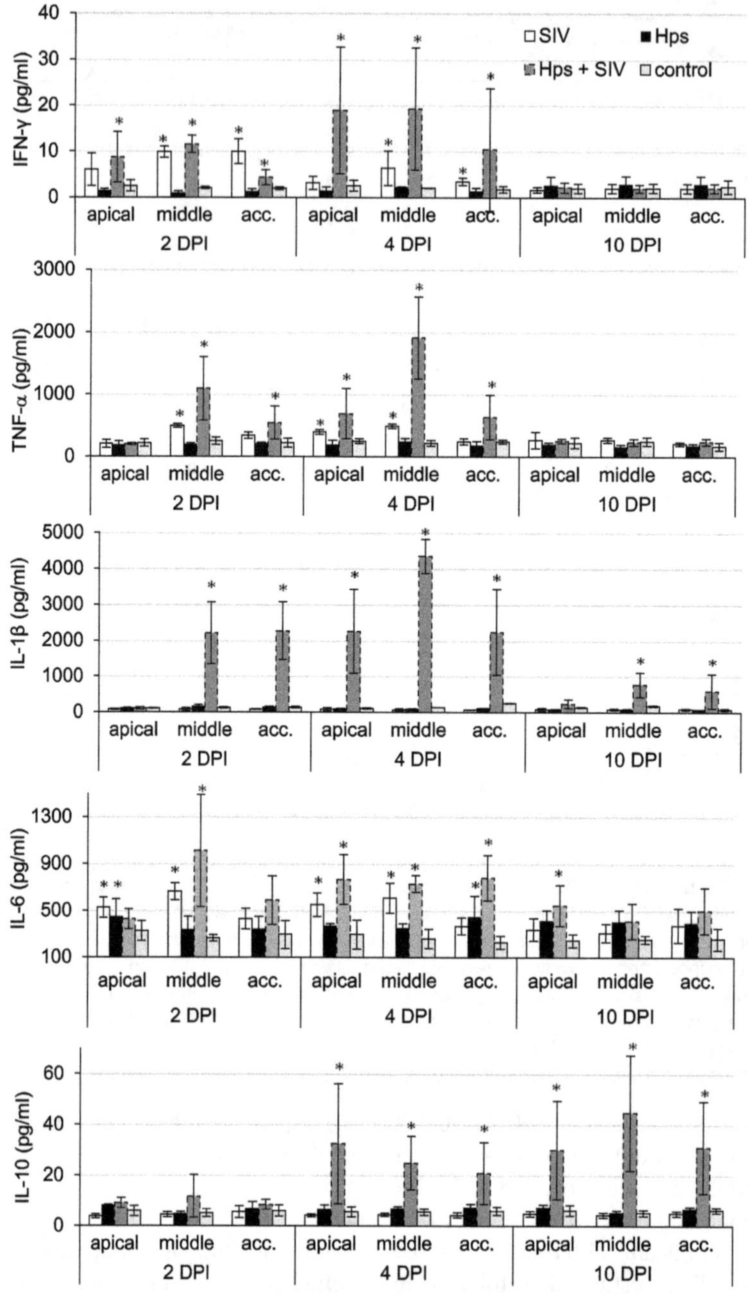

Fig. 11 Quantification of cytokines in lung tissue of pigs single or dual inoculated with swine influenza virus (SIV) and/or *Haemophilus parasius* (Hps) (mean±SD). acc-accessory lobe; * - significant differences compared to control pigs (within the same day, at the same part of the lung)

phagocytic function of alveolar macrophages) [23–26]. Furthermore, it has been shown that damage caused by SIV in the respiratory tract (i.e. loss of cilia, extrusion of mucus, exudation, necrosis and metaplasia of airway epithelium), can reduce the ability of the host to clear the bacterial superinfection [2, 21]. *Hps* is one of the pathogens which may complicate swine influenza and be one of the etiological agents of PRDC [2, 3, 8, 27].

The mechanism by which SIV affects the host's susceptibility as well as its immune response to secondary bacterial infections has not been fully elucidated. Previous research reviled that interactions among multiple pathogens can lead to an exacerbated inflammatory response and increased severity of infections [12, 28–30]. For example, gross lesions in the lungs and magnitude of APP response in pigs co-infected with SIV and *Pasteurella multocida* were more intensive compared to animals infected only with SIV or *Pasteurella multocida* [28]. Similar results were observed in pigs co-inoculated with SIV and *A. pleuropneumoniae* [19]. Co-infection with SIV and *A. pleuropneumoniae* potentiated the severity of lung lesions caused by SIV and enhanced virus replication in the lung and nasal SIV shedding. Enhanced SIV replication contributed to a more severe clinical course of the disease as well as earlier and higher magnitude immune and inflammatory responses [19]. Loving et al. [12] reported that SIV infection increased *Bordetella bronchiseptica* (Bb) colonization and increased the production of proinflammatory cytokines likely to exacerbate lung lesions. Pulmonary lesions in the co-infected pigs were more intense compared to SIV-only or Bb-only groups. The type I interferon, IL-1β and IL-8 were also significantly elevated in lungs of co-infected pigs.

There is limited data on the influence of SIV and *Hps* coinfection on the clinical course, kinetics of the immune and inflammatory response, as well as pathogen load and shedding [13]. Both microorganisms are frequently isolated from respiratory tract of pigs in the field conditions [1, 27]. A previous study [13], investigating the role of prior SIV infection on the *Hps* colonization, revealed that *Hps* colonization was higher in the nose and lungs of SIV/*Hps* pigs compared to *Hps*-only pigs. These results indicate that SIV infection contributes to enhance bacterial colonization. In SIV/*Hps* pigs IL-8, IL-6 and IL-1β protein levels were increased in the tracheal wash and bronchoalveolar lavage fluid (BALF), and BALF cells IL-8, IL-6 and IL-1β mRNA expression levels were significantly increased over SIV-only and Hps-only pigs.

Based on the results of our study it could be stated that *Hps* did not cause significant lesions in the lung unless pigs were co-infected with SIV. No significant macroscopic lung lesions after experimental infection with *Hps* has been also reported previously [8]. In the same study *Hps* was not isolated from *Hps*-single infected pigs. In our experiment we had been able to isolate of *Hps* in the case of 3 out of 11 *Hps*-single inoculated pigs, but in group co-inoculated with SIV the isolation was successful in 8 out of 11 animals. In the remaining groups (SIV and control) *Hps* was not isolated from lung. Typical systemic lesions of polyserositis were found in only one pig from co-inoculated group. In the present study no significant differences between gross lung lesions has been found between groups single or dually inoculated with SIV but in both groups lung score was significantly higher than in *Hps*-single inoculated group. In addition, more severe clinical signs were observed in dual inoculated pigs compared to single *Hps*- but not SIV-inoculated animals. The more severe clinical course of the infection was probably a consequence of more severe lung lesions present in pigs inoculated with SIV or SIV and *Hps*. Enhanced lung lesions in pigs single or dual inoculated with SIV could be a result of stronger replication of infective agents and more severe local inflammatory responses. Similarly as in the previous study [12] establishing that the titre of Bb was higher in the respiratory tract of SIV/Bb co-infected pigs, we found that SIV enhanced *Hps* colonization of the lung. In accordance to other experiment [19] the significantly higher SIV titre in the nasal swabs and lung was observed in co-inoculated pigs. Simultaneously, no effect of SIV on the *Hps* shedding has been found. These findings suggest that *Hps* can facilitate SIV replication in the respiratory tissue of dual inoculated pigs.

The significant influence of both pathogens on the systemic inflammatory response has been also found in the present study. In the groups inoculated with bacteria (single or dual) the APP response was in general higher than in virus-single inoculated animals. These findings are in accordance with the results of previous studies with various respiratory pathogens of swine [12, 19, 31, 32].

Conclusions

The results of our study revealed that coinfection with SIV and *Hps* modulates inflammatory responses, clinical course of disease and pathogen load within the respiratory tract in pigs. Co-infection with SIV potentiates the severity of lung lesions and facilitated *Hps* replication in the porcine lung. Furthermore, *Hps* influenced the SIV nasal shedding. Enhanced *Hps* and SIV replication, together with stronger systemic and local inflammatory response contributed to a more severe clinical signs, as well as stronger and earlier immune response in co-inoculated animals compared to single inoculated pigs. Moreover, we confirmed the previous evidence [8] that single-*Hps* infection does not produce significant pneumonic lesions but it should be in mind that other strains of *Hps* may produce lesions different from that reported in the present study.

Methods

Virus

The virus used in experiment (avian-like H1N1 A/Poland/Swine/14131/2014 (SIV)), had been isolated from the lung of pig suffering from acute swine influenza. This strain is representative H1N1 SIVs circulating recently in Poland. The stock used for nasal inoculation represented the third passage in eggs. The virus titre was evaluated in Madin-Darby canine kidney (MDCK) cells (ATCC).

Bacteria

Strain of *Hps*, previously isolated in National Veterinary Research Institute was selected for the experimental infections (isolate PIWetHps192/2015). Strain originating from lung of pig from Polish herd and the analysis of the 16S rRNA gene sequences [33] revealed 99% similarity to *Hps* isolate CN9–2 described by Olvera et al. [34] (classified as moderate virulent serovar 15).

To prepare the inoculum, the strain was streaked onto a pleuropneumonia-like organism (PPLO) agar (Becton Dickinson, USA), supplemented with 10 μg/ml of β-NAD

(Sigma-Aldrich, Germany), 1 mg/ml glucose (Avantor Performance Materials, Poland) and 5% horse serum (Sigma-Aldrich, Germany), which was incubated for 24 h at 37 °C in an atmosphere of 8% CO2. Colonies were harvested and suspended in phosphate-buffered saline (PBS) (Life Technologies, USA) to 0.5 McFarland turbidity (which corresponds with approximately 1.5×10^8 colony forming units (CFU)/ml). A plate count was also performed to quantify the accurate number of viable bacteria (final result 1.2×10^8 CFU/ml of *Hps* strain).

Experimental design

Thirty seven 6-week-old piglets bought from a commercial farm, both sexes, were used in the study (as research animals). Piglets were randomly allocated to 4 groups (*Hps* ($n = 11$); *Hps* + SIV (n = 11); SIV (n = 11); control ($n = 4$) (a sample size calculation based on a resource equation method). The sourced herd was seronegative to P, pseudorabies virus and *Mycoplasma hyopneumoniae.* No evidence of streptococcosis, pleuropneumoniae, Glässers disease and atrophic rhinitis was recorded based on clinical, serological (detection of dermonecrotoxin specific antibodies and antibodies to ApxIV) and pathological examinations (turbinate lesions, polyserositis, polyarthritis, serofibrinous or fibrino-purulent exudate on mucosal surface, arthritis, meningitis). Before the start of the study all piglets were free of influenza A virus and *Hps* antibodies as determined by haemagglutination inhibition assays (HI) using A/Poland/Swine/14131/2014 (H1N1), A/swine/England/96 (H1N2), A/swine/Flanders/1/98 (H3N2), pdm-like H1N1 (A/swine/Poland/031951/12) and Swinecheck® HPS ELISA test (Biovet, Canada).

During the experiment research animals were housed on a (Biosafety Level-3) BSL3 animal facility in four independent units. Animal use and handling protocols were approved by II Local Ethical Commission for the Animal Experiments of University of Life Sciences in Lublin (number of approval: 77/2014).

The animals were acclimatized to BSL3 hygienic conditions for 7 days before commencing the experiment. On day 0, piglets from SIV and *Hps* + SIV groups were inoculated intranasally (IN) with SIV ($10^{6.8}TCID_{50}$ in 3 ml of PBS. Piglets from *Hps* and *Hps* + SIV groups were inoculated IN with *Hps* (3.6×10^8 CFU *Hps* in 3 ml of PBS. Four mock-inoculated pigs served as controls.

Pigs were examined daily from day - 7 to 10 post inoculation (DPI) or until euthanasia (at 2 and 4 DPI). Animals were observed and scored for the respiratory signs as follows: respiratory rate: 0 – normal (<34 breaths/min), 1 – slightly elevated (35–40 breaths/min), 2 – moderately elevated (41–45 breaths/min), slight abdominal breathing, 3 – clearly elevated (>46 breaths/min), distinct abdominal breathing; nasal discharge 0 – absent, 1 present; coughing 0 – absent, 1 present; sneezing 0 – absent, 1 present, anorexia 0 – absent, 1 present [17]. Rectal temperature was also measured daily. Hyperthermia was recorded when the rectal temperature reached 40 °C. If the fever was observed 1 additional point was added to the clinical score. All scores per topic were accumulated for a final clinical score calculated for each pig (0–8).

Sample collection

Nasal swabs were collated daily from all animals (at –7, 0 (inoculation), 1, 2, 3, 4, 5, 6, 7, 8, 9 and 10 DPI). Blood samples were collected at –7, 0 (inoculation), 1, 2, 3, 5, 7 and 10 DPI. Three piglets per inoculated groups were euthanized at 2 and 4 DPI. The remaining inoculated as well as control pigs were euthanized and necropsied at 10 DPI. Complete necropsy was done on each animal, with special emphasis on the respiratory tract. Lung lesions were scored using the method developed by Madec and Kobisch [35] according to the scheme presented in details previously [19]. Samples from lung (apical, middle, caudal right lobes and accessory lobe) were collected for further analyses.

Laboratory examination

Pathogen shedding and load

SIV titration (nasal swabs, lung tissue) in Madin-Darby canine kidney cells (MDCK) (ATCC) were performed in duplicate as described previously [17].

For determination the quantity of *Hps* in samples collected from piglets (nasal swabs and lung tissue fragments) the quantitative real-time PCR was used (all samples were tested in duplicate) [36]. It targets the 392–466 bp region of the infB gene of *Hps*. Nasal swabs were placed into centrifuge tubes (2 ml), suspended in 1 ml of PBS and after 10 min vortexed for 30 s. The liquid was collected to the new tube (1.5 ml) and suspensions were centrifuged at 3000 *g* during 3 min. The supernatant was discarded and the remaining pellet was resuspended in 100 µl of TRIS buffer (10 mM Tris–HCl pH 8.5) and vortexed for an additional 30 s. Homogenates (50% wt/vol) of middle right lobe (the main site of gross lesions observed in the present study) were prepared in PBS. DNA was extracted from thus prepared samples using the Genomic Mini DNA isolation kit (A&A Biotechnology, Poland) according to the manufacturer instructions. DNA was stored at –70 °C for further analysis.

Serum analyses

All sera were examined using HI assays (SIV) against challenge strain and ELISA test against *Hps* as directed by the manufacturer (Swinecheck®HPS, Biovet, Canada). The presence or absence of antibodies to investigated antigen (Ag) was determined by calculating the ELISA ratio. ELISA ratio (Er) was calculated according to the following formula:

$$\mathrm{Er} = \frac{\text{OD of test serum from wells with Ag-OD of test serum from wells without Ag}}{\text{mean OD } (+) \text{ from wells with Ag-mean OD } (+) \text{ from wells without Ag}}$$

(+) - positive control

Antibodies against SIVs were measured using a HI assay, performed according to the standard procedure, using 0.5% chicken erythrocytes and 4HA units of challenge strains [37]. All sera were tested in serial twofold dilutions, starting at 1:20. For estimates of the prevalence of antibodies, titres ≥20 were considered positive [38]. For statistical analyses the titres lower than 20 was set as 5.

Acute phase proteins (C-reactive protein (CRP, haptoglobin (Hp), serum amyloid A (SAA) and pig major acute phase protein (Pig-MAP)) were examined using ELISA assays according to producer's recommendations (Pig C-reactive protein ELISA and Pig haptoglobin ELISA from Life Diagnostics, USA; Pig-MAP KIT ELISA from Acuvet Biotech S.L., Spain; Phase Serum Amyloid A Assay from Tridelta Development Ltd. County Kildare, Ireland). All serum samples were tested in duplicate.

Lung proinflammatory cytokine levels

Lung tissues were collected from pigs during necropsy and prepared in PBS (pH 7.4) [12, 16]. 1.0 g of the lung tissue fragments were suspended in 1 ml of PBS, respectively (1:1 *w*/*v*), and frozen before being homogenized. After homogenization, with the use of tissue homogenizer X620 (CAT, Germany), the samples were centrifuged at 3000 *g* for 10 min. The supernatants were collected and stored at −80°C before cytokines analysis was performed using ELISA assay. The ELISA kits specific for porcine cytokines: IL-10, IFN-γ and TNF-α were bought from Invitrogen Corporation (Camarillo, USA), and these used for IL-1β were bought from RayBiotech, Inc. (Norcross, USA). The concentration of IL-6 was determined with the use of IL-6 Pig ELISA Kit from Abcam (Cambridge, UK). All tests were performed in duplicate according to the manufacturers' recommendations. The quantity of the cytokines was calculated based on standard curve for each cytokine with the use of FindGraph software.

Statistical analysis

The data were subjected to the W. Shapiro-Wilk's test of normality and the Levene'a test of equal variances with STATISTICA 8.0 (StatSoft). Differences between means were tested for statistical significance by a nonparametric Kruskal - Wallis test with post hoc multiple comparisons for comparison of all pairs. The Friedman test was used to compare observations repeated on the same subjects. For analysis of correlation the Spearman Rank correlation test was used. For all analyses, $p < 0.05$ was considered statistically significant.

Abbreviations

Ag: Antigen; APP: Acute phase proteins 19; CFU: Colony forming unit; CRP: C-reactive protein; DPI: Day post infection; Er: ELISA ratio; HI: Haemagglutination inhibition; Hp: Haptoglobin; Hps: *Haemophilus parasuis*; IFN-γ: Interferon gamma; IL: Interleukin; OD: Optical density; PBS: Phosphate buffered saline; Pig-MAP: Pig major acute phase protein; Pm: *Pasteurella multocida*; PRDC: Porcine respiratory disease complex; PRRSV: Porcine reproductive and respiratory syndrome virus; SAA: Serum amyloid A; SIV: Swine influenza virus; TCID50: 50% tissue culture infective dose; TNF-α: Tumor necrosis factor alfa

Acknowledgments

The authors wish to thank Ewelina Stasiak and Barbara Frącek for technical assistance.

Funding

This work was supported by The National Science Centre (DEC-2014/13/B/NZ6/02566) and by KNOW (Leading National Research Centre) Scientific Consortium, "Healthy Animal - Safe Food", a decision of Ministry of Science and Higher Education, No. 05–1/KNOW2/2015 (K/02/1.1; K/02/5.0). The funders of the study had no role in study design or conclusion of present study.

Authors' contributions

MPM designed the experiments and analyzed the experimental data and performed statistical analysis. AD, EC-D, KK and MPM performed the experiments (inoculation, necropsy, clinical examination, preparation the serum and tissue samples, laboratory examination). MPM and ZP prepared the manuscript and supervised the experiment. All authors have read and approved the final manuscript.

Consent for publication

Not applicable.

Competing interests

None of the authors of this paper has a relationship with other people or organisations that could influence or bias the content of the paper. The authors declare that they have no competing interests.

References

1. Fablet C, Marois C, Dorenlor V, Eono F, Eveno E, Jolly JP, Le Devendec L, Kobisch M, Madec F, Rose N. Bacterial pathogens associated with lung lesions in slaughter pigs from 125 herds. Res Vet Sci. 2012;93(2):627–30.
2. Opriessnig T, Gimenez-Lirola LG, Halbur PG. Polymicrobial respiratory disease in pigs. Anim Health Res Rev. 2011;12(2):133–48.
3. Choi YK, Goyal SM, Joo HS. Retrospective analysis of etiologic agents associated with respiratory diseases in pigs. Can Vet J. 2003;44(9):735–7.
4. Truszczyński M, Pejsak Z. Contribution of Pasteurella multocida to the porcine respiratory disease complex. Medycyna Weterynaryjna. 2010;66(8):512–5.
5. de la Fuente AJ M, Gutierrez Martin CB, Perez Martinez C, Garcia Iglesias MJ, Tejerina F, Rodriguez Ferri EF. Effect of different vaccine formulations on the development of Glasser's disease induced in pigs by experimental Haemophilus parasuis infection. J Comp Pathol. 2009;140(2–3):169–76.

6. Simon-Grifé M, Martín-Valls GE, Vilar MJ, Busquets N, Mora-Salvatierra M, Bestebroer TM, Fouchier R, Martín M, Mateu E, Casal J. Swine influenza virus infection dynamics in two pig farms; results of a longitudinal assessment. Vet Res. 2012;43(1):24.
7. Brockmeier SL, Halbur PG, Thacker EL. Porcine respiratory disease complex. In: GJ BKA, editor. Polymicrobial diseases. Washington (DC): ASM Press; 2002.
8. Vahle JL, Haynes JS, Andrews JJ. Experimental reproduction of Haemophilus parasuis infection in swine: clinical, bacteriological, and morphologic findings. J Vet Diagn Investig. 1995;7(4):476–80.
9. Oliveira S, Pijoan C. Haemophilus parasuis: new trends on diagnosis, epidemiology and control. Vet Microbiol. 2004;99(1):1–12.
10. Rapp-Gabrielson VJ, Gabrielson DA. Prevalence of Haemophilus parasuis serovars among isolates from swine. Am J Vet Res. 1992;53(5):659–64.
11. Jablonski A, Zebek S, Kolacz R, Pejsak Z. Usefulness of PCR/RFLP and ERIC PCR techniques for epidemiological study of Haemophilus parasuis infections in pigs. Pol J Vet Sci. 2011;14(1):111–6.
12. Loving CL, Brockmeier SL, Vincent AL, Palmer MV, Sacco RE, Nicholson TL. Influenza virus coinfection with Bordetella bronchiseptica enhances bacterial colonization and host responses exacerbating pulmonary lesions. Microb Pathog. 2010;49(5):237–45.
13. Loving C, Brockmeier S, Vincent A. Prior swine influenza virus infection enhances pulmonary responses to secondary Haemophilus parasuis infection. In: Proceedings of the Pig Veterinary Society International Congress. Perry: IPVS; 2010. p. 264.
14. Oliveira S, Galina L, Blanco I, Canals A, Pijoan C. Naturally-farrowed, artificially-reared pigs as an alternative model for experimental infection by Haemophilus parasuis. Can J Vet Res. 2003;67(2):146–50.
15. Barigazzi G, Valenza F, Bollo E. Anatomohistopathological features related to Haemophilus parasuis infection in pigs. In: Proceedings of the Pig Veterinary Society International Congress. IPVS: Bangkok; 1994. p. 235.
16. Pomorska-Mol M, Markowska-Daniel I, Kwit K, Czyzewska E, Dors A, Rachubik J, Pejsak Z. Immune and inflammatory response in pigs during acute influenza caused by H1N1 swine influenza virus. Arch Virol. 2014;159(10):2605–14.
17. Pomorska-Mol M, Kwit K, Markowska-Daniel I, Kowalski C, Pejsak Z. Local and systemic immune response in pigs during subclinical and clinical swine influenza infection. Res Vet Sci. 2014;97(2):412–21.
18. Pomorska-Mol M, Markowska-Daniel I, Kwit K, Stepniewska K, Pejsak Z. Profile of the porcine acute-phase proteins response following experimental co-infection with H3N2 swine influenza virus and Pasteurella multocida. Biomarkers. 2015;20(3):189–95.
19. Pomorska-Mól M, Dors A, Kwit K, Kowalczyk A, Stasiak E, Pejsak Z. Kinetics of single and dual infection of pigs with swine influenza virus and Actinobacillus pleuropneumoniae. Vet Microbiol. 2017;201:113–20.
20. Pomorska-Mól M, Markowska-Daniel I, Kwit K, Urbaniak K, Pejsak Z. Correlation between serum acute phase proteins, lung pathology and disease in pigs after H3N2 swine influenza virus and Bordetella bronchiseptica experimental co-infection. BULL VET INST PULAWY 2015;59:1-7.
21. Brown IH. The epidemiology and evolution of influenza viruses in pigs. Vet Microbiol. 2000;74(1–2):29–46.
22. van Reeth K, Nauwynck H. Proinflammatory cytokines and viral respiratory disease in pigs. Vet Res. 2000;31(2):187–213.
23. Avadhanula V, Rodriguez CA, Devincenzo JP, Wang Y, Webby RJ, Ulett GC, Adderson EE. Respiratory viruses augment the adhesion of bacterial pathogens to respiratory epithelium in a viral species- and cell type-dependent manner. J Virol. 2006;80(4):1629–36.
24. Astry CL, Jakab GJ. Influenza virus-induced immune complexes suppress alveolar macrophage phagocytosis. J Virol. 1984;50(2):287–92.
25. Didierlaurent A, Goulding J, Patel S, Snelgrove R, Low L, Bebien M, Lawrence T, van Rijt LS, Lambrecht BN, Sirard JC, et al. Sustained desensitization to bacterial toll-like receptor ligands after resolution of respiratory influenza infection. J Exp Med. 2008;205(2):323–9.
26. Azoulay-Dupuis E, Lambre CR, Soler P, Moreau J, Thibon M. Lung alterations in guinea-pigs infected with influenza virus. J Comp Pathol. 1984;94(2):273–83.
27. Fablet C, Marois-Crehan C, Simon G, Grasland B, Jestin A, Kobisch M, Madec F, Rose N. Infectious agents associated with respiratory diseases in 125 farrow-to-finish pig herds: a cross-sectional study. Vet Microbiol. 2012;157(1–2):152–63.
28. Pomorska-Mol M, Markowska-Daniel I, Kwit K, Stepniewska K, Pejsak Z. C-reactive protein, haptoglobin, serum amyloid a and pig major acute phase protein response in pigs simultaneously infected with H1N1 swine influenza virus and Pasteurella multocida. BMC Vet Res. 2013;9:14.
29. Pomorska-Mol M, Markowska-Daniel I, Kwit K. Acute phase protein response in pigs experimentally co-infected with swine influenza virus and Bordetella bronchiseptica. Cen Eur J Immunol. 2012;37(3):221–6.
30. Brockmeier SL, Loving CL, Nicholson TL, Palmer MV. Coinfection of pigs with porcine respiratory coronavirus and Bordetella bronchiseptica. Vet Microbiol. 2008;128(1–2):36–47.
31. Thacker EL, Thacker BJ, Janke BH. Interaction between Mycoplasma hyopneumoniae and swine influenza virus. J Clin Microbiol. 2001;39(7):2525–30.
32. Thacker EL, Halbur PG, Ross RF, Thanawongnuwech R, Thacker BJ. Mycoplasma hyopneumoniae potentiation of porcine reproductive and respiratory syndrome virus-induced pneumonia. J Clin Microbiol. 1999;37(3):620–7.
33. Olvera A, Calsamiglia M, Aragon V. Genotypic diversity of Haemophilus parasuis field strains. Appl Environ Microbiol. 2006;72(6):3984–92.
34. Olvera A, Cerdà-Cuéllar M, Nofrarías M, Revilla E, Segalés J, Aragon A: Dynamics of Haemophilus parasuis genotypes in a farm recovered from an outbreak of Glässer's disease. 2007, 123(1–3):230–237.
35. Madec F, Kobisch M. Bilan lésionnel des porcs charcutiers à l'abattoir. Journées de la Recherche Porcine en France. 1982;14:405–12.
36. Turni C, Pyke M, Blackall PJ. Validation of a real-time PCR for Haemophilus parasuis. J Appl Microbiol. 2017;108(4):1323–31.
37. Pomorska-Mol M, Markowska-Daniel I, Pejsak Z. Acute phase protein response during subclinical infection of pigs with H1N1 swine influenza virus. Vet Microbiol. 2012;159(3–4):499–503.
38. Pomorska-Mol M, Czyzewska-Dors E, Kwit K, Wierzchoslawski K, Pejsak Z. Ceftiofur hydrochloride affects the humoral and cellular immune response in pigs after vaccination against swine influenza and pseudorabies. BMC Vet Res. 2015;11:268.

16

Effect of herd size on subclinical infection of swine in Vietnam with influenza A viruses

Nobuhiro Takemae[1,2], Yugo Shobugawa[3], Phuong Thanh Nguyen[4], Tung Nguyen[5], Tien Ngoc Nguyen[5], Thanh Long To[6], Phuong Duy Thai[4], Tho Dang Nguyen[6], Duy Thanh Nguyen[4], Dung Kim Nguyen[4], Hoa Thi Do[6], Thi Quynh Anh Le[4], Phan Truong Hua[4], Hung Van Vo[4], Diep Thi Nguyen[5], Dang Hoang Nguyen[6], Yuko Uchida[1,2], Reiko Saito[3] and Takehiko Saito[1,2,7*]

Abstract

Background: Influenza A viruses of swine (IAV-S) cause acute and subclinical respiratory disease. To increase our understanding of the etiology of the subclinical form and thus help prevent the persistence of IAV-S in pig populations, we conducted active virologic surveillance in Vietnam, the second-largest pig-producing country in Asia, from February 2010 to December 2013.

Results: From a total of 7034 nasal swabs collected from clinically healthy pigs at 250 farms and 10 slaughterhouses, we isolated 172 IAV-S from swine at the weaning and early-fattening stages. The isolation rate of IAV-S was significantly higher among pigs aged 3 weeks to 4.5 months than in older and younger animals. IAV-S were isolated from 16 large, corporate farms and 6 family-operated farms from among the 250 farms evaluated. Multivariate logistic regression analysis revealed that "having more than 1,000 pigs" was the most influential risk factor for IAV-S positivity. Farms affected by reassortant IAV-S had significantly larger pig populations than did those where A(H1N1)pdm09 viruses were isolated, thus suggesting that large, corporate farms serve as sites of reassortment events.

Conclusions: We demonstrate the asymptomatic circulation of IAV-S in the Vietnamese pig population. Raising a large number of pigs on a farm has the strongest impact on the incidence of subclinical IAV-S infection. Given that only some of the corporate farms surveyed were IAV-S positive, further active monitoring is necessary to identify additional risk factors important in subclinical infection of pigs with IAV-S in Vietnam.

Keywords: Active surveillance, Influenza A virus, Pig, Pig farm, Vietnam

Background

Influenza A viruses of swine (IAV-S) are important infectious agents that contribute to porcine respiratory disease complex [1–4]. Pigs infected with IAV-S typically demonstrate depression, anorexia, and labored abdominal breathing [5], and IAV-S frequently are isolated from pigs showing acute clinical signs [3]. The high morbidity rate associated with IAV-S, which reaches approximately 100 % among pigs kept together in the same pig pen or farm, causes heavy economic losses in the pig industry because of high medication costs and decreased weight gain [6]. In addition, our previous active surveillance of IAV-S in clinically healthy pigs in Thailand revealed that subclinical infection frequently affects pigs in the weaning and early-fattening stages on farrow-to-finish pig farms [7]. This finding suggests that IAV-S exist either in a subclinical form or in an epizootic form that causes the typical respiratory syndrome in pigs [8–11]. However, the dynamics of subclinical IAV-S in pig populations are not yet well understood, largely because most IAV-S surveillance is conducted passively—that is, by using samples submitted to a laboratory after outbreaks of respiratory disease.

* Correspondence: taksaito@affrc.go.jp
[1]Influenza and Prion Diseases Research Center, National Institute of Animal Health, NARO, Ibaraki, Japan
[2]Thailand-Japan Zoonotic Diseases Collaboration Center, Bangkok, Thailand
Full list of author information is available at the end of the article

According to serosurveillance data from Canada [12], seroprevalence for the H1N1 subtype was 61.1 % among 65 sow herds and 24.3 % among 72 finisher herds. In addition, an estimated 49.8 % of the finisher herds in the United States are infected with IAV-S [13]. Serologic studies on IAV-S in Canada [12], Belgium [1], France [4], Spain [14, 15], Malaysia [16], and England [17] have found that "high number of pigs per farm or pen", followed by "importation or purchase of pigs" and "proximity of the farm to other pig farms", are the key risk factors for increased rates of seropositivity against IAV-S. In addition, "way of the moving pigs on the farms" and "lack of all-in–all-out management" have been suggested as risk factors for H1N1 and H1N2 IAV-S, respectively [4]. Despite these studies, how IAV-S persist in pig populations during the intervals between disease outbreaks remains unclear, because serosurveillance cannot reveal the dynamics of infection with either subclinical or epizootic IAV-S.

IAV-S in Vietnam have not been studied thoroughly, even though Vietnam is considered a high-priority target country for improvements in IAV-S monitoring, given that its pig and poultry populations are large [18]. Vietnam was the second-largest producer of pork in Asia in 2012 [19], and about 85 % of the country's total pig production comes from smallholders rearing fewer than 20 sows [20, 21]. In addition, these smallholders often concurrently raise multiple types of livestock, including pigs and poultry—a practice considered to support the interspecies transmission of influenza viruses as well as genetic reassortment between avian and mammalian influenza viruses [22]. Furthermore, large-scale production by commercial producers rose from 2 % to 17 % of the total pig product in the 2000s [21, 23], resulting in an increase of about 7 million pigs in Vietnam [19]; thus, industrialized production is gradually replacing traditional, small-farm production.

We have been monitoring Vietnamese IAV-S at the various types of pig holdings, including large- and small-scale farms and slaughterhouses, since February 2010 and have reported subclinical infections with novel reassortant H3N2 and H1N2 IAV-S and A(H1N1)pdm09 viruses in Vietnamese pigs from 2010 to 2011 [24, 25]. The reassortant H3N2 and H1N2 IAV-S affected corporate, large-scale farms, whereas the A(H1N1)pdm09 viruses were present on both large-scale farms and family-operated small farms. Overall, most of the farms that we investigated earlier had neither of these viruses. These findings prompted us to consider that management procedures might affect the incidence of subclinical IAV-S infection on pig farms in Vietnam. In addition, we surmised that risk factors for subclinical infection might differ between the enzootic strains in pig populations and the A(H1N1)pdm09 viruses, which were recently reintroduced into pig populations from humans [26]. To answer these questions, we collected information related to pig husbandry methods, including the number of pigs, biosecurity level, and type of operation, through interviews with farmers when we collected samples between February 2010 and December 2013 for virus isolation. We applied univariate and logistic regression analysis to the husbandry and virologic surveillance data to identify factors involved in the enzooticity of IAV-S in Vietnamese pigs.

Methods

Sample collection

We collected nasal swabs 17 times in total from pig farms in northern and southern Vietnam from February 2010 to December 2013. Nasal swab samples were collected twice or three times in a year during the period. We collected a total of 6659 nasal-swab samples from clinically healthy pigs on a total of 250 pig farms located in 10 provinces where pig farming was prevalent, comprising 3 provinces (Bac Ninh, Hanoi, and Nam Dinh) in the northern region and 7 provinces (Ba Ria Vung Tau, Binh Duong, Dong Nai, Long An, Ho Chi Minh, Soc Trang, and Tien Giang) in the southern region. Farms were recruited to include a variety of farms differing in total number of pigs reared and operation type to reflect the whole situation of Vietnamese pig industry. Owners' consent was obtained upon enrolment. Previous history of influenza or respiratory disease was not considered as a condition for the enrollment. The first five collection events occurred during or before February 2011; nasal swabs were collected from groups of suckling pigs, weanling pigs, fattening pigs, mature sows, and adult boars. During the remaining twelve samplings, we sampled weanling and fattening pigs only. Of the 250 farms, 55 were visited more than once (2 to 6 times) and during different periods. We collected 14 to 30 nasal swabs from each farm at each visit, thus allowing us to detect at least one infected pig when the disease prevalence was 7.5 % to 20 % at 95 % confidence [27]. If a small farm had fewer than 14 pigs, nasal swabs were collected from all available pigs.

During December 2010, we visited 10 slaughterhouses located in Ho Chi Minh, Binh Duong, and Long An provinces and collected 375 nasal swabs in total. At each slaughterhouse we collected nasal swabs from 20 to 75 finishing pigs (age, approximately 6 months); samples were collected from as many pigs as possible at each slaughterhouse at each sampling time. In the same way as for the samples taken from pig farms, all of the samples from slaughterhouse pigs were collected from animals that lacked clinically evident respiratory disease.

Ethical approval was not required for this study, because taking a nasal swab does not cause pain and lasting harm to a pig. Informed consent was obtained from all participating pig farm/slaughter house owners.

Virus isolation and characterization

Nasal swab samples were collected from pigs by using flocked swabs with a plastic handle (Ex Swab 001, Denka Seiken, Tokyo, Japan). The swab was inserted 7 to 10 cm from the external naris, and the nasopharynx was rubbed several times with the swab. Each sample-bearing swab was placed immediately into a 15-ml tube containing 2 ml transport medium (MEM containing penicillin [1000 unit/ml], streptomycin [1000 µg/ml], Fungizone [25 µg/ml] (Thermo Fisher Scientific, Waltham, MA, USA), 0.01 M HEPES, and 0.5 % bovine serum albumin) and kept at 4 °C. After centrifugation at 1400 × *g* for 5 min, the supernatant fluid was aliquoted and kept at −80 °C until use. Pooled supernatant (2 to 5 nasal swabs per pool) was screened by real-time PCR using SYBR Premix Ex Taq (Takara Bio, Shiga, Japan) with primers targeting the M gene of influenza A viruses, as previously described [24]. When a pooled sample was positive by PCR, the nasal swabs represented in the pooled samples were individually passed over a 0.45-µm pore-size filter (Millipore, Billerica, MA, USA) and the filtered materials was inoculated into floating MDCK cells. To prepare floating MDCK cells, monolayers of MDCK cells were washed 3 times with sterile PBS to eliminate residual fetal calf serum; 0.05 % trypsin–EDTA solution (Thermo Fisher Scientific) was then added and the trypsinized cells were collected into maintenance MEM containing penicillin (100 units/ml), streptomycin (100 µg/ml), Fungizone (2.5 µg/ml), gentamicin (100 µg/ml), and 0.4 % bovine serum albumin. After centrifugation at 400 × *g* for 5 min, the cells were resuspended at a concentration of 1.0×10^6 cells/ml in maintenance MEM containing 5.0 µg/ml TPCK–trypsin (Thermo Fisher Scientific), and 1.6 ml was dispensed into each Nunc cell-culture tube (flat surface area 5.5 cm^2) (Thermo Fisher Scientific). A 160-µl aliquot of the original nasal swab was inoculated into the resuspended MDCK cells and incubated for 4 days at 37 °C in 5 % CO_2. When viruses were not isolated from the PCR-positive swab using floating MDCK cells, the original materials were inoculated into embryonated chicken eggs and/or primary cultures of porcine alveolar epithelial cells as previously described [25, 28]. Hemagglutination (HA) activity was tested by using 0.55 % red blood cells from guinea pigs or chickens as previously described [28]. If HA activity was not observed after the first passage, the supernatant fluids collected were inoculated into each substrate once more.

Nucleotide sequences of the viruses isolated were determined by direct sequencing of PCR products as previously described [25] and by next-generation sequencing (NGS) (Miseq, Illumina, San Diego, CA, USA). cDNA libraries for NGS were prepared by using a NEBNext Ultra RNA Library Prep Kit for Illumina (NEB, Ipswich, MA, USA). The libraries prepared were sequenced by using a Miseq Reagent Kit V2 (Illumina), and the fragments obtained were mapped to the reference sequences of influenza A viruses by using Genomics Workbench software (CLC Bio, Aarhus, Denmark). The sequences obtained were used as query sequences in BLAST searches, then the genetic origins of each segment were determined based on the genetic lineages of the strains with the highest identity of the known lineage, such as A(H1N1)pdm09, North American Triple reassortant, and human seasonal lineages and so on. The nucleotide sequences obtained in the present study have been deposited in GISAID Epiful database (http://www.gisaid.org), strain IDs are available on Additional file 1.

Statistical analysis

The age and production stage of the pigs from which the nasal swabs were collected were recorded during the visit. In addition, epidemiologic data (including farm type, number of pigs, availability of disinfection facilities, other animals on farm, operation type, the type of pig house, introduction of pigs from other farms, vaccine history, and so on; Additional file 2) were collected as variables for statistical analysis by interviewing the farmers on each farm. The variables were defined as follows: farm type ("corporate farm" managed by a company or "family-operated" farm managed by owner's family); numbers of pigs (numbers of sows, suckling pigs, weanling pigs, fattening pigs, and boars); disinfection facility (availability of shower or tank for humans or vehicles at the farm entrance); other animals on farm (poultry, cats, dogs, cattle, etc. kept or not kept); operation type (farrow-to-finish or wean-to-finish or farrow-to-wean, or a combination of these three operation types); type of pig house (windowless or open-sided or semi-open-sided; open- and semi-open-sided pig houses allow wildlife such as birds to enter easily); introduction of pigs from other farms (pigs for breeding purchased or produced on the premises); vaccine history (types of vaccines used on farms, e.g., classic swine fever, foot-and-mouth disease, porcine reproductive and respiratory syndrome, Aujeszky's disease, *Mycoplasma* spp.); respiratory disease histories in pigs or working staff (respiratory symptoms observed in pigs or working staff within the 6 months before our sampling); and presence of livestock farms within 100 m.

Influenza positivity was confirmed through virus isolation. The age and stage distributions of the pigs investigated were assessed by Fisher's exact test to identify the age or production group most susceptible to subclinical infection with IAV-S. A farm was considered positive when at least one virus was isolated from the nasal swabs tested. Differences in management procedures between influenza-positive and influenza-negative farms were assessed by using a logistic regression model in univariate analysis. IAV-S positivity or negativity was set as the dependent variable, and all variables describing farm characteristics were evaluated individually in regression models; selected variables were evaluated simultaneously in multivariate analysis. Independent variables were identified by calculating Pearson's correlation coefficient, then variables with a high correlation coefficient (>0.6) were excluded to avoid multicollinearity. Finally, variables among influenza-positive farms were analyzed to reveal whether risk factors for subclinical infection with IAV-S differed among strains. All of the statistical procedures were performed in STATA SE version 12 (LightStone, Tokyo, Japan).

Results

The 250 farms analyzed comprised 45 corporate farms, 189 family-operated farms (including smallholders), and 16 farms for which no information regarding farm type was obtained. The largest farm had 82,700 pigs, and the smallest farm had 6 pigs (median, 72); 2 farms did not report the number of pigs. Among the 250 farms were 133 farrow-to-finish farms that maintained sows and fed the offspring until they reached market weight, 30 wean-to-finish farms that purchased weanling piglets and raised them to finishing, and 8 farrow-to-wean farms from which piglets were sold after they were weaned; the remaining 79 farms used a combination of these three operation types. Vaccines against swine influenza were not available in Vietnam; the most common vaccines used at the farms were for classic swine fever (75.6 % of the farms investigated), foot-and-mouth disease (52.0 %), and porcine reproductive and respiratory syndrome (29.2 %). Dogs and poultry (chickens or ducks) were the other animals most commonly kept on pig farms (60.4 %). In addition, 27 farms reported respiratory symptoms in pigs, represented by coughing and nasal discharge, within the 6 months before our sampling; 5 of these 27 farms reported concurrent respiratory symptoms in working staff.

The number of pigs slaughtered daily ranged from 70 to 900 (median, 117.5) at the 10 slaughterhouses investigated. Finishing pigs were slaughtered within 6 to 48 h after arriving at a slaughterhouse from a pig farm. Of the 10 slaughterhouses, 8 processed pigs only; both pigs and cattle were killed at the remaining 2 slaughterhouses.

A total of 172 IAV-S—43 A(H1N1)pdm09, 47 H1N2, and 82 H3N2 subtype—were isolated from the 6659 nasal swabs collected from clinically healthy pigs at pig farms (Table 1). No viruses were isolated from the 375 nasal swabs collected at slaughterhouses. Virus isolation rates differed significantly between production stages (Fisher's exact test: $P < 0.001$): 62.2 % of the viruses were isolated from weanling pigs compared with 37.8 % from fattening pigs (Table 1). Pigs from which IAV-S were isolated ranged in age from 3 weeks to 4.5 months (median, 1.5 months); no viruses were isolated from suckling pigs younger than 3 weeks or older than 6 months, including finishing pigs, sows, and boars.

At least one IAV-S was isolated from each of 22 of the 250 farms tested, including 16 corporate farms housing 1392 to 82,700 pigs (median, 4205) and 6 family-operated farms with 20 to 654 pigs (median, 45). Univariate analysis regarding farm management practices between the 22 IAV-S-positive farms and the 228 IAV-S-negative farms revealed that the factors of farm type, total number of pigs, availability of a shower-in facility for humans, presence of a disinfection facility for vehicles, and presence of other animals on the farm were significantly associated with IAV-S subclinical infection (Table 2). The likelihood of IAV-S positivity was significantly increased when a farm was a corporate rather than a family-owned operation ($P < 0.001$) and when it had more than 1000 pigs compared with fewer than 50 pigs ($P < 0.001$). In addition, the availability of disinfection facilities for either humans or vehicles at the farm entrance increased the likelihood of IAV-S subclinical infection ($P < 0.001$). The likelihood of IAV-S positivity was also significantly increased in farms where disease histories in pigs ($P = 0.002$) and staffs ($P = 0.032$) had been observed within 6 months before sampling (Table 2). In contrast, pig farms that also had poultry (chicken, duck), dogs, cats, cattle, or other animals had a significantly lower odds ratio than did the farms that reared pigs only ($P = 0.005$). No correlations were found between the likelihood of IAV-S subclinical infection and presence of pig and/or other livestock farms within 100 m.

The subsequent regression multivariate analysis showed that the factor "total number of pigs" on the pig farm was significantly associated with subclinical infection with IAV-S (Table 3). Specifically, the likelihood of IAV-S positivity was 25.54 times higher for farms with 1000 pigs or more than for those with fewer than 1000 pigs ($P < 0.001$) (Table 3). The four variables included in the regression analysis—"type of operation", "total number of pigs", "type of pig house", and "other animals on farm"—were selected on the basis of the Pearson correlation analysis (see Additional file 3). Because "total number of pigs" was highly associated with "corporate farms", "shower-in facility for humans", and "disinfection facility for vehicles", those three variables were excluded from the multivariate model. In addition the presence of other animals was negatively associated with the total number of pigs (Additional file 3). We therefore could not rule out the possibility that the presence of other animals were confounded with the total number of pigs.

Table 1 Specimen collection and IAV-S isolated from different pig production stages and age groups in Vietnam

		IAV-S positive		IAV-S negative		P value[a]	Number of IAV-S in each subtype		
		number	%	number	%		H1N1	H1N2	H3N2
Stage	Suckling pig	0	0	290	4.2	<0.001	0	0	0
	Weanling pig	107	62.2	3268	47.6		19	17	71
	Fattening pig	65	37.8	2671	38.9		23	32	10
	Finishing pig[b]	0	0	375	5.5		0	0	0
	Sow	0	0	240	3.5		0	0	0
	Boar	0	0	18	0.3		0	0	0
Age	0 to <1 month old	22	12.8	467	6.8	<0.001	0	7	15
	1 to <2 months old	80	46.5	2593	37.8		17	12	51
	2 to <3 months old	46	26.7	2030	29.6		14	20	12
	3 to <6 months old	24	14.0	1139	16.6		11	10	3
	>6 months old	0	0	633	9.2		0	0	0
Number of viruses isolated		172					42	49	81

[a]Fisher's exact test
[b]Samples from finishing pigs were collected at slaughterhouses

However, because "other animals on farm" had been considered as a risk factor for IAV-S infection in other previous study [16], we used this variate in the multivariate analysis. As the result, it did not turn out that it has effect on the IAV-S positivity in our multivariate analysis (Table 3).

All of the genetic origins of each segment of the isolates in this study showed more than 97 % identities with strains whose genetic origins had been defined in previous studies. All of the segments of the H1N1 isolates were derived from A(H1N1)pdm09 viruses (Fig. 1). In contrast, the H1N2 and H3N2 IAV-S isolated in this study were reassortants that had at least two genes derived from enzootic strains in the Vietnamese pig population (Fig. 1) [24, 29]. In particular, 113 IAV-S (87 %) out of 130 H1N2 and H3N2 isolates were reassortants between endemic strains and A(H1N1)pdm09 viruses (Fig. 1). To examine whether the risk factors for IAV-S subclinical infection differed among strains, we compared management practices between A(H1N1)pdm09-positive farms and farms positive for endemic IAV-S. One corporate farm where both A(H1N1)pdm09 virus and an enzootic strain were isolated was included as being both A(H1N1)pdm09v-positive and enzootic-positive (Table 4). This comparison revealed that two variables—"total number of pigs" and "other animals on farm"—differed significantly between the two kinds of farms (Fisher's exact test: $P < 0.01$) (Table 4). That is, farms with 1,000 pigs or more had a significantly higher risk of infection by endemic strains infection than did the farms where A(H1N1)pdm09 viruses were isolated. No enzootic strains were isolated from family-operated farms with fewer than 50 pigs, whereas A(H1N1)pdm09 viruses were isolated from 4 family-operated farms. All 8 farms from which A(H1N1)pdm09 viruses were isolated were rearing other animals in addition to pigs. In contrast, the 9 farms, out of 15 farms positive for enzootic IAV-S, were raising only pigs.

Discussion

To date, few studies [30–32] have addressed the subclinical forms of IAV-S, because the presence of IAV-S on a farm has been demonstrated mainly through passive or serologic surveillance efforts. Our active virologic monitoring indicates that IAV-S have spread subclinically in the Vietnamese pig population. One important finding of our study is that, in Vietnam, IAV-S are more prevalent on farms with 1000 pigs or more than on smaller farms. Modern industrialized farms have emerged in Vietnam since 2000 and have gradually replaced the traditional, small, family-run farms [21, 23], as has occurred in the United States and in European countries over the last several decades [31, 33]. Rearing a large number of pigs on a farm is recognized as one of the most influential risk factors for IAV-S seropositivity in sows and fattening pigs [1, 4, 12, 17]. Our current results coincide with these previous findings, although the earlier serologic studies did not differentiate between subclinical infections and typical, clinical infections in pigs [1, 4, 12, 17]. Housing large numbers of susceptible pigs closely together likely provides appropriate conditions for IAV-S to circulate continuously in the pig population on a farm [12, 31]. In addition, the intensification of husbandry practices associated with large-scale farms might increase the frequency of movement of workers and vehicles to and within a farm, thus increasing the risk of pathogen transmission [34].

We isolated A(H1N1)pdm09 viruses from both corporate and family-run farms. This result is consistent

Table 2 Differences in farm characteristics between IAV-S-positive and IAV-S-negative farms

Variable		IAV-S-positive farms, no.	(%)	IAV-S-negative farms, no.	(%)	Odds ratio	95 % CI	*p* value[a]
Farm type[b]	Family-operated farm	6	(27.3 %)	183	(86.3 %)		reference	
	Corporate farm	16	(72.7 %)	29	(13.7 %)	16.83	6.09 to 46.52	<0.001
Total number of pigs	<50	4	(18.2 %)	108	(47.8 %)		reference	
	50 to 500	1	(4.5 %)	83	(36.7 %)	0.33	0.04 to 2.97	0.319
	501 to 1000	1	(4.5 %)	14	(6.2 %)	1.93	0.20 to 18.50	0.569
	≧1000	16	(72.7 %)	21	(9.3 %)	20.57	6.25 to 67.70	<0.001
Shower-in facility for humans[c]	No	5	(26.3 %)	195	(85.9 %)	17.06	reference	
	Yes	14	(73.7 %)	32	(14.1 %)		5.75 to 50.62	<0.001
Disinfection facility for vehicles[c]	No	7	(31.8 %)	194	(85.8 %)	12.99	reference	
	Yes	15	(68.2 %)	32	(14.2 %)		4.92 to 34.34	<0.001
Other animals on farm[d]	No	9	(42.9 %)	33	(16.1 %)	0.26	reference	
	Yes	12	(57.1 %)	172	(83.9 %)		0.10 to 0.66	0.005
Type of operation	Not farrow-to-finish[e]	5	(22.7 %)	91	(39.9 %)		reference	
	Including farrow-to-finish	17	(77.3 %)	137	(60.1 %)	2.26	0.81 to 6.34	0.12
Type of pig house[f]	Open- or semi-open-sided house	20	(90.9 %)	178	(78.1 %)	0.36	reference	
	Windowless	2	(9.1 %)	50	(21.9 %)		0.08 to 1.58	0.173
Introduction of pigs	No	1	(5.6 %)	30	(19.7 %)	4.18	reference	
	Yes	17	(94.4 %)	122	(80.3 %)		0.54 to 32.67	0.173
Vaccination[g]	No	1	(5.3 %)	32	(15.1 %)	3.20	reference	
	Yes	18	(94.7 %)	180	(84.9 %)		0.41 to 24.82	0.266
Respiratory diseases history in pig[h]	No	15	(68.2 %)	208	(91.2 %)		reference	
	Yes	7	(31.8 %)	20	(8.8 %)	4.85	1.77 to 13.29	0.002
Respiratory diseases history in working staff[h]	No	20	(90.9 %)	225	(98.7 %)		reference	
	Yes	2	(9.1 %)	3	(1.3 %)	7.50	1.18 to 47.54	0.032
Livestock farm within 100 m[i]	No	14	(68.2 %)	116	(91.2 %)		reference	
	Yes	6	(31.8 %)	111	(8.8 %)	0.45	0.17 to 1.21	0.112
Pig farm within 100 m	No	14	(68.2 %)	157	(91.2 %)	0.96	reference	
	Yes	6	(31.8 %)	70	(8.8 %)		0.35 to 2.61	0.938

[a]Logistic regression analyses were performed to calculate odds ratio of IAV-S-positive vs -negative farms for each variable
[b]Corporate farm managed by a company, and family-operated farm managed by owner's family
[c]Disinfection facilities for humans or vehicles at the farm entrance
[d]Poultry (chickens, ducks), dogs, cats, cattle, etc
[e]Farrow-to-wean or wean-to-finish farms
[f]Windowless house or (semi-) open-sided house
[g]Vaccines for diseases other than swine influenza. Swine influenza vaccine is not available in Vietnam
[h]Respiratory symptoms observed in pigs or working staff within the 6 months before our sampling
[i]Presence of livestock farms including pig farm within 100 m

with other reports, such as those of the large, corporate farms in the United States [26] and Canada [35], as well as small family-operated farms in Peru [36] and Canada [37]. According to the genetic analysis, Vietnamese H1N1 isolates in this study showed the high identity with A(H1N1)pdm09 viruses, reflecting viral transmission from humans to pigs, as has been seen in many other countries [35, 38–40]. Such human-to-pig transmission of A(H1N1)pdm09 viruses increases global public health concerns, because reassortment with enzootic IAV-S could generate influenza A viruses with novel gene combinations in the pig population. Pigs are highly susceptible to A(H1N1)pdm09 viruses [41], and our data suggest that efforts to prevent the introduction of these strains into farms have not been effective. According to the NCBI Influenza Virus Resource, A(H1N1)pdm09 viruses had been isolated from pigs in 34 countries as of 2015 [42]. Unsurprisingly, many novel reassortants

Table 3 Logistic estimates for IAV-S positivity according to selected variables

Variable		*P*	Odds ratio	95 % CI
Total number of pigs	<1000		reference	
	≧1000	<0.001	25.54	7.42 to 87.98
Type of operation	Not farrow-to-finish		reference	
	Including farrow-to-finish	0.85	0.89	0.24 to 3.24
Type of pig house	Open-sided or semi-open-sided house		reference	
	Windowless	0.26	0.36	0.06 to 2.10
Other animals on farm	No		reference	
	Yes	0.55	0.70	0.21 to 2.29
Constant		<0.001	0.13	

between A(H1N1)pdm09 viruses and the enzootic IAV-S have arisen in many countries and regions [43–49]. One such example with public health implications is a novel reassortant H3N2v, which is a triple-reassortant H3N2 IAV-S that contains an M gene from an A(H1N1)pdm09 virus. The H3N2v isolate was first identified from human in the United States in July 2011, and more than 300 human cases have been reported, although human-to-human transmission is limited [50].

According to the results of BLAST searches, most of the H1N2 and H3N2 IAV-S that we isolated were reassortants between enzootic strains in Vietnamese pigs and A(H1N1)pdm09 viruses. In particular, 97 % of these reassortants (125 isolates) were isolated from farms with 1,000 pigs or more. To our knowledge, eight out of 12 genotypes of H1N2 and H3N2 subtypes are never reported outside Vietnam (Fig. 1) [44, 51–55]. These findings suggests that large-scale farms provide an environment that is more conducive than that of small-scale farms for IAV-S to exchange their gene segments with each other and with other viruses. Subclinical infections likely spread more slowly than does the epidemic form that leads to acute respiratory disease on a farm [11, 12]. If so, subclinical infections with IAV-S warrant increased attention to prevent the generation of novel viruses, because prolonged virus circulation would increase the opportunity for reassortment events. We recently reported that numerous IAV-S with various gene constellations arose in weanling pigs co-infected with H1N1 and H3N2 IAV-S on a large, corporate farm [56]. In particular, plaque purification assays of nasal swabs revealed that at least 16 different constellations of gene segments emerged within a single co-infected pig that lacked clinical signs.

Young pigs of the weaning and early-fattening stages appear to play an important role in the interepizootic survival of IAV-S. High virus-isolation rates from clinically healthy pigs have been obtained from those aged 4

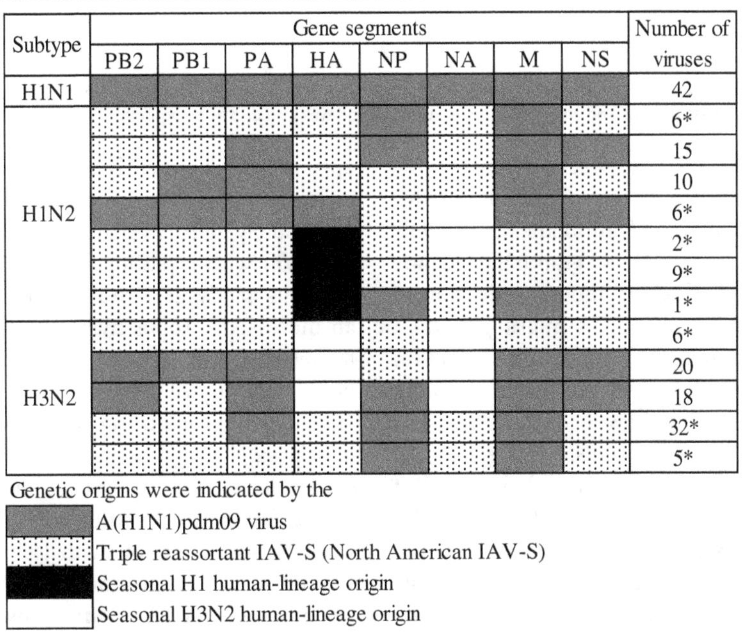

Fig. 1 Gene constellations of the IAV-S identified. Gene segments derived from A(H1N1)pdm09 viruses are represented as gray squares; those from enzootic strains are represented as stippled (North American triple-reassortant IAV-S), black (human, seasonal, H1 origin), and white (human, seasonal, H3 origin) squares. PB2, polymerase gene 2; PB1, polymerase gene 1; PA, polymerase gene A; HA, hemagglutinin gene; NP, nucleoprotein gene; NA, neuraminidase gene; M, matrix gene; and NS, non-structural gene. The numbers of the isolates in each genotype are indicated in the rightmost column. Asterisks indicate the novel genotypes found in this study

Table 4 Differences in farm characteristics between A(H1N1)pdm09v-positive and enzootic IAV-S-positive farms[a]

Variable		A(H1N1)pdm09v-positive farms, no. (%)	Enzootic IAV-S-positive farms, no. (%)	*P* value*
Total number of pigs	<50	4 (50.0 %)	0 (0.0 %)	
	50 to 500	0 (0.0 %)	1 (6.7 %)	
	500 to 1000	0 (0.0 %)	1 (6.7 %)	
	>1000	4 (50.0 %)	13 (86.7 %)	0.01
Other animals on farm	No	0 (0.0 %)	9 (60.0 %)	
	Yes	8 (100.0 %)	5 (33.3 %)	
	No answer	0 (0.0 %)	1(6.7 %)	0.01
Farm type	Family-operated farm	4 (50.0 %)	2 (13.3 %)	
	Corporate farm	4 (50.0 %)	13 (86.7 %)	0.13
Shower-in facility for humans	No	3 (37.5 %)	2 (13.3 %)	
	Yes	5 (62.5 %)	10 (66.7 %)	
	No answer	0 (0.0 %)	3 (20.0 %)	0.24
Disinfection facility for vehicles	No	3 (37.5 %)	4 (26.7 %)	
	Yes	5 (62.5 %)	11 (73.3 %)	0.66
Type of operation	Not farrow-to-finish	3 (37.5 %)	2 (13.3 %)	
	Including farrow-to-finish	5 (62.5 %)	13 (86.7 %)	0.30
Type of pig house	Open-sided or semi-open-sided house	8 (100.0 %)	13 (86.7 %)	
	Windowless	0 (0.0 %)	2 (13.3 %)	0.53
Introduction of pigs from external source	No	0 (0.0 %)	1 (6.7 %)	
	Yes	7 (87.5 %)	11 (73.3 %)	
	No information	1 (12.5 %)	3 (20.0 %)	1.00
Vaccination	No	0 (0.0 %)	1 (6.7 %)	
	Yes	5 (62.5 %)	14 (93.3 %)	
	No answer	3 (37.5 %)	0 (0.0 %)	0.03

*Fisher's exact test was applied to compare proportions between A(H1N1)pdm09v positive- and enzootic IAV-S-positive- farms
[a]One farm from which both A(H1N1)pdm09 virus and an enzootic strain were isolated was included as being both A(H1N1)pdm09v-positive and enzootic-positive

to 12 weeks in Thailand [7, 47], 12 weeks in Japan [57], and 4 to 12 weeks in the current study. These ages coincide with the waning of maternal antibodies in piglets; maternal antibodies against IAV-S gradually decline through 10 weeks of age [11]. Continuous production of susceptible piglets on large-scale farms might provide a chain of naïve hosts to maintain subclinical infection with IAV-S. In fact, recurrent IAV-S infections in young pigs on large commercial farms have been reported. For example, on a 300-sow farrow-to-finish swine farm in Spain, a specific IAV-S repeatedly affected a group of pigs over the course of 6 months, and this particular strain was the isolate most frequently found when the pigs were tested as 3- and 7-week-olds [10]. Interestingly, three of the pigs examined were infected with the same subtype strain twice on two different occasions during the 6-month period. Our previous active surveillance in Thailand alternately isolated H1N1 and H3N2 IAV-S from weanling pigs (age 4 to 8 weeks) at a 17-month interval [7]. In addition to young pigs, sows appear to be frequently infected with IAV-S, perhaps because they typically are the only group with any longevity (usually 4 to 6 years) on a farm; the likelihood of infection with a pathogen increases with time [15]. Our previous study and those of others have demonstrated an increased seropositivity rate against IAV-S in sows at farrow-to-finish farms [7, 12, 15, 58]. However, we did not isolate any IAV-S from clinically healthy sows in our current study or during our previous active surveillance in Thailand and Vietnam [7, 24, 47]. Therefore, how sows are involved in asymptomatic circulation of IAV-S on pig farms remains unclear.

Subclinical infection with IAV-S is currently not considered to have a pronounced negative effect on growth performance on pig farms. However, Er et al. [59] recently demonstrated that subclinical infection of pigs on Norwegian farms with A(H1N1)pdm09 viruses reduced both feed conversion efficiency and average daily growth. Interestingly, the adverse effect lasted longer than the viral shedding period (about 7 days). Specifically, pigs infected when they weighed 33 to 60 kg required 8.0 kg more feed to reach 100 kg bodyweight than did unexposed pigs. Consequently, the infected pigs took longer to reach market weight [55]. Although our current investigation did not directly address such adverse effects of subclinical infection in Vietnamese pigs, similar effects might be presumed.

In contrast to the situation on farms from which we isolated enzootic strains, the farms that harbored A(H1N1)pdm09 viruses were more likely to have kept animals other than pigs. Having mammalian pets on a farm was a risk factor for IAV-S seropositivity on Malaysian pig farms [16]. However, whether these other animals serve as "couriers" for spreading influenza A viruses within a farm is unclear, although A(H1N1)pdm09 viruses have a wide host range among mammals [41], including dogs [60] and cats [61]. In addition, we could not rule out the possibility that 'presence of other animals' is confounded with the number of pigs as concerned in the univariate analysis. Further study would be needed to understand a role of the presence of other animals in pig farms.

Introduction of pigs from outside a farm is another important risk factor for seropositivity against IAV-S in pigs [5, 12, 15, 16]. Many outbreaks of swine influenza are clearly related to the introduction of infected pigs [62]. However, our analysis failed to reveal a significant relationship between subclinical infection with IAV-S and the introduction of pigs, although 17 of the 22 IAV-S-positive farms had obtained gilts or weanling pigs from external sources. This discrepancy may be explained in part by the fact that 32 % (80 farms) of the farms had not recorded their purchase histories; these missing values consequently were excluded from our statistical analysis. Evaluating the effect of the introduction of pigs on subclinical infection with IAV-S on pig farms merits increased attention. Interestingly, 90 % of IAV-S positive farms (20 farms) had open- or semi-open-sided houses although it did not show significant P value compared with the positive farms having windowless pig houses, suggesting that the type of pig house may be worthy of attention in future studies. Although involvement of seasonality, presence of other respiratory pathogens, and humidity or temperature of barns, that were considered as risk factors for the IAV-S occurrence by previous studies [1, 4, 62], was unable to be evaluated in this study, those could be risk factors even in subclinical infections of IAV-S in pig farms and further study on those variables would provide useful information.

Conclusions

Taken together, our findings demonstrate the asymptomatic circulation of IAV-S in the Vietnamese pig population. Raising a large number of pigs on a farm has the strongest impact on the incidence of subclinical IAV-S infection, although not all the large-scale farms we evaluated suffered from subclinical IAV-S infection. In fact, 29 of the 37 large, corporate farms in our surveillance yielded no IAV-S, raising the possibility that risk factor(s) for subclinical infection other than a large number of pigs exist within this type of farm. Further active surveillance to define risk factors for subclinical infection with IAV-S in Vietnam would provide early detection of a virus with pandemic potential and would also mitigate economic losses in the pig industry.

Additional files

Additional file 1: Isolate_IDs and virus names deposited in GISAID Epiful database. (XLS 48 kb)

Additional file 2: Farm and sample information sheets used in the interviews with farm owners in this study. (DOC 107 kb)

Additional file 3: Pearson correlation matrix for the variables investigated. Pearson's correlation coefficient was used to identify independent variables collected in this study. (XLS 45 kb)

Acknowledgements

We thank all of the pig farmers who participated in this study and the staff of the Sub-Department of Animal Health of Bac Ninh, Ba Ria Vung Tau, Binh Duong, Dong Nai, Long An, Hanoi city, Ho Chi Minh city, Nam Dinh, Soc Trang, and Tien Giang provinces in Vietnam for coordinating and supporting the collection of pig nasal swabs. This research is supported by the Japan Initiative for Global Research Network on Infectious Diseases (J-GRID) from Ministry of Education, Culture, Sport, Science & Technology in Japan, and Japan Agency for Medical Research and Development (AMED).

Authors' contributions

NT designed the study, collected samples, isolated and characterized viruses, and drafted the manuscript; TS designed and coordinated the study and drafted the manuscript; YS and RS participated in the statistical analysis; PDT, DTN, TQAL, PTH, and HW, participated in the collection of the samples in 7 provinces in the southern region, and conducted virus isolation. HTD, DTN and, DHN participated in the collection of the samples in 3 provinces in the northern region, and conducted virus isolation; PTN and DKN coordinated the surveillance and collected epidemiological data in southern region. TN, TLT, TDN coordinated the surveillance and collected epidemiological data in the northern region; and TNN and YU helped to coordinate for this project; All authors have read and approved the manuscript.

Competing interests

The authors declare that they have no competing interests.

Author details

[1]Influenza and Prion Diseases Research Center, National Institute of Animal Health, NARO, Ibaraki, Japan. [2]Thailand–Japan Zoonotic Diseases Collaboration Center, Bangkok, Thailand. [3]Division of International Health, Graduate School of Medical and Dental Sciences, Niigata University, Niigata, Japan. [4]Department of Animal Health, Center for Veterinary Diagnostics, Regional Animal Health Office No. 6, Ho Chi Minh City, Vietnam. [5]Department of Animal Health, Epidemiology Division, Hanoi, Vietnam. [6]Department of Animal Health, National Centre for Veterinary Diagnostics, Hanoi, Vietnam. [7]United Graduate School of Veterinary Sciences, Gifu University, Gifu, Japan.

References

1. Maes D, Deluyker H, Verdonck M, Castryck F, Miry C, Vrijens B, et al. Herd factors associated with the seroprevalences of four major respiratory pathogens in slaughter pigs from farrow-to-finish pig herds. Vet Res. 2000;31:313–27.

2. Deblanc C, Gorin S, Quéguiner S, Gautier-Bouchardon AV, Ferré S, Amenna N, et al. Pre-infection of pigs with Mycoplasma hyopneumoniae modifies outcomes of infection with European swine influenza virus of H1N1, but not H1N2, subtype. Vet Microbiol. 2012;157:96–105.
3. Fablet C, Marois-Créhan C, Simon G, Grasland B, Jestin A, Kobisch M, et al. Infectious agents associated with respiratory diseases in 125 farrow-to-finish pig herds: A cross-sectional study. Vet Microbiol. 2012;157:152–63.
4. Fablet C, Simon G, Dorenlor V, Eono F, Eveno E, Gorin S, et al. Different herd level factors associated with H1N1 or H1N2 influenza virus infections in fattening pigs. Prev Vet Med. 2013;112:257–65.
5. Olsen CW, Brown IH, Easterday BC, Van Reeth K, Swine influenza. In: Straw DJ, Zimmerman JJ, d'Alaaire S, Taylor DJ, editors. Diseases of swine. 9th ed. Oxford: Blackwell Publishing; 2006. p. 469–82.
6. Bennett R, Ijpelaar J. Updated estimates of the costs associated with thirty four endemic livestock diseases in Great Britain: A note. J Agr Econ. 2005;56:135–44.
7. Takemae N, Parchariyanon S, Ruttanapumma R, Hiromoto Y, Hayashi T, Uchida Y, et al. Swine influenza virus infection in different age groups of pigs in farrow-to-finish farms in Thailand. Virol J. 2011;8:537.
8. Elbers ARW, Tielen MJM, Cromwijk WAJ, Hunneman WA. Variation in seropositivity for some respiratory disease agents in finishing pigs: Epidemiological studies on some health parameters and farm and management conditions in the herds. Vet Q. 1992;14:8–13.
9. Brown IH. The epidemiology and evolution of influenza viruses in pigs. Vet Microbiol. 2000;74:29–46.
10. Simon-Grife M, Martin-Valls G, Vilar M, Busquets N, Mora-Salvatierra M, Bestebroer T, et al. Swine influenza virus infection dynamics in two pig farms; results of a longitudinal assessment. Vet Res. 2012;43:24.
11. Loeffen WLA, Nodelijk G, Heinen PP, van Leengoed LAMG, Hunneman WA, Verheijden JHM. Estimating the incidence of influenza-virus infections in Dutch weaned piglets using blood samples from a cross-sectional study. Vet Microbiol. 2003;91:295–308.
12. Poljak Z, Dewey CE, Martin SW, Christensen J, Carman S, Friendship RM. Prevalence of and risk factors for influenza in southern Ontario swine herds in 2001 and 2003. Can J Vet Res. 2008;72:7–17.
13. Bush EJ, Thacker EL, Swenson SL. National seroprevalence of PRRS, mycoplasma, and swine influenza virus. Am Assoc Swine Vet. 2003; 491–4. https://www.aphis.usda.gov/animal_health/nahms/swine/downloads/swine2000/Sero_PRRS.pdf.
14. Fraile L, Alegre A, López-Jiménez R, Nofrarías M, Segalés J. Risk factors associated with pleuritis and cranio-ventral pulmonary consolidation in slaughter-aged pigs. Vet J. 2010;184:326–33.
15. Simon-Grife M, Martin-Valls GE, Vilar MJ, Garcia-Bocanegra I, Mora M, Martin M, et al. Seroprevalence and risk factors of swine influenza in Spain. Vet Microbiol. 2011;149:56–63.
16. Suriya R, Hassan L, Omar AR, Aini I, Tan CG, Lim YS, et al. Seroprevalence and Risk Factors for Influenza A Viruses in Pigs in Peninsular Malaysia. Zoonoses Public Health. 2008;55:342–51.
17. Mastin A, Alarcon P, Pfeiffer D, Wood J, Williamson S, Brown I, et al. Prevalence and risk factors for swine influenza virus infection in the English pig population. PLOS Currents Influenza. 2011. doi:10.1371/currents.RRN1209.
18. Vincent A, Awada L, Brown I, Chen H, Claes F, Dauphin G, et al. Review of influenza A virus in swine worldwide: A call for increased surveillance and research. Zoonoses Public Health. 2014;61:4–17.
19. FAO. FAOSTAT data. http://faostat.fao.org/. Accessed 20 Dec 2014.
20. Que NN. Pig systems in Asia and the Pacific: How can research and development enhance benefits to the poor? In: Proceedings of the regional workshop. Bangkok: Thailand: International Livestock Research Institute; 2006.
21. Dzung NM. Pig production and marketing in Vietnam. http://www.angrin.tlri.gov.tw/English/2014Swine/p145-152.pdf. Accessed 22 Jul 2015.
22. Shortridge KF, Stuart-Harris CH. An influenza epicentre? Lancet. 1982;320:812–3.
23. Cameron RDA. A review of the industrialisation of pig production worldwide with particular reference to the Asian region. http://www.fao.org/ag/againfo/themes/documents/pigs/A%20review%20of%20the%20industrialisation%20of%20pig%20production%20worldwide%20with%20particular%20reference%20to%20the%20Asian%20region.pdf. Accessed 22 Jul 2015.
24. Ngo LT, Hiromoto Y, Pham VP, Le HT, Nguyen T, Le VT, et al. Isolation of novel triple-reassortant swine H3N2 influenza viruses possessing the hemagglutinin and neuraminidase genes of a seasonal influenza virus in Vietnam in 2010. Influenza Other Respi Viruses. 2011;6:6–10.
25. Takemae N, Nguyen T, Ngo LT, Hiromoto Y, Uchida Y, Pham VP, et al. Antigenic variation of H1N1, H1N2 and H3N2 swine influenza viruses in Japan and Vietnam. Arc Virol. 2013;158:859–76.
26. Nelson MI, Stratton J, Killian ML, Janas-Martindale A, Vincent AL. Continual Reintroduction of Human Pandemic H1N1 Influenza A Viruses into Swine in the United States, 2009 to 2014. J Virol. 2015;89:6218–26.
27. Michael T. Veterinary Epidemiology. 2nd ed. Oxford: Blackwell Science Ltd; 1995.
28. Takemae N, Ruttanapumma R, Parchariyanon S, Yoneyama S, Hayashi T, Hiramatsu H, et al. Alterations in receptor binding properties of swine influenza viruses of H1 subtype after isolation in embryonated chicken eggs. J Gen Virol. 2010;91:938–48.
29. Takemae N, Ngo TL, Nguyen T, Pham PV, Do TH, Le TV, et al. Patterns of genetic reassortment between endemic swine influenza viruses and pandemic A(H1N1)2009 viruses in Vietnamese pig population. In: Options for the Control of Influenza VIII Conference. Cape Town, South Africa: 2013. p. 633–4
30. Simon G, Larsen Lars E, Dürrwald R, Foni E, Harder T, Van Reeth K, et al. European Surveillance Network for Influenza in Pigs: Surveillance Programs, Diagnostic Tools and Swine Influenza Virus Subtypes Identified in 14 European Countries from 2010 to 2013. PLoS One. 2014;9:e115815.
31. Krueger WS, Gray GC. Swine Influenza Virus Infections in Man. Curr Top Microbiol Immunol. 2013;370:201–25.
32. Corzo CA, Culhane M, Juleen K, Stigger-Rosser E, Ducatez MF, Webby RJ, et al. Active surveillance for influenza A virus among swine, Midwestern United States, 2009–2011. Emerg Infect Dis. 2013;19:954–60.
33. European Commission. Eurostat. http://ec.europa.eu/eurostat. Accessed 27 Jun 2015.
34. Jones BA, Grace D, Kock R, Alonso S, Rushton J, Said MY, et al. Zoonosis emergence linked to agricultural intensification and environmental change. Proc Natl Acad Sci U S A. 2013;110:8399–404.
35. Forgie SE, Keenliside J, Wilkinson C, Webby R, Lu P, Sorensen O, et al. Swine Outbreak of Pandemic Influenza A Virus on a Canadian Research Farm Supports Human-to-Swine Transmission. Clin Infect Dis. 2011;52:10–8.
36. Tinoco YO, Montgomery JM, Kasper MR, Nelson MI, Azziz-Baumgartner E, Gilman RH, et al. Transmission dynamics of pandemic influenza A(H1N1)pdm09 virus in humans and swine in backyard farms in Tumbes, Peru. Influenza Other Respir Viruses. 2015:in press.
37. Weller CB, Cadmus KJ, Ehrhart EJ, Powers BE, Pabilonia KL. Detection and isolation of Influenza A virus subtype H1N1 from a small backyard swine herd in Colorado. J Vet Diagn Invest. 2013;25:782–4.
38. Howden KJ, Brockhoff EJ, Caya FD, McLeod LJ, Lavoie M, Ing JD, et al. An investigation into human pandemic influenza virus (H1N1) 2009 on an Alberta swine farm. Can Vet J. 2009;50:1153–61.
39. Pereda A, Cappuccio J, Quiroga MA, Baumeister E, Insarralde L, Ibar M, et al. Pandemic (H1N1) 2009 Outbreak on Pig Farm, Argentina. Emerg Infect Dis. 2010;16:304–7.
40. Vijaykrishna D, Smith GJD, Pybus OG, Zhu H, Bhatt S, Poon LLM, et al. Long-term evolution and transmission dynamics of swine influenza A virus. Nature. 2011;473:519–22.
41. Keenliside J. Pandemic Influenza A H1N1 in Swine and Other Animals. Curr Top Microbiol Immunol. 2013;370:259–71.
42. NCBI. Influenza Virus Resource. http://www.ncbi.nlm.nih.gov/genomes/FLU/FLU.html. Accessed 22 June 2015.
43. Vijaykrishna D, Poon LLM, Zhu HC, Ma SK, Li OTW, Cheung CL, et al. Reassortment of pandemic H1N1/2009 influenza A virus in swine. Science. 2010;328:1529.
44. Ducatez MF, Hause B, Stigger-Rosser E, Darnell D, Corzo C, Juleen K, et al. Multiple reassortment between pandemic (H1N1) 2009 and endemic influenza viruses in pigs, United States. Emerg Infect Dis. 2011;17:1624–9.
45. Starick E, Lange E, Grund C, Grosse BE, Dohring S, Maas A, et al. Reassortants of pandemic influenza A virus H1N1/2009 and endemic porcine HxN2 viruses emerge in swine populations in Germany. J Gen Virol. 2012;93:1658–63.
46. Howard WA, Essen SC, Strugnell BW, Russell C, Barrass L, Reid SM, et al. Reassortant pandemic (H1N1) 2009 virus in pigs, United Kingdom. Emerg Infect Dis. 2011;17:1049–52.
47. Hiromoto Y, Parchariyanon S, Ketusing N, Netrabukkana P, Hayashi T, Kobayashi T, et al. Isolation of the Pandemic (H1N1) 2009 virus and its reassortant with an H3N2 swine influenza virus from healthy weaning pigs in Thailand in 2011. Virus Res. 2012;169:175–81.
48. Sreta D, Tantawet S, Na Ayudhya SN, Thontiravong A, Wongphatcharachai M, Lapkuntod J, et al. Pandemic (H1N1) 2009 virus on commercial swine farm, Thailand. Emerg Infect Dis. 2010;16:1587–90.

49. Kanehira K, Takemae N, Uchida Y, Hikono H, Saito T. Reassortant swine influenza viruses isolated in Japan contain genes from pandemic A(H1N1) 2009. Microbiol Immunol. 2014;58:327–41.
50. MA J, Epperson S, Biggerstaff M, Allen D, Balish A, Barnes N, et al. Outbreak of Variant Influenza A(H3N2) Virus in the United States. Clin Infect Dis. 2013;57:1703–12.
51. Kong W, Wang F, Dong B, Ou C, Meng D, Liu J, et al. Novel reassortant influenza viruses between pandemic (H1N1) 2009 and other influenza viruses pose a risk to public health. Microb Pathog. 2015;89:62–72.
52. Baudon E, Poon LL, Dao TD, Pham NT, Cowling BJ, Peyre M, et al. Detection of Novel Reassortant Influenza A (H3N2) and H1N1 2009 Pandemic Viruses in Swine in Hanoi, Vietnam. Zoonoses Public Health. 2015;62:429–34.
53. Nonthabenjawan N, Chanvatik S, Chaiyawong S, Jairak W, Boonyapisusopha S, Tuanudom R, et al. Genetic diversity of swine influenza viruses in Thai swine farms, 2011–2014. Virus Genes. 2015;50:221–30.
54. Rajão DS, Gauger PC, Anderson TK, Lewis NS, Abente EJ, Killian ML, et al. Novel Reassortant Human-Like H3N2 and H3N1 Influenza A Viruses Detected in Pigs Are Virulent and Antigenically Distinct from Swine Viruses Endemic to the United States. J Virol. 2015;89:11213–22.
55. Liang H, Lam TT-Y, Fan X, Chen X, Zeng Y, Zhou J, et al. Expansion of Genotypic Diversity and Establishment of 2009 H1N1 Pandemic-Origin Internal Genes in Pigs in China. J Virol. 2014;88:10864–74.
56. Abe H, Mine J, Parchariyanon S, Takemae N, Boonpornprasert P, Ubonyaem N, et al. Co-infection of influenza A viruses of swine contributes to effective shuffling of gene segments in a naturally reared pig. Virology. 2015:in press.
57. Ozawa M, Matsuu A, Yonezawa K, Igarashi M, Okuya K, Kawabata T, et al. Efficient isolation of swine influenza viruses by age-targeted specimen collection. J Clin Microbiol. 2015;53:1331–8.
58. Markowska-Daniel I, Stankevicius A. Seroprevalence of antibodies against swine influenza virus in pigs of different age. Bull Vet Inst Pulawy. 2005;49:3–7.
59. Er C, Lium B, Tavornpanich S, Hofmo PO, Forberg H, Hauge AG, et al. Adverse effects of Influenza A(H1N1)pdm09 virus infection on growth performance of Norwegian pigs - a longitudinal study at a boar testing station. BMC Vet Res. 2014;10:284.
60. Song D, Kim H, Na W, Hong M, Park S-J, Moon H, et al. Canine susceptibility to human influenza viruses (A/pdm 09H1N1, A/H3N2 and B). J Gen Virol. 2015;96:254–8.
61. Campagnolo ER, Rankin JT, Daverio SA, Hunt EA, Lute JR, Tewari D, et al. Fatal pandemic (H1N1) 2009 influenza A virus infection in a Pennsylvania domestic cat. Zoonoses Public Health. 2011;58:500–7.
62. Easterday BC, Van Reeth K, Swine influenza. In: Straw BE, D'Allaire S, Mengling WL, Taylor DJ, editors. Diseases of Swine. 8th ed. Iowa: Iowa State University Press; 1999. p. 277–90.

17

The molecular characteristic analysis of PRRSV GSWW/2015 strain and its pathogenicity to pigs

Weijie Bai, Zhijia Wang, Pu Sun, Jing Zhang, Huifang Bao, Yimei Cao, Yanyan Chang, Zaixin Liu, Dong Li* and Zengjun Lu*

Abstract

Background: Porcine reproductive and respiratory syndrome (PRRS) is a severe disease, causing great economic losses to the pig industry. The causative agent, porcine reproductive and respiratory syndrome virus (PRRSV) is highly variable. Since the emergence of highly pathogenic PRRSV (HP-PRRSV) in China in 2006, this virus strain has undergone extensive variation. To investigate the genetic variation and pathogenicity of currently isolated PRRSV GSWW/2015 strain, its whole genome was sequenced and analyzed for the specific variation in NSP2, GP3 and GP5 regions. Pigs were challenged with the isolated virus to investigate its pathogenicity.

Methods: The PRRSV GSWW/2015 strain was isolated by seeding the viral material in Marc-145 cells. The virus specific cytopathic effect (CPE) was confirmed by indirect immunofluorescent assay (IFA) and PCR to detect the virus protein and RNA. Nine pairs of primers were designed to obtain the complete genome by PCR. All PCR fragments were cloned into T-vector for sequencing. The genetic variation of GSWW/2015 strain was analyzed by multiple sequence alignments. Nineteen PRRSV-free piglets were intranasally challenged with 10^8 copies of GSWW virus, while seven piglets were housed together as contact-infected control. Clinical signs were recorded daily after challenge. Blood samples were obtained every week and the viral titer was detected by quantitative real-time PCR (qRT-PCR). The PRRSV specific antibody was detected by LSI ELISA kit.

Results: The complete genome of PRRSV GSWW/2015 strain (GenBank accession number KX767091) was obtained. The whole genome of this strain shares 88.5 and 60.6% identity with VR-2332 and LV respectively, indicating that it belongs to the North American type (NA-type). Sequence alignments revealed that GSWW/2015 strain has a discontinuous deletion of 30 amino acids in NSP2, which is similar with HP-PRRSV. Some amino acids mutations can be observed in antigenic epitope regions of GP3 and GP5 compared with earlier strains of HP-PRRSV. Some piglets showed typical clinical signs of PRRSV after challenge. Only four pigs showed viremia within 3 days after challenge, most pigs showed peaked viremia after 21–28 days including 7 contact-infected pigs. Two pigs were detected to be positive for antibody to PRRSV at 14 days post infection (DPI), and 11 pigs (11/26) show seroconversion for PRRSV at 49 DPI. Twelve piglets died of PRRSV infection within two months.

Conclusions: The genome of PRRSV GSWW/2015 strain shows the features of HP-PRRSV with 30 discontinuous amino acids deletion in NSP2 and some new amino acid mutations in epitope regions of GP5 and GP3, which might alter the antigenicity of the virus. Furthermore, the virus showed high virulence to piglets as reported in HP-PRRSV, and induced long-lasting viremia and low level of antibody responses. This work further enriched our knowledge on PRRSV evolution and pathogenicity.

Keywords: PRRSV GSWW/2015 strain, Genetic variation, Pathogenicity, Viremia

* Correspondence: lidong@caas.cn; luzengjun@caas.cn
State Key Laboratory of Veterinary Etiologic Biology, Lanzhou Veterinary Research Institute, Chinese Academy of Agricultural Sciences, Lanzhou 730046, Gansu, China

Background

PRRS is one of the most devastating swine diseases, which has caused enormous economic losses to global pig industry [15]. PRRS first emerged in Western Europe and North America in the 1990s and now has become an endemic disease worldwide [3, 19]. The pathogenic PRRSV mainly causes reproductive failure in sows and respiratory disorder in all-age pigs. PRRSV is an enveloped RNA virus and classified as a member of the order *Nidovirales*, family *Arteriviridae*, which also contains equine arteritis virus (EAV), lactate dehydrogenase-elevating virus (LDV) and simian hemorrhagic fever virus (SHFV) [5]. Due to the genetic and antigenic differences, PRRSV can be divided into two major genotypes: the European type (EU-type, type 1) and North American type (NA-type, type 2). Representative strains of the two genotypes are LV and VR-2332 respectively, sharing only approximately 55–70% nucleotide and 50–80% amino acid similarity [10]. In 2016, the International Committee on Taxonomy of Viruses split PRRSV into two new species defined as porcine reproductive and respiratory syndrome virus 1 (PRRSV-1) and porcine reproductive and respiratory syndrome virus 2 (PRRSV-2). The single positive-stranded PRRSV genome is approximately 15 kb in length and contains ten open reading frames (ORF): ORF1a, ORF1b, ORF2a, ORF2b, ORFs 3–5, ORF5a and ORFs 6–7 [13]. ORF1a and ORF1b encode replication-related polymerase proteins, which are cleaved into at least 16 nonstructural proteins (nsp): nsp1α, nsp1β, nsp2, nsp2NF, nsp2TF, nsp3–6, nsp7α, nsp7β and nsp8–12. The 3′-end of the viral genome contains eight ORFs encoding structural proteins, including GP2a,E, GP3, GP4, GP5, GP5a, M and N. Within PRRSV genome, nsp2 undergoes remarkable genetic variation associated with natural mutations and deletions. GP3 and GP5 are also highly variable among structural proteins. Therefore, nsp2, GP3 and GP5 are often used for phylogenetic analysis for the genetic variation and molecular epidemiology.

In 2006, a highly pathogenic PRRS (HP-PRRS) emerged in China with characteristics of high fever, increased morbidity and mortality [17]. The agent, HP-PRRSV had a unique discontinuous deletion of 30 amino acids in nsp2 and has become a dominant strain prevalent in the field. To learn the evolution of the currently circulated strains in China, one PRRSV strain named GSWW/2015 was isolated from the lung tissue of a sick pig collected from a farm in Gansu Province in 2015. The complete genome of GSWW/2015 was obtained and compared with 34 reference strains. Amino acid sequences of nsp2, GP3 and GP5 were analyzed in detail to study the genetic variation of this virus isolate. Furthermore, the pathogenicity of this virus strain was investigated by infection of piglets with cell-cultured virus material. This research provides further information on the understanding of the evolution and pathogenicity of currently circulated high virulent PRRSV.

Methods

Clinical samples

The pigs in one farm in Wuwei county, Gansu Province of China were suspected to be infected by PRRSV in 2015. According to the farmer's description, some pigs showed typical clinical signs of PRRSV infection, such as high fever, blue ears, anhelation and eventual death. The lung tissue was collected from a dead pig by a local veterinarian and then sent to our lab for further confirmation of PRRSV infection. Then the lung tissue was homogenized in Dulbecco's modified Eagle's medium (DMEM, Gibco) for RNA extraction and virus isolation.

RT-PCR detection of the virus RNA in viral material

Total RNA was extracted from tissue homogenates by the RNeasy Mini Kit (QIAGEN, Germany). Then the cDNA was synthesized by reverse transcription with the Superscript reverse transcriptase (Invitrogen, USA) using the oligo(dT) primer. PCR was performed using a pair of specific primers to amplify a 375 bp conserve gene fragment in M protein (forward: 5`-CCTTCGGGTACATG ACATTCGT-3`; Reverse: 5`-TTGCTGCTTGCCGT TGTTATT-3`). The PCR products were analyzed by agarose gel electrophoresis to confirm the existence of virus RNA.

Virus isolation

The tissue homogenates were centrifuged at 12,000 g for 20 min. The supernatant was passed through a 0.22-μm filter and then added on Marc-145 cell monolayer. After incubation for 1 h at 37 °C, the medium was replaced with new DMEM containing 2% fetal bovine serum (FBS, Gibco) and antibiotics (50 μg/ml penicillin, 50 μg/ml streptomycin, 100 μg/ml neomycin) at 37 °C for 3–5 days. The culture supernatant was harvested and freeze-thawed for three times when cytopathic effects (CPE) appeared. The supernatant was then transferred to Marc-145 cells for virus propagation and stored at – 70 °C as viral stocks.

Indirect fluorescent antibody assay (IFA)

Marc-145 cells were incubated with the isolated virus for 1 h at 37 °C and then maintained in DMEM with 2% FBS and antibiotics. At 48 h post-infection, cells were washed with PBS and then fixed with methanol-acetone (1:1) for 15 min at room temperature. Cells were washed with PBS for three times and then incubated with monoclonal antibody (Mab) SR30 (RTI, 1:500) against PRRSV N protein for 1 h. After washing with PBS for 5 times, cells were incubated with FITC-conjugated goat anti-mouse secondary antibody (Molecular Probes, 1:100) for 1 h. Then cells were washed 5 times with PBS and staining was visualized with a fluorescent microscope.

The whole genome sequencing

Nine pairs of primers were designed based on HP-PRRSV strain SHH (Accession number EU106888) to amplify the full-length genome of GSWW strain (Table 1). The PCR products were purified and cloned into pEASY-T1 vector. For each fragment, at least 3 positive bacteria colonies were selected for plasmid extraction and sequencing to get the correct genome information. Recombinant plasmids were sent to TaKaRa (Dalian, China) for sequencing.

Genetic variation analysis of GSWW/2015 strain

The correct genome sequence of GSWW/2015 strain was obtained by incorporation of the consistent sequencing results of different colonies of different fragments. The whole genome of GSWW/2015 was aligned with 34 PRRSV reference strains (Table 2) and a phylogenetic tree was constructed using MEGA5.2 based on the neighbor-joining method. Bootstrap values were calculated on 1000 replicates. The variation of different coding and non-coding regions of GSWW/2015 was analyzed by comparison with corresponding parts of VR-2332, LV, CH-1a and HUN4 strains by ClustalW in Lasergene software (Version 7.1). The amino acid variation of part of Nsp2, GP3 and GP5 was shown in detail by aligned with 34 reference strains.

The pathogenicity of PRRSV GSWW/2015 strain to pigs

To investigate the pathogenicity of PRRSV GSWW strain, 26 four-week-old piglets (Large White) approximately 20 kg were selected for this challenge experiment. We did not perform a sample size calculation. All pigs came from a pig farm in a mountain village in Zhuanglang county of Gansu province where PRRS has not been reported before. All pigs were twice detected to be negative for antibody against PRRSV. All pigs were transported to our Animal Biosafety Level 3 Laboratory in Lanzhou Veterinary

Table 2 Thirty-four PRRSV reference strains used for sequence alignment

No.	Strains	GenBank No.	No.	Isolates	GenBank No.
1	VR-2332	PRU87392	18	CG	EU864231
2	MLV	AF066183	19	GDQY2	GU454850
3	CH-1a	AY032626	20	SHH	EU106888
4	BJ-4	AF331831	21	08HuN	GU169411
5	S1	DQ459471	22	08SDWF	GU168569
6	HB-1sh	AY150312	23	GDBY1	GQ374442
7	HB-2sh	AY262352	24	KP	GU232735
8	CH2002	EU880438	25	WUH2	EU678352
9	CH2003	EU880440	26	WUH3	HM853673
10	CH2004	EU880439	27	YN2008	EU880435
11	HN1	AY457635	28	GS2008	EU880431
12	CC1	EF153486	29	XL2008	EU880436
13	Em2007	EU262603	30	09HUB5	GU168568
14	CH-1R	EU807840	31	09HUB7	GU168567
15	HUN4	EF635006	32	HLJHL	HM189676
16	JXA1	EF112445	33	SX-1	GQ857656
17	JXwn06	EF641008	34	SX2009	FJ895329

Table 1 Primers for PCR of the complete genome of PRRSV GSWW/2015 strain

Fragment	Sequence of primers(5′-3′)	Position in genome
A	ATGACGTATAGGTGTTGGCTCTATG	1–1518
	GGAAATGCAGTGCCAACCACARTTC	
B	ACTTCTCYGTTAAGGAGAGTTGGAT	1175–4216
	GATACAGTCTGCAACAATGCCAAGCCTAAGCA	
C	GTTACAGTTACCCATTCTTCGG	3911–5191
	GAGGTACCCAAACATAACTAGC	
D	CCTTGGTCGTTTTGATTTTTGT	5081–6304
	AAGATAGCACAAACATCCCAAAG	
E	GGCAGTCACATAATTAAAGACACAT	6061–7292
	TGGACCTCCTCATAAAACACAT	
F	ATTCCGGTGATGTGTTTTATGAGGAGGT	7262–10,030
	ACATCACCATCCTGGACYTGTTGAAG	
G	TTACCACACCCACTTCCACCAGCATTG	9604–12,066
	AGAGGCTTTGCATAGACCCCATTTCATTTCAATTCA	
H	TGAATTGAAATGAAATGGGGTCTATGCAAAGCCTCT	11,973–14,584
	CGGCATCTGGAGGTGATGAATTTCCAGGTTTCTAT	
I	CCTTCGGGTACATGACATTCGT	14,543–15,347
	TTTTTTTTTTTTTTTTTTTTTTTTTTTTTAATTWCGG	

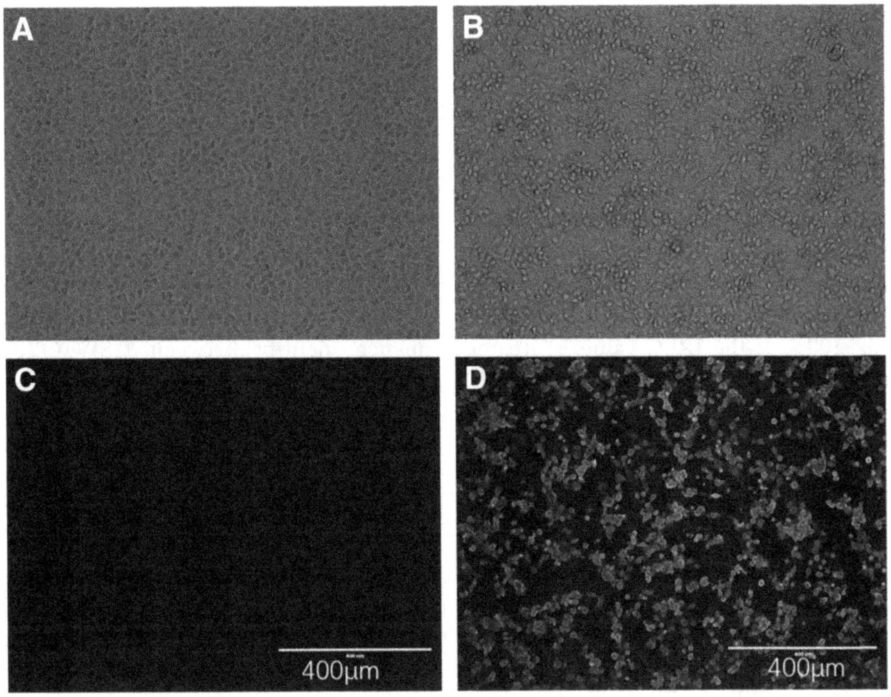

Fig. 1 Isolation and Identification of PRRSV virus in Marc-145 cells. **a** showed normal cell; **b** showed the CPE after inoculation of viral material; **c** showed the normal cell after incubation with SR30 monoclonal antibody by IFA; **d** showed the positive results after reaction with SR30 antibody by IFA

Research Institute. The pigs were divided evenly into 2 groups and raised in 2 rooms approximately 20 square meters for one week before challenge. Nine and ten piglets in 2 rooms were intranasally challenged with 10^8 copies of GSWW/2015 virus, and seven piglets were kept in the same room as contact-infection control. Whole blood samples were collected before challenge and at 4, 7, 14, 21, 28, 35, 42, 49, 56, 63 days post infection (DPI) for viremia detection. The serum samples were also collected before infection and at every week point until 125 DPI for antibody detection. At the end of experiment, the piglets were anaesthetized intramuscularly with 15 mg/kg ketamine (Ursotamin, Serumwerk-Bernburg AG, Bernburg, Germany) and 2 mg/kg azaperon (Stresnil, Janssen-Cilag GmbH, Baar, Switzerland) prior to euthanization by the i.v. administration of 200 mg/kg pentobarbital (Pentobarbital 10%, NAF Apotek, Oslo). Then the piglets were humanly bled to death.

Quantitative real-time PCR of the viremia levels

The whole blood samples were used to extract the viral RNA by Trizol, and the virus RNA copies were detected by Real-time RT-PCR method as described by Liu et al. [12] (2010, in Chinese). The quantitative PCR primers and probe are as following: Forward: 5'-CGGCAAATG ATAACCACGC-3′, Reverse: 5'-TTCTGCCACCCAAC

Table 3 Homology of the different parts of genome and proteins of GSWW/2015 compared with representative strains of PRRSV

	HUN4	CH-1a	VR-2332	LV
Complete	96.9	93.5	88.5	60.6
5′ UTR	99.5	97.3	92.0	62.0
ORF1a	96.3	92.2	86.3	57.3
ORF1b	96.9	94.4	90.2	63.3
ORF2	98.1	95.3	93.3	66.0
ORF3	97.0	94.1	87.8	64.8
ORF4	97.4	95.0	89.2	67.4
ORF5	97.0	92.9	87.7	64.1
ORF6	99.6	97.3	95.2	69.5
ORF7	99.5	96.2	93.5	68.7
3'UTR	98.4	95.3	92.0	74.6
NSP2	93.0	84.3	73.0	37.5
GP2	96.1	93.8	92.6	61.8
GP3	94.5	90.6	85.0	55.7
GP4	97.8	97.2	89.9	70.8
GP5	95.5	90.5	87.5	58.2
M	99.4	97.7	97.7	80.3
N	100.0	95.1	95.1	65.0

Notes:Different ORF and UTR regions are analyzed based on the nucleotide sequence. NSP2, GP2-5, M and N protein are analyzed by deduced protein sequences

ACGAG-3′; TaqMan probe: 5′-FAM-TGTGCCG TTR ACCGTAGTGGAGCC-TAMRA-3′.

PRRSV specific antibody detection by LSI ELISA

PRRSV antibody in serum samples were detected by a commercial ELISA kit (LSI Vet™ Porcine PRRS/US-Serum) from LSI company of France. This kit is based on the principle of an indirect ELISA. The assays were performed according to the manufacturers' specifications. Antibody value (IRPC value) was expressed as the following formula: IRPC = (OD sample-OD NC)/(OD PC-OD NC) × 100%. If the IRPC value is greater than 0.2, the sample is judged to be positive for PRRSV antibody; Otherwise, the sample is judged to be negative for PRRSV antibody.

Results

Virus isolation and identification

The causative agent was confirmed to be PRRSV by RT-PCR and IFA. One specific DNA band of approximately 375 bp was amplified as expected. After inoculation of Marc145 cells with the viral material prepared with lung tissue, the typical CPE of PRRSV infection can be observed within 72 h after 2 passages (Fig. 1a, b). PRRSV antigen was also detected in Marc145 cells after incubation with SR30 Mab recognizing Nucleoprotein N (Fig. 1a-d). The results indicated the PRRSV strain was isolated by direct inoculation of Marc-145 cells with viral material. The virus strain was designated as PRRSV GSWW/2015.

Full-length genomic sequence of PRRSV GSWW/2015

The full-length genome of GSWW/2015 was 15,319 nucleotides in length, excluding the poly (A) tail. The sequence identity between GSWW/2015 and other 4 representative PRRSV strains are listed in Table 3. The complete genome of GSWW/2015 strain shares 93.5, 96.9, 88.5 and 60.6% identity with CH-1a (the first PRRSV strain isolated in China in 1996), HUN4 [18] (a representative strain of HP-PRRSV), VR-2332 (NA-type) and LV (EU-type), respectively. The results indicate that GSWW strain belongs to the NA-type. The 5′-UTR, 3′-UTR, ORF1a, ORF 1b exhibited 62.0–99.5%, 74.6–98.4%, 57.3–96.3% and 63.3–96.9% sequence identity with 4 different reference strains, respectively (Table 3). Nsp2 was the most variable non-structural protein with

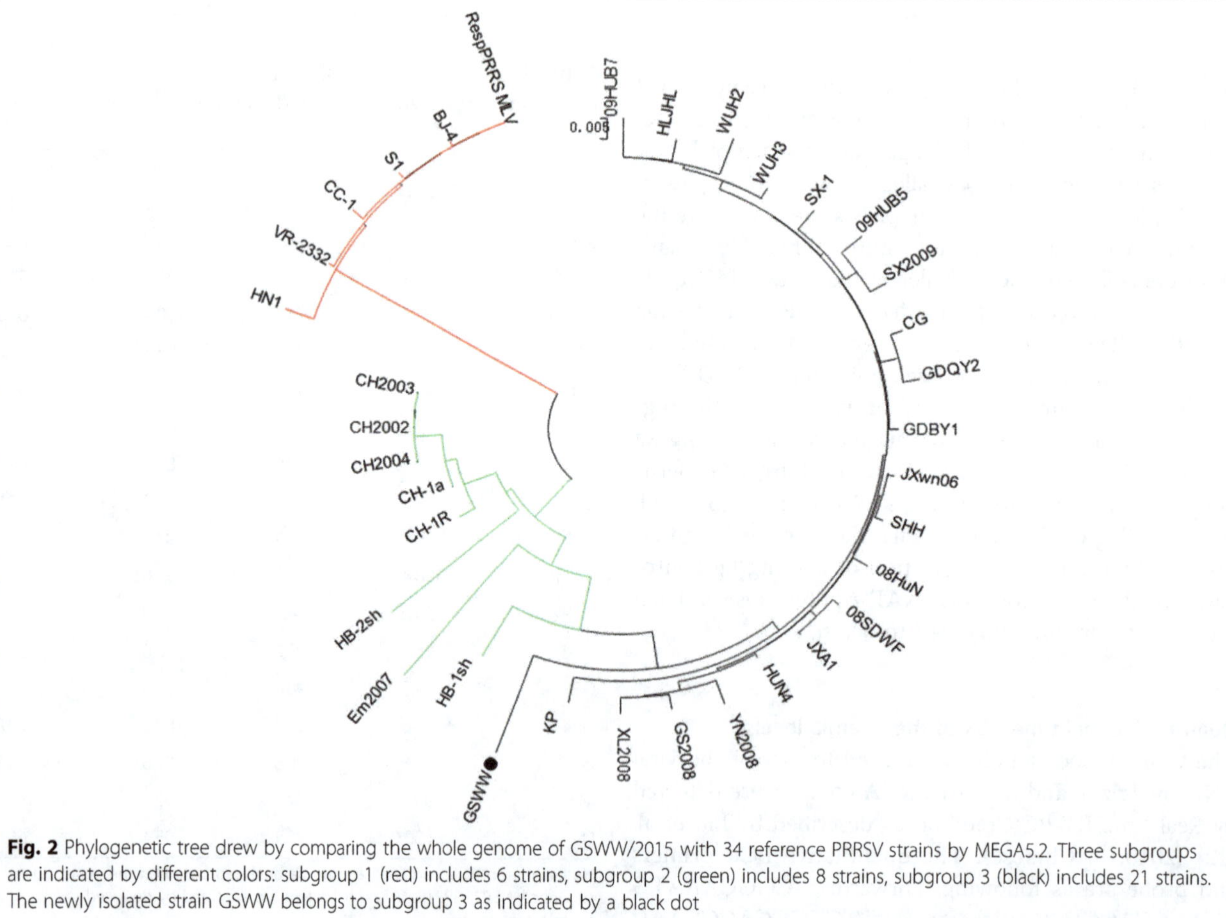

Fig. 2 Phylogenetic tree drew by comparing the whole genome of GSWW/2015 with 34 reference PRRSV strains by MEGA5.2. Three subgroups are indicated by different colors: subgroup 1 (red) includes 6 strains, subgroup 2 (green) includes 8 strains, subgroup 3 (black) includes 21 strains. The newly isolated strain GSWW belongs to subgroup 3 as indicated by a black dot

37.5–93.0% amino acid identity compared with 4 reference strains. GP3 and GP5 exhibited 55.7–94.5% and 58.2–95.5% amino acid identity respectively, indicating they were the most variable structural proteins. The N protein of GSWW strain was identical with HUN4 strain. The M protein was the most conserved structural protein sharing 80.3–99.4% amino acid identity with other 4 reference strains (Table 3).

Phylogenetic analysis

A phylogenetic tree was constructed based on the complete genome sequences of GSWW and 34 PRRSV reference strains (Fig. 2). Phylogenetic analysis revealed that the NA-type PRRSV was divided into three subgroups. Subgroup 1 comprised 6 strains: VR-2332, RespPRRS MLV, BJ-4, S1, HN1 and CC1. Subgroup 2 included CH-1a, Em2007, HB-1sh, HB-2sh, CH-1R, CH2002, CH2003 and CH2004. Subgroup 3 consisted of 21 HP-PRRSV strains including GSWW/2015 strain, and the representative strains were HUN4, JXA1 and JXwn06.

Amino acid variation of NSP2, GP3 and GP5 proteins

To explore the genetic variation in specific proteins, amino acid sequences of Nsp2, GP3 and GP5 were aligned with 34 PRRSV reference strains (Fig. 3). The NSP2 region of GSWW/2015 strain shows a discontinuous deletion of 30-aa at positions 480 and 534–562, which is a typical feature of HP-PRRSV strains emerged in China since 2006 [17]. The amino acid sequence of NSP2 shows 91.6–93.2% similarity with other HP-PRRSV strains indicating a remarkable genetic variation in this protein.

Two antigenic epitopes (^{67}YEPGRSLW^{74} and ^{74}WCRIGHDRCGED^{85}) in GP3 had been described previously [20]. GP3 of GSWW/2015 strain shows some accumulated mutations in these two epitopes. Two unique amino acid mutations (E^{68}N and G^{70}A) in the epitope (^{67}YEPGRSLW^{74}) were observed compared with other HP-PRRSV strains, while another two amino acid mutations (Y^{67}L and L^{73}F) were the same with other HP-PRRSV strains. In the epitope (^{74}WCRIGHDRCGED^{85}), GSWW/2015 strain shows one specific amino acid mutations (Y^{79}H). Some other specific mutations can also be observed at positions A/T^{30}N, F^{43}Y and L/P^{58}Q (Fig. 4). The influence of these changes on the antigenicity of GP3 need to be further investigated.

The amino acid mutations were described here for GSWW/2015 in the primary neutralizing epitope (PNE) (^{37}SHF/LQLIYNL^{45}) and the decoy epitope (^{27}V/ALVN^{30}) of GP5 protein [16]. Two amino acid mutations (A/V^{26}T, L^{28}P) specific for GSWW/2015 were observed in the decoy epitope region compared with other HP-PRRSV strains and subgroup 1 and 2 isolates. One

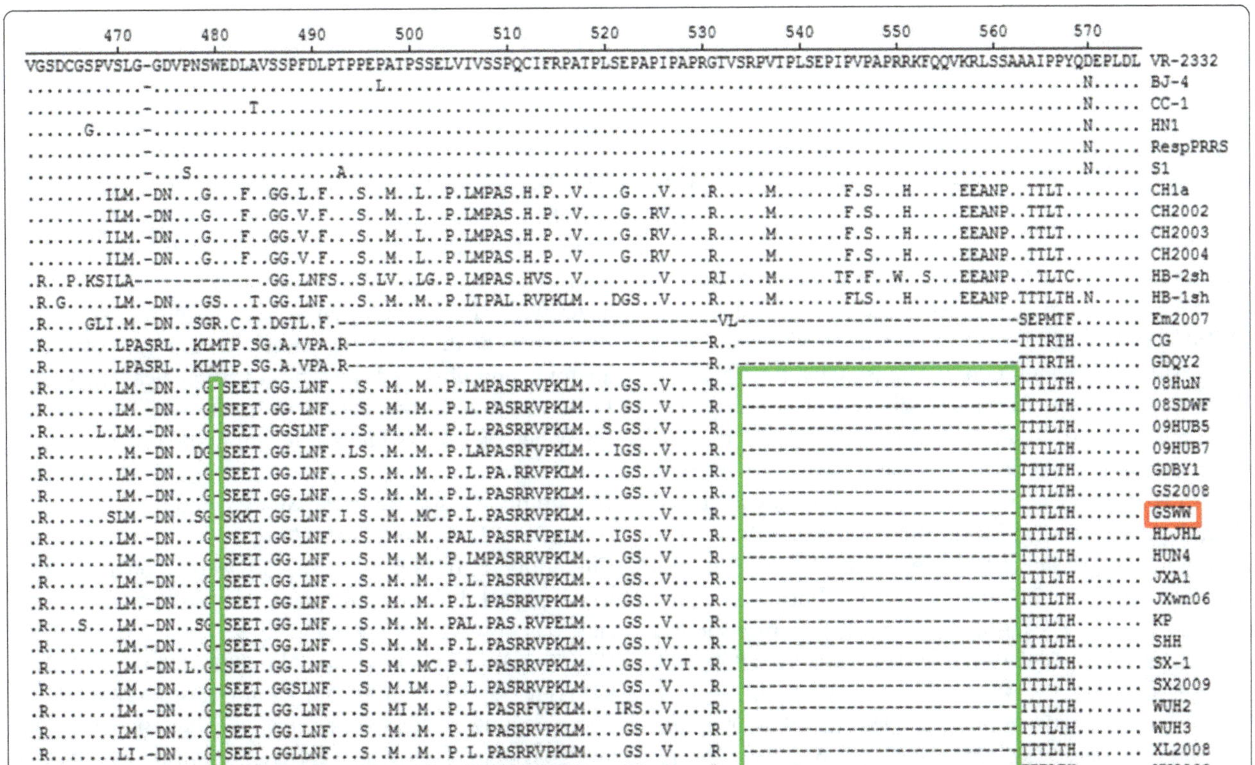

Fig. 3 High variable regions in NSP2 of GSWW/2015 compared with 34 reference PRRSV strains. A discontinuous deletion of 30-aa (positions 480 and 534–562) were indicated by two green boxes in HP-PRRSV emerged in China in 2006

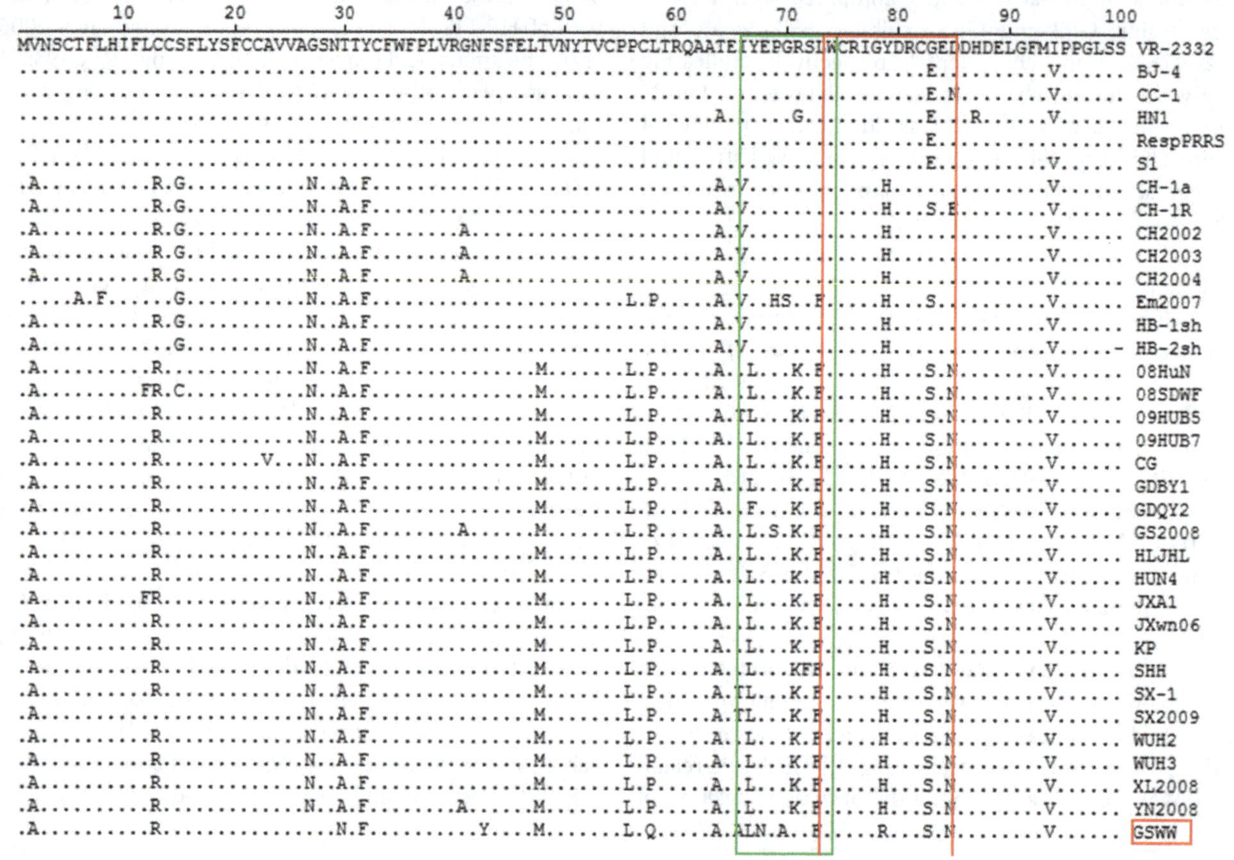

Fig. 4 GP3 protein of GSWW/2015 compared with 34 reference PRRSV strains. Two antigenic epitopes (^{67}YEPGRSLW^{74} and ^{74}WCRIGHDRCGED^{85}) in GP3 were indicated in green and red boxes

N-linked glycosylation site (N-X-S/T) is absent at position 35 ($N^{34}S$) of GSWW/2015 strain compared with other HP-PRRSV (Fig. 5).

The pathogenicity of PRRSV GSWW/2015 strain to pigs

Nineteen pigs were challenged by airway inoculation of PRRSV GSWW/2015 strain. Two infected piglets died early without obvious clinical signs. One pig (No.974) showed viremia on day 4 and died on day 7 (Fig. 6e). One pig (No.970) died on day 28 without obvious viremia (Fig. 6e) but seroconversion was observed after 14 DPI (Fig. 7e). The other 24 piglets gradually appeared clinical signs of typical PRRS, such as fever, lethargy and emaciation, some showed blue ears, anhelation. Five pigs (No. 956, 980, 975, 927 and 299) showed peaked viremia at 7 and 14 DPI (Fig. 6a-h), and the other 19 pigs showed peaked viremia at 21 DPI (7 pigs, No. 984, 902, 955, 943, 999, 982 and 992), 28 DPI (6 pigs, No. 907, 932, 989, 959, 909 and 954), 35 DPI (4 pigs, No. 945, 987, 994, 990) and 42 DPI (2 pigs, No. 946, 988), respectively. Seven contact-infected pigs showed peaked viremia after 14 DPI. The viremia lasted for one month in most pigs, however virus activity could be detected in herd level during the whole period of experiment. Fourteen piglets (No. 907, 999, 975, 927, 946, 988, 932, 943, 990, 955, 984, 992, 299 and 959) showed high level of viremia and died gradually at 35 to 118 DPI (Figs. 6 and 7). The rest 10 pigs (No. 956, 980, 902, 994, 945, 954, 987, 989, 909 and 982) were anaesthetized and humanely bled to death at the end of the experiment. Dead pigs were proceeded pathologic anatomy and observed the typical pathological changes of PRRS, such as consolidation of lungs, swelling and diffusely hemorrhage in lungs and lymph nodes.

The antibody response to PRRSV detected by a commercial ELISA kit (LSI ELISA)

The antibody responses to PRRSV were shown in Fig. 7 for all pigs at different time point. The earliest seroconversion was observed in two pigs No. 956 and 970 at 14 DPI (Fig. 7a, e), and then 5 pigs (No. 299, 980, 959, 975 and 943) (Fig. 7a, d, e, f) at 28 DPI. There were another 12 pigs (No. 984, 992, 902, 954, 932, 946, 989, 945, 909, 982, 987 and 994) gradually became serological positive for PRRSV antibody during 42~ 125 DPI (Fig. 7a-h). Seven pigs (No. 974, 927, 955, 988, 999, 990 and 907) with high level viremia after virus infection did not show seroconversion

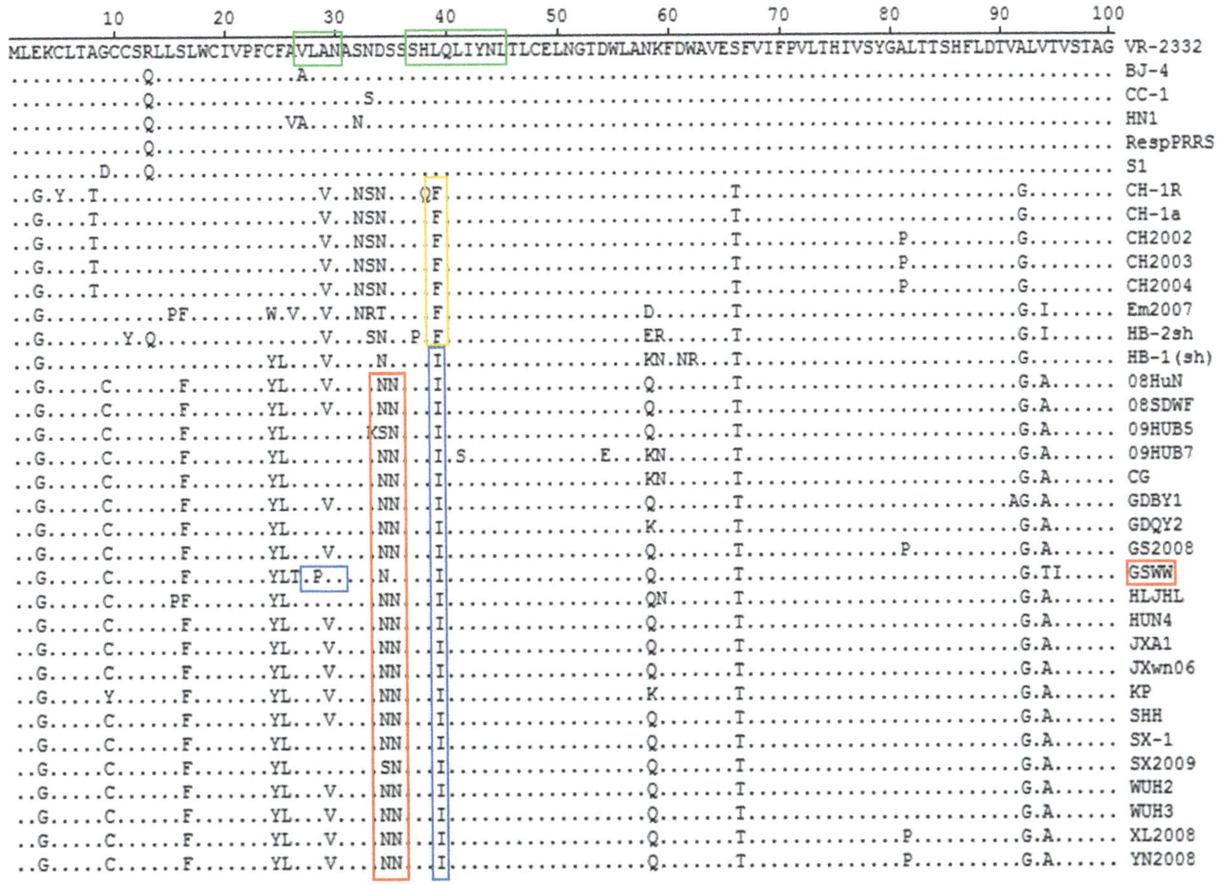

Fig. 5 Part of GP5 protein of GSWW/2015 compared with 34 reference PRRSV strains. The primary neutralizing epitope (PNE) (^{37}SHF/LQLIYNL^{45}) and the decoy epitope (^{27}V/ALVN^{30}) are indicated by two green boxes. The putative N-linked glycosylation sites are indicated by a red box. The decoy epitope of GSWW/2015 strain has one unique amino acid mutation (L^{28}P) and one N-linked glycosylation site is absent at position 35 compared with other HP-PRRSV strains

for PRRSV antibody because of death before 70 DPI including 4 contact-infected pigs (Fig. 7g, h).

Discussion

PRRS is considered one of the most important diseases affecting Chinese pig industry. In 1995, PRRSV was first isolated in China. Several PRRSV strains were subsequently isolated and sequenced in the following years, including BJ-4, HB-1(sh)/2002 and HB-2(sh)/2002. In 2006, a large-scale HP-PRRS outbreak was reported in China with characteristics of high morbidity and mortality. Studies indicated that HP-PRRSV originated from CH-1a-like virus and experienced gradually genetic variation and accumulation in genomic sequences [2]. HP-PRRSV rapidly became the dominant strains prevailing in the field.

In this study, we isolated a new highly pathogenic PRRSV strain (designated as GSWW/2015) circulated in north-western region of China as confirmed by RT-PCR, IFA and animal challenge experiments. The complete genome was sequenced and compared with 34 reference strains. Phylogenic analysis showed that the GSWW/2015 belongs to subgroup 3 of NA-type PRRSV as HP-PRRSV strain. Subgroup 1 and 2 isolates were classical PRRSV. VR-2332 and CH-1a were the representative strains of subgroup 1 and 2, respectively. In addition, we analyzed the genetic variation in different regions of genome by comparison of GSWW/2015 with four representative strains. NSP2 is the highest variable region, and then GP3 and GP5 proteins (Table 3). It is still not clear of the mechanism for PRRSV to maintain this highly variable feature in NSP2 region.

NSP2 experiences remarkable genetic variation and contains natural insertions and deletions in the hypervariable region [8, 14]. Given the tolerance of insertions and deletions in the nonessential region, NSP2 is considered a potential candidate gene for genetic modifications [9]. The natural deletion of 12 amino acids in NSP2 was first found in HB-2(sh)/2002 strain [11]. The 30-aa deleted region of HP-PRRSV contained B-cell epitopes [7] and T-cell epitopes [6]. The deletion of 30-aa in NSP2 was considered the genetic marker of HP-PRRSV, but it was not related to

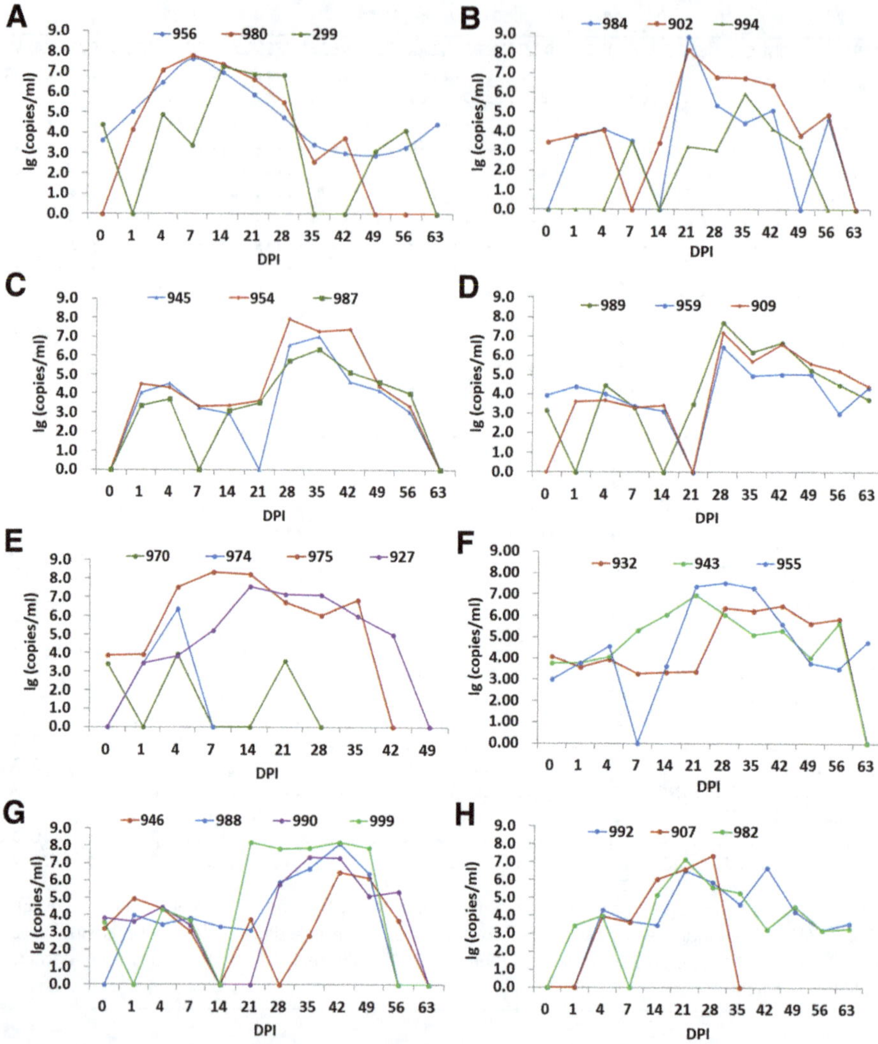

Fig. 6 Viremia levels in blood detected by qRT-PCR. **a-f** showed the results of pigs infected by airway; **g**, **h** showed the results of 7 contact-infected pigs

the increased virulence [21]. It is similar with other HP-PRRSV strains for GSWW/2015 strain to contain a discontinuous deletion of 30 amino acids in NSP2.

GP5 is a major inducer of neutralizing antibodies in vivo. The decoy epitope in GP5 was hypervariable and highly immunodominant, while the PNE was conserved among PRRSV isolates and was not immunodominant. Thus, antibody to the decoy epitope is dominant and responses are early after PRRSV infection, while antibody to PNE is delayed or at a very low level [16]. Sequence alignments showed that the GP5 decoy epitope of GSWW/2015 strain had one unique amino acid mutation ($L^{28}P$), which is different from other HP-PRRSV strains listed in this paper. In the PNE, residues ^{38}HLQLIYN^{44} were considered as the main recognition site for neutralizing antibodies. The residue of L39 in subgroup 1 changed to I/F39 in subgroup 2 and HP-PRRSV including GSWW/2015 strain, which may influence the binding of neutralizing antibodies. In addition, several putative N-linked glycosylation sites were in the ectodomain of GP5. N44 glycosylation site located in the PNE is critical for the recovery of infectious PRRSV. N33 and N51 mutations enhanced viral sensitivity to neutralization antibody. GSWW strain had one amino acid mutation at position 35 ($N^{35}D$) which is different from other HP-PRRSV strains and similar with earlier PRRSV stains in subgroup 2. It had been reported that the glycosylation was related with viral immune evasion and minimized neutralizing antibody response against the PNE [1].

GP3 is the most variable structural protein as showed by comparing GP3 protein of GSWW/2015 with other representative PRRSV strains. Although antibody to GP3 is produced at a very low level, it may play an important role in neutralization and clearance of virus [4]. There

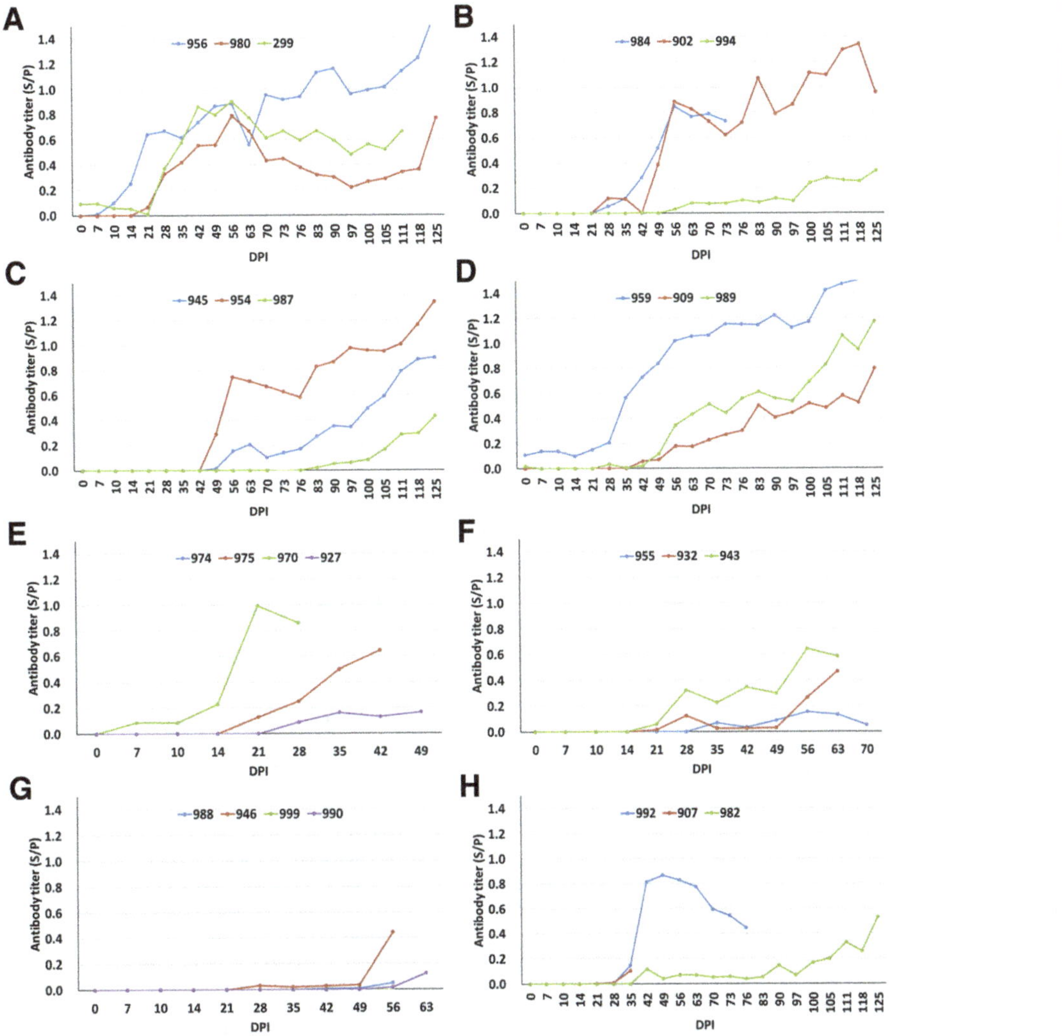

Fig. 7 Antibody responses to PRRSV detected by LSI ELISA kit. **a-f** showed the results of pigs inoculated by airway; **g**, **h** showed the results of 7 contact-infected pigs. Antibody titer greater than 0.2 were judged to be positive for PRRSV antibody

are more amino acids mutations observed in GP3 of GSWW/2015 strain compared with other HP-PRRSV strains, including $E^{68}N$, $G^{70}A$, $K^{71}R$ in epitope ^{67}YEPGR/KSLW^{74} and $H^{79}R$ in epitope ^{74}WCRIGY/HDRCGED/N^{85} [20], as well as changes at A/$T^{30}N$, $F^{43}Y$, L/$P^{58}Q$. The biological meaning of these mutations need to be further illustrated.

Considering the fundings, size of the pig farm and capacity of our P3 lab, we thought 26 piglets were enough to investigate the characteristics of the virus. Pig challenge experiment showed that GSWW/2015 is a highly pathogenic PRRSV strain. After challenge, most piglets showed fever and obvious clinical signs, such as listlessness and anorexia. The clinical signs became more severe over the next few days with lethargy and emaciation. Fourteen piglets died gradually at 35 to 118 DPI, which showed high level of viremia and developed enlarged tonsil, swelling and diffuse consolidation and hemorrhage in lung and lymph nodes. Some piglets showed viremia early on day 1 (No.946 and 956), day 4 (No.299, 974, 975 and 980) and day 7 (No.943), while some showed viremia late on day 14 (No.907 and 982), day 21 (No.902 and 984 etc) and day 28 (No.945 and 954 etc). Contact-infected pigs (Fig. 7g, h) showed viremia later than airway inoculated pigs except for one pig No. 946. Most pigs inoculated by airway or contact-infected showed peaked viremia after 2–3 weeks of exposure. This may reflect a complex situation for PRRSV infection in pig herd. The viral titer in blood could reach up to 10^8 copies/ml. The viremia lasted over a month individually, but overall the viremia lasted over two months because the piglets developed viremia at different time.

The antibody responses to PRRSV were overall delayed and not sufficient. Seven pigs that showed high level of viremia after infection did not show seroconversion for

PRRSV antibody until death (Fig. 7g, h). Two pigs (No. 987 and 994) that showed peaked viremia at 28 and 42 DPI developed detectable antibody to PRRSV at 111 and 100 DPI (Fig. 7c, b). These results indicate that serological method seem not to be so sensitive for detection of PRRSV infection.

Conclusions

GSWW/2015 strain is a highly pathogenic PRRSV strain circulated in north-western of China. This virus strain displays a unique discontinuous deletion of 30-aa in NSP2 and accumulated amino acids changes in GP3 and GP5, which might alter the antigenicity of the virus. Furthermore, GSWW/2015 strain can induce high level of viremia and persistent infection in individual and herd level. Antibody response to PRRSV is delayed compared with detection of viremia for diagnosis of virus infection. The correlation between long-lasting viremia and low level of antibody responses needs to be further investigated.

Abbreviations

CPE: Cytopathic effect; EAV: Equine arteritis virus; HP-PRRSV: Highly pathogenic porcine reproductive and respiratory syndrome virus; IFA: Indirect immunofluorescent assay; LDV: Lactate dehydrogenase-elevating virus; NSP: Non-structural protein; PRRS: Porcine reproductive and respiratory syndrome; PRRSV: Porcine reproductive and respiratory syndrome virus; qRT-PCR: Quantitative real-time PCR; SHFV: Simian hemorrhagic fever virus

Acknowledgements

The authors are grateful to be supported by State Key Laboratory of Veterinary Etiologic Biology, Lanzhou Veterinary Research Institute, CAAS.

Funding

This study was funded by a Sci-Tech Supporting Program of Gansu province of China (1504NKCA057) and Gansu Youth research program (1208RJAY079). Design of the study, collection, analysis, and interpretation of data and the writing of the manuscript were not influenced by the funding body.

Authors' contributions

WJB participated in the sequence analysis and animal experiment, and drafted the manuscript. ZJW, PS and JZ obtained the sequence of GSWW strain and worked for the variation analysis. HFB, YMC and YYC conducted the qRT-PCR, ELISA detection and analysis of the data. DL, ZJL and ZXL participated in the experiment design and revision of the manuscript. All authors contributed to the final editing and approval of the manuscript.

Consent for publication

Not applicable.

Competing interests

The authors declare that they have no competing interests.

References

1. Ansari IH, Kwon B, Osorio FA, Pattnaik AK. Influence of N-linked glycosylation of porcine reproductive and respiratory syndrome virus GP5 on virus infectivity, antigenicity, and ability to induce neutralizing antibodies. J Virol. 2006;80:3994–4004.
2. An TQ, Tian ZJ, Xiao Y, Li R, Peng JM, Wei TC, Zhang Y, Zhou YJ, Tong GZ. Origin of highly pathogenic porcine reproductive and respiratory syndrome virus, China. Emerg Infect Dis. 2010;16:365–7.
3. Benfield DA, Nelson E, Collins JE, Harris L, Goyal SM, Robison D, Christianson WT, Morrison RB, Gorcyca D, Chladek D. Characterization of swine infertility and respiratory syndrome (SIRS) virus (isolate ATCC VR-2332). J Vet Diagn Investig. 1992;4:127–33.
4. Cancel-Tirado SM, Evans RB, Yoon KJ. Monoclonal antibody analysis of porcine reproductive and respiratory syndrome virus epitopes associated with antibody-dependent enhancement and neutralization of virus infection. Vet Immunol Immunopathol. 2004;102:249–62.
5. Cavanagh D. Nidovirales: a new order comprising Coronaviridae and Arteriviridae. Arch Virol. 1997;142:629–33.
6. Chen Z, Lawson S, Sun Z, Zhou X, Guan X, Christopher-Hennings J, Nelson EA, Fang Y. Identification of two auto-cleavage products of nonstructural protein 1 (nsp1) in porcine reproductive and respiratory syndrome virus infected cells: nsp1 function as interferon antagonist. Virology. 2010;398:87–97.
7. de Lima M, Pattnaik AK, Flores EF, Osorio FA. Serologic marker candidates identified among B-cell linear epitopes of Nsp2 and structural proteins of a north American strain of porcine reproductive and respiratory syndrome virus. Virology. 2006;353:410–21.
8. Fang Y, Kim DY, Ropp S, Steen P, Christopher-Hennings J, Nelson EA, Rowland RR. Heterogeneity in Nsp2 of European-like porcine reproductive and respiratory syndrome viruses isolated in the United States. Virus Res. 2004;100:229–35.
9. Fang Y, Rowland RR, Roof M, Lunney JK, Christopher-Hennings J, Nelson EA. A full-length cDNA infectious clone of north American type 1 porcine reproductive and respiratory syndrome virus: expression of green fluorescent protein in the Nsp2 region. J Virol. 2006;80:11447–55.
10. Forsberg R. Divergence time of porcine reproductive and respiratory syndrome virus subtypes. Mol Biol Evol. 2005;22:2121–34.
11. Gao ZQ, Guo X, Yang HC. Genomic characterization of two Chinese isolates of porcine respiratory and reproductive syndrome virus. Arch Virol. 2004;149: 1341–51.
12. Liu CL, Zhang JW, Wei ZZ, Yuan SS. Development and application of TaqMan fluorescent qualitative RT-PCR method for PRRSV. Chinese Journal of Preventive Veterinary Medicine. 2010;32(11):858–61.
13. Meulenberg JJ, Petersen den Besten A, de Kluyver E, van Nieuwstadt A, Wensvoort G, Moormann RJ. Molecular characterization of Lelystad virus. Vet Microbiol. 1997;55:197–202.
14. Nelsen CJ, Murtaugh MP, Faaberg KS. Porcine reproductive and respiratory syndrome virus comparison: divergent evolution on two continents. J Virol. 1999;73:270–80.
15. Neumann EJ, Kliebenstein JB, Johnson CD, Mabry JW, Bush EJ, Seitzinger AH, Green AL, Zimmerman JJ. Assessment of the economic impact of porcine reproductive and respiratory syndrome on swine production in the United States. J Am Vet Med Assoc. 2005;227:385–92.
16. Ostrowski M, Galeota JA, Jar AM, Platt KB, Osorio FA, Lopez OJ. Identification of neutralizing and nonneutralizing epitopes in the porcine reproductive and respiratory syndrome virus GP5 ectodomain. J Virol. 2002;76:4241–50.
17. Tian K, Yu X, Zhao T, Feng Y, Cao Z, Wang C, Hu Y, Chen X, Hu D, Tian X. Emergence of fatal PRRSV variants: unparalleled outbreaks of atypical PRRS in China and molecular dissection of the unique hallmark. PLoS One. 2007;2:e526.
18. Tong GZ, Zhou YJ, Hao XF, Tian ZJ, An TQ, Qiu HJ. Highly pathogenic porcine reproductive and respiratory syndrome, China. Emerg Infect Dis. 2007;13:1434–6.
19. Wensvoort G, Terpstra C, Pol JM, terLaak EA, Bloemraad M, de Kluyver EP, Kragten C, van Buiten L, den Besten A, Wagenaar F. Mystery swine disease in the Netherlands: the isolation of Lelystad virus. Vet Q. 1991;13:121–30.
20. Zhou YJ, An TQ, He YX, Liu JX, Qiu HJ, Wang YF, Tong GZ. Antigenic structure analysis of glycosylated protein 3 of porcine reproductive and respiratory syndrome virus. Virus Res. 2006;118:98–104.
21. Zhou L, Zhang J, Zeng J, Yin S, Li Y, Zheng L, Guo X, Ge X, Yang H. The 30-amino-acid deletion in the Nsp2 of highly pathogenic porcine reproductive and respiratory syndrome virus emerging in China is not related to its virulence. J Virol. 2009;83:5156–67.

18

Development of a novel oil-in-water emulsion and evaluation of its potential adjuvant function in a swine influenza vaccine in mice

Jinqiu Zhang[1], Jinfeng Miao[2], Xiangan Han[3], Yu Lu[1*], Bihua Deng[1], Fang Lv[1], Yanhong Zhao[1], Chan Ding[3] and Jibo Hou[1]

Abstract

Background: Vaccination is the principal strategy for prevention and control of diseases, and adjuvant use is an effective strategy to enhance vaccine efficacy. Traditional mineral oil-based adjuvants have been reported with post-immunization reactions. Developing new adjuvant formulations with improved potency and safety will be of great value.

Results: In the study reported herein, a novel oil-in-water (O/W) Emulsion Adjuvant containing Squalane (termed EAS) was developed, characterized and investigated for swine influenza virus immunization. The data show that EAS is a homogeneous nanoemulsion with small particle size (~ 105 nm), low viscosity (2.04 ± 0.24 cP at 20 °C), excellent stability (at least 24 months at 4 °C) and low toxicity. EAS-adjuvanted H3N2 swine influenza vaccine was administrated in mice subcutaneously to assess the adjuvant potency of EAS. The results demonstrated that in mice EAS-adjuvanted vaccine induced significantly higher titers of hemagglutination inhibition (HI) and IgG antibodies than water-in-oil (W/O) vaccines or antigen alone, respectively, at day 42 post vaccination (dpv) ($P < 0.05$). EAS-adjuvanted vaccine elicited significantly stronger IgG1 and IgG2a antibodies and higher concentrations of Th1 (IFN-γ and IL-2) cytokines compared to the W/O vaccine or antigen alone. Mice immunized with EAS-adjuvanted influenza vaccine conferred potent protection after homologous challenge.

Conclusion: The O/W emulsion EAS developed in the present work induced potent humoral and cellular immune responses against inactivated swine influenza virus, conferred effective protection after homologous virus challenge and showed low toxicity in mice, indicating that EAS is as good as the commercial adjuvant MF59. The superiority of EAS to the conventional W/O formulation in adjuvant activity, safety and stability will make it a potential veterinary adjuvant.

Keywords: Swine influenza virus, Oil-in-water emulsion, H3N2 vaccine, Adjuvant

* Correspondence: luyu@jaas.ac.cn
[1]National Research Center for Veterinary Vaccine Engineering and Technology of China, Jiangsu Academy of Agricultural Sciences, Nanjing 210014, China
Full list of author information is available at the end of the article

Background

Vaccination is the principal strategy for prevention and control of diseases, and adjuvant use is an effective strategy to enhance vaccine efficacy. Emulsions have a long history as adjuvants for both human and animal vaccines. However, traditional oil-based emulsion adjuvants, such as Freund's complete or incomplete adjuvant, have been reported with post-immunization reactions. Developing new adjuvant formulations with improved potency and safety will be of great value.

Swine influenza is an acute respiratory disease of pigs mainly caused by the influenza A virus. Although mortality is usually low, swine influenza may result in poor growth, weight loss, immunosuppression of infected pigs and economic loss in the pig industry [1]. Furthermore, it has been hypothesized that pigs can serve as an intermediate host for the adaptation of avian influenza viruses to humans or as mixing vessels for the generation of reassortant viruses [2–4]. Vaccination is the primary strategy for prevention and control of swine influenza in China and other countries. However, previous studies demonstrate that commercial vaccines in a water-in-oil (W/O) formulation is not highly effective in preventing vaccinated pigs from wild-type virus infection [5, 6]. In addition, post-immunization reactions associated with mineral oil-based adjuvants have been reported, such as edema, abscess/granuloma formation or necrosis at injection sites, which render pork unfit for consumption and greatly limits the wide application of these vaccines [7]. Hence, developing new adjuvant formulations with improved potency and safety will be of great value and impact both in the swine industry and for global public health. In this study, swine influenza virus was used as a model antigen to investigate the new adjuvant's immunogenicity.

The most successful adjuvants of influenza vaccines for human use are squalene-based oil-in-water emulsions, such as MF59 (Novartis) and ASO3 (GlaxoSmithKline). A number of clinical trials indicate that squalene-in-water emulsions outperform aluminum salts or W/O emulsions at increasing vaccine immunogenicity and affording cross-reactivity without causing unacceptable adverse reactions [8–11]. Squalene or squalane (hydrogenated form of squalene) has been used as an alternative to mineral oil for its tolerance and investigated extensively in vaccine adjuvant applications. In the current study, a new squalane-in-water (O/W) emulsion, termed EAS, was developed for veterinary vaccines. We describe the main physicochemical characteristics, stability and tolerability of the new O/W emulsion adjuvant. Then, vaccine supplemented with EAS was used to immunize mice subcutaneously to assess its capacity to induce a specific immune response. Our results show that EAS-adjuvanted H3N2 swine influenza vaccine can induce significantly higher antibody titers than W/O vaccines in mice, and elicit a mixed Th1/Th2 response. Compared to the conventional W/O formulation adjuvant, EAS was shown to be a better candidate for swine influenza immunization due to its superiority in adjuvant efficacy, stability and safety.

Results

Characterization of the O/W emulsion EAS

A novel emulsion formulation containing squalane, PEG-PPG-PEG, soy lecithin and carbopol was prepared. Particle size, polydispersity index, zeta potential, viscosity, conductivity and pH value of the developed emulsion EAS were measured (Table 1). The mean particle size of the EAS emulsion was ~ 105 nm, with a low polydispersity index (Table 1 and Fig. 1a). TEM analysis was performed to investigate the morphology of emulsion droplets (Fig. 1b). Images from the O/W emulsion showed a characteristic spherical shape, and the diameter of emulsion droplets was in agreement with DLS measurements as described above. The zeta potential value of these emulsions was about − 38 mV, higher than the common slightly negative charge usually reported for other O/W emulsions [12]. EAS had a viscosity of 2.04 ± 0.24 cP at 20 °C. Conductivity measurements demonstrated that EAS is an oil-in-water system [13].

Stability of the O/W emulsion EAS

The stability of EAS at different storage temperatures was monitored by visual inspection and particle sizing change. At 4 °C, the emulsion had minimal changes in particle size, zeta potential, pH value and viscosity over 24 months (Table 2). At elevated temperatures (25 or 37 °C) the samples demonstrated stability over 6-month or 3-month durations, respectively. The samples stored at 25 or 37 °C had an increase in particle size after 6 months or 3 months, respectively. Thereafter, visible evidence of coalescence or phase separation of the oil and aqueous phases gradually emerged. Overall, results provided in Table 2 support the long-term stability of EAS at 4 °C.

Toxicity evaluation of EAS

To assess EAS tolerability in animals, the local reactogenicity of different formulations was monitored at injection sites for edema or erythema and animals were observed for health problems following injection. There were not any changes at the sites of injection in the PBS group (Fig. 2a). No systemic effects or gross lesions were noted post-administration of the EAS and MF59 formulations (Fig. 2 b and c). When

Table 1 Characteristics of the O/W emulsion adjuvant (values are shown as means± SD, $n = 3$)

Visual appearance	Particle size (Dv50; nm)	Polydispersity index (PDI)	Zeta potential (mV)	Viscosity (cP)	Conductivity (mS/cm)	pH
Milky-white liquid	105 ± 2	0.12 ± 0.03	− 38.8 ± 0.2	2.04 ± 0.24	−0.0269 ± 0.0017	6.80 ± 0.02

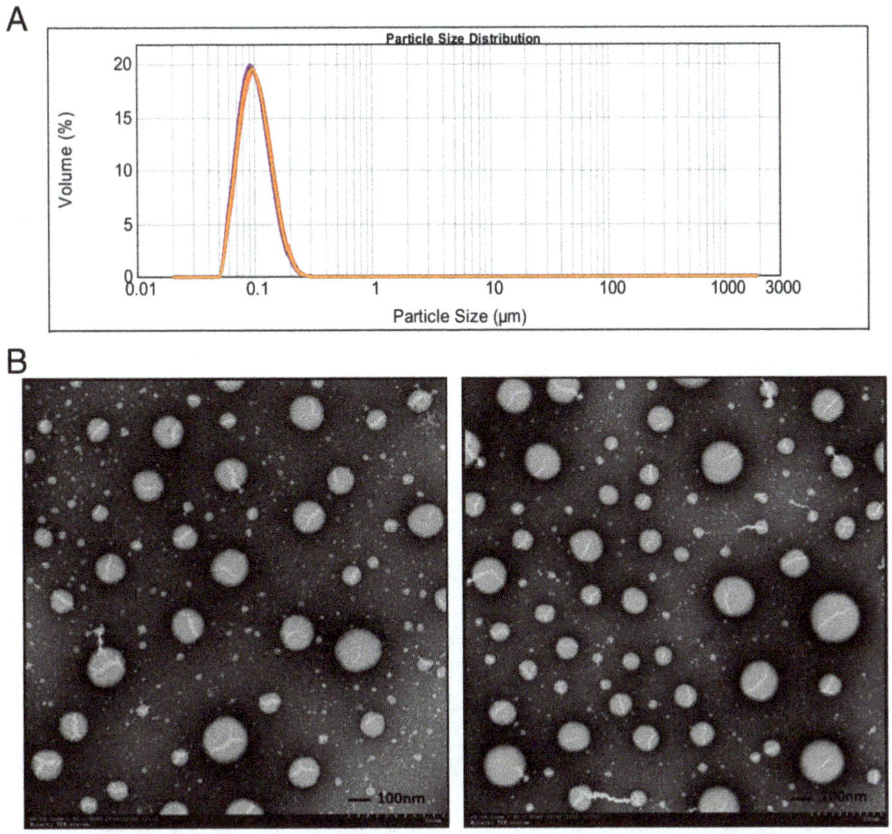

Fig. 1 The particle size distribution and TEM images of EAS. **a**: Nine total measurements were made on 3 separate samples from the same batch of EAS as measured by dynamic light scattering. **b**: Cryo-transmission electron microscopy of two samples of EAS. Bar represents 100 nm

administered with the W/O formulation, mild to serious reactions, such as edema, abscesses, granulomas and nodules were present at injection sites (Fig. 2d).

Histological analysis was used to evaluate the toxicity of the different formulations. No pathologic changes were observed in control group (Fig. 2e), whereas inflammation, as evidenced by hyperplasia of connective tissue (thick arrow), folliculus pili and hair papilla (ellipse); by infiltrating PMNs (thin arrow) were present in tissue after injection with W/O emulsion (Fig. 2h). The pathologic changes in

Table 2 Heat Stability Study of EAS at 4 °C, 25 °C and 37 °C (values are shown as means ±SD, $n = 3$)

EAS		Time (months)							
		T0	1	3	6	9	12	18	24
4 °C	Particle size	104 ± 2	104 ± 2	101 ± 3	105 ± 1	104 ± 2	105 ± 2	107 ± 2	106 ± 2
	Zeta potential	−38.8 ± 0.1	−38.3 ± 0.4	− 38.5 ± 0.2	− 38.8 ± 0.2	− 38.7 ± 0.2	−38.5 ± 0.2	− 38.7 ± 0.02	−38.3 ± 0.3
	pH	6.8 ± 0.1	6.7 ± 0.2	6.8 ± 0.1	6.6 ± 0.3	6.8 ± 0.1	6.8 ± 0.1	6.7 ± 0.3	6.7 ± 0.2
	Viscosity	2.01 ± 0.14	2.01 ± 0.21	1.90 ± 0.17	1.94 ± 0.17	2.04 ± 0.15	2.11 ± 0.01	1.99 ± 0.04	2.03 ± 0.12
25 °C	Particle size	104 ± 2	103 ± 3	109 ± 1	114 ± 2	141 ± 9	ND	ND	ND
	Zeta potential	−38.3 ± 0.1	−38.4 ± 0.5	−38.7 ± 0.3	−38.5 ± 0.5	−35.4 ± 0.4	ND	ND	ND
	pH	6.8 ± 0.2	6.5 ± 0.3	6.8 ± 0.1	6.5 ± 0.3	6.6 ± 0.2	ND	ND	ND
	Viscosity	2.01 ± 0.05	2.04 ± 0.01	2.24 ± 0.23	2.17 ± 0.05	2.43 ± 0.22	ND	ND	ND
37 °C	Particle size	105 ± 2	107 ± 2	115 ± 2	157 ± 12	ND	ND	ND	ND
	Zeta potential	−38.6 ± 0.3	−38.4 ± 0.2	−36.9 ± 0.3	−35.8 ± 0.4	ND	ND	ND	ND
	pH	6.8 ± 0.2	6.5 ± 0.3	6.6 ± 0.2	6.7 ± 0.2	ND	ND	ND	ND
	Viscosity	2.03 ± 0.11	2.11 ± 0.18	2.34 ± 0.19	2.55 ± 0.38	ND	ND	ND	ND

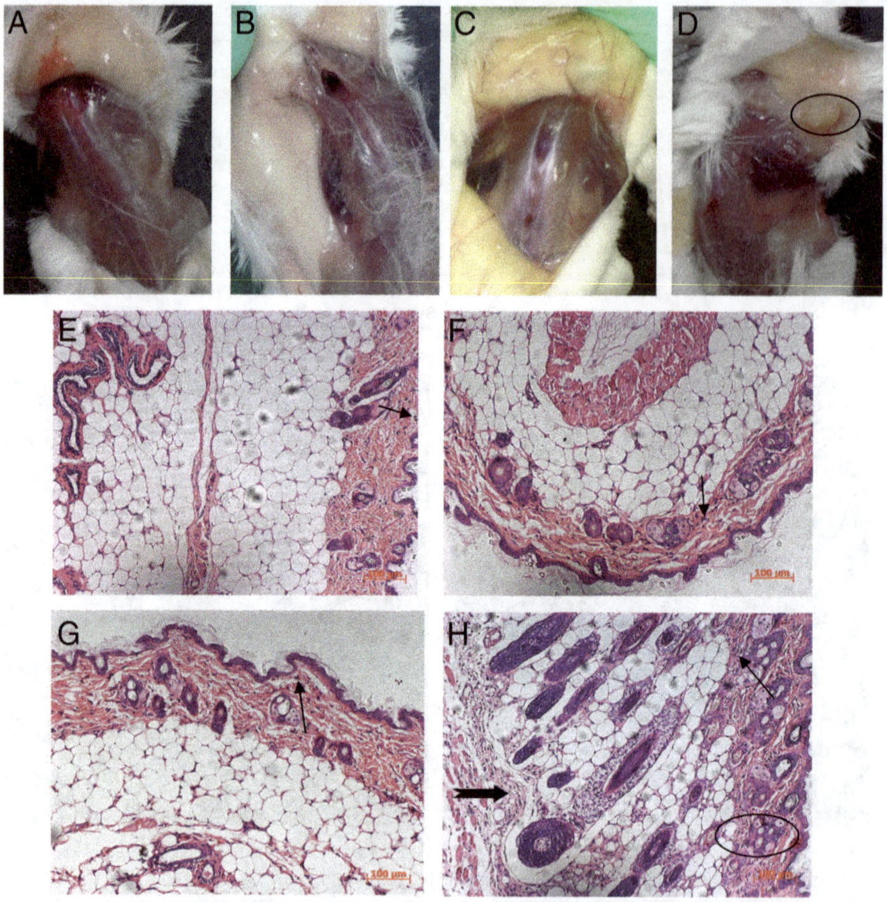

Fig. 2 Toxicity analysis of EAS. **a** to **d**: the local reactogenicity of different formulations at the sites of injection. The subcutaneous injection sites of each formulation in female BALB/c mice were observed 72 h after administration. **a**: PBS control; **b**: EAS; **c**: MF59; **d**: W/O formulation. **e** to **h**: the histology of the subcutaneous injection sites of mice (H.E. × 100).The tissues excised from the sites of administration 72 h after the injection of each sample were fixed in 10% formalin and embedded in paraffin for histologic examination. Hematoxylin and eosin stained slides were prepared using standard methods. **e**: PBS control; **f**: EAS; **g**: MF59; **h**: W/O formulation

the EAS and MF59 emulsion groups were mild and there were no significant differences between these two groups (Fig. 2 f and g).

EAS-adjuvanted vaccine induces a high serum HI antibody response

Mice were immunized with swine influenza antigen incorporated into different adjuvants. Sera samples were collected 3 weeks after the first and second immunization. The haemagglutination inhibition (HI) assay was used to evaluate the anti-HA antibody response. As shown in Fig. 3a, all adjuvant formulations induced significantly higher HI titers than the non-adjuvanted vaccine group at days 21 and 42 post-vaccination (dpv) ($P < 0.05$)). EAS induced significantly higher HI titers than the W/O formulation at 42dpv ($P < 0.05$)), although there were no statistically significant difference between them at 21dpv ($P > 0.05$). Minimal differences in antibody responses were observed between animals immunized with EAS and MF59 adjuvant at 21 and 42dpv ($P > 0.05$).

EAS-adjuvanted vaccine induces high titers of humoral immune reactive antibody

Humoral immune responses induced by different formulations were detected by measuring H3N2 specific IgG antibodies of vaccinated mice using ELISA. All adjuvant formulations elicited significantly higher total IgG titers compared to antigen alone at both 21 and 42dpv ($P < 0.05$, Fig. 3b). EAS and MF59 vaccinated groups had significantly higher total IgG titers than the W/O formulation at 3 weeks after the first and second immunizations ($P < 0.05$). But there were no statistical differences between EAS and MF59 vaccinated groups ($P > 0.05$). Anti-flu IgG1 and IgG2a serum levels were determined to indicate the different qualitative response types induced by various formulations. As shown in Fig. 3c, all adjuvant formulations significantly increased antigen-specific IgG1 antibodies compared to antigen alone both at 21 and 42dpv

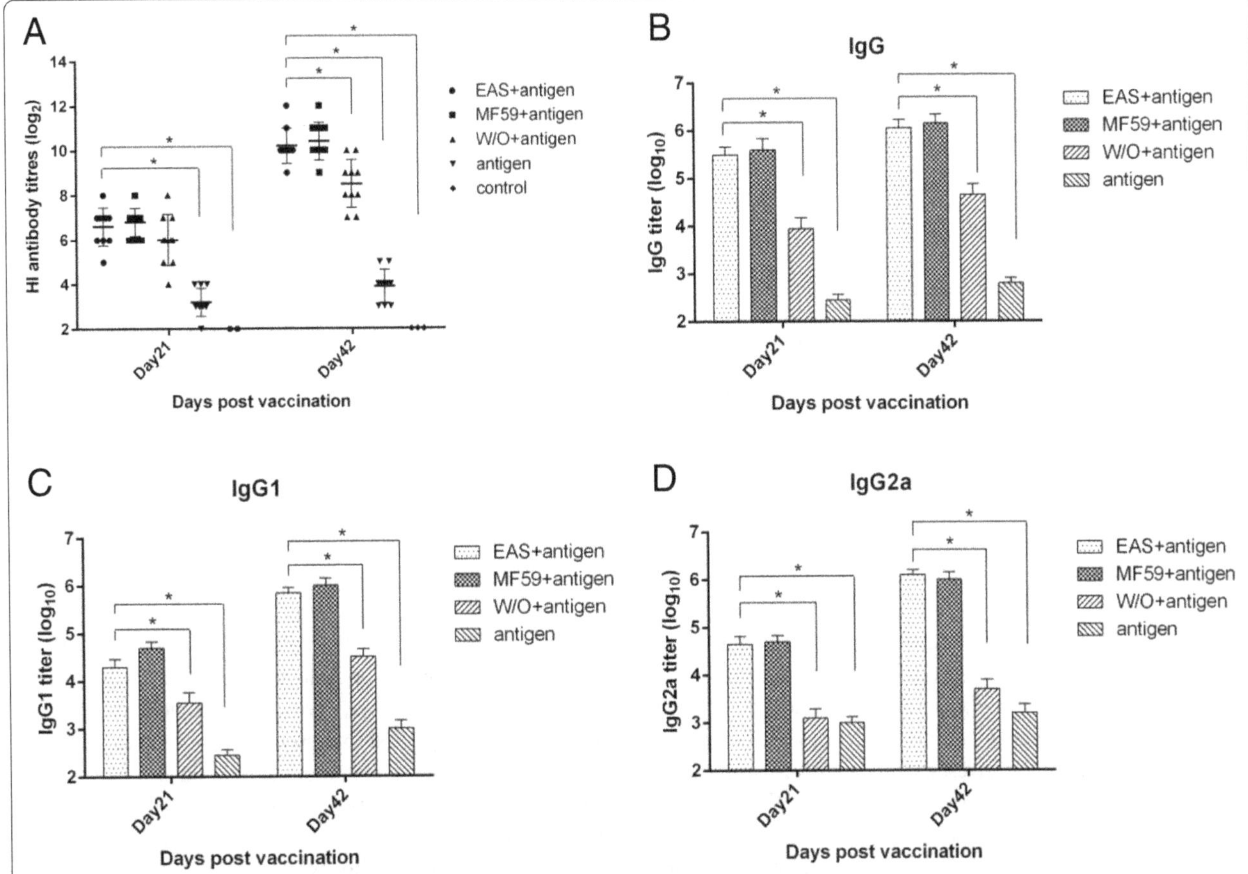

Fig. 3 HI antibody titers and antigen (A/swine/Shandong/3/2005)-specific antibodies (IgG, IgG1 and IgG2a) in BALB/c mice after immunization with various formulations. Mice received two immunizations at 3 weeks intervals and sera were collected on days 21 and 42 after primary immunization. Data are shown as individual data points or means ±SD. Asterisks indicate statistically significant differences ($P < 0.05$) between groups

($P < 0.05$). However, only EAS- or MF59-adjuvanted antigen significantly amplified IgG2a responses compared to the W/O formulation or antigen alone after primary or booster immunization ($P < 0.05$, Fig. 3d).

EAS-adjuvanted vaccine elicits high concentrations of cytokines and a mixed Th1/Th2 profile

The concentration of cytokines in supernatants of ex vivo stimulated splenocytes was measured by radioimmunoassay. No or very low levels of cytokines were detected in the supernatant of splenocytes from control mice. Splenocytes from mice immunized with EAS-adjuvanted vaccine secreted significantly higher levels of Th1 cytokines (IFN-γ and IL-2) compared to the W/O formulation or antigen alone group 48 h after stimulation ($P < 0.05$, Fig. 4). Additionally, higher levels of Th2 cytokines (IL-4 and IL-5) were detected in the EAS-adjuvanted vaccine group compared to the other vaccine groups, although there was no significant difference between them ($P > 0.05$). Cytokine profiles after 48 h of stimulation were similar between EAS and MF59 vaccine groups.

EAS-adjuvanted vaccine confers effective protection against homologous virus challenge

All mice survived and no obvious clinical signs were observed after challenge. Virus was not detected in the lungs of immunized mice at 5 dpi except the antigen alone vaccinated group or mock vaccinated group (Table 3). The immunized mice in EAS, MF59 and W/O group showed slight and transient body weight loss (1%~ 2%) on 2 dpi, and then recovered quickly from 4 dpi. In antigen alone immunized group, mice showed mild weight loss (less than 5%), then they recovered gradually and regained their body weight on 8 dpi. In contrast, mock vaccinated mice displayed significant and progressive weight loss, which lasted 2 weeks, and the worst weight loss with 10.5% decline occurred on 6 dpi (Fig. 5).

Discussion

For farm and laboratory animals, the most commonly used emulsion adjuvants are mineral (paraffin) oil-based Freund's complete or incomplete adjuvant. Although these W/O emulsions have adjuvant effects in veterinary vaccines, they are too

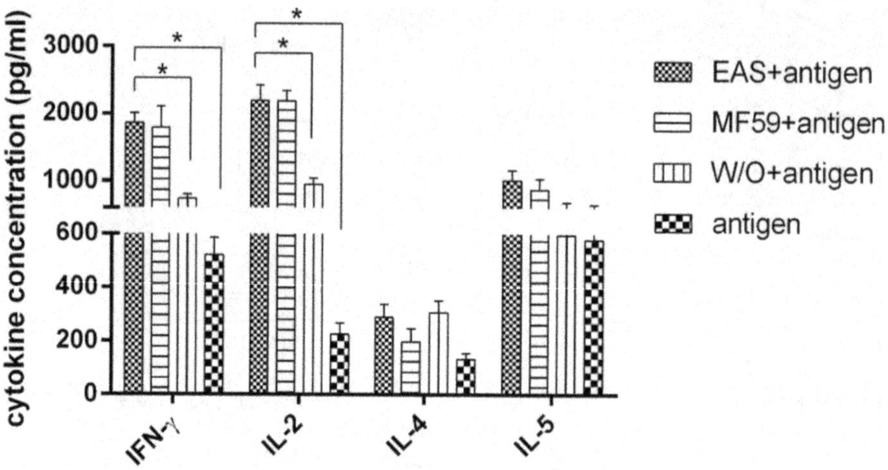

Fig. 4 The cytokine response induced in the spleen of BALB/c mice after immunization with various formulations. Mice ($n = 3$) received 2 immunizations at 3 weeks intervals and splenocytes were collected at day 21 after booster immunization. The cell supernatant was analyzed for influenza-induced IFN-γ, IL-2, IL-4 and IL-5 by radioimmunoassay after 48 h of stimulation. Data are shown as means ± SD. Asterisks indicate statistically significant differences ($P < 0.05$) between groups

reactogenic for routine use [14]. O/W emulsion, owing to the generally lower concentration of oils and better safety and tolerability profiles, will likely be preferred for the next generation of adjuvants. The objective of this study was to develop a novel O/W emulsion and investigate its adjuvant potential in inactivated swine influenza vaccine. DLS and TEM analyses document that EAS is a homogeneous nanoemulsion with small particle size (~ 105 nm) and a low polydispersity index (0.159 ± 0.036). The low viscosity (2.04 ± 0.24 cP at 20 °C) was expected because of the small average diameter of the droplets. The small average diameter and low viscosity of EAS will be of benefit following sterile filtration and parenteral administration.

The adjuvant potential of EAS was investigated and compared with the W/O formulation and MF59 adjuvant in mice immunized with inactivated swine influenza virus. The results showed that mice immunized subcutaneously twice with EAS-adjuvanted vaccine had significantly higher titers of HI and IgG antibodies than the W/O formulation or antigen alone ($P < 0.05$), but there was no difference between the EAS-adjuvanted group and MF59-adjuvanted group ($P > 0.05$). Remarkably, data from many previous studies indicates that the size of adjuvant particles has an important effect on adjuvant activity and the type of evolving immune responses. For example, Li et al. showed that smaller OVA-conjugated nanoparticles (~ 230 nm) induced stronger OVA-specific antibody and cellular immune responses than the larger OVA-nanoparticles (~ 780 nm) when subcutaneously injected into mice [15]. Foged et al. [16] and Kanchan et al. [17] also showed that smaller particles (< 500 nm) were more efficiently internalized by DCs and macrophages than larger particles (> 1 μm). Moreover, the particle size of MF59 (~ 160 nm) was optimized in the preparation process by microfluidizer and was crucial to its maximal adjuvant effect for a wide range of antigens in many clinical and pre-clinical studies [18]. Since the mean particle size of EAS was less than 200 nm, we presume that it may have similar effect on its adjuvant efficacy. The correlation between the particle size of EAS and its adjuvant activity will be defined in further studies.

Immunity to influenza is dependent on both antibody and cell mediated immune responses, and both are critical to inducing protective immunity [19–22]. Oil in water adjuvants including MF59 and AS03 were shown to significantly

Table 3 Lung virus isolation from mice of different groups challenge with the homologous virus

Group	Number of mice carrying H3N2 virus in lung post challenge/total number (Positive rate)
EAS + antigen	0/5
MF59 + antigen	0/5
W/O + antigen	0/5
antigen	1/5
mock	4/5

Mice were challenged intranasally with 0.2×10^5 EID50 of the H3N2 subtype virus strain A/swine/Shandong/3/2005 two weeks after the second immunization. Five mice of each group were euthanized at 5 days post infection (dpi), and whole lungs were collected and homogenized in PBS. The homogenates were centrifuged and the supernatant from each sample was collected for passage in 10-day-old specific pathogen free (SPF) embryonated chicken eggs. The allantoic fluid was harvested and tested for hemagglutinin activity

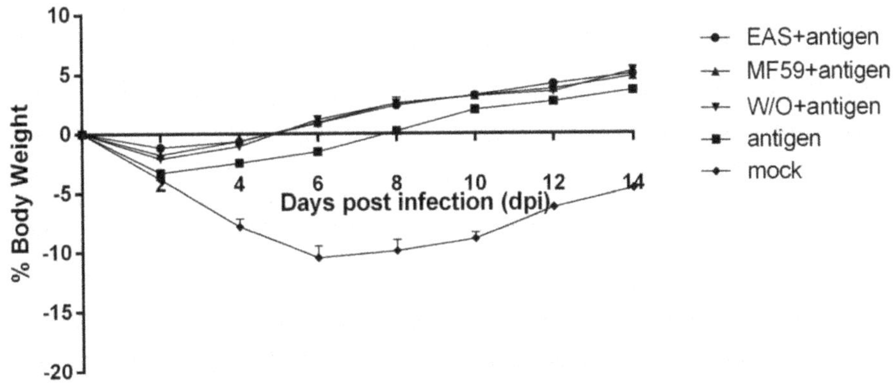

Fig. 5 Weight changes of mice after homologous virus challenge. Mice were challenged intranasally with 0.2×10^5 EID50 of the H3N2 subtype virus strain A/swine/Shandong/3/2005 two weeks after the second immunization. The survival rate, clinical signs and bodyweight of the challenged mice were monitored for 14 days after the challenge. Data are shown as means ± SD. Asterisks indicate statistically significant differences ($P < 0.05$) between groups

improve humoral and T cell responses against human or avian influenza [8–11]. In the current study, although all vaccinated mice induced amplified H3N2 specific ELISA antibodies, only the EAS and MF59 vaccinated groups induced both strong IgG1 and IgG2a antibodies, while the W/O formulation or antigen alone induced predominantly IgG1 antibodies. The predominance of IgG2a isotypes indicates skewing towards Th1 responses, which promotes efficient generation of cytotoxic T cells resulting in faster virus clearance and recovery after viral infection [23–25]. These results demonstrate that EAS induces a balanced IgG1/IgG2a response and a mixed Th1/Th2 response, which is important for protective immunity against influenza. Furthermore, the cytokine profile from the supernatants of ex vivo stimulated cells showed that the EAS-adjuvanted vaccine induced significantly higher levels of Th1 cytokines compared to the W/O formulation or antigen alone, implying an effective stimulation of the innate immune system and consequent facilitation of enhanced immunity to influenza, as did MF59. Moreover, no virus was detected in the lungs of immunized mice at day 5 post infection except the antigen alone vaccinated group or mock vaccinated group, showing that EAS-adjuvanted vaccine, as well as MF59-adjuvanted vaccine and the conventional W/O vaccine could provide effective protection against homologous challenge. Taken together, EAS-adjuvanted vaccine enhanced HI titers, induced virus-specific cell-mediated immune response and provided potent protection against virus challenge. EAS could be a promising candidate adjuvant for veterinary vaccine. Remarkably, although the adjuvant effect of MF59 was due to the fully formulated emulsion [18, 26, 27], we presume that some component of EAS might induce a comparable adjuvant effect. Specifically, carbopol-based adjuvant suspensions have been evaluated in veterinary vaccines against several pathogens [28, 29], and the non-ionic block polymer pluronic® L121 (similar to pluronic® L31 in chemical structure) has been reported to contribute to the potent adjuvant efficacy of the Syntex adjuvant formulation (SAF) [30, 31]. We presume that these ingredients may account for the enhanced immune response of the EAS formulation. Research on the mechanism of action of EAS is ongoing.

For an emulsion to be used for parenteral administration, stability is one of the most important parameters. Many factors are associated with the stability of emulsions, such as initial particle size, uniformity, surface tension and interface charge [32–34]. Emulsions with smaller initial particle size are more stable than those with larger particles [35]. For instance, the small droplet size of MF59 emulsion enhances emulsion stability for at least 2 years at 2–8 °C [26, 36]. Moreover, higher zeta potential is closely related to a higher surface charge of colloidal particles and thus has more charge repulsion, which is another indication of the stability of colloidal systems [35, 37]. The zeta potential of EAS was about − 38 mV, significantly higher than the common value of − 20 to − 30 mV reported for other O/W emulsions [37]. This might be due to the use of soy lecithin and carbopol 971P, which contains various anionic fractions. These negatively charged components usually account for a major proportion of surface charge and hence are of great importance to the stability of emulsions. In the current study, EAS was stable for 24 months and did not present any significant physical alteration or phrase separation over the storage period at 4 °C. We presume that the small particle size, low polydispersity index and high zeta potential may contribute to its excellent stability.

Beside the potent adjuvant efficacy and superior stability of EAS, safety is another major concern when considering new adjuvant formulations for vaccine applications. The local reactogenicity and tolerability of EAS was assessed in mice by visual inspection and histological analysis. Although mild inflammatory reactions were present in mice injected with EAS, there were no obvious health problems or gross lesions. However, mice injected with the W/O formulation, had adverse reactions at injection sites. The safety profile of EAS should be further tested in pigs or other farm animals in the near future. Moreover, during pandemic, it is very often that antigen is in short and it is important to have an adjuvant to save lots of antigens. Thus, dose-dependent tests are needed. And, it will be also nice to examine whether this adjuvant enhances long-term protection, cross-protection of vaccine and whether the adjuvant will enhance the immunity itself, and so on. These will be investigated in the further study.

Conclusion

Developing new adjuvant formulations with improved potency, enhanced safety and low viscosity will be of great value for swine industry. The O/W emulsion EAS developed in the present work induced potent humoral and cellular immune responses against inactivated swine influenza virus, conferred effective protection after homologous virus challenge and showed low toxicity in mice, indicating that EAS is as good as the commercial adjuvant MF59. The superiority of EAS to the conventional W/O formulation in adjuvant activity, safety and stability will make it a potential veterinary adjuvant.

Methods

Adjuvant components and virus

Squalane (vegetable-based) was purchased from Croda Ltd., Shanghai, China. Polyoxyethylene 20 sorbitan monooleate (polysorbate 80) and Poloxamer 407 were purchased from Sigma-Aldrich (St. Louis, MO, USA). Poly (ethylene glycol) -block-poly (propylene glycol) -block-poly (ethylene glycol) (PEG-PPG-PEG Pluronic® L-31) was obtained from BASF Corporation, USA. Soy lecithin (PC~ 70%) was purchased from Shanghai Tywei Pharmaceutical Co., Ltd. (Shanghai, China). Polyethylene glycol 400 monooleate (PEG400MO) was purchased from Xinchang pharmaceutical Co., Ltd. (Zhejiang, China). Carbomer 971P was obtained from Lubrizol (Wickliffee, OH, USA). A/swine/Shandong/3/2005 (H3N2 subtype) was isolated from pigs with respiratory disease on farms in eastern China [38]. Viruses were propagated in the allantoic cavities of 10-day-old embryonated specific-pathogen-free (SPF) chicken eggs or in Madin-Darby canine kidney cells (MDCK). The infective allantoic fluid was aliquoted and stored at – 80 °C.

Preparation of emulsion

The recipe of the emulsion adjuvant was as described in the Chinese patent license with registration number 201310021011.3. Briefly, the lipophilic emulsifiers, PEG-PPG-PEG Pluronic® L-31 and soy lecithin were fully dissolved in the oil phase (squalane) and the hydrophilic emulsifiers, polysorbate 80, Poloxamer 407, and PEG400MO were fully dissolved in the water phase (PBS, pH 7.4) containing carbopol 971P. The oil phase was added to the aqueous phase with a high-shear mixer (MICCRA D-9, Nordrhein-Westfalen, Germany) at 11,000 rpm for 15 min to yield a coarse emulsion. The coarse emulsion was immediately processed through a High Pressure Homogenizer (ATS engineering, Shanghai, China) for six cycles at 1000 bar. Finally, the emulsion was filter-sterilized by 0.22 μm filtration (Millipore AS, Oslo, Norway) and adjusted to pH 6.8. Emulsion adjuvant containing squalane was named EAS.

Characterization of emulsion

Emulsion particle sizing was determined via dynamic light scattering (DLS) with a Mastersizer 2000 (Malvern Instruments, Worcestershire, UK). The size and homogeneity of oil droplets in EAS were observed by transmission electron microscopy (TEM) with a JEM-1230 (JEOL Ltd., Tokyo, Japan), as described previously [39]. Zeta potential was determined on a Zetasizer Nano-ZS 90 (Malvern Instruments Corp., UK). The dynamic viscosity of EAS was measured at 25 °C using a digital viscometer (DV-II + Pro, Brookfield Engineering Laboratory, Middleboro, MA, USA).

For stability analysis, filter sterilized EAS samples were stored at 4, 25 and 37 °C over 24 months. Colloidal stability of emulsion was assessed by visual inspection and particle sizing change. Laser light diffraction techniques were used for size measurements because of their wide range of particle sizing, enabling the detection of larger droplets that may appear as a result of emulsion destabilization.

Preparation of vaccine

The H3N2 subtype swine influenza vaccine was prepared as an O/W form. In brief, the H3N2 subtype virus strain A/swine/Shandong/3/2005 was propagated in allantoic cavities of 10-day-old specific pathogen free (SPF) embryonated chicken eggs. The viral-laden allantoic fluids (1024 HA units per 0.1 ml) were purified by centrifugation (28,000×g, 30 min, 4 °C) and inactivated with 0.5% (*v*/v) β-propiolactone at 37 °C for 24 h. Equal volumes of purified virus and EAS were thoroughly mixed on a shaker to manufacture an O/W emulsion vaccine. MF59 emulsion adjuvant and MF59-adjuvanted vaccine was also prepared according to the protocol published for MF59 [26]. Briefly, MF59, consisting of 5% squalene (v/v), 0.5% Tween80 (v/v), 0.5% Span 85 (v/v) (Sigma, St. Louis, MO, USA) in 20 mM citrate buffer, was prepared by homogenization at 12,000 psi with a Microfluidizer (model 110Y; Microfluidics, Newton, MA). The emulsion was sterilized by 0.22 μm filtration. MF59-adjuvanted vaccine was prepared by thoroughly mixing of purified virus and MF59 at a ratio of 1:1 (v/v). Conventional vaccine in a water-in-oil form (W/O vaccine) was prepared as previously described and used as a control [40]. For W/O emulsion vaccine, the purified virus was emulsified in Marcol 52 mineral oil (ESSO, Paris, France) at a ratio of 1:3 (v/v, virus to adjuvant).

Toxicity analysis
Female BALB/c mice (18-22 g) purchased from Beijing Merial Vital Laboratory Animal Technology Co., Ltd. (Beijing, China) were housed under specific pathogen-free conditions. Mice from each group ($n = 3$) were inoculated subcutaneously with 200 µl of EAS, MF59 or W/O emulsion. Mice in the control group received the same amount of PBS. The tissues excised from the sites of administration 72 h after injection were fixed in 10% formalin and embedded in paraffin for histologic examination. Hematoxylin and eosin stained slides were prepared using standard methods [41].

Immunization of mice
Female BALB/c mice (18-22 g) purchased from Beijing Merial Vital Laboratory Animal Technology Co., Ltd. (Beijing, China) were housed under specific pathogen-free conditions. Mice from each group ($n = 20$) were injected subcutaneously twice with 200 µl of O/W emulsion vaccines (containing 1024 HA units) or 400 µl of W/O vaccine (containing 1024 HA units) at 3 weeks intervals. Mice in the control group received immunizations with 200 µl of PBS. Sera were collected 3 weeks after the first and second immunization.

Hemagglutination inhibition titer (HI)
To determine hemagglutination-inhibition (HI) titers, sera were first treated with receptor-destroying enzyme (RDE) (DenkaSeiken, Tokyo, Japan) by incubation overnight at 37 °C to eliminate hemagglutination non-specific inhibitors in serum samples. Then, sera were heated at 56 °C for 30 min to inactivate the receptor-destroying enzyme. Sera were serially (1:2) diluted, mixed with 4HA units of influenza virus, and incubated for 30 min at room temperature prior to adding 1% chicken red blood cells. HI titers are defined as the highest serum dilution completely inhibiting hemagglutination.

Elisa
Influenza virus-specific antibodies (IgG, IgG1 and IgG2a) were quantified using an ELISA assay, as previously described [42] except that plates were coated with inactivated whole H3N2 influenza virus antigen (2 µg/ml). The titers of IgG, IgG1 and IgG2a were calculated using a four-parameter logistic equation (Softmax software, Molecular Devices). The inflection point of the titration curve was taken as titer value.

Ex vivo re-stimulation of splenocytes
Antigen-specific T cell responses were measured following re-stimulation of splenocytes with whole β-propiolactone-inactivated H3N2 influenza virus. Briefly, splenocytes were isolated from immunized mice and cultured in RPMI-1640 supplemented with 10% fetal bovine serum, 100 U/ml penicillin, and 0.1 mg/ml streptomycin. Splenocytes (2×10^6cells/well) were then stimulated with inactivated H3N2 influenza virus (2 µg/ml). Forty-eight hours later, cytokines (IL-2, IL-4, IL-5, IFN-γ) were measured from supernatants by radioimmunoassay. Commercial kits were purchased from the Institute of Radiation of Science and Technology Development Center of the General Hospital of People's Liberation Army (Beijing, China). The assay was conducted according to the manufacturer's protocol. All samples were assayed in triplicate.

Virus challenge of immunized mice
Mice were challenged intranasally with 0.2×10^5 EID50 of the H3N2 subtype virus strain A/swine/Shandong/3/2005 two weeks after the second immunization. Five mice of each group were euthanized at day 5 post infection (dpi), and whole lungs were collected and homogenized in PBS. The homogenates were centrifuged and the supernatant from each sample was collected for passage in 10-day-old specific pathogen free (SPF) embryonated chicken eggs. The allantoic fluid was harvested and tested for hemagglutinin activity. The survival rate, clinical signs and bodyweight of the remaining mice were monitored for 14 days after the challenge.

Statistical analyses
Data were expressed as individual data points or means ± standard deviation (SD). Differences were evaluated by one-way analysis of variance (ANOVA) followed by post-hoc tests. Differences were considered significant at a P-value < 0.05.

Ethics statement
Protocols involving mice were approved by the Institutional Animal Care and Use Committee and were conducted following the guidelines of the Institutional Biosafety Committee at the Jiangsu Academy of Agriculture Sciences. Efforts were made to minimize animal suffering. All the animals were euthanized after the study in a chamber with carbon dioxide (BIOSCAPE, CO_2 – box model L). The animals were placed into CO_2 – box and 100% carbon dioxide was imported. The following ratios of CO_2/O_2% vol/min were applied for induction 5/95% vol/min and for euthanasia 100/0% vol/min. The secondary physical method of euthanasia was performed by decapitation. In the progress, the animals were unconscious.

Abbreviations
DLS: Dynamic light scattering; dpv: Days post-vaccination; EAS: Emulsion Adjuvant containing Squalane; HI: Hemagglutination inhibition titer; MDCK: Madin-Darby canine kidney; O/W: Oil in water; PEG400MO: Polyethylene glycol 400 monooleate; PEG-PPG-PEG: Poly (ethylene glycol) -block-poly (propylene glycol) -block-poly (ethylene glycol); polysorbate 80: Polyoxyethylene 20 sorbitan monooleate; RDE: Receptor-destroying enzyme; SD: Standard deviation; SPF: specific-pathogen-free; TEM: Transmission electron microscopy; W/O: Water in oil

Acknowledgments
The authors wish to express their thanks to Dr. Howard Gelberg (Oregon State University) for manuscript editing.

Funding
This work was supported by the National Natural Science Foundation of China (No. 31772701, 31672515, 31472164), the Special Fund for Independent Innovation of Agricultural Science and Technology in Jiangsu Province of China (No. cx (17) 3027). The article processing charge was covered by National Natural Science Foundation of China (No. 31772701) and the Special Fund for Independent Innovation of Agricultural Science and Technology in Jiangsu Province of China (No. cx (17) 3027).

Authors' contributions
Conceived and designed the experiments: JQZ, JFM, YL and JBH. Performed the animal experiments: JQZ, JFM, XGH, BHD and FL. Analyzed the data: YHZ and CD. Wrote and revised the manuscript: JQZ and JFM. All authors read and approved the final manuscript.

Consent for publication
Not applicable.

Competing interests
The authors declare that they have no competing interests.

Author details
[1]National Research Center for Veterinary Vaccine Engineering and Technology of China, Jiangsu Academy of Agricultural Sciences, Nanjing 210014, China. [2]College of Veterinary Medicine, Nanjing Agricultural University, Nanjing 210095, China. [3]Shanghai Veterinary Research Institute, Chinese Academy of Agricultural Sciences, Shanghai 200241, China.

References
1. Brockmeier S L, Register K B, Nicholson T L, et al. Bordetellosis Diseases of swine. 10th ed. Wiley-Blackwell. 2012:670–79.
2. Crisci E, Mussá T, Fraile L, Montoya M. Review: influenza virus in pigs. Mol Immunol. 2013;55:200–11.
3. Pearce MB, Jayaraman A, Pappas C, Belser JA, Zeng H, Gustin KM, Maines TR, Sun X, Raman R, Cox NJ, Sasisekharan R, Katz JM, Tumpey TM. Pathogenesis and transmission of swine origin a (H3N2) v influenza viruses in ferrets. Proc Natl Acad Sci U S A. 2012;109:3944–9.
4. Yassine HM, Al-Natour MQ, Lee CW, Saif YM. Interspecies and intraspecies transmission of triple reassortant H3N2 influenza a viruses. Virol J. 2007;4: 129. https://doi.org/10.1186/1743-422X-4-129.
5. Van Reeth K, Ma W. Swine influenza virus vaccines: to change or not to change-that's the question. Curr Top Microbiol Immunol. 2013;370:173–200.
6. Aucouturier J, Dupuis L, Ganne V. Adjuvants designed for veterinary and human vaccines. Vaccine. 2001;19:2666–72.
7. Petrovsky N, Aguilar JC. Vaccine adjuvants: Current state and future trends. Immunol Cell Biol. 2004;82:488–96.
8. Dell'Era L, Corona F, Daleno C, Scala A, Principi N, Esposito S. Immunogenicity, safety and tolerability of MF59-adjuvanted seasonal influenza vaccine in children with juvenile idiopathic arthritis. Vaccine. 2012;30:936–40.
9. Stephenson I, Bugarini R, Nicholson KG, Podda A, Wood JM, Zambon MC, Katz JM. Cross-reactivity to highly pathogenic avian influenza H5N1 viruses after vaccination with nonadjuvanted and MF59-adjuvanted influenza a/ duck/Singapore/97 (H5N3) vaccine: a potential priming strategy. J Infect Dis. 2005;191:1210–5.
10. Morel S, Didierlaurent A, Bourguignon P, Delhaye S, Baras B, Jacob V. Adjuvant system AS03 containing α-tocopherol modulates innate immune response and leads to improved adaptive immunity. Vaccine. 2011;29:2461–73.
11. Vesikari T, Richardus JH, Berglund J, Korhonen T, Flodmark CE, Lindstrand A, Silfverdal SA, Bambure V, Caplanusi A, Dieussaert I, Roy-Ghanta S, Vaughn DW. Immunogenicity and safety of a trivalent inactivated influenza vaccine in children 6 months to 17 years of age, previously vaccinated with an AS03-adjuvanted a (H1N1) Pdm09 vaccine: two open-label, randomized trials. Pediatr Infect Dis J. 2015;34:774–82.
12. Orr MT, Fox CB, Baldwin SL, Sivananthan SJ, Lucas E, Lin S, Phan T, Moon JJ, Vedvick TS, Reed SG, Coler RN. Adjuvant formulation structure and composition are critical for the development of an effective vaccine against tuberculosis. J Control Release. 2013;172:190–200.
13. Lawrence MJ, Rees GD. Microemulsion-based media as novel drug delivery systems. Adv Drug Deliv Rev. 2000;45:89–121.
14. Stills HF Jr. Adjuvants and antibody production: dispelling the myths associated with freund's complete and other adjuvants. ILAR J. 2005;46:280–93.
15. Li X, Sloat BR, Yanasarn N, Cui Z. Relationship between the size of nanoparticles and their adjuvant activity: data from a study with an improved experimental design. Eur J Pharm Biopharm. 2011;78:107–16.
16. Foged C, Brodin B, Frokjaer S, Sundblad A. Particle size and surface charge affect particle uptake by human dendritic cells in an in vitro model. Int J Pharm. 2005;298:315–22.
17. Kanchan V, Panda AK. Interactions of antigen-loaded polylactide particles with macrophages and their correlation with the immune response. Biomaterials. 2007;28:5344–57.
18. O'Hagan DT, Ott GS, De Gregorio E, Seubert A. The mechanism of action of MF59-an innately attractive adjuvant formulation. Vaccine. 2012;30:4341–8.
19. Cox F, Baart M, Huizingh J, Tolboom J, Dekking L, Goudsmit J, Saeland E, Radošević K. Protection against H5N1 influenza virus induced by matrix-M adjuvanted seasonal virosomal vaccine in mice requires both antibodies and T cells. PLoS One. 2015; 10(12):e0145243. https://doi.org/10.1371/journal.pone.0145243.
20. Kulkarni RR, Rasheed MA, Bhaumik SK, Ranjan P, Cao W, Davis C, Marisetti K, Thomas S, Gangappa S, Sambhara S, Murali-Krishna K. Activation of the RIG-I pathway during influenza vaccination enhances the germinal center reaction, promotes T follicular helper cell induction, and provides a dose-sparing effect and protective immunity. J Virol. 2014;88:13990–4001.
21. Chua BY, Wong CY, Mifsud EJ, Edenborough KM, Sekiya T, Tan AC, Mercuri F, Rockman S, Chen W, Turner SJ, Doherty PC, Kelso A, Brown LE, Jackson DC. Inactivated influenza vaccine that provides rapid, innate-immune-system-mediated protection and subsequent long-term adaptive immunity. MBio. 2015;6(6):e01024–15.
22. Cox RJ, Brokstad KA, Ogra P. Influenza virus: immunity and vaccination strategies. Comparison of the immune response to inactivated and live, attenuated influenza vaccines. Scand J Immunol. 2004;59:1–15.
23. Thomas PG, Keating R, Hulse-Post DJ, Doherty PC. Cell-mediated protection in influenza infection. Emerg Infect Dis. 2006;12:48–54.
24. Hovden AO, Cox RJ, Haaheim LR. Whole influenza virus vaccine is more immunogenic than split influenza virus vaccine and induces primarily an IgG2a response in BALB/c mice. Scand J Immunol. 2005;62(1):36–44.
25. Moran TM, Park H, Fernandez-Sesma A, Schulman JL. Th2 responses to inactivated influenza virus can be converted to Th1 responses and facilitate recovery from heterosubtypic virus infection. J Infect Dis. 1999;180(3):579–85.
26. Ott G, Barchfeld GL, Chernoff D, Radhakrishnan R, van Hoogevest P, Van Nest G. MF59. Design and evaluation of a safe and potent adjuvant for human vaccines. Pharm Biotechnol. 1995;6:277–96.
27. Calabro S, Tritto E, Pezzotti A, Taccone M, Muzzi A, Bertholet S, De Gregorio E, O'Hagan DT, Baudner B, Seubert A. The adjuvant effect of MF59 is due to the oil-in-water emulsion formulation, none of the individual components induce a comparable adjuvant effect. Vaccine. 2013;31:3363–9.
28. Mair KH, Koinig H, Gerner W, Höhne A, Bretthauer J, Kroll JJ, Roof MB, Saalmüller A, Stadler K, Libanova R. Carbopol improves the early cellular immune responses induced by the modified-life vaccine Ingelvac PRRS® MLV. Vet Microbiol. 2015;176:352–7.
29. Holmes MA, Townsend HG, Kohler AK, Hussey S, Breathnach C, Barnett C, Holland R, Lunn DP. Immune responses to commercial equine vaccines against equine herpesvirus-1, equine influenza virus, eastern equine encephalomyelitis, and tetanus. Vet Immunol Immunopathol. 2006;111:67–80.
30. Hjorth RN, Bonde GM, Piner ED, Goldberg KM, Levner MH. The effect of Syntex adjuvant formulation (SAF-m) on humoral immunity to the influenza virus in the mouse. Vaccine. 1997;15:541–6.
31. Hunter RL. Overview of vaccine adjuvants: present and future. Vaccine. 2002;20:S7–12.
32. Silva AL, Marcelino HR, Verissimo LM, Araujo IB, Agnez-Lima LF, do Egito ES. Stearylamine-containing cationic nanoemulsion as a promising carrier for gene delivery. J Nanosci Nanotechnol. 2016;16:1339–45.
33. Kulkarni CV, Moinuddin Z, Agarwal Y. Effect of fullerene on the dispersibility of nanostructured lipid particles and encapsulation in sterically stabilized emulsions. J Colloid Interface Sci. 2016;480:69–75.

34. Kim YH, Koczo K, Wasan DT. Dynamic film and interfacial tensions in emulsion and foam systems. J Colloid Interface Sci. 1997;187:29–44.
35. Yue H, Ma G. Polymeric micro/nanoparticles: particle design and potential vaccine delivery applications. Vaccine. 2015;33:5927–36.
36. O'Hagan DT, Ott GS, Nest GV, Rappuoli R, Giudice GD. The history of MF59(®) adjuvant: a phoenix that arose from the ashes. Expert Rev Vaccines. 2013;12:13–30.
37. Fox CB, Baldwin SL, Duthie MS, Reed SG, Vedvick TS. Immunomodulatory and physical effects of oil composition in vaccine adjuvant emulsions. Vaccine. 2011;29:9563–72.
38. Qi X, Jiao Y, Pan H, Cui L, Fan W, Huang B, Shi Z, Wang H. Genetic analysis and rescue of a triple-reassortant H3N2 influenza a virus isolated from swine in eastern China. Virol Sin. 2009;24:52–8.
39. Cai W, Deng W, Yang H, Chen X, Jin F. A propofol microemulsion with low free propofol in the aqueous phase: formulation, physicochemical characterization, stability and pharmacokinetics. Int J Pharm. 2012;436:536–44.
40. Tang Y, Lu J, Wu P, Liu Z, Tian Z, Zha G, Chen H, Wang Q, Wang Q, Hou F, Kang SM, Hou J. Inactivated vaccine with adjuvants consisting of pattern recognition receptor agonists confers protection against avian influenza viruses in chickens. Vet Microbiol. 2014;172:120–8.
41. Miao J, Zhang J, Zheng L, Yu X, Zhu W, Zou S. Taurine attenuates Streptococcus uberis-induced mastitis in rats by increasing T regulatory cells. Amino Acids. 2012;42:2417–28.
42. Mantile F, Trovato M, Santoni A, Barba P, Ottonello S, De Berardinis P, Prisco A. Alum and squalene-oil-in-water emulsion enhance the titer and avidity of anti-Aβ antibodies induced by multimeric protein antigen (1-11) E2, preserving the Igg1-skewed isotype distribution. PLoS One. 2014;9(7): e101474. https://doi.org/10.1371/journal.pone.0101474.

19

African swine fever virus does not express viral microRNAs in experimentally infected pigs

Fernando Núñez-Hernández[1], Gonzalo Vera[2], Armand Sánchez[2,3], Fernando Rodríguez[1] and José I. Núñez[1*]

Abstract

Background: African swine fever virus (ASFV) is the etiological agent of African swine fever (ASF), a re-expanding devastating and highly lethal hemorrhagic viral disease. microRNAs (miRNAs) are a new class of small non-coding RNAs that regulate gene expression post-transcriptionally. The discovery of virus specific miRNAs has increased both in number and importance in the past few years. We have recently described the differential expression of several porcine miRNAs during in vivo infection with attenuated and virulent ASFV strains. Here, we have extended these studies trying to identify the presence of viral miRNAs encoded by ASFV in an in vivo infection in pigs.

Results: Sixteen small RNA libraries were analyzed from spleen and submandibular lymph nodes obtained from eight pigs, seven infected with either the virulent E75 ASFV strain or its attenuated counterpart E75CV1, or from pigs surviving E75CV1-infection and challenged with BA71 (heterologous challenge) and one non infected as negative control. Samples were recovered at different times post-infection. Libraries were analyzed by next-generation sequencing. Some viral miRNA candidates were initially identified, which did not correspond to porcine miRNAs. Further structural analyses were carried out in order to confirm if they met the conformational requirements to be considered a viral miRNA.

Conclusions: The analysis of sixteen small RNA libraries prepared from two different tissues obtained from pigs experimentally infected with E75, E75CV1 or with E75CV1 plus BA71, revealed the presence of six potential miRNA sequences but none of them met the requirements to be considered as viral miRNAs. Thus, we can conclude that ASFV does not express miRNAs in vivo, at least under the experimental conditions described here.

Keywords: African swine fever virus, microRNA, Viral miRNA

Background

African swine fever (ASF) is a contagious disease that affects domestic and wild pigs caused by ASF virus (ASFV) belonging to the *Asfarviridae* family, genus *Asfivirus*. ASFV is a large icosahedral, enveloped, double stranded (ds) DNA virus ranging from 170 to 193 kb [1]. ASFV is today considered one of the main biological threats for pigs world-wide, causing enormous economical loss in affected countries. Endemic since its origin in several areas of sub-Saharan Africa, ASFV re-entered the European continent in 2007, expanding to surrounding areas and reaching the European Union (EU) borders in 2014. Since then, the virus reached some Eastern European Union countries and in 2017, ASFV was reported in Czech Republic and Romania [2]. Lack of vaccines or treatments complicates its control [3], therefore gaining knowledge about ASFV pathogenesis is valuable for the future development of anti-ASFV strategies. The viral particle, with a diameter of 200 nm, has three concentric wraps with an additional external membrane obtained when coming out by budding from the infected cell. Between 150 and 175 ORFs have been identified but the functions for half of them still remain unknown. Sixteen different genomes have been identified and fully sequenced from pigs, wild boars and ticks and 23 genotypes have been so far described [4]. The virus infects monocytes and macrophages, key cell players for the immune

* Correspondence: joseignacio.nunez@irta.cat
[1]Institut de Recerca i Tecnologia Agroalimentàries (IRTA)-Centre de Recerca en Sanitat Animal (CReSA), Campus de la Universitat Autònoma de Barcelona, Bellaterra, Barcelona, Spain
Full list of author information is available at the end of the article

system. In addition, it has been observed that virus replicates in endothelial cells, hepatocytes, renal tubular epithelial cells and neutrophils, mainly at late stages of an acute ASFV-infection. miRNAs are a new class of small non-coding RNAs with posttranscriptional regulation functions of gene expression. miRNAs play an increasing role in many biological processes [5]. The study of miRNA-mediated host-pathogen interactions has emerged in the last decade mainly due to the important role that miRNAs play in antiviral defense [6]. In addition, miRNAs encoded by viruses have been identified to be involved in the infection process. To date, the microRNA database, miRBase [7], shows 308 precursors and 502 mature viral miRNAs have been identified. Viruses encoding miRNAs has been identified in several families, as *Herpesviridae, Polyomaviridae, Adenoviridae, Papillomaviridae, Baculoviridae, Ascoviridae* and *Iridoviridae* [8–10]. All of them are DNA viruses, with an essential nuclear phase in their replication cycle, necessary for canonical miRNA biogenesis. In addition, *Ascovirus* and *Iridovirus*, together with *Asfivirus*, belong to the monophyletic superfamily of nucleocytoplasmic large DNA viruses (NCLDV). Thus, ASFV was a good candidate for a virus capable of encoding miRNAs. On the other hand, recently, our group has identified differential expression of porcine miRNAs in pigs after the infection with ASFV [11].

Considering this background, the aim of the present study was to explore if ASFV can encode viral miRNAs in an experimental infection in its natural host by using high-throughput sequencing. To this end, in order to characterize the potential presence of ASFV-specific miRNAs, in silico prediction was carried out to determine if the ASFV genomes of two different ASFV strains with different degrees of virulence, encode possible miRNA precursors. Subsequently, to explore whether the possible miRNAs candidates are present in the ASFV, small RNA libraries from target tissues were constructed and analyzed.

Methods

In silico prediction

The Vmir prediction algorithm [12] was used to predict the presence of hairpin structures in the ASFV genomes from: strain E75 (Genbank accession number FN557520) [1] and BA71 (Genbank accession number KP055815) [13]. The sequence of the non-pathogenic BA71V (Genbank accession number NC_001659) [14], highly adapted to Vero cells, was additionally included in the study. Computational prediction was conducted by using Vmir of viral miRNAs, setting as conditions a hairpin size from 50 to 100 nt and a window count of 15.

Samples analyzed

In order to explore whether these candidates were present in the ASFV genome, samples from spleen and submandibular lymph node (SLN) from seven 8-week-old Landrace X Large White male pigs were used. The animals were acquired from Hypor (A Coruña, Spain), and were fed ad libitum with conventional compound feed for growing pigs. The animals were intramuscularly inoculated in the neck with the virulent ASFV strains: BA71 or E75 or with the attenuated E75CV1, obtained by adaptation of E75 after three passages in Vero cell lineage. The same dose, 10^4 hemadsorbing units (HAU_{50}), was used for each virus. One non-infected pig was included as negative control. All samples used are summarized in Table 1, noticing that some of the samples were previously used to successfully identify the expression of cellular miRNAs during the ASFV infection in vivo [11]. The potential presence of viral miRNAs in ASFV-infected pigs was analyzed by high-throughput sequencing of small RNA libraries prepared from two tissues recovered in three conditions: i) The animals infected with virulent strain E75 necropsied at 3 and 7 dpi, ii) The animals infected with the attenuated strain E75CV1 and necropsied at 3 and 31 dpi, iii) The animals infected with the attenuated strain E75CV1 and re-inoculated at 31 dpi with the virulent strain BA71 and necropsied at 38 dpi. As negative control, small RNA libraries were sequenced from a non-infected animal at 0 dpi.

The time points chosen for each experimental infection were selected taking into account previous results [15] and covering acute and chronic phases of infection with different ASFV strains. Euthanasia was performed

Table 1 Summary of the animals, samples and viral strains used in this study

Animal number	Tissue	ASFV strain/inoculation			Necropsy (dpi)
		E75	E75CV1	BA71[a]	
1	Spleen	+			3
	SLN	+			3
2	Spleen	+			7
	SLN	+			7
3	Spleen		+		3
	SLN		+		3
4	Spleen		+		3
	SLN		+		3
5	Spleen		+		31
	SLN		+		31
6	Spleen		+	+	38
	SLN		+	+	38
7	Spleen		+	+	38
	SLN		+	+	38
8	Spleen				0
	SLN				0

[a]Re-inoculated animals with 10^4 HAU of the BA71 strain at day 31

according to European Directive 2010/63/EU, using a pentobarbital overdose of 60–100 mg/kg administered via the anterior vena cava.

All animal experiments were carried out in the BSL3 facilities at CReSA, and all animal managements were performed in accordance with the guidelines of the Good Experimental Practices. All procedures were approved by the Ethical and Animal Welfare Committee of the Universitat Autònoma de Barcelona with the permit number DMAH-5796.

Real-time PCR

SYBR Green quantitative PCR (qPCR) was used with the following oligonucleotides: pF1 primer (5′ CCTCGGCGA GCGCTTTATCAC 3′) and pR2 (5′ GGAAACTCA TTCACCAAATCCTT 3′), designed in a highly conserved region within the p72 ORF [16]. qPCR mix contained 480 nM each primer, 12.5 μl of Power SYBR®Green PCR Master Mix (Thermo Fisher Scientific) and 2.5 μl of template. Nanopure autoclaved water was added to final volume of 25 μL. Amplification were carried out with these conditions: 10 min at 95 °C, 2 min at 50 °C and 40 cycles of 15 s at 95 °C and 1 min at 60 °C. Triplicates of each sample were used for the qPCR.

Small RNA library construction

Total RNA extractions were carried out in order to construct small RNA libraries from spleen and SLN samples from the animals infected with E75CV1 necropsied at 31 dpi, the E75CV1-infected animals and re-inoculated at 31 dpi with BA71, necropsied at 38 dpi, and from one non-infected animal as described in [17] with some modifications. A total of 8 small RNA libraries were constructed in a two-step ligation procedure with the 3′ and 5′ adaptors from IDT technologies. Briefly, reverse transcription (RT) was carried out with primer mir5 and PCR amplification with primers A5 and B3 (which included multiplex identifiers at the 5′ end) containing sequences complementary to the 3′ and 5′ adaptors used for miRNA library construction. Ion Torrent adapters were ligated to PCR products and libraries were then amplified with Ion Torrent primers. Libraries were sequenced following the manufacturer's protocol with Ion PGM™ sequencer (Thermo Fisher Scientific, Massachusetts, USA) at DNA sequencing facilities at CRAG (Centre de Recerca en Agrigenòmica, Universitat Autònoma de Barcelona, Spain). On the other hand, cellular miRNAs expression has been previously detected using some of these libraries thus ensuring that they are valid for the present study.

Sequence processing scheme and analysis

Strict quality parameters of the individual nucleotide sequence reads has been applied and only those with the Phread base quality scores of Q > 30 in all its bases have been used. Primer sequences were removed and only those insert sequences between 15 and 29 nucleotides were used for further analysis. Sequences aligned with *Sus scrofa* genome were analyzed in [11] since they are porcine miRNAs. Local Blast against ASFV genomes was carried out and Mfold [18] was used in order to evaluate the secondary structure and free energy for the potential miRNA candidates. Likewise, candidates were blasted to the output of Vmir hairpin ASFV structures. In addition, candidates were checked with the algorithm developed in miREval 2.0 for detecting novel miRNAs [19].

Results

The in silico prediction allowed the identification of 415 miRNA candidates in the E75 strain with a score higher than 100 (Fig. 1), in the case of BA71, 391 candidates with a score higher than 100 were identified (Fig. 2) and in the case of BA71V, 366 candidates were identified in the same conditions (data not shown).

In the animal infection, the pigs inoculated with the virulent strains E75 and BA71 developed typical clinical signs, while the pigs inoculated with the attenuated E75CV1 strain developed mild or no clinical signs [15]. Quantitative PCR was performed from the samples of spleen and SLN from all the animals. Those animals inoculated with E75 showed low Ct values at 7 dpi coinciding with the peak of virus replication and ASF clinical signs, while in contrast, inoculation of the same dose of the homologous attenuated E75CV1 strain showed no amplification. The animals infected with E75CV1 and re-inoculated with the BA71 virulent strain showed amplification levels similar to those found after E75 infection, correlating with the lack of cross-protection observed for these two strains [15]. As expected, the negative control animal did not show any specific PCR amplification (Table 2).

Total RNAs from SLN and spleen were used to construct small RNA libraries from the selected animals. High-throughput sequencing provided 272,967 reads from the eight new libraries that, in addition to eight previously sequenced libraries with 301,802 reads, provided a total of 574,769 reads from the sixteen libraries (Table 3). New sequencing data were submitted to ENA database [20] with the accession numbers ERX1811688–95. When trimmed to filter sequences ranging from 15 to 29 nucleotides, a total of 169,511 reads were obtained. After the identification of host miRNAs by comparing with miRBase [7], sequences were blasted to ASFV. Reads were blasted to the E75 and BA71 isolates considering only sequences with 100% of alignment and identity rendering 9 hits with the ASFV genome (Table 3). An increased number of mismatches in the extremes

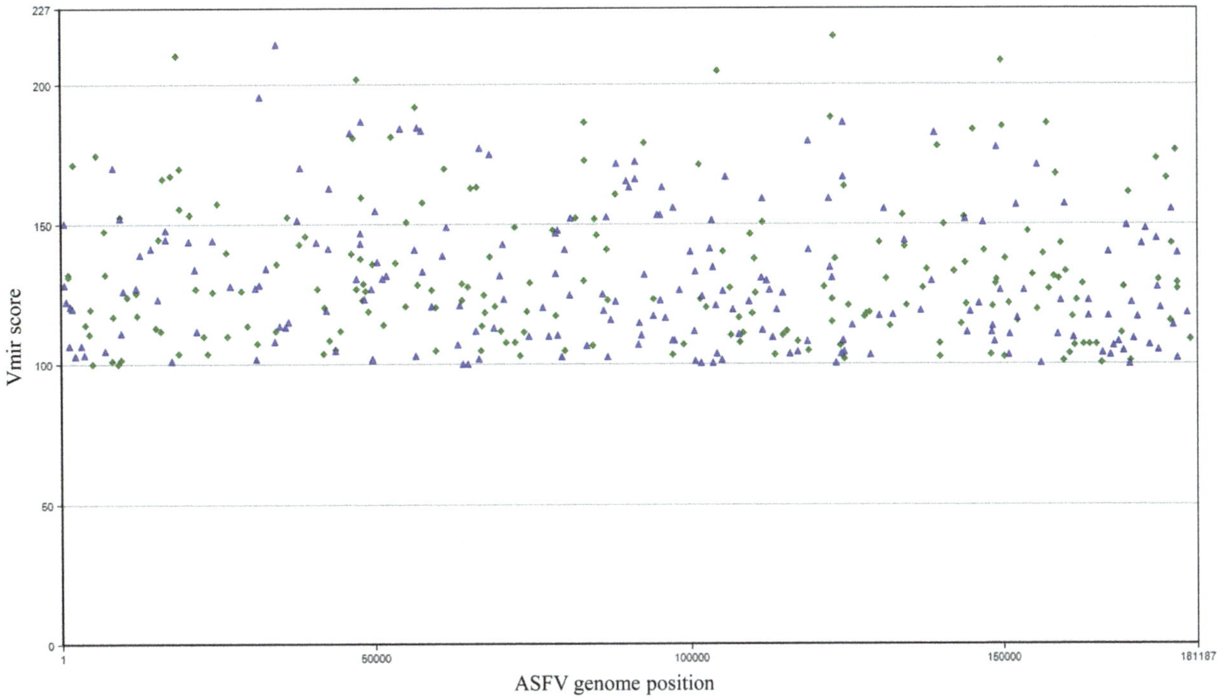

Fig. 1 Hairpin structures predicted for ASFV genome of E75 isolate (Genbank accession number FN557520). Predictions have been done by using Vmir with score higher than 100, hairpin size from 50 to 100 and window count of 15. Green diamonds and blue triangles indicate stem-loop structures in direct or reverse orientation, respectively

due to miRNA variability (isomiRs) [21] were allowed. The search rendered 31 hits. This processing allowed the identification of 40 viral genome hits with 8 unique sequences when allowing 100% homology (Tables 3 and 4) and 23 unique sequences when allowing < 100% homology (Tables 3 and 5). From these sequences, 25 candidates were obtained when grouped by isomiRs and 6 candidates when copy number (CN) was ≥2.

Sequences were blasted to the output of Vmir hairpins from E75, BA71 and BA71V. In addition, candidates were evaluated with miREval 2.0 software with no positive results. Therefore, after the analysis of the complementarity of the candidates with the Vmir prediction and the checking with miREval, together with the analysis with Mfold of their secondary structure and the free minimum energy of their folding, none of the candidates

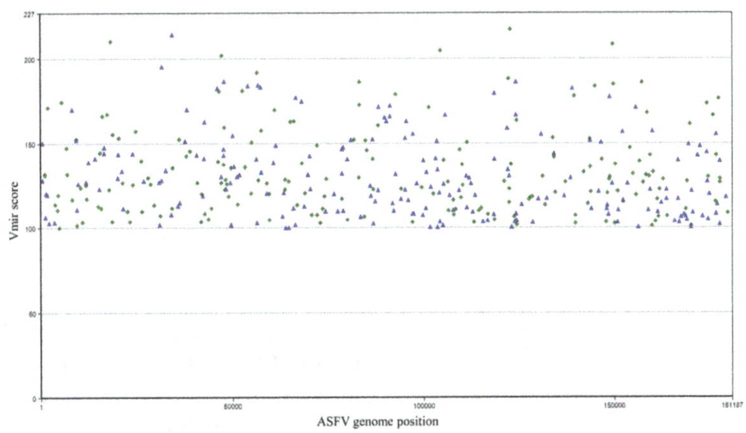

Fig. 2 Hairpin structures predicted for ASFV genome of BA71 isolate (Genbank accession number KP055815). Predictions have been done by using Vmir with score higher than 100, hairpin size from 50 to 100 and window count of 15. Green diamonds and blue triangles indicate stem-loop structures in direct or reverse orientation, respectively

Table 2 qPCR from spleen and SLN of the eight animals in the in vivo infection

Tissue	Animal number							
	1	2	3	4	5	6	7	8
Spleen	31.99	27.81	–	–	–	24.84	27.3	–
SLN	27.71	24.6	–	–	–	25.17	28.11	–

Ct values from animals inoculated with the E75 virulent strain at 3 and 7 dpi (animals 1 and 2); animals inoculated with the E75CV1 attenuated strain and necropsied at 7 and 31 dpi (animals 3, 4 and 5); animals re-inoculated at 31 dpi and necropsied at 38 dpi (animals 6 and 7) and negative control animal sacrificed at 0 dpi (animal 8)

could be considered as a viral miRNA as they failed to fulfill the necessary requirements.

Discussion

In a previous study carried out by our group, it was described that there is in vivo upregulation and downregulation of several porcine miRNAs after infection with ASFV [11]. Using the small RNA libraries obtained for this purpose plus new small RNA libraries constructed in this work, we have studied the capability of E75, BA71 and E75CV1 isolates of ASFV to express viral miRNAs in vivo by using high-throughput sequencing.

The genomic characteristics of ASFV fit with the requirements of a virus to be able to encode viral miRNAs because it is a DNA virus with a nuclear phase [22, 23] and the in silico prediction carried out in this work found several potential hairpins to be virus- encoded miRNAs. In addition, 16 viral miRNAs have been identified in Singapore grouper iridovirus (SGIV) [24] and in tiger frog virus (TFV) [25] both members of the *Iridoviridae* family. Likewise, virus encoded miRNAs have been identified in ascovirus which infects mosquitoes [26]. In this last case, a viral miRNA reduces DNA polymerase I levels by transcriptional degradation and modulates the ascovirus replication. All these viruses belong, as the asfivirus, to the monophyletic superfamily of nucleocytoplasmic large DNA viruses (NCLDV), reinforcing that

Table 3 Summary of the high-throughput reads, blast and candidates for viral miRNAs discovery

Total reads	574,769
Trimmed not- empty reads (15–29 nt)	169,511
Blast ASFV 100%	9
Unique sequences 100%	8
Blast ASFV < 100%	31
Unique sequences < 100%	23
Total unique sequences	31
Viral miRNA candidates[a]	25
Viral miRNA candidates CN ≥ 2	6
Candidate + Mfold structure/ ASFV miRNAs	–

[a] Viral candidates copy number (CN) after sequence association by isomiRs

ASFV is a good candidate to explore virus encoded miRNAs.

There is no clear knowledge about when viral miRNAs are expressed at highest levels after infection according to Cullen [27], who showed the variability of the viral miRNAs expression with time among different viruses. Therefore, we have analyzed samples from the infected animals at different times points post-infection in addition to different viruses with different virulence and the animals infected with an attenuated strain and re-inoculated with a heterologous virulent strain in order to increase the spectrum of conditions. Besides, although E75 and BA71 are classified in the West African-European cluster, the percentage of identity at genome level is 88.5%, the lower identity among viruses included in this cluster [1]. ASFV produces lytic infection. Nevertheless, although most virus-encoded miRNAs have been related to persistent infections, viral miRNAs have also been detected during lytic infection [9, 17].

After the identification of porcine miRNAs expressed in ASFV-infected animals [11], high-throughput sequencing revealed other potential miRNAs sharing identity with the viral genome. Out of a total of 40, six with a copy number ≥ 2 were selected for further analysis. These candidates were blasted against the Vmir hairpins prediction from E75 and BA71 genomes. Also, BA71V, a highly adapted strain in Vero cells, was included in the analysis in order to avoid the loss of candidates because of the possibility of genome variability in cell culture passages [13]. However, it was observed that none of the candidates matched any of the predicted hairpins, had appropriate secondary structure, or minimum free energy, showing that the candidates did not have the necessary characteristics to be identified as viral miRNAs. The candidate ASFV-C9, which presents the higher CN (9), mapped into the early structural protein p22 [28]. p22 is a target gene of miR-30e-5p, a differentially expressed (DE) miRNA described in our previous work [11]. This would explain why a higher number of sequences have been found. On the other hand, all isomiRs were blasted to miRBase, and none of them were identified as host miRNA. Therefore, ASFV-C9 with all other sequences can be considered as degradation products of viral RNA. Being aware of the reduced number of animals used, different tissues were used to generate a total of 14 RNA libraries, number that exceeds the majority of similar studies so far published, normally ranging from 1 to 4 and carried out in cell culture, and not in the natural host [29–32].

Although DNA viruses have the potential to encode viral miRNAs, this characteristic does not imply the viral miRNAs expression of these viruses. For example, the herpesvirus family have the highest viral miRNAs encoding rates, and almost each member is capable to codify miRNAs. However, there are members of this family as the varicella zoster virus (VZV) and other human neurotropic

Table 4 Candidates obtained with a 100% of identity with the ASFV genome and their copy number (CN)

Candidate ID	Candidate sequences blast vs ASFV = 100%	Candidates CN
ASFV-C1	GAGACCAAGAACCTGGGCA	2
ASFV-C2	ATGTGCCCTGGTCCCGTAGGAGTG	1
ASFV-C3	CGTCTGGGAGAAATGGAGCA	1
ASFV-C4	CACCGTGTGGATGCCCAGGG	1
ASFV-C5	GAGCTCGTGACCATTGAA	1
ASFV-C6	GGTTCACTGGTGTCCATGAT	1
ASFV-C7	ATGATCGTAGCATTTGGTGTA	1
ASFV-C8	GGCGAGTCACTTGGTTTGCT	1

herpesviruses (HSV1 and HSV2) [33], which do not encode viral miRNAs. The knowledge of why some viruses encode miRNAs and why some phylogenetically related viruses do not, can be of great relevance for the fields of virology and RNAi [10].

In this study, we have found that ASFV, under these experimental conditions, does not express viral miRNAs like other viruses such as Cowpox virus or Porcine circovirus type 2 (PCV2) [34, 35]. Interestingly, in a recent and exhaustive work carried out by Jaing et al. about gene expression in blood of ASFV-infected pigs, wherein some DE host miRNA have been identified, viral miRNAs are not described [36]. In the literature, there are examples in which were indicated that certain viruses encode miRNAs that were initially considered as non coding miRNAs, e.g. human papillomavirus [37]. Therefore, studies with higher number of reads, together with analysis of the presence of viral miRNAs in cell culture and other in vivo conditions should be considered before fully discounting if ASFV expresses miRNAs.

Table 5 Candidates obtained with less than 100% of identity with the ASFV genome and their copy number (CN) grouped by isomiRs

Candidate ID	Candidate sequences blast vs ASFV < 100%	IsomiRs CN	Candidates CN
ASFV-C9	TCTCCCAACCTGTACAGT	4	9
	TCTCCCAACCTGTACAGGT	1	
	CTCCCAACCTGTACAGT	3	
	TCGTCCCAACCTGTACAGT	1	
ASFV-C10	TGAGGTAGTAGGTTGTGT	2	4
	TGAGGTAGTAGGTTGTGTG	2	
ASFV-C11	CGCTGCGGGTGTGGTGGGCC	1	2
	CGCTGCGGGTGTGGTGG	1	
ASFV-C12	TGTGCAAATCTATGCAAAAC	2	2
ASFV-C13	GGTAGTAGGTTGTGTGGTT	1	2
	GGTAGTAGGTTGTGTGGAT	1	
ASFV-C14	AGGGCACCAAGGTAAC	1	1
ASFV-C15	ACGCCCTGGGGCCTATGAG	1	1
ASFV-C16	TCGCTGCGGGTGTGGTGGG	1	1
ASFV-C17	CCGCTGCGGGATGAAC	1	1
ASFV-C18	GGGAAAATCCACGGCCCTGC	1	1
ASFV-C19	TGTATGGAGGCCCTTTTT	1	1
ASFV-C20	CTCCTGGGGCCGCACTCTC	1	1
ASFV-C21	TTCACTGCCCTGATCCTCT	1	1
ASFV-C22	GCGACCCGTCAAGTCCAACAG	1	1
ASFV-C23	GTCGGAGCCTGAGCCGGGAG	1	1
ASFV-C24	CCCCCACACAGTTTGAC	1	1
ASFV-C25	TCTCCCAATCCTTGCCAGT	1	1

Conclusions

In the present work, we can conclude that African swine fever virus does not express viral miRNAs in the in vivo conditions studied here. This finding is contrary to what happens with other large DNA viruses and can be relevant to the biology of this important pathogen.

Abbreviations

ASF: African swine fever; *ASFV*: African swine fever virus; *CN*: Copy number; *DE*: Differentially expressed; *DPI*: Days post-infection; *ENA*: European nucleotide database; *HTS*: High-throughput sequencing; *NCLDV*: Nucleocytoplasmic large DNA virus; *OIE*: World Organization for Animal Health; *SLN*: Submandibular lymph node

Acknowledgements

Authors thank all the personnel from the animal facilities at CReSA. IRTA is supported by CERCA Programme / Generalitat de Catalunya.

Funding

This work was supported by the projects AGL2010–22358-C02 and AGL2013–48998-C2–1-R from MINECO (Spanish government). FN-H is the recipient of a PhD fellowship FI-DGR (AGAUR) from Generalitat de Catalunya.

Authors' contributions

JIN, AS and FR conceived, designed and coordinated this study. FN-H and JIN performed the experiments and analyzed the data. GV performed the NGS data analysis. JIN and FN-H wrote the paper with significant contributions from FR. All authors read and approved the final manuscript.

Consent for publication

Not applicable.

Competing interests

The authors declare that they have no competing interests.

Author details

[1]Institut de Recerca i Tecnologia Agroalimentàries (IRTA)-Centre de Recerca en Sanitat Animal (CReSA), Campus de la Universitat Autònoma de Barcelona, Bellaterra, Barcelona, Spain. [2]Centre de Recerca en Agrigenòmica (CRAG), Consorci CSIC-IRTA-UAB-UB, Bellaterra, Barcelona, Spain. [3]Departament de Ciència Animal i dels Aliments, Universitat Autònoma de Barcelona (UAB), Bellaterra, Barcelona, Spain.

References

1. de Villiers EP, Gallardo C, Arias M, da Silva M, Upton C, Martin R, Bishop RP. Phylogenomic analysis of 11 complete African swine fever virus genome sequences. Virology. 2010;400(1):128–36.
2. World Organisation for Animal Health, OIE [http://www.oie.int].
3. Arias M, de la Torre A, Dixon L, Gallardo C, Jori F, Laddomada A, Martins C, Parkhouse RM, Revilla Y, Rodriguez FAJ, et al. Approaches and perspectives for development of African swine fever virus vaccines. Vaccines (Basel). 2017;5(4):e35.
4. Achenbach JE, Gallardo C, Nieto-Pelegrin E, Rivera-Arroyo B, Degefa-Negi T, Arias M, Jenberie S, Mulisa DD, Gizaw D, Gelaye E, et al. Identification of a new genotype of African swine fever virus in domestic pigs from Ethiopia. Transbound Emerg Dis. 2017;64(5):1393–404.
5. Tufekci KU, Meuwissen RL, Genc S. The role of microRNAs in biological processes. Methods Mol Biol. 2014;1107:15–31.
6. Umbach JL, Cullen BR. The role of RNAi and microRNAs in animal virus replication and antiviral immunity. Genes Dev. 2009;23(10):1151–64.
7. Griffiths-Jones S, Grocock RJ, van Dongen S, Bateman A, Enright AJ. miRBase: microRNA sequences, targets and gene nomenclature. Nucleic Acids Res. 2006;34(Database issue):D140–4.
8. Grundhoff A, Sullivan CS, microRNAs V-e. Virology. 2011;411(2):325–43.
9. Sullivan CS, Grundhoff AT, Tevethia S, Pipas JM, Ganem D. SV40-encoded microRNAs regulate viral gene expression and reduce susceptibility to cytotoxic T cells. Nature. 2005;435(7042):682–6.
10. Kincaid RP, Sullivan CS. Virus-encoded microRNAs: an overview and a look to the future. PLoS Pathog. 2012;8(12):e1003018.
11. Nunez-Hernandez F, Perez LJ, Munoz M, Vera G, Accensi F, Sanchez A, Rodriguez F, Nunez JI. Differential expression of porcine microRNAs in African swine fever virus infected pigs: a proof-of-concept study. Virol J. 2017;14(1):198.
12. Grundhoff A. Computational prediction of viral miRNAs. Methods Mol Biol. 2011;721:143–52.
13. Yanez RJ, Rodriguez JM, Nogal ML, Yuste L, Enriquez C, Rodriguez JF, Vinuela E. Analysis of the complete nucleotide sequence of African swine fever virus. Virology. 1995;208(1):249–78.
14. Rodríguez JM, Moreno LT, Alejo A, Lacasta A, Rodríguez F, Salas ML. Genome sequence of African swine fever virus BA71, the virulent parental strain of the nonpathogenic and tissue-culture adapted BA71V. PLoS One. 2015;10(11):e0142889.
15. Lacasta A, Monteagudo PL, Jimenez-Marin A, Accensi F, Ballester M, Argilaguet J, Galindo-Cardiel I, Segales J, Salas ML, Dominguez J, et al. Live attenuated African swine fever viruses as ideal tools to dissect the mechanisms involved in viral pathogenesis and immune protection. Vet Res. 2015;46:135.
16. Zsak L, Borca MV, Risatti GR, Zsak A, French RA, Lu Z, Kutish GF, Neilan JG, Callahan JD, Nelson WM, et al. Preclinical diagnosis of African swine fever in contact-exposed swine by a real-time PCR assay. J Clin Microbiol. 2005;43(1): 112–9.
17. Timoneda O, Nunez-Hernandez F, Balcells I, Munoz M, Castello A, Vera G, Perez LJ, Egea R, Mir G, Cordoba S, et al. The role of viral and host microRNAs in the Aujeszky's disease virus during the infection process. PLoS One. 2014;9(1):e86965.
18. Zuker M. Mfold web server for nucleic acid folding and hybridization prediction. Nucleic Acids Res. 2003;31(13):3406–15.
19. Gao D, Middleton R, Rasko JE, Ritchie W. miREval 2.0: a web tool for simple microRNA prediction in genome sequences. Bioinformatics. 2013;29(24): 3225–6.
20. European Nucleotide Database [http://www.ebi.ac.uk/ena].
21. Neilsen CT, Goodall GJ, Bracken CP. IsomiRs--the overlooked repertoire in the dynamic microRNAome. Trends Genet. 2012;28(11):544–9.
22. Van Etten J. Lesser known large dsDNA viruses. Preface. Curr Top Microbiol Immunol. 2009;328:v–vii.
23. Ballester M, Rodríguez-Cariño C, Pérez M, Gallardo C, Rodríguez JM, Salas ML, Rodriguez F. Disruption of nuclear organization during the initial phase of African swine fever virus infection. J Virol. 2011;85(16):8263–9.
24. Yan Y, Cui H, Jiang S, Huang Y, Huang X, Wei S, Xu W, Qin Q. Identification of a novel marine fish virus, Singapore grouper iridovirus-encoded microRNAs expressed in grouper cells by Solexa sequencing. PLoS One. 2011;6(4):e19148.
25. Yuan J-M, Chen Y-S, He J, Weng S-P, Guo C-J, He J-G. Identification and differential expression analysis of MicroRNAs encoded by Tiger frog virus in cross-species infection in vitro. Virology J. 2016;13:73.
26. Hussain M, Taft RJ, Asgari S. An insect virus-encoded microRNA regulates viral replication. J Virol. 2008;82(18):9164–70.
27. Cullen BR. How do viruses avoid inhibition by endogenous cellular microRNAs? PLoS Pathog. 2013;9(11):e1003694.
28. Camacho A, Vinuela E. Protein p22 of African swine fever virus: an early structural protein that is incorporated into the membrane of infected cells. Virology. 1991;181(1):251–7.
29. Anselmo A, Flori L, Jaffrezic F, Rutigliano T, Cecere M, Cortes-Perez N, Lefevre F, Rogel-Gaillard C, Giuffra E. Co-expression of host and viral microRNAs in porcine dendritic cells infected by the pseudorabies virus. PLoS One. 2011;6(3):e17374.
30. Glazov EA, Horwood PF, Assavalapsakul W, Kongsuwan K, Mitchell RW, Mitter N, Mahony TJ. Characterization of microRNAs encoded by the bovine herpesvirus 1 genome. J Gen Virol. 2010;91(Pt 1):32–41.
31. Burnside J, Bernberg E, Anderson A, Lu C, Meyers BC, Green PJ, Jain N, Isaacs G, Morgan RW. Marek's disease virus encodes MicroRNAs that map to meq and the latency-associated transcript. J Virol. 2006;80(17):8778–86.
32. Levy CS, Hopkins J, Russell GC, Dalziel RG. Novel virus-encoded microRNA molecules expressed by ovine herpesvirus 2-immortalized bovine T-cells. J Gen Virol. 2012;93(Pt 1):150–4.

33. Umbach JL, Nagel MA, Cohrs RJ, Gilden DH, Cullen BR. Analysis of human alphaherpesvirus microRNA expression in latently infected human trigeminal ganglia. J Virol. 2009;83(20):10677–83.
34. Skalsky RL, Cullen BR. Viruses, microRNAs, and host interactions. Annu Rev Microbiol. 2010;64:123–41.
35. Nunez-Hernandez F, Perez LJ, Vera G, Cordoba S, Segales J, Sanchez A, Nunez JI. Evaluation of the capability of the PCV2 genome to encode miRNAs: lack of viral miRNA expression in an experimental infection. Vet Res. 2015;46:48.
36. Jaing C, Rowland RRR, Allen JE, Certoma A, Thissen JB, Bingham J, Rowe B, White JR, Wynne JW, Johnson D, et al. Gene expression analysis of whole blood RNA from pigs infected with low and high pathogenic African swine fever viruses. Sci Rep. 2017;7(1):10115.
37. Qian K, Pietila T, Ronty M, Michon F, Frilander MJ, Ritari J, Tarkkanen J, Paulin L, Auvinen P, Auvinen E. Identification and validation of human papillomavirus encoded microRNAs. PLoS One. 2013;8(7):e70202.

20

Highly sensitive electrochemical biosensor based on redox - active monolayer for detection of anti-hemagglutinin antibodies against swine-origin influenza virus H1N1 in sera of vaccinated mice

Edyta Mikuła[1], Cristiane Erdmann Silva[2], Edyta Kopera[3,4], Konrad Zdanowski[3,5], Jerzy Radecki[1] and Hanna Radecka[1*]

Abstract

Background: In this work, we report an electrochemical biosensor for the detection of anti-hemagglutinin antibodies against the swine virus H1N1 present in mice sera immunized with mixture of His_6-H1 HA in monomeric and oligomeric form. The oriented immobilization of the recombinant His-tagged hemagglutinin (His_6-H1 HA) consists of: (i) formation of a mixed layer of 4-mercaptobutanol (MBT) and the thiol derivative of dipyrromethene (DPM); (ii) complexation of Cu (II) by DPM; (iii) immobilization of His_6-H1 HA via coordination bonds between Cu (II) sites from DPM–Cu (II) complex and imidazole nitrogen atoms of a histidine tag; (iv) filling free spaces with bovine serum albumin. The interactions between recombinant His_6- H1 HA covalently attached to the electrode surface and the anti-hemagglutinin H1 antibodies present in mice sera were explored with Osteryoung square-wave voltammetry.

Results: This analytical device was able to detect the antibodies present in vaccinated mice sera diluted from 1×10^9 to 1×10^8 fold.

Conclusions: The unprecedented sensitivity of described biosensor is much better than widely use ELISA test and other analytical methods for determination of antibodies against the influenza A viruses. It has been proved that redox active DPM-Cu (II) monolayer is a universal platform suitable for stable and oriented immobilization of any His-tagged sensing elements. Thus, this universal layer could be a base of numerous analytical devices suitable for detection of antibodies against different viruses.

Keywords: Detection of antibodies in mice sera, Avian swine virus, Histidine-tagged hemagglutinin monomer, Electrochemical biosensor

Background

Influenza viruses induce annual epidemics and casual pandemics that have claimed the lives of millions. Their very high seasonal variation makes effective vaccination and environment control very challenging [1–5]. The twenty-first century pandemic resulted from an influenza A (H1N1) virus that quickly spread worldwide and was reported in 214 countries in various states, claiming many victims [6–8]. In April 2009, a pandemic H1N1 influenza virus emerged, rapidly spread and resulted in launching the pandemic scheme worldwide [4, 9–11]. The virus was circulating in the pig population prior to its transmission to humans [12, 13]. The recent study showed that dogs may play critical roles in influenza virus transmission to human [3]. These animals living so close to people may generate potential public health risk. H1N1 virus is special for its high transmission speed, although its lethality and virulence are temperate. After the WHO statement of the post-pandemic

* Correspondence: h.radecka@pan.olsztyn.pl
[1]Institute of Animal Reproduction and Food Research of Polish Academy of Sciences, Tuwima 10, 10-748 Olsztyn, Poland
Full list of author information is available at the end of the article

period since August 10, 2010, the influenza A (H1N1) virus continued to circulate as a casual virus [14].

There are many cases to emergence of swine-origin H1N1 viruses that have transmitted to and prevalence among humans, subsequent in outbreaks internationally [15, 16]. However, transmission of the virus from pigs to humans does not always ultimately cause flu, sometimes results only in the creation of antibodies in the blood [17]. Record of these outbreaks and real-time monitoring of the evolution of this virus are important for the infectious disease control programs and for better understanding of the factors that specify viral pathogenicity and transmissibility.

In swine, fatality is usually low (around 1–4%), but the virus can cause weight loss and poor growth, leading to the economic loss [18].

Vaccination helps prevent influenza morbidity and mortality. Effective vaccines induce protective immunity which is correlated with the presence of virus-specific antibodies in serum that are directed against the external coat proteins of the virion, hemagglutinin (HA) and, to a lesser extent, neuraminidase (NA). The level of HA-specific antibodies correlate with the vaccine protective efficacy [19–21].

Several methods for determination of antibodies against influenza virus are routinely used in serological analysis. Among them Hemagglutination Inhibition (HI) assay is the most frequently applied to detect antibodies that inhibit the interaction of influenza HA with receptors on red blood cells or cultured cells. It is an indirect assay in which the highest dilution of serum that prevents hemagglutination is called the HI titer of the serum [19, 20, 22]. Another common serological assay to measure the total serum antibodies against specific influenza antigen is ELISA test [23, 24]. All of these assays although routinely used possess some drawbacks. Their main disadvantages are the need of large sample volume and specialized equipment. In addition, they are not adequate for the construction of simple, disposable pocket like sensors for a wide application range.

Therefore, the development of effective influenza vaccines, as well as methods for viruses and antibodies detection are still challenging tasks for scientists.

The electrochemical biosensors are promising alternative to currently used detection systems. The low sample consumption, high sensitivity, selectivity, compatibility with modern micro-fabrication technologies and good possibility for miniaturization are the main reasons to attract the powerful interests which is confirmed by increasing number of publications [25–27].

The immobilization of either antibody or antigen on the sensor surface is a key step in the fabrication of most immunosensors.

One of the very frequently applied immobilization method is based on non-specific physical adsorption onto gold nano particles as well as carbon nanotubes [28–33]. The application of reaction between amino or carboxylic groups present in the protein structure with complementary reactive groups chemically attached onto solid support using EDC/NHS coupling ensure more stable sensing element immobilization. Unfortunately, the right orientation of sensing element on the sensor surface is not fully guarantee using EDC/NHS approach. This problem could be solved using antibodies F (ab') fragments which could be self-assembled on the nano-gold surfaces through covalent bonds between Au and disulfide or thiol groups from hinge region of immunoglobulin. Such approach guarantee right antibodies orientation [34, 35].

The application of His-tag chemistry for immobilization bioanalytical active molecules on the surface of redox active monolayers deposited on the gold electrodes has solicited vivid interest among scientists. This method allows to keep the stable and oriented immobilization of sensing element onto solid support with maintaining their biological activity [36, 37]. In this type electrochemical biosensors, the procedure for immobilization of the specific recognition elements involved the interaction between transition metal centers forming complexes on the electrode surface and nitrogen atoms from the histidine–tag present. The formation of antigen-antibody complex at the electrode; aqueous sample interface affects the accessibility of ions from supporting electrolyte towards the redox centres embedded into sensing layers. The outcome of this phenomenon are changes of redox centres characteristics, which is the base of electrochemical signal generation [36]. The application of His-tag chemistry allows to keep the stable and oriented immobilization of sensing element onto solid support with maintaining their biological activity [37, 38]. Moreover, using this type of biosensors, the presence of electroactive markers in the sample solution is not required. This is very crucial for analytical procedures involving naturally occurring molecules, whose properties might be influenced by redox markers.

In our previously published paper [36], we have proposed the redox active layer consisted with dipyrromethene (DPM)–Cu (II) complex for stable and oriented immobilization of histidine – tagged fragment of avian influenza H5N1 virus. This sensor was suitable for selective and sensitive detection of antibodies against avian influenza virus type H5N1 present in hen sera.

Thus, we have applied the same approach in the research presented in order to evaluate immunization efficiency of his-tagged recombinant hemagglutinin derived from H1N1 used for mice vaccination. The hemagglutinin (HA) from the H1N1pdm09 influenza virus (His_6-H1 HA) attached to the DPM-Cu (II) redox active layer deposited on gold electrode was applied as a sensing element responsible for detection antibodies present in mice sera vaccinated with mixture of His$_6$-H1 HA in monomeric and oligomeric form.

Results

Characterization of biosensor based on redox active DPM-cu (II) monolayer

The process of the biosensor formation is shown in Fig. 1.

This strategy has been already applied for biosensor assembly destined for detection of antibodies against H5N1 viruses present in vaccinated hen sera [36]. Briefly, in the first step, on the Au electrode surface a mixed DPM and MBT voltammograms of a gold electrode modified by MBT. Then, Cu (II) was complexed by DPM attached to the surface of the electrode. Using such modification conditions, Cu (II) surface coverage in the range $7.35 \pm 0.4 \times 10^{-11}$ mol cm^{-1} was obtained [38].

Next, the recombinant histidine-tagged hemagglutinin, in monomeric form was immobilized by means of coordination bonds between Cu (II) centres and the nitrogen atoms of imidazole present in His$_6$-H1 HA. This methodology allows for secure immobilization of sensing elements with keeping their right position. BSA was used to stop up any remaining free spaces on the gold electrode surface in order to abolish undefined binding.

The immobilization of His$_6$-H1 HA on the surface of a DPM–Cu (II) monolayer was examined by Osteryoung square-wave voltammetry. This technique allows to quantify the difference between the oxidation and reduction peak current in order to remove the capacitive current [39]. The DPM-Cu (II) redox peak current was visible at 267 mV ± 5 mV. The complexation reaction between Cu (II) and His$_6$-H1 HA-monomer generated the drop of Cu (II) redox peaks current about 34 ± 6% (Fig. 2).

The detection of the anti-hemagglutinin antibodies in mice sera using electrodes incorporated with His$_6$-H1 HA-monomer

The presented biosensor was applied for determination anti-hemagglutinin H1 monoclonal antibodies present in mice sera vaccinated with mixture of monomeric and oligomeric form H1 HA. The reproducibility of proposed sensor was estimated based on potential of peak redox Cu (II)/Cu (I) current as well as its intensity measured in buffer free of analyte. These values have been calculated for 60 gold electrodes modified with MBT/DPM-Cu (II)-His$_6$-H1HA. Obtained values 251 mV ± 19 mV and 1.67 ± 0.25 μA proved the good reproducibility of proposed sensor fabrication. A properly constructed biosensors were used once to measure antibodies concentration in the series of diluted mice sera. Next, the electrodes were cleaning, modified and again used for the measurements.

The samples of blood from vaccinated mice were taken after: the first dose 1 × 25 μg of HA, the second dose 2 × 25 μg and the third dose 3 × 25 μg. The samples of blood from non-vaccinated mice, was taken at the same time interval, but the animals received only saline and adjuvant. The His$_6$ -monomeric of H1 HA attached to the electrode surface (Fig. 1) was responsible for the detection of anti-H1 HA antibodies. The

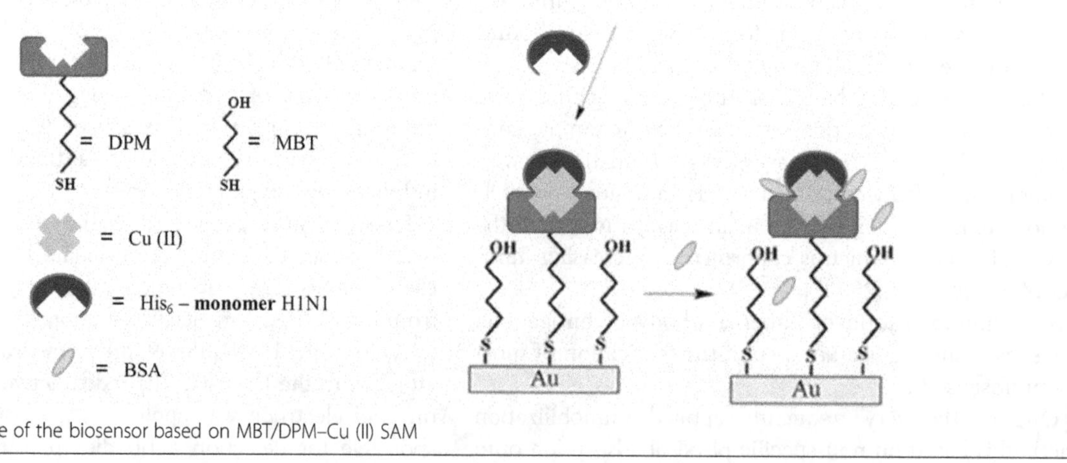

Fig. 1 The scheme of the biosensor based on MBT/DPM–Cu (II) SAM

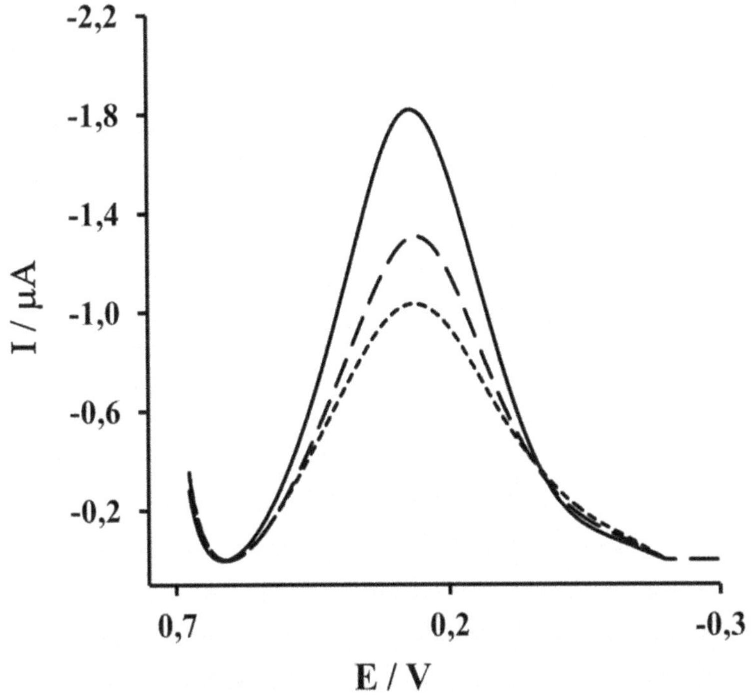

Fig. 2 Square wave voltammograms of a gold electrode modified by MBT/DPM–Cu (II) (solid line), after immobilization of His$_6$-H1 HA monomer (dashed lines); and after filling free spaces with bovine serum albumin (finely dashed lines). Measurement conditions: 0.01 M PBS (pH 7.4), scan rate 100mVs^{-1}

formation of antigen – antibody complex at the electrode surface caused a decrease of the Cu (II)/Cu (I) redox current vs. decrease of vaccinated sera dilution (Figs. 3a and 4a). The immunological response caused by monomeric form of H1 HA was selective. In sera from un-vaccinated mice the specific anti-H1 HA antibodies were not detected (Fig. 3b).

The immune-response towards His$_6$-H1 HA–monomer were dose depended. After first antigen dose, the moderate responses were observed. The calibration slopes obtained for the sera taken from vaccinated and unvaccinated mice were similar (Fig. 4a). The substantial increase of antibodies level in vaccinated mice sera was observed after the third antigen dose. This was confirmed

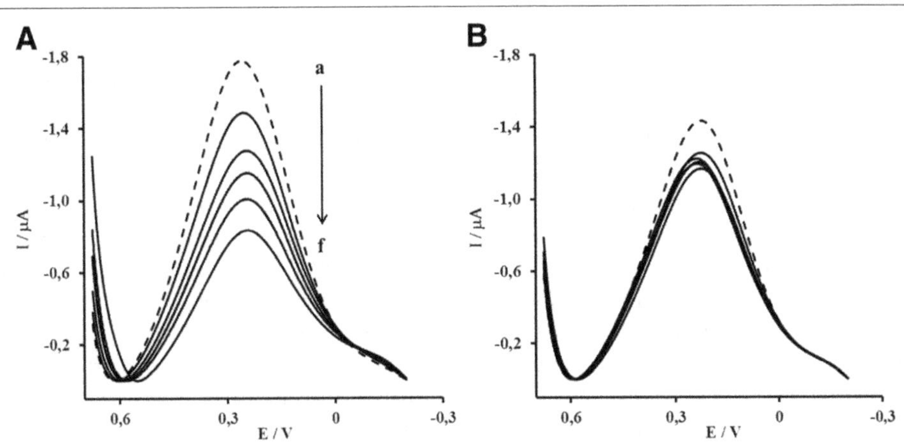

Fig. 3 The representative OSWV responses obtained for electrodes modified with Au-MBT/DPM–Cu (II)–His$_6$–H1 HA monomer in the presence of: **(a)** sera from mice after third dose 3 × 25 µg of H1HA, **(b)** sera from mice after third dose of saline and adjuvant. The sera were diluted with PBS pH 7.4 in the range from (a) 0.000 (only buffer -dashed line, (b) 1 × 10^{10}, (c) 5 × 10^9, (d) 1 × 10^9, (e) 5 × 10^8, (f) 1 × 10^8 Measuring conditions: electrodes modified with: Au-MBT/DPM–Cu (II)–His$_6$–H1 HA monomer, electrolyte: PBS buffer pH = 7.4 (buffer composition: 0.1368 M NaCl, 0.0027 M KCl, 0.0101 M Na_2HPO_4, 0.0018 M KH_2PO_4).

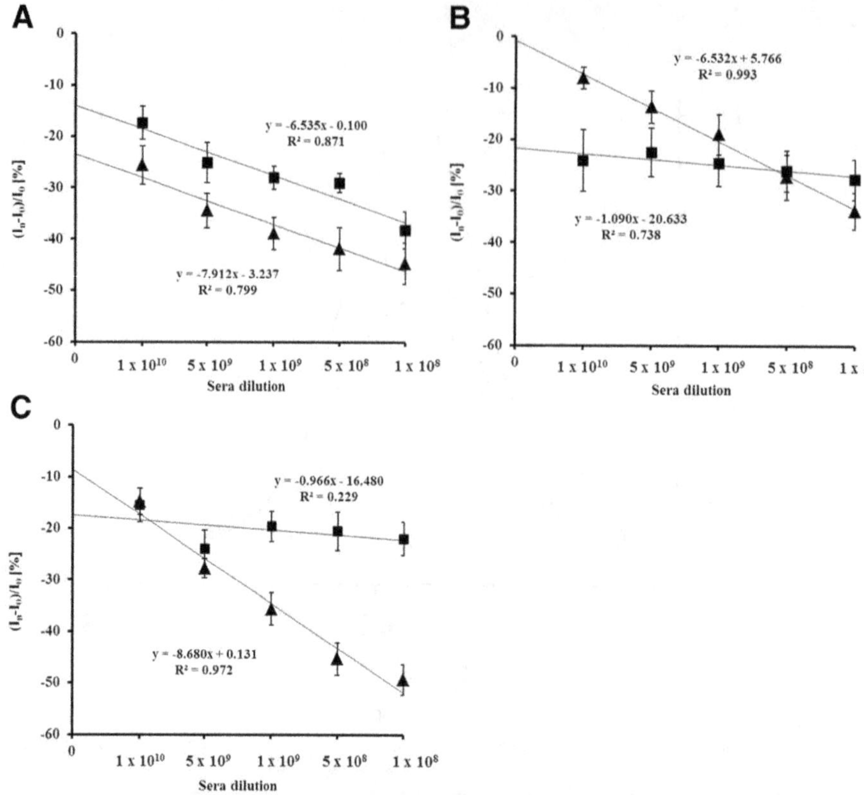

Fig. 4 The relationship of relative Cu (II)/Cu (I) redox current decrease vs. dilution of: (▲) sera from a vaccinated mice; (■) sera from a non-vaccinated mice after: (**a**) the first dose 1 × 25 μg, (**b**) the second dose 2 × 25 μg, (**C**) the third dose 3 × 25 μg of H1 HA or saline and adjuvant mixture. Measuring conditions: see Fig. 3 caption. I_0–Cu (II)/Cu (I) redox current measured in the presence of buffer; I_i– Cu (II)/Cu (I) redox current measured in the presence of a particular sera dilution

by the highest calibration slope of – 8.680 (Fig. 4c). The moderate responses, with slope of – 0.966, recorded in the presence of sera taken from mice treated only with saline and adjuvant confirm the specificity of immunization caused by monomeric form of H1 HA (Fig. 4c).

Discussion

The proposed electrochemical biosensor allows for successful discrimination between sera of un-vaccinated and vaccinated mice against swine virus H1N1. This is evidence that immunosensor performance is not affected by matrix mice sera components, which is very crucial from analytical point of view.

The biosensor was able to detect the antibodies present in vaccinated mice sera diluted from 1×10^9 to 1×10^8 fold. This unprecedented sensitivity is several magnitude (10^7) better than sensitivity widely use ELISA test for the same subtype viruses H1N1. The antibodies against influenza A/H1N1 have been detected in human and swine serum diluted only 1: 200 or 1:2000, respectively [40, 41].

The sera dilution range suitable for biosensor presented is also superior in the comparison to dilution range used for the detection of other types of viruses [36, 42–46] (Table 1).

Why electrochemical immunosenors are superior in the comparison to the other transduces? There are several reasons such as: the direct conversion of binding event between antibody and antigen to an electronic signal, an excellent detection limits, small analyte volumes (in μL level), ability to be used in turbid biofluids, suitability for rapid measurements and easy miniaturization. It should be also underlined that immunosensor proposed is based on only primary antibody. The lack of the necessity of using the secondary antibody makes immunosensor fabrication simpler and cheaper in the comparison of "sandwich type" immunosensor.

Taking into account the above advantages, the electrochemical immunosensor proposed could be used as the alternative tool for widely used ELISA for control of the presence of H1N1 virus.

Conclusions

The biosensor based on DPM-Cu (II) redox active monolayer deposited on gold electrode surface was suitable for oriented and stable immobilization of His_6–

Table 1 Analytical methods used for determination of antibodies against the influenza A viruses

Measurement technique	Sensing element	Analyte	Determination in real samples	References
OSWV	Recombinants hemagglutinin from the avian influenza virus type H5N1	Anti-hemagglutinin H5 monoclonal antibodies	Hen serum diluted $1{:}7\times10^{6}$	[36]
ELISA	HA_{50-274}-H1N1 in E.coli	A/H1N1/2009 antibodies	Human serum diluted 1:200 in PBS	[41]
ELISA	Influenza H1N1 X-53 antigenically identical to A/NewJersey/11/76	Antibodies against influenza A/H1N1	Swine serum diluted 1:2000 in 2% fish gelatin-tween-PBS	[42]
ELISA	Influenza H5N1 A/Chicken/ HongKong/YU22 antigen	Human H5 antibodies	Human serum diluted 1:1280	[43]
EIS	Peptide chains connecting amino acid sequence 98–106 (YPYDVPDYA) of HA	HA-antibody	Not determined	[44]
ELISA	Influenza H5N1 A/Hong Kong/156/97	Antibody to avian influenza A (H5N1)	Human serum diluted 1: 409600	[45]
Western blot assay	Recombinant HA protein from A/Hong Kong/156/97	Antibody to avian influenza A (H5N1)	Human serum diluted 1: 100	[45]
Modified hemagglutination inhibition (HI) test	Horse erythrocytes and hemagglutinating units of virus type H7N7	Antibodies against the avian influenza A (H7N7) virus	Human serum diluted 1: 640	[46]
EIS	Recombinants hemagglutinin from the avian influenza virus type H5N1	Anti-hemagglutinin H5 monoclonal antibodies	Hen serum diluted $1{:}7\times10^{7}$	[47]
OSWV	Recombinant His-tagged HA subtype H1N1- monomer from the H1N1 pdm09 influenza virus	Anti-hemagglutinin antibodies against the swine virus H1N1	Mice sera diluted 1×10^{9}–1×10^{8}	This work

H1 HA-monomer resposible for detection of anti-hemagglutinin antibodies against swine virus present in vacinnted mice sera.

The bisosensor was able to detect the presence of antibodies of sera sample dilluted 10^9 fold. This remarkable sensistivity is a few order of magnitude better than widely used ELISA test. It is worst to underline, that only 10 µl sample volume is necessary to perform of analyse.

It has been proved that redox active DPM-Cu (II) monolayer is a univerasl platform suitable for stable and oriented immobilistion of any His-tagged sensing elements. Thus, this layer could be a base of numerous analytical devices suitable for detection of antibodies against different viruses.

Methods

Materials and chemicals

DPM was synthesized by ProChimia Surfaces Company (Sopot, Poland). 4-Mercapto-1-butanol (MBT), phosphate buffer saline (PBS) components (137 mM NaCl, 2.7 mM KCl, 1.8 mM Na_2HPO_4, 10 mM KH_2PO_4), copper (II) acetate, and chloroform were obtained from Sigma-Aldrich (Poznań, Poland). Alumina 0.3 and 0.05 µm were purchased from Buehler (Lake Bluff, IL, USA). Sulphuric acid, potassium hydroxide, and methanol were supplied by POCh (Gliwice, Poland). Bovine serum albumin (BSA) was purchased from Invitrogen Life Technologies (Darmstadt, Germany).

The recombinant H1 HA antigen (mixture of monomer and oligomer) used in this study was based on the sequence of the H1N1pdm09 (A/H1N1/Gdańsk/036/2009) and produced in *Pichia pastoris*. It contains a His_6-tag at the N terminus. Plasmid pPICZαA (Invitrogen) and plasmid pJET/H1 carrying H1N1 virus hemagglutinin gene (A/H1N1/Gdansk/036/2009, kindly gifted by prof. Bogusław Szewczyk, UG, Poland) have been used for construction of expression vector pPICZαA/H1. *Pichia pastoris* cells of strains KM 71 (his4, aox1:ARG4, arg4) (Invitrogen) were transformed with recombinant plasmids by electroporation. The presence of recombinant protein both in medium and cells (control), was detected by SDS-PAGE and Western blotting. The H1 protein (with His-tag at the N-terminus) was purified was purified by affinity chromatography using Ni-NTA agarose (Qiagen, Germany), and its purity was analysed using 4–12% SDS-PAGE (Bio-Rad, Poland). After dialysis against PBS, pH 7.4, the protein was lyophilized and stored at – 20 °C. Oligomeric status of H1 HA protein was analysed on a Superdex-200 10/300 GL column (GE Healthcare, Poland), pre-equilibrated with 10 mM Tris pH 7.8 with 200 mM NaCl. Molecular weight marker standards (Bio-Rad, Poland) were used for column calibration providing the generation of standard curves to identify the molecular weights of the protein forms present in samples. The protein elution was monitored at 280 nm.

All aqueous solutions were prepared using Milli-Q water, with resistivity 18.2 MΩ·cm (Millipore, Darmstadt, Germany). Reagents and solvents were of analytical grade and used without further purification. Experiments were carried out at room temperature unless stated otherwise.

Immunization procedure

Healthy adult female mice BALB/c (6–7 weeks old) were provided from the Animal House of Mossakowski Medical Center, Polish Academy of Sciences. The mice were housed in the individually ventilated cage (IVC) systems with controlled humidity of 55+/– 2%, a temperature of 22+/– 20C and 12-h light/dark cycle. All mice were allowed free access to food and water. After acclimatization mice were used for generating the experimental procedures. The experimental protocol was approved by the Local Ethics Committee. Procedures were adhered to guidelines published in the European directive 2010/63/UE on the protection of animals used for scientific purposes.

Seven-week old, pathogen-free, female Balb/c mice were used for vaccination. The experimental groups consisted of 10 mice. The control group was administered adjuvant only. The recombinant antigen suspended in saline solution supplemented with Alhydrogel (aluminum hydroxide) was administered subcutaneously (sc) into the neck skin fold at the dose of 25 μg. There were three injections (first application of antigen and/or adjuvant + two booster shots) at an interval of three weeks between each dose in order to monitor immunological response. Control mice received only a specific adjuvant. Blood samples were taken two weeks after each injection in order to determine the level of antibodies. Sera samples, taken from individual groups at each time point of experiment were pooled and (serially) diluted in 0.01 M PBS buffer (taking into account a molar concentration of phosphate ions). Sera were stored at – 20 °C.

All the animals were euthanized at the end of procedures in a chamber with carbon dioxide (BIOSCAPE, CO_2 – box model L). The following ratios of CO_2/O_2% vol/min were applied for induction 5/95% vol/min and for eutanasia 100/0% vol/min. BIOSCAPE, CO_2 – box model L2 meets all established recommendations and statutory provisions for euthanasia of small rodents using CO_2 according to Annex IV of European directive 2010/63/UE, a secondary physical method of euthanasia was cervical dislocation. Euthanasia in the chamber BIOSCAPE CO_2 model

L2 does not require earlier anaesthesia because mice are anaesthetised in the chamber during the first part of euthanasia process.

Preparation of biosensor—Successive steps of gold electrode modification

The biosensors were prepared according to procedure previously reported [36]. Briefly, clean gold electrodes were immersed in mixed solution of 10^{-5} M of DPM and 10^{-3} M of 4-mercapto-1-butanol (MBT) in dichloromethane at 4 °C for 3 h. Next, after washing with dichloromethane and dichloromethane-methanol solution (1:1), the electrodes were dipped in 1 mM copper (II) acetate solution in dichloromethane-methanol mixture (1,1) for 1 h. The tubes containing electrodes were sealed with teflon tape to avoid solvent evaporation. Then, the electrodes were washing in dichloromethane-methanol solution, next methanol and in the end TRIS buffer. Next, 10 μL of 10 μg/ml His_6- H1 HA in monomeric form dissolved TRIS buffer (10 mM, pH 7.6) were placed on the gold surfaces for 2 h. After that the electrodes were washing with TRIS buffer. Next, 10-μl droplets of BSA solution in a concentration of 1% (m/v) were applied on the surface of each electrodes and left for 30 min. After deposition of the BSA, the electrodes were washed and stored at 4 °C in TRIS buffer, pH 7,6 until used. Next, 10 μL aliquots of the respective dilutions of the mouse sera (10-fold serial dilutions in the range from 1×10^9 to 1×10^8) in 0.01 M PBS buffer were deposited onto the electrode surface for 30 min. The electrodes were covered by Eppendorf tubes in order to protect against evaporation and air pollution. After 30 min. of incubation at room temperature, the electrodes were rinsed with 3 mL of 0.01 M PBS, pH 7.4 in order to remove the unbound antibodies.

Osteryoung Square wave voltammetry (OSWV) measurements

All Osteryoung Square Wave Voltammetry (OSWV) measurements were performed with a potentiostat–galvanostat AutoLab (Eco Chemie, Utrecht, The Netherlands) as stated by procedure already published [47]. Briefly, the following electrodes were used: a gold working electrode, an Ag/AgCl reference electrode and a Pt counter electrode. The potential was scanning from + 0.7 V to – 0.3 V, with a step potential of 0.001 V, a square-wave frequency of 25 Hz, and amplitude of 0.05 V. PBS buffer with the following composition: 0.1368 M NaCl, 0.0027 M KCl, 0.0101 M Na_2HPO_4, 0.0018 KH_2PO_4 was used as the basic electrolyte.

Abbreviations

BSA: Bovine serum albumin; DPM: thiol derivative of dipyrromethene; EDC/NHS: 1-Ethyl-3-(3-dimethylaminopropyl) carbodiimide/N-hydroxysuccinimide; EIS: Electrochemical impedance spectroscopy; ELISA: Enzyme-linked immunosorbent assay; HA: Hemagglutinin; His_6-H1 HA: Recombinant His-tagged hemagglutinin; MBT: 4-mercapto-1-butanol; OSWV: Osteryoung Square Wave Voltammetry; PBS: Phosphate buffer saline; SAM: Self-assembled monolayers; WHO: World Health Organization

Acknowledgements

Not Applicable.

Funding

The design of the study and collection, analysis, and interpretation of data were supported by the National Centre for Research and Development

(NCBiR) under grant no. PBS2/A7/14/ 2014 and Institute of Animal Reproduction and Food Research, Polish Academy of Sciences, Olsztyn, Poland. Cristiane Andreia Erdmann was supported by National Council of Scientific and Technological Development-Brazil (CNPq), with a fellowship within the program Science without Borders. The article processing charge was covered by the KNOW Consortium: "Healthy Animal - Safe Food" (Ministry of Sciences and Higher Education; Dec: 05–1/KNOW2/2015).

Authors' contributions

HR design of research plan, control of all experiments, interpretation of electrochemical and analytical results, manuscript preparation and revising; JR design of research plan, interpretation of electrochemical and analytical results, manuscript preparation and revising; EM preforming of the experimental work, data analysing, results disscusion, manuscript preparation and revising; CES preforming of the experimental work, data analysing; EK design of research plan, interpretation of data, manuscript revising; KZ production and purification of protein, mice immunization, getting the sera for analysis, acquisition and interpretation of data. All authors read and approved the final manuscript.

Consent for publication

Not applicable.

Competing interests

The authors declare that they have no competing interests.

Author details

[1]Institute of Animal Reproduction and Food Research of Polish Academy of Sciences, Tuwima 10, 10-748 Olsztyn, Poland. [2]Universidade Estadual de Ponta Grossa - UEPG, Setor de Ciências Exatas e da Terra, Departamento de Química, Av. Carlos Cavalcanti, 4748, CEP 84030-900, Ponta Grossa/ PR, Brazil. [3]Institute of Biochemistry and Biophysics of Polish Academy of Sciences, Pawińskiego 5a, 02-106 Warsaw, Poland. [4]Research and Development Center, Olimp Laboratories, Pustynia, Dębica, Poland. Institute of Chemistry, University of Natural Sciences and Humanities, 3 Maja 54, 08-110 Siedlce, Poland.

References

1. Neumann G, Noda T, Kawaoka Y. Emergence and pandemic potential of swine-origin H1N1 influenza virus. Nature. 2009;459:931–9.
2. Su S, Gu M, Liu D, Cui J, Gao GF, Zhou J, Liu X. Epidemiology, Evolution, and Pathogenesis of H7N9 influenza viruses in five epidemic waves since 2013 in China. Trends Microbiol. 2017;9:713–28.
3. Li G, Wang R, Zhang C, Wang S, He W, Zhang J, Liu J, Cai Y, Zhou J, Su S. Genetic and evolutionary analysis of emerging H3N2 canine influenza virus. Emerg Microbes Infect. 2018;7:73.
4. Al Khatib HA, Al Thani AA, Yassine HM. Evolution and dynamics of the pandemic H1N1 influenza hemagglutinin protein from 2009 to 2017. Arch Virol. 2018; 163(11):3035-3049; doi:org/https://doi.org/10.1007/s00705-018-3962-z.
5. Suptawiwata O, Kongchanagulb A, Boonarkartc C, Auewarakul P. H1N1 seasonal influenza virus evolutionary rate changed over time. Virus Res. 2018;250:43–50.
6. Dawood FS, Iuliano AD, Reed C, Meltzer MI, Shay DK, Cheng PY, Bandaranayake D, Breiman RF, Brooks WA, Buchy P, Feikin DR, Fowler KB, Gordon A, Hien NT, Horby P, Huang QS, Katz MA, Krishnan A, Lal R, Montgomery JM, Molbak K, Pebody R, Presanis AM, Razuri H, Steens A, Tinoco YO, Wallinga J, Vong S, Bresee J, Widdowson MA. Estimated global mortality associated with the first 12months of 2009 pandemic influenza a H1N1 virus circulation: a modelling study. Lancet Infect Dis. 2012;12:687–95.
7. Prokopyeva EA, Sobolev IA, Prokopyev MV, Shestopalov AM. Adaptation of influenza a (H1N1) pdm09 virus in experimental mouse models. Infect Genet Evol. 2016;39:265–71.
8. Pandemic (H1N1) 2009 update-102. In: World Health Organization, 2010a. http://www.who.int/csr/don/2010_05_28/en/ . Accessed 17 June 2015.
9. Bai L, Cao B, Wang C. Influenza a pandemic (H1N1) 2009 virus infection. Chin Med J. 2011;124:3399–402.
10. Nelson MI, Gramer MR, Vincent AL, Holmes EC. Global transmission of influenza viruses from humans to swine. J Gen Virol. 2012;93:2195–203.
11. Arunorat J, Charoenvisal N, Woonwong Y, Kedkovid R, Jittimanee S, Sitthicharoenchai P, Kesdangsakonwut S, Poolpermd P, Thanawongnuwech R. Protection of human influenza vaccines against a reassortant swine influenza virus of pandemic H1N1 origin using a pig model. Res Vet Sci. 2017;114:6–11.
12. Forrest HL, Webster RG. Perspectives on influenza evolution and the role of research. Anim Health Res Rev. 2010;11:3–18.
13. Peiris JS, Poon LL, Guan Y. Emergence of a novel swine-origin influenza a virus (S-OIV) H1N1 virus in humans. J Clin Virol. 2009;45:169–73.
14. H1N1 in Post-pandemic Period. In: World Health Organization; 2010b. http://www.who.int/mediacentre/news/statements/2010/h1n1_vpc_20100810/en/. Accessed 17 June 2015.
15. Byahatti SM, Dandagi GL. An insight into the swine-influenza A(H1N1) virus infection in humans. Lung India. 2011;28(1):34–38.
16. Rewar S, Mirdha D, Rewar P. Treatment and prevention of pandemic H1N1 influenza. Ann Glob Health. 2015;81:645–53.
17. Wu J, Yi L, Ni H, Zou L, Zhang H, Zeng X, Liang L, Li L, Zhong H, Zhang X, Lin J, Kea C. Anti-Human H1N1pdm09 and swine H1N1 Virus Antibodies among Swine Workers in Guangdong Province. China Sci Rep. 2015;5:1–9.
18. Kothalawala H, Toussaint MJ, Gruys E. An overview of swine influenza. Vet Q. 2006;28:46–53.
19. Arya SK, Kongsuphol P, Wong CC, Polla LJ, Park MK. Label free biosensor for sensitive human influenza virus hemagglutinin specific antibody detection using coiled-coil peptide modified microelectrode array based platform. Sens Actuators B Chem. 2014;194:127–33.
20. Carney PJ, Lipatov AS, Monto AS, Donis RO, Stevens J. Flexible label-free quantitative assay for antibodies to influenza virus hemagglutinins. Clin Vaccine Immunol. 2010;17:1407–16.
21. Kamikawa TL, Mikolajczyk MG, Kennedy M, Zhang P, Wang W, Scott DE. Nanoparticle-based biosensor for the detection of emerging pandemic influenza strains. Biosens Bioelectron. 2010;26:1346–52.
22. Huang Y, Anderson SA, Forshee RA, Yang H. A modified dose–response model that describes the relationship between haemagglutination inhibition titre and protection against influenza infection. J Appl Microbiol. 2017;124:294–301.
23. Lebarbenchon C, Brown JD, Luttrell MP, Stallknecht DE. Comparison of two commercial enzyme-linked immunosorbent assays for detection of influenza a virus antibodies. JVet Diagn Investig. 2012;24:16–165.
24. Moreno A, Lelli D, Brocchi E, Sozzi E, Vinco LJ, Grilli G, Cordioli P. Monoclonal antibody-based ELISA for detection of antibodies against H5 avian influenza viruses. J Virol Methods. 2013;187:424–30.
25. Rapp BE, Gruhl FJ, Länge K. Biosensors with label-free detection designed for diagnostic applications. Anal Bioanal Chem. 2010;398:2403–12.
26. Palchetti I, Mascini M. Electroanalytical biosensors and their potential for food pathogen and toxin detection. Anal Bioanal Chem. 2008;391:455–71.
27. Radecka H, Radecki J. Electrochemical sensors for detections of influenza viruses: fundamentals and applications. In: Baddour MM, editor. Steps forwards in diagnosing and controlling influenza: InTechOpen Limited, The Shard, 25th floor, 32 Lodon Bridge Street, London: SE 19SG-United Kingdom. 2016. p. 47–59.
28. Luckarift HR, Ivnitski DM, Lau C, Khripin C, Atanassov P, Johnson GR. Gold-decorated carbon composite electrodes for enzymatic oxygen reduction. Electroanalysis. 2012;24:931–7.
29. Zhang Z, Zhang R, Li C, Yuan L, Li P, Yao L, Liu S. Nitrogen-droped carbon hollow spheres for immobilization, direct electrochemistry, and biosensing of protein. Electroanalysis. 2012;24:1424–30.
30. Serafín V, Eguílaz M, Agüí L, Yáñez-Sedeño P, Pingarrón JM. An electrochemical immunosensor for testosterone using gold nanoparticles-carbon nanotubes composite electrodes. Electroanalysis. 2011;23:169–76.
31. Grosan CB, Varodi C, Vulcu AL, Olenic L, Pruneanu S, Almasan V. Structural and electrochemical characterization of novel leucine-gold nanoparticles modified electrode. Electrochim Acta. 2012;63:146–52.

32. Farka Z, Juřík T, Kovář D, Trnková L, Skládal P. Nanoparticle-based immunochemical biosensors and assays: recent advances and challenges. Chem Rev. 2017;117:9973–10042.
33. Wąsowicz M, Viswanathan S, Dvornyk A, Grzelak K, Kłudkiewicz B, Radecka H. Comparison of electrochemical immunosensor based on gold nano materials and immunoblot techniques for detection of histidine-tagged proteins in culture medium. Biosens Bioelectron. 2008;24:284–9.
34. Iwata R, Satoh R, Iwasaki Y, Akiyoshi K. Covalent immobilization of antibody fragments on well-defined polymer brushes via site-directed method. Colloids Surf, B. 2008;62:288–98.
35. Wąsowicz M, Milner M, Radecka D, Grzelak K, Radecka H. Immunosensor incorporating anti-his (C-term) IgG F (ab') fragments attached to gold nanorods for detection of his-tagged proteins in culture medium. Sensors. 2010;10:5409–24.
36. Jarocka U, Sawicka R, Stachyra A, Góra-Sochacka A, Sirko A, Zagórski-Ostoja W, Sączyńska V, Porębska A, Dehaen W, Radecki J, Radecka H. A biosensor based on electroactive dipyrromethene – cu (II) layer deposited onto gold electrodes for the detection of antibodies against avian influenza virus type H5N1 in hen sera. Anal Bioanal Chem. 2015;407:7807–14.
37. Ta DT, Guedens W, Vranken T, Vanschoenbeek K, Redeker ES, Michiels L, Adriaensens P. Enhanced biosensor platforms for detecting the atherosclerotic biomarker VCAM1 based on bioconjugation with uniformly oriented VCAM1-targeting nanobodies. Biosensors. 2016;6:34.
38. Kurzątkowska K, Jankowska A, Wysłouch Cieszyńska A, Zhukova L, Puchalska M, Dehaen W, Radecka H, Radecki J. Voltammetric detection of the S100B protein using his-tagged RAGE domain immobilized onto a gold electrode modified with a dipyrromethene–cu (II) complex and different diluents. J Electroanal Chem. 2016;767:76–83.
39. Bard JA, Faulkner LR. Electrochemical methods. 2nd ed. New York, USA: John Wiley & Sons, Inc.; 2001.
40. Alvarez MM, López-Pacheco F, Aguilar-Yañez JM, Portillo-Lara R, Mendoza-Ochoa GI, García-Echauri S, Freiden P, Schultz-Cherry S, Zertuche-Guerra MI, Bulnes-Abundis D, Salgado-Gallegos J, Elizondo-Montemayor L, Hernández-Torre M. Specific recognition of influenza a/H1N1/2009 antibodies in human serum: a simple virus-free ELISA method. PLoS One. 2010;5:10176.
41. Lee BW, Bey RF, Baarsch MJ, Emery DA. Subtype specific ELISA for the detection of antibodies. J Virol Methods. 1993;45:121–36.
42. Stelzer-Braid S, Wong B, Robertson P, Lynch GW, Laurie K, Shaw R, Bar I, Selleck PW, Baleriola C, Escott R, Katsoulotos G, Rawlinson WD. A commercial ELISA detects high levels of human H5 antibody but cross-reacts with influenza a antibodies. J Clin Virol. 2008;43:241–3.
43. Arya SK, Kongsuphol P, Chung Won C, Polla LJ, Park MK. Label free biosensor for sensitive human influenza virus hemagglutinin specific antibody detection using coiled-coil peptide modified microelectrode array based platform. Sensors Actuators B Chem. 2014;194:127–33.
44. Rowe T, Abernathy RA, Hu-Primmer J, Thompson WW, Lu X, Lim W, Fukuda K, Cox NJ, Katz JM. Detection of antibody to avian influenza a (H5N1) virus in human serum by using a combination of serologic assays. J Clin Virol. 1999;37:937–43.
45. Meiner A, Bosman A, Van de Kamp EE, Wilbrink B, Beest Holle M, Koopmans M. Measurement of antibodies to avian influenza virus a (H7N7) in humans by hemagglutination inhibition test. J Virol Methods. 2006;132:113–20.
46. Jarocka U, Sawicka R, Góra-Sochacka A, Sirko A, Zagórski-Ostoja W, Radecki J, Radecka H. Electrochemical immunosensor for detection of antibodies against influenza a virus H5N1 in hen serum. Biosens Bioelectron. 2014;55:301–6.
47. Mikuła E, Sulima M, Marszałek I, Wysłouch Cieszyńska A, Verwilst P, Dehaen W, Radecki J, Radecka H. Oriented immobilization of his-tagged protein on a redox active thiol derivative of DPTA-cu (II) layer deposited on a gold electrode—the base of electrochemical biosensors. Sensors. 2013;13:11586–602.

21

Development and application of an indirect ELISA for the detection of antibodies to porcine epidemic diarrhea virus based on a recombinant spike protein

Huixing Lin[1], Hong Zhou[1], Lu Gao[1], Bin Li[2], Kongwang He[2] and Hongjie Fan[1,3*]

Abstract

Background: As the major causative agent of swine viral diarrhea, porcine epidemic diarrhea virus (PEDV) has caused massive losses to the economies of swine raising countries. Accordingly, the serological detection of corresponding antibodies would be beneficial to diagnose PEDV indirectly to control the disease. In this study, an indirect enzyme-linked immunosorbent assay (ELISA) based on the recombinant truncated spike (S) protein of PEDV was developed and validated.

Results: The reaction conditions of the developed indirect ELISA were optimized. This indirect ELISA was compared to indirect immunoinfluscent assay (IFA), and the overall coincidence rate was 96.74% based on testing 368 clinical serum samples with different PEDV antibody levels. No cross-reactivity with other common swine pathogens was detected for the developed S1 indirect ELISA. Finally, the S1 indirect ELISA was applied to detect serum antibodies of 3304 field samples collected from different pig farms in eastern China, and it presented an overall substantial agreement on the PEDV infection status.

Conclusions: This established S1 indirect ELISA is capable of detecting serum antibodies against PEDV, and due to its high sensitivity and specificity, it could be applied for serological evaluation and indirect diagnosis of PEDV infection.

Keywords: Porcine epidemic diarrhea virus, Spike protein, ELISA

Background

Porcine epidemic diarrhea (PED) is a highly contagious swine enteritis caused by porcine epidemic diarrhea virus (PEDV), which belongs to the order *Nidovirales* and family *Coronaviridae*. The typical symptoms of PED are diarrhea, vomiting, and dehydration, which can be especially dangerous to suckling piglets [1, 2]. The mortality of neonatal piglets younger than 5 days old can approach 100% [3–5]. PED first appeared in Britain in 1971, followed by an outbreak of diarrhea in several pig farms in Belgium in 1977 [6]. These outbreaks led to identification of a coronavirus-like particle named CV777, which is now recognized as the classic PEDV strain. In recent years, PED epidemics have become prevalent in swine-raising countries in Asia, including South Korea, China, Japan, and Vietnam, and can cause enormous economic loss [7, 8].

PEDV is a single-stranded RNA virus composed primarily of four structural proteins: the spike protein (S, 180–220 kDa), membrane protein (M, 27–32 kDa), envelope protein (E, 7 kDa) and nucleocapsid protein (N, 55–58 kDa). S protein is located on the surface of the virus particle. It is categorized as a type I membrane fusion protein and has the significant biological effect of binding to target cell receptors and entering the cell

* Correspondence: fhj@njau.edu.cn
[1]MOE Joint International Research Laboratory of Animal Health and Food Safety, College of Veterinary Medicine, Nanjing Agricultural University, Nanjing 210095, China
[3]Jiangsu Co-Innovation Center for the Prevention and Control of Important Animal Infectious Diseases and Zoonoses, Yangzhou University, Yangzhou 225009, China
Full list of author information is available at the end of the article

through plasma membrane fusion [9, 10]. The S protein has higher antigenicity than any of the other PEDV proteins, and anti-S antibodies detected in PEDV-infected pigs persist longer than anti-N antibodies [11]. The S protein can be separated into the S1 (1–789 aa) subunit and the S2 (790–1383 aa) subunit [12]. The S1 subunit is the extracellular domain and can recognize and bind to target cell receptors [13], and it is closely linked to the formation of neutralizing antibodies. Therefore, this study selected a gene fragment within the S1 subunit as a coating antigen to develop an indirect enzyme-linked immunosorbent assay (ELISA) method for the detection of PEDV antibodies.

Methods

Materials

The PEDV YC2014 strain was isolated on a breeding farm in Yancheng city in 2014 (GenBank: KU252649.1). The prokaryotic expression vector pET-28a(+) was purchased from BioVector NTCC Inc. (Beijing, China). The HRP-goat anti-pig IgA, HRP-goat anti-pig IgG, and FITC-goat anti-pig IgA was purchased from Abcam plc. (Shanghai, China). The standard PEDV negative serum were collected from specific pathogen free (SPF) pigs. The standard PEDV positive serum were collected from experimentally PEDV immunized SPF pigs, at 7, 14, 21, 28, 35, 42 and 49 day post-inoculation (dpi). These standard serum were identified of PEDV-specific antibodies positive by both indirect immunoinfluscent assay (IFA) and seroneutralization assay (SN) as previously described [14, 15]. The swine PoRV antibody ELISA kit and the swine TGEV ELISA kit were obtained from Ingenasa (Madrid, Spain).

Construction of the recombinant plasmid

The gene sequence of truncated spike protein (named *S1*) was amplified from the genomic RNA of PEDV YC2014 strain (Genbank: KU252649.1) by reverse-transcriptase (RT)-PCR. The forward primer was 5' CGCGGATCCGTCACTAGGTGCCAGTCCACTATTAA-3'and the reverse primer was 5'-CCCAAGCTTTCAATTGTAAATATCCACTTTAAGAAAACAATAA-3′. Underlined portions represent *Bam*H I and *Hind* III restriction sites, respectively. The target gene was 1068 bp in length and subcloned into the prokaryotic expression vector pET-28a(+), then transformed into a strain of competent *E. coli* cells, DH5α. Transformed colonies were selected from Luria-Bertani (LB) agar plates containing kanamycin (50 μg/mL) and were identified by PCR. The resulting recombinant expression plasmid was named 28a-S1 and was identified by double enzyme digestion and DNA sequence analysis. Subsequently, the recombinant expression plasmid 28a-S1 was transformed into *E. coli* BL21 (DE3).

Expression and purification of the recombinant protein S1

The positive transformants were cultured in LB medium containing 50 μg/mL kanamycin with vigorous shaking at 37 °C until the 600 nm optical density (OD_{600}) of bacteria cultures reached approximately 0.5. Then, by adding isopropyl-β-D-thiogalactopyranoside (IPTG), the recombinant protein S1 was induced for 6–8 h at 37 °C. The expression of recombinant proteins was analyzed by 12% (*v*/v) sodium dodecyl sulfate-polyacrylamide gel electrophoresis (SDS-PAGE) and the gels were stained with coomassie brilliant blue. Induced cells were pelleted and washed in phosphate-buffered saline (PBS) three times, then lysed by sonication in an ice-water bath. The lysed cells were centrifuged at 12,000 g for 10 min, then the precipitate (inclusion body) was dissolved with binding buffer containing 8 M urea. The supernatant and the precipitate were then subjected to SDS-PAGE analysis. The recombinant protein was purified through affinity chromatography using a Ni-NTA spin column following the manufacturer's recommendations.

Western blotting

Purified recombinant protein S1 was subjected to 12% (*v*/v) SDS-PAGE, and the gel was prepared for western blotting as follows. Recombinant proteins separated in the gel were electrically transferred to a nitrocellulose membrane and the membrane was blocked overnight at 4 °C with Tris-buffered saline containing Tween-20 (TBST) which contained 5% (*w*/*v*) skimmed milk powder. The composition of TBST is as follows: 20 mM Tris-HCl, 150 mM NaCl, and 0.05% Tween-20. The membrane was then incubated with pig anti-PEDV polyclonal antibody (1:300 dilution in blocking buffer) for 1 h at 37 °C on a plate shaker. Following this incubation, the membrane was washed three times with TBST buffer and reacted with HRP-goat anti-pig IgG (1:2000 dilution in TBST) at 37 °C for 45 min. After three washes, the final color reaction was developed with a solution of 3,3′-Diaminobenzidine (DAB).

Recombinant protein S1 indirect ELISA

Conventional indirect ELISA was performed with the following steps. ELISA plates with 96 wells (Costar, USA) were coated with 100 μL purified recombinant S1 protein in bicarbonate buffer (pH = 9.6) for 2 h at 37 °C. Then, plates were washed three times with PBST (PBS containing 0.05% Tween-20) and blocked with 5% skimmed milk in PBS for 2 h at 37 °C. After plates were washed, 100 μL porcine serum samples diluted in PBS containing 5% (*w*/*v*) skimmed milk was added and incubated for 45 min at 37 °C. Plates were washed four times and reacted with 100 μL diluted secondary antibody (HRP-goat anti-pig IgA or HRP-goat anti-pig IgG) for

30 min at 37 °C for the purpose of detecting IgA or IgG against PEDV in serum samples. Plates were then washed four times and 100 μL tetramethylbenzidine (TMB) substrate solution was added to each well for a chromogenic reaction at room temperature for 15 min in complete darkness. The color reaction was stopped by the addition 50 μL of 2 M H_2SO_4 to each well. Finally, the OD_{450} was measured and recorded immediately using an Infinite 200 PRO microplatereader (Tecan, Männedorf, Switzerland).

The optimal dilution of recombinant protein S1 and standard serum was determined by a checkerboard titration based on the method mentioned above. Briefly, the concentration of S1 protein was gradually reduced in the following series: 10, 7.5, 5, 2.5, 1.0, and 0.5 μg/mL. The standard PEDV positive and negative serum were serially diluted in a 2-fold series from 1:20 to 1:320. When the OD_{450} ratio of positive serum to negative serum was highest, and the OD_{450} of positive serum was closest to 1.0, the corresponding dilutions of coated antigen and serum sample were considered optimal. In addition to optimal protein dilution, the coating conditions, blocking solution, and reaction time of various materials was explored. Furthermore, the optimal concentration of HRP-goat anti-pig IgA was tested using the following dilutions: 1:2000, 1:5000, 1:10000, 1:15000, and 1:20000.

Determination of the cut-off value

Two hundred and seventy serum samples were collected for the purpose of determining the positive-negative cut-off value, of which 90 serum samples were collected from 90 SPF pigs, 180 serum samples were collected from grow-finish pigs from five farms between 2009 and 2012. These five farms were located in areas with no previous history of enteric signs compatible with viral diarrhea, and were PEDV RNA negative by real-time RT-PCR based on a single collection. These serum samples were confirmed PEDV-negative by both IFA and SN assays as previously described [14, 15], and then were used to define the cut-off value in the S1 indirect ELISA. The OD_{450} value of these PEDV-negative serum samples obtained in this S1 indirect ELISA were recorded to calculate the cut-off value. The mean OD_{450} value of these negative samples (N) + 3 × standard deviations (SD) was defined as the cut-off value. Serum samples showing OD_{450} value greater than or equal to this cut-off were considered PEDV-seropositive.

Assessment of S1 indirect ELISA

To assess the accuracy of this developed S1 indirect ELISA, 368 serum samples from different pig farms were tested using this ELISA method. As a comparison, IFA was applied to test these samples and act as a reference method to distinguish positive or negative samples. Briefly, Vero cells grown on 96-well plates were infected with the PEDV YC2014 strain at multiplicity of infection (m. o. i) of 5. At 48 h post-infection, cells were washed three times with PBST and fixed with cold methanol for 10 min at – 20 °C. Cells were then washed three times with PBST and blocked with 10% bovine serum albumin (BSA) at 37 °C for 1 h. After been double diluted for six consecutive dilutions in dilution buffer (1% BSA in PBST), the 368 serum samples with varied PEDV antibody status were added in the wells of 96-well plate, and were incubated for 1 h at 37 °C. After three washes with PBST, cells were treated with a FITC-conjugated goat anti-pig IgA (Thermo Scientific) at a 1:500 dilution with PBS for 30 min at 37 °C. After a final four washes with PBST, all wells were examined using fluorescence microscopy (Axio Observer Z1, Zeiss, Germany). The PEDV antibody titers of the serum samples were expressed as the highest dilution of serum samples producing green fluorescent in the wells of 96-well plates.

The results of this two methods were compared, and the sensitivity and specificity of detection were calculated to evaluate the accuracy of the S1 indirect ELISA. Sensitivity was defined as the ratio of positive tests from the developed S1 indirect ELISA to the positive tests from the IFA. Specificity was defined as the ratio of negative tests from the developed ELISA to the negative tests from the reference IFA.

Serum cross-reactivity of S1 indirect ELISA to other pathogens

To validate the cross-reactivity, this S1 indirect ELISA was utilized to test porcine serum positive for other swine pathogens, namely, porcine transmissible gastroenteritis virus (TGEV), swine rotavirus (PoRV), porcine kobuvirus (PKV), porcine bocavirus (PBoV), porcine norovirus (PNoV), porcine circovirus type 2 (PCV2), porcine reproductive and respiratory syndrome virus (PRRSV), and enterotoxigenic *E. coli* (ETEC), *Jerson Prand* of the small intestine, *Clostridium Welchii* Type C. The positive sera were prepared by our lab, by immunizing the specific pathogen free (SPF) piglets with purified virus or bacteria. Thirty positive serum samples for each virus were tested, and each sample was repeated in triplicate.

Determination of repeatability of S1 indirect ELISA

To test the repeatability of this ELISA, 255 serum samples with different PEDV antibody levels were chosen. For inter-assay variability, each sample was tested in 5 replicates on plates of different occasions. For intra-assay variability, each sample was tested in 5 replicates on plates within the same occasion. The results were presented as the coefficient of variation (CV), which is the ratio of the standard deviation (SD) to the mean OD_{450} value of each group of samples (S). A CV value criterion of 10% was used to meet the repeatability requirement of the test.

PEDV antibody detection of field serum samples

This S1 indirect ELISA was applied to seroepidemiological analysis of a total of 3304 clinical swine serum samples collected from thirty seven farms in eastern China. The PEDV infection status of a given farm was determined based on demonstration of PEDV RNA in fecal samples by real-time RT-PCR and presence of enteric signs [16]. One thousand one hundred and twenty five serum samples were collected from nursery and grow-finish pigs from ten farms between 2011 and 2015 at 3–6 weeks after the start of PEDV outbreaks in these farms. Four hundred and eighty two serum samples were collected from nursery and grow-finish pigs from five farms between 2012 and 2015. These five farms were located in areas with no previous history of enteric signs compatible with viral diarrhea, were PEDV RNA negative by real-time RT-PCR based on a single collection, and were considered non-exposed to PEDV. Three hundred and forty four serum samples from nursery pigs without PEDV exposure were collected from six farms between 2011 and 2015. These samples were confirmed to be positive for anti-PoRV antibodies (3 farms, $n = 149$) or anti-TGEV antibodies (3 farms, $n = 195$) by both IFA and commercial ELISA kits (obtained from Ingenasa). One thousand three hundred and fifty three porcine serum samples with unknown PEDV exposure status were randomly selected from sixteen farms from nursery and grow-finish pigs between 2011 and 2014.

Results

Subcloning, inducible expression and purification of recombinant S1 protein

The gene of PEDV truncated S1 fragment (67–1134 nt) was amplified by RT-PCR (Fig. 1a). A 1068 bp PCR product was obtained and subcloned to prokaryotic

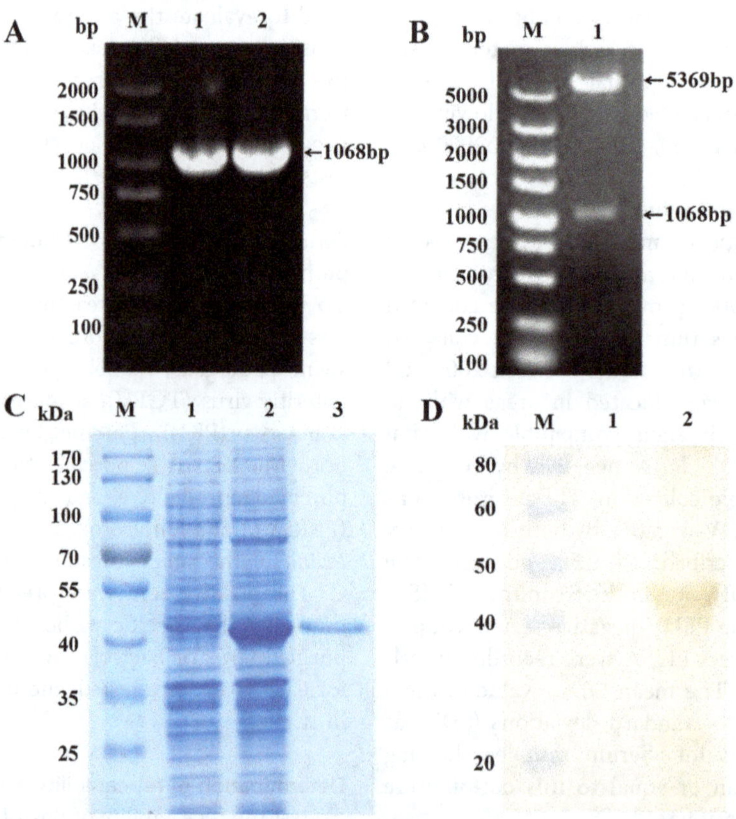

Fig. 1 Amplification, SDS-PAGE and western blotting analysis of the recombinant protein S1. **a** RT-PCR amplification of the truncated S1 gene fragment. Lane M, DL2000 DNA marker. Lane 1 and 2, the truncated S1 gene fragment. **b** Identifiction of the recombinant expression plasmid 28a-S1 by double enzyme digestion. Lane M, DL5000 DNA marker. Lane 1, the recombinant expression plasmid 28a-S1 digested by *Bam*H I/*Sal* I. **c** SDS-PAGE analysis of S1 protein. Lane M, prestained protein molecular weight standard. Lane 1, transformed cells of BL21/pET-28a(+) after IPTG induction for 6 h. Lane 2, transformed cells of BL21/28a-S1 after IPTG induction for 6 h. Lane 3, purified recombinant protein S1 by affinity chromatography of Ni-NTA spin column. **d** Western blotting analysis of S1 protein. Lane M, prestained protein molecular weight standard. Lane 1, *E. coli* BL21 with empty vector pET-28a(+) reacted with polyclonal mouse anti-PEDV antibody. Lane 2, purified S1 protein reacted with polyclonal mouse anti-PEDV antibody. A prominent band with the expected size 42 kDa appeared after incubation

expression vector pET-28a(+), and the inserted gene was sequenced to ensure the correctness of the reading frame. As shown by SDS-PAGE (Fig. 1c), the recombinant protein S1 was expressed in the form of inclusion body, resulting in a 6 × His-tag fusion protein whose molecular mass was approximately 42 kDa. Sonicated lysates from recombinant *E. coli* were harvested, and the precipitate was dissolved in 8 M urea and purified by affinity chromatography of Ni^{2+}-NTA agarose. The immunoreactivity of S1 protein was examined by western blotting. An obvious band revealed that S1 protein was specifically bound by pig anti-PEDV polyclonal antibody (Fig. 1d).

Optimization of S1 indirect ELISA

As expected with checkerboard titration, with concentrations of antigen and serum regularly decreasing, absorbance values of corresponding samples declined. The optimal dilution of coated antigen S1 protein was measured at 0.25 μg/well (2.5 μg/mL), and optimal serum sample dilution was 1:40 (Table 1). Furthermore, other reaction conditions of the developed ELISA were optimized. In brief, the optimum coating condition was 2 h at 37 °C. The best blocking solution was selected as 5% skimmed milk in PBS. The optimal reaction times for serum, secondary antibodies, and TMB solution were 45 min, 30 min and 15 min, respectively. Finally, the best working dilution of the HRP-goat anti-pig IgA was 1:10,000.

Determination of the cut-off threshold value

To determine the cut-off value of the S1 indirect ELISA, 270 PEDV-seronegative samples, verified by both IFA and SN assays, were tested by this ELISA method. The average optical density of these negative serum samples (N) was calculated as 0.185, and the standard deviation (SD) of these samples was 0.0337. Consequently, the cut-off threshold value of S1 indirect ELISA was calculated to be 0.286, indicating that the sample $OD_{450} \geq 0.286$ was identified as PEDV-seropositive and vice versa.

S1 indirect ELISA validation

This developed S1 indirect ELISA was applied to 368 serum samples with varied PEDV antibody status (Table 2). In these samples, the S1 indirect ELISA detected 213 PEDV-positive samples, of which 206 tested PEDV-positive by IFA. On the other hand, of the remaining 155 samples that tested PEDV-seronegative by this S1 indirect ELISA, 150 of them were tested PEDV-negative by IFA. Hence, the sensitivity of S1 indirect ELISA was 96.71% among PEDV-seropositive individuals, and the specificity was 96.77% among PEDV-seronegative individuals using IFA as standard evaluation method. In summary, the overall coincidence rate of the S1 indirect ELISA to IFA was 96.74%.

Cross-reactivity of S1 indirect ELISA

To test the cross-reactivity of this S1 indirect ELISA, other viruses known to cause swine diarrhea were examined. The average OD_{450} of positive serum samples for TGEV, PoRV, PKV, PBoV, PNoV, PCV2, PRRSV, ETEC, *Jerson Prand* of the small intestine, and *Clostridium Welchii* Type C were 0.193, 0.121, 0.098, 0.147, 0.150, 0.182, 0.178, 0.188, 0.145 and 0.124, respectively. The results showed that these serum samples were PEDV-seronegative and non-cross-reactive with this S1 indirect ELISA, indicating that the established ELISA was an effective method for detecting PEDV antibodies.

Table 1 Checkerboard titration of the recombinant protein S1

OD450 ratio (P/N)		Dilution of serum sample				
P/N		1:20	1:40	1:80	1:160	1:320
Concentrations of antigen (μg/mL)	10	1.233/0.185	0.980/0.100	0.730/0.082	0.551/0.052	0.401/0.041
		6.665	9.80	8.902	10.596	9.780
	7.5	1.118/0.150	0.942/0.092	0.631/0.075	0.459/0.047	0.309/0.029
		7.453	10.239	8.413	9.766	10.655
	5.0	1.102/0.141	0.854/0.077	0.591/0.067	0.388/0.042	0.228/0.022
		7.816	11.091	8.821	9.238	10.364
	2.5	1.032/0.120	0.832/0.073	0.547/0.063	0.335/0.040	0.195/0.019
		8.600	11.397	8.683	8.375	10.263
	1.0	0.927/0.112	0.753/0.071	0.473/0.057	0.316/0.037	0.183/0.017
		8.277	10.606	8.298	8.541	10.765
	0.5	0.818/0.103	0.714/0.068	0.447/0.055	0.292/0.033	0.171/0.016
		7.942	10.500	8.127	8.848	10.688

Table 2 Comparison of the S1 indirect ELISA with the IFA

		IFA results		
		Positive	Negative	Total
S1 indirect ELISA results	Positive	206	7	213
	Negative	5	150	155
	Total	211	157	368
Data analysis	Sensitivity	96.71%		
	Specificity		96.77%	
	Coincidence rate			96.74%

The repeatability of S1 indirect ELISA

Intra-assay variability of the S1 indirect ELISA was assessed by testing 255 swine serum samples, each with 5 replicates. This analysis produced CVs ranging from 2.2–3.7%, with an average value of 2.8%. Inter-assay variability of four batches using identical samples produced CVs ranging from 2.6–4.5%, with an average value of 3.2%. The results demonstrated that this ELISA method yielded low levels of variation, and its repeatability was in the credible range.

PEDV antibody detection of field serum samples

This S1 indirect ELISA method was used on 3304 swine serum samples of different PEDV exposure status collected from 37 farms (Table 3). In the 10 farms from which 1125 samples were collected during the PEDV outbreaks between 2011 and 2015, 1027 samples were tested PEDV antibody positive, the positive detection varied from 78 to 100% between 10 farms. In the 5 PEDV non-exposed farms from which 482 samples were collected between 2012 and 2015, 31 samples were tested PEDV antibody positive, the positive detection varied from 5.1 to 7.8% between 5 farms. Among PoRV or TGEV antibody positive serum samples, 16/149 anti-PoRV antibody positive sample and 27/195 anti-TGEV antibody positive samples were tested PEDV antibody positive. In the 16 farms from which 1353 samples with unknown PEDV exposure status were collected between 2011 and 2014, 491 samples were tested PEDV antibody positive, the positive detection varied from 15 to 47% between 16 farms.

Comparation of IgA with IgG in the sera of PEDV immunized pigs

This S1 indirect ELISA was applied to test the sera of PEDV immunized pigs at 7, 14, 21, 28, 35, 42 and 49 day post-inoculation (dpi). The results (Fig. 2) showed that, both the IgA and the IgG were positive at 7 dpi. At early infection stage (7 dpi), the IgA titer was significantly higher than the IgG titer; at 14 dpi the IgA titer was equivalent to the IgG titer; and after 21 dpi, the IgA titer was significantly lower than the IgG titer. The IgG could exist in the sera of infection recovered stage for more time than IgA.

Discussion

Since December 2010, a large-scale outbreak of diarrhea has been observed in swine farms in China. Accumulated evidence indicates that this large-scale outbreak of diarrhea were caused by highly virulent PEDV variants [17, 18]. Serological assays can quickly detect large numbers of samples with both high sensitivity and specificity. Several indirect ELISA have been developed based on either whole PEDV preparations or recombinant viral proteins [19–21]. The S protein of PEDV has numerous epitopes and highly antigenic index regions that induce the production of neutralizing antibodies [10, 22, 23], and anti-S antibodies detected in PEDV-infected pigs persist longer than anti-N antibodies [11], thus, we choose S protein as the diagnostic antigen.

The recombinant S1 protein was applied to establish an indirect ELISA, and its reaction conditions were optimized. As PEDV is an enteric virus, it directly infects and damages enterocytes. Mucosal IgA, but not systemic IgG, plays a crucial role in protection [24, 25]. In this research, the titers of IgA in the serum were tested for serological evaluation and indirect diagnosis of PEDV infection. Of the 1125 serum samples which were PEDV exposed, the overall positive rate of the antibody is 91.29%, which were varied from 78 to 100% between 10 farms. Of the 482 serum samples which were PEDV non-exposed, the overall positive rate of the antibody is 6.43%, which were varied from 5.1 to 7.8% between 5 farms. The evaluated ELISA presented an overall substantial agreement on the PEDV infection status of the field swine serum samples.

Table 3 Detection rates of anti-PEDV antibodies in field serum samples

PEDV exposure	PoRV/TGEV exposure	No. samples	No. positive	Positive rate
Exposed	Non-exposed	1125	1027	91.29%
Non-exposed	Non-exposed	482	31	6.43%
Non-exposed	Exposed	149	16	10.74%
Non-exposed	Exposed	195	27	13.85%
Unknown	Unknown	1353	491	36.29%

Samples were collected from farms with known or unknown PEDV exposure as determined by real-time RT-PCR of fecal samples

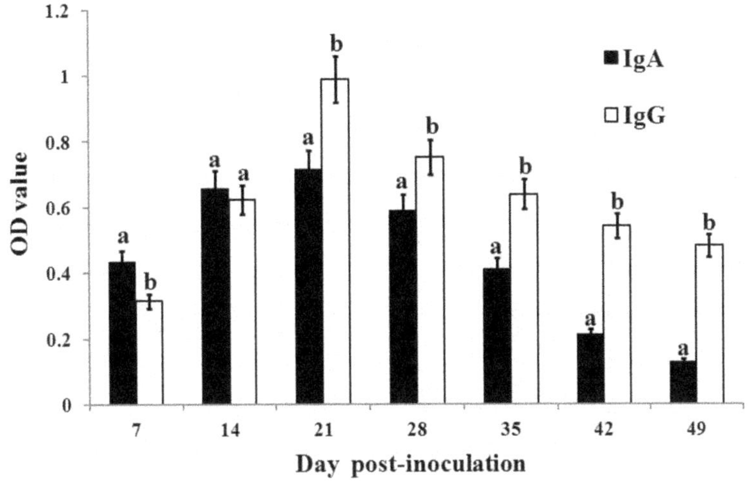

Fig. 2 Determination of IgA and IgG in the sera of PEDV immunized pigs. The sera of PEDV immunized pigs were tested by this S1 indirect ELISA at 7, 14, 21, 28, 35, 42 and 49 day post-inoculation (dpi). Both the IgA and the IgG were positive at 7 dpi. The IgG could exist in the sera for longer time than IgA. Different letters (**a**, and **b**) indicate significant difference between the groups

The intra- and inter-assay variability tests proved that this ELISA method had good repeatability. When testing other positive serum related to swine viral pathogens, this established ELISA demonstrated no cross-reactivity to them. Further, the overall rate of coincidence of this ELISA was calculated at 96.74% compared with IFA, proving that the diagnostic sensitivity and specificity of this ELISA method were favorable.

Of the numerous pathogens which can cause swine viral diarrhea, PEDV, TGEV, and PoRV account for the largest proportion [26]. In the present study, 16/149 anti-PoRV antibody positive sample and 27/195 anti-TGEV antibody positive samples were tested PEDV antibody positive, which indicated there may be co-infection of PEDV and other virus.

Conclusions

In conclusion, this established S1 indirect ELISA is capable of detecting serum antibodies against PEDV, and due to its high sensitivity and specificity, it could be applied for serological evaluation and indirect diagnosis of PEDV infection.

Abbreviations

CV: Coefficient of variation; ELISA: Enzyme-linked immunosorbent assay; IFA: Indirect immunoinfluscent assay; PEDV: Porcine epidemic diarrhea virus (PEDV); SD: Standard deviation; SN: Seroneutralization assay; TMB: Tetramethylbenzidine

Funding

This study was supported by the National Key Research and Development Program of China (2018YFD0500100), the National Natural Science Foundation of China (31702278, 31672574), the Jiangsu Agricultural Science and Technology Innovation Fund (CX(15)1056), the Postdoctoral Fund of Jiangsu Province (1501030C) and the Priority Academic Program Development of Jiangsu Higher Education Institutions (PAPD).

Authors' contributions

HL, KH and HF designed the study. HL, HZ, LG and BL performed and collected data from experiment and analyzed data. HL, HZ wrote the manuscript. All authors read and approved the final manuscript.

Ethics approval

This study was performed in accordance with the recommendations in the Guide for the Care and Use of Laboratory Animals of the Ministry of Health, China. All experimental protocols were approved by the Institutional Animal Care and Use Committee of Nanjing Agricultural University (No. SYXK2015–0057) and performed accordingly. Samples were collected only from animals for laboratory analyses, avoiding unnecessary pain and suffering of the animals. The owners gave their written consent for sample collection, and the locations where we sampled are not privately owned or protected in any way. The studies did not involve endangered or protected species.

Consent for publication

Not applicable.

Competing interests

The authors declare that they have no competing interests.

Author details

[1]MOE Joint International Research Laboratory of Animal Health and Food Safety, College of Veterinary Medicine, Nanjing Agricultural University, Nanjing 210095, China. [2]Institute of Veterinary Medicine, Jiangsu Academy of Agricultural Sciences, Nanjing 210014, China. [3]Jiangsu Co-Innovation Center for the Prevention and Control of Important Animal Infectious Diseases and Zoonoses, Yangzhou University, Yangzhou 225009, China.

References

1. Hanke D, Pohlmann A, Sauter-Louis C, Hoper D, Stadler J, Ritzmann M, Steinrigl A, Schwarz BA, Akimkin V, Fux R, et al. Porcine epidemic diarrhea in Europe: in-detail analyses of disease dynamics and molecular epidemiology. Viruses. 2017;9(7):177.
2. Curry SM, Gibson KA, Burrough ER, Schwartz KJ, Yoon KJ, Gabler NK. Nursery pig growth performance and tissue accretion modulation due to porcine epidemic diarrhea virus or porcine deltacoronavirus challenge. J Anim Sci. 2017;95(1):173–81.
3. Kim O, Chae C. In situ hybridization for the detection and localization of porcine epidemic diarrhea virus in the intestinal tissues from naturally infected piglets. Vet Pathol. 2000;37(1):62–7.

4. Li B, Du L, Yu Z, Sun B, Xu X, Fan B, Guo R, Yuan W, He K. Poly (d,l-lactide-co-glycolide) nanoparticle-entrapped vaccine induces a protective immune response against porcine epidemic diarrhea virus infection in piglets. Vaccine. 2017;35(50):7010–7.
5. Annamalai T, Lin CM, Gao X, Liu X, Lu Z, Saif LJ, Wang Q. Cross protective immune responses in nursing piglets infected with a US spike-insertion deletion porcine epidemic diarrhea virus strain and challenged with an original US PEDV strain. Vet Res. 2017;48(1):61.
6. Wood EN. An apparently new syndrome of porcine epidemic diarrhoea. Vet Rec. 1977;100(12):243–4.
7. Chung HC, Nguyen VG, Moon HJ, Lee JH, Park SJ, Lee GE, Kim HK, Noh YS, Lee CH, Goede D, et al. Isolation of porcine epidemic diarrhea virus during outbreaks in South Korea, 2013-2014. Emerg Infect Dis. 2015;21(12):2238–40.
8. Fan JH, Zuo YZ, Li JH, Pei LH. Heterogeneity in membrane protein genes of porcine epidemic diarrhea viruses isolated in China. Virus Genes. 2012;45(1):113–7.
9. Supekar VM, Bruckmann C, Ingallinella P, Bianchi E, Pessi A, Carfi A. Structure of a proteolytically resistant core from the severe acute respiratory syndrome coronavirus S2 fusion protein. Proc Natl Acad Sci U S A. 2004; 101(52):17958–63.
10. Chang SH, Bae JL, Kang TJ, Kim J, Chung GH, Lim CW, Laude H, Yang MS, Jang YS. Identification of the epitope region capable of inducing neutralizing antibodies against the porcine epidemic diarrhea virus. Molecules and cells. 2002;14(2):295–9.
11. Knuchel M, Ackermann M, Muller HK, Kihm U. An ELISA for detection of antibodies against porcine epidemic diarrhoea virus (PEDV) based on the specific solubility of the viral surface glycoprotein. Vet Microbiol. 1992;32(2):117–34.
12. Sun DB, Feng L, Shi HY, Chen JF, Liu SW, Chen HY, Wang YF. Spike protein region (aa 636789) of porcine epidemic diarrhea virus is essential for induction of neutralizing antibodies. Acta Virol. 2007;51(3):149–56.
13. Deng F, Ye G, Liu Q, Navid MT, Zhong X, Li Y, Wan C, Xiao S, He Q, Fu ZF, et al. Identification and comparison of receptor binding characteristics of the spike protein of two porcine epidemic diarrhea virus strains. Viruses. 2016;8(3):55.
14. Paudel S, Park JE, Jang H, Shin HJ. Comparison of serum neutralization and enzyme-linked immunosorbent assay on sera from porcine epidemic diarrhea virus vaccinated pigs. The Veterinary quarterly. 2014;34(4):218–23.
15. Lin H, Chen L, Gao L, Yuan X, Ma Z, Fan H. Epidemic strain YC2014 of porcine epidemic diarrhea virus could provide piglets against homologous challenge. Virol J. 2016;13:68.
16. Kim SH, Kim IJ, Pyo HM, Tark DS, Song JY, Hyun BH. Multiplex real-time RT-PCR for the simultaneous detection and quantification of transmissible gastroenteritis virus and porcine epidemic diarrhea virus. J Virol Methods. 2007; 146(1–2):172–7.
17. Li W, Li H, Liu Y, Pan Y, Deng F, Song Y, Tang X, He Q. New variants of porcine epidemic diarrhea virus, China, 2011. Emerg Infect Dis. 2012;18(8):1350–3.
18. Li Z, Chen F, Yuan Y, Zeng X, Wei Z, Zhu L, Sun B, Xie Q, Cao Y, Xue C, et al. Sequence and phylogenetic analysis of nucleocapsid genes of porcine epidemic diarrhea virus (PEDV) strains in China. Arch Virol. 2013;158(6):1267–73.
19. Oh JS, Song DS, Yang JS, Song JY, Moon HJ, Kim TY, Park BK. Comparison of an enzyme-linked immunosorbent assay with serum neutralization test for serodiagnosis of porcine epidemic diarrhea virus infection. J Vet Sci. 2005; 6(4):349–52.
20. Thachil A, Gerber PF, Xiao CT, Huang YW, Opriessnig T. Development and application of an ELISA for the detection of porcine deltacoronavirus IgG antibodies. PLoS One. 2015;10(4):e0124363.
21. Gerber PF, Gong Q, Huang YW, Wang C, Holtkamp D, Opriessnig T. Detection of antibodies against porcine epidemic diarrhea virus in serum and colostrum by indirect ELISA. Vet J. 2014;202(1):33–6.
22. Cruz DJ, Kim CJ, Shin HJ. Phage-displayed peptides having antigenic similarities with porcine epidemic diarrhea virus (PEDV) neutralizing epitopes. Virology. 2006;354(1):28–34.
23. Sun D, Feng L, Shi H, Chen J, Cui X, Chen H, Liu S, Tong Y, Wang Y, Tong G. Identification of two novel B cell epitopes on porcine epidemic diarrhea virus spike protein. Vet Microbiol. 2008;131(1–2):73–81.
24. Jung K, Saif LJ. Porcine epidemic diarrhea virus infection: etiology, epidemiology, pathogenesis and immunoprophylaxis. Vet J. 2015; 204(2):134–43.
25. Poonsuk K, Gimenez-Lirola LG, Zhang J, Arruda P, Chen Q, Correa da Silva Carrion L, Magtoto R, Pineyro P, Sarmento L, Wang C, et al. Does circulating antibody play a role in the protection of piglets against porcine epidemic diarrhea virus? PLoS One. 2016;11(4):e0153041.
26. Lin CM, Gao X, Oka T, Vlasova AN, Esseili MA, Wang Q, Saif LJ. Antigenic relationships among porcine epidemic diarrhea virus and transmissible gastroenteritis virus strains. J Virol. 2015;89(6):3332–42.

Spatial multi-criteria decision analysis to predict suitability for African swine fever endemicity in Africa

William A de Glanville[1,3*], Laurence Vial[2], Solenne Costard[1,4], Barbara Wieland[1] and Dirk U Pfeiffer[1]

Abstract

Background: African swine fever (ASF) is endemic in several countries of Africa and may pose a risk to all pig producing areas on the continent. Official ASF reporting is often rare and there remains limited awareness of the continent-wide distribution of the disease.
In the absence of accurate ASF outbreak data and few quantitative studies on the epidemiology of the disease in Africa, we used spatial multi-criteria decision analysis (MCDA) to derive predictions of the continental distribution of suitability for ASF persistence in domestic pig populations as part of sylvatic or domestic transmission cycles. In order to incorporate the uncertainty in the relative importance of different criteria in defining suitability, we modelled decisions within the MCDA framework using a stochastic approach. The predictive performance of suitability estimates was assessed via a partial ROC analysis using ASF outbreak data reported to the OIE since 2005.

Results: Outputs from the spatial MCDA indicate that large areas of sub-Saharan Africa may be suitable for ASF persistence as part of either domestic or sylvatic transmission cycles. Areas with high suitability for pig to pig transmission ('domestic cycles') were estimated to occur throughout sub-Saharan Africa, whilst areas with high suitability for introduction from wildlife reservoirs ('sylvatic cycles') were found predominantly in East, Central and Southern Africa. Based on average AUC ratios from the partial ROC analysis, the predictive ability of suitability estimates for domestic cycles alone was considerably higher than suitability estimates for sylvatic cycles alone, or domestic and sylvatic cycles in combination.

Conclusions: This study provides the first standardised estimates of the distribution of suitability for ASF transmission associated with domestic and sylvatic cycles in Africa. We provide further evidence for the utility of knowledge-driven risk mapping in animal health, particularly in data-sparse environments.

Keywords: African swine fever, Knowledge-driven risk mapping, Multi-criteria decision analysis

Background

African swine fever (ASF) is a severe and highly contagious viral infection of domestic pigs. Outbreaks have been reported from almost all the countries of Africa that occur on or below the equator, as well as several countries of West Africa and the islands of Madagascar and Cape Verde [1,2]. The disease can impose severe limitations on pig production in endemic countries, as well as in adjoining areas, which may be at high risk of virus introduction [3,4]. The ASF virus (ASFV) has repeatedly spread outside Africa via the movement of pigs or pig products and continues to pose a considerable threat to pig production in the wider world [1].

Conditions leading to ASF endemicity in domestic pigs in Africa are not fully understood but are likely to vary on a regional basis. In parts of eastern and southern Africa, for example, cycles involving wild suids, such as warthogs (*Phacochoerus africanus*) and soft tick vectors of the *Ornithodoros moubata* complex provide a reservoir of ASFV for domestic pigs [5]. Such 'sylvatic' cycles may allow the disease to persist in pig populations, even in areas with low pig population density. In parts of

* Correspondence: w.a.de-glanville@sms.ed.ac.uk
[1]The Royal Veterinary College, Hawkshead Lane, Hatfield, Hertfordshire AL9 7TA, UK
[3]Current address: Centre for Immunity, Infection and Evolution (CIIE), Ashworth Laboratories, University of Edinburgh, Edinburgh, UK
Full list of author information is available at the end of the article

West Africa, on the other hand, sylvatic cycles have been infrequently described and endemicity is more likely to be the result of sustained virus transmission within high density and highly connected pig populations [2,6-8]. Factors contributing to the transmission of ASF in these 'domestic' pig cycles may include the use of free-ranging husbandry methods, the movement of infected pigs between farms and to markets, and the feeding of contaminated domestic waste to pigs [1]. African swine fever endemicity in domestic pig populations in Africa may therefore be the result of cycles involving repeated virus introduction from wild suid reservoirs, sustained virus spread within domestic pig populations, or a combination of both.

Risk maps can be used to provide a visual representation of the spatial distribution of the risk of an event, and have been advocated as having a role in the development of targeted disease surveillance and control activities [9,10]. Disease risk maps are traditionally developed as an extension of a statistical modelling process in which geographically explicit predictor variables are used to estimate the probability of disease occurrence [11-13]. Such 'data-driven' methods are limited to those areas in which surveillance activities have effective coverage, or in which epidemiological studies can provide adequate data to describe the distribution of a disease. In areas where these data are unavailable, as is often the case for animal diseases in developing countries, a more pragmatic approach to risk mapping has been proposed [14,15]. 'Knowledge-driven' risk mapping is one such approach that uses literature based-evidence or expert opinion, rather than a empirical exploration of available data, to describe the relative importance of risk factors for a disease [16]. In data sparse environments, this evidence can be integrated into a formal decision making process to predict the suitability of a geographic area for disease occurrence based on the presence of the identified risk factors.

The likelihood of infectious disease occurrence is typically influenced by multiple interacting factors. Knowledge-driven disease risk mapping should therefore be performed as part of a formal and systematic evaluation framework that takes into account the relative contribution each factor makes to the overall estimation of suitability. Multi-criteria decision analysis (MCDA), a methodology that allows the analysis of complex decision problems involving conflicting criteria, has previously been used within a geographic information system (GIS) for this purpose [14,15,17,18]. Broadly, MCDA allows the prioritisation of the criteria that influence a decision, and provides a framework by which users can reach a decision that reflects these priorities. In the context of risk mapping, 'criteria' are risk factors for an undesirable event, such as disease occurrence, while the 'decision' relates to the estimation of suitability of an area for the event, and therefore the relative likelihood that it can occur.

In the absence of available (or reliable) disease data to adequately describe the distribution of ASF in domestic pigs in Africa, we used a spatial MCDA to predict suitability for repeated introduction of the virus into pig populations from sylvatic reservoirs and suitability for sustained spread within domestic pig populations. African swine fever has a complex epidemiology with multiple pathways for introduction and spread [1]. There remains considerable uncertainty about the relative importance of these different transmission routes, and the risk factors that influence them, particularly in Africa where few quantitative epidemiological studies have been performed. In order to incorporate some of this uncertainty into the MCDA procedure, we used a probabilistic framework that describes the contribution each risk factor makes to suitability of an area for ASF persistence in domestic pig populations via sylvatic or domestic transmission cycles.

Methods

Multi-criteria decision analysis (MCDA)

The MCDA procedure used in this study involved the following general steps (modified from Store and Kangas [19]):

1. *Assessment of the suitability structure*: identifying risk factors for ASF transmission and determining their importance in relation to the objective(s).
2. *Producing spatial layers*: raw data acquisition and transformation to the appropriate GIS layers.
3. *Cartographic modelling*: combining risk factor layers based on the suitability structures defined.
4. *Validation*: comparison of suitability predictions with available disease data.

Assessment of the suitability structure

Probable risk factors for ASF transmission in Africa

On the basis of a literature review, risk factors were identified that are expected to influence the suitability of an area for repeated transmission of ASF into domestic pig populations from sylvatic reservoirs (the 'sylvatic' cycle) *(objective 1)* or suitability for sustained transmission of ASF within domestic pig populations (the 'domestic' cycle) (*objective 2*). Repeat transmission via either cycle could be expected to lead to ASF persistence and endemicity. Risk factors for ASFV transmission, and the availability of evidence to support their role in the epidemiology of the disease, have been extensively reviewed in a number of recent papers [1,2,5,7,20], and we thus provide only a summary of the literature.

Warthogs (*Phacochoerus africanus)* have long been recognised as a major reservoir of ASFV for domestic pigs in Africa and outbreaks are frequently reported when pigs are reared in areas in which warthogs are common [5]. The transmission of ASFV from infected warthogs to domestic pigs typically occurs via *Ornithodoros* spp. tick vectors [21], although transmission may also occur as a result of contact with contaminated wild suid carcasses [22]. Free-living bushpigs (*Potamochoerus porcus* and *P. larvatus*) and giant forest hogs (*Hylochoerus meinertzhageni*) have also been found to be infected with ASFV [5] and may therefore act as a reservoir in areas in which they occur. The epidemiological significance of bushpigs or giant forest hogs, and the extent to which these species interact with *Ornithodoros* spp. ticks in the transmission of ASFV to domestic pigs, has not been fully determined, but is generally considered to be small in comparison to warthogs [5,20].

As well as parasitising wild suids, *Ornithodoros* spp. inhabit cracks and crevices in pig pens and people's homes, where they may feed on domestic pigs [23]. Some *Ornithodoros* spp. ticks have been shown to be capable of transovarial, transtadial and sexual transmission of ASFV [24], and can survive for long periods without feeding [25]. These tick vectors may therefore contribute to the persistence of ASF within domestic pig populations, even in the absence of wild suid reservoirs and, occasionally, in the long term absence of viraemic domestic pig hosts [26]. *Ornithodoros* spp., which occur widely in sub-Saharan Africa [23,27-29], are thought to contribute to disease endemicity in Malawi [30], but little evidence has been found for a role for soft tick vectors in domestic (or sylvatic) cycles in West Africa [31], and few studies have been conducted in the rest of sub-Saharan Africa.

The role of pig population density has not, to our knowledge, been determined for ASF in Africa, although it was found to be a predictor of disease risk during recent outbreaks in Russia [32]. High pig or pig farm density has been shown to be associated with infection risk for a variety of viral pig diseases [33,34] and the risk of introduction of infection from wildlife has been related to higher domestic animal density more generally [35].

Infected pigs can shed ASFV for several weeks, hence pig movement between farms, to markets and to slaughter is likely to be a major route by which the virus spreads within domestic pig populations [1], although there have been relatively few studies to quantify the importance of these factors in Africa [6,8,36]. A higher density of road networks was found to increase ASF risk in Russia [32], further highlighting the probable importance of trade on disease transmission as part of the domestic cycle.

Given the available information, we identified the following risk factors as potentially contributing to the suitability of an area for objective 1 ('sylvatic cycles'): occurrence of warthogs; occurrence of bushpigs; occurrence of giant forest hogs; occurrence of *Ornithodoros* tick spp.; pig population density. The following factors were considered important in describing the suitability of an area for objective 2 ('domestic cycles'): proximity to major market centres, acting as a proxy for trade in pigs and their products; pig population density; and the occurrence of *Ornithodoros* tick spp.

Suitability structure

Warthogs, bushpigs and giant forest hogs are likely to have variable importance in the epidemiology of ASF in Africa, with each interacting differently with *Ornithodoros* spp. and pig population density in the transmission of the disease to domestic pigs [5]. The suitability of an area for the introduction of ASF from wildlife reservoirs (*objective 1*) was therefore considered using the hierarchical approach shown in Figure 1. For this, the likelihood of introduction of ASF from each species was assessed separately based on the interaction between wild suid habitat suitability (as a proxy for probability that the wild suid species occurs in an area), *Ornithodoros* spp. habitat suitability (as a proxy for the probability tick vectors occur in an area) and pig population density. The overall suitability could then be considered as the weighted average of the individual suitabilities for each wild suid species, with weights assigned based on the perceived importance of each species in the transmission of ASF to domestic pigs. The suitability of an area for sustained spread within domestic pig populations considered the interaction between pig population density, *Ornithodoros* spp. habitat suitability (as a proxy for the probability tick vectors occur in an area) and proximity to major market centres.

As well as these 'suitability' criteria (i.e. risk factors), possible constraints on the suitability of an area for sustained transmission of ASFV through sylvatic or domestic cycles were identified. For *objective 1*, constraints on the suitability of an area for the introduction of ASF from each wild suid species were considered to be those areas in which warthogs, bushpigs or giant forest hogs were presumed to be entirely absent (i.e. outside the species' usual range). For both objectives, areas of Africa in which domestic pigs are absent were considered to constrain suitability for sustained ASF transmission via either cycle.

Estimating criteria weights

Comparing risk factors

A pairwise comparison approach [37] was used to define the relative importance of each of the identified suitability criteria (risk factors) in relation to objective 1 or 2. Each criterion was compared with each of the other criteria for each objective, and assigned a score using the preference statements described in Table 1. Hence, risk factor *y* could be considered equally to extremely more (less) important when compared to risk factor *z* in relation to the objective of interest. To approximate the uncertainty that existed in these estimates of relative importance, a Betapert distribution was created for each pairwise comparison using the @Risk add-on for Microsoft

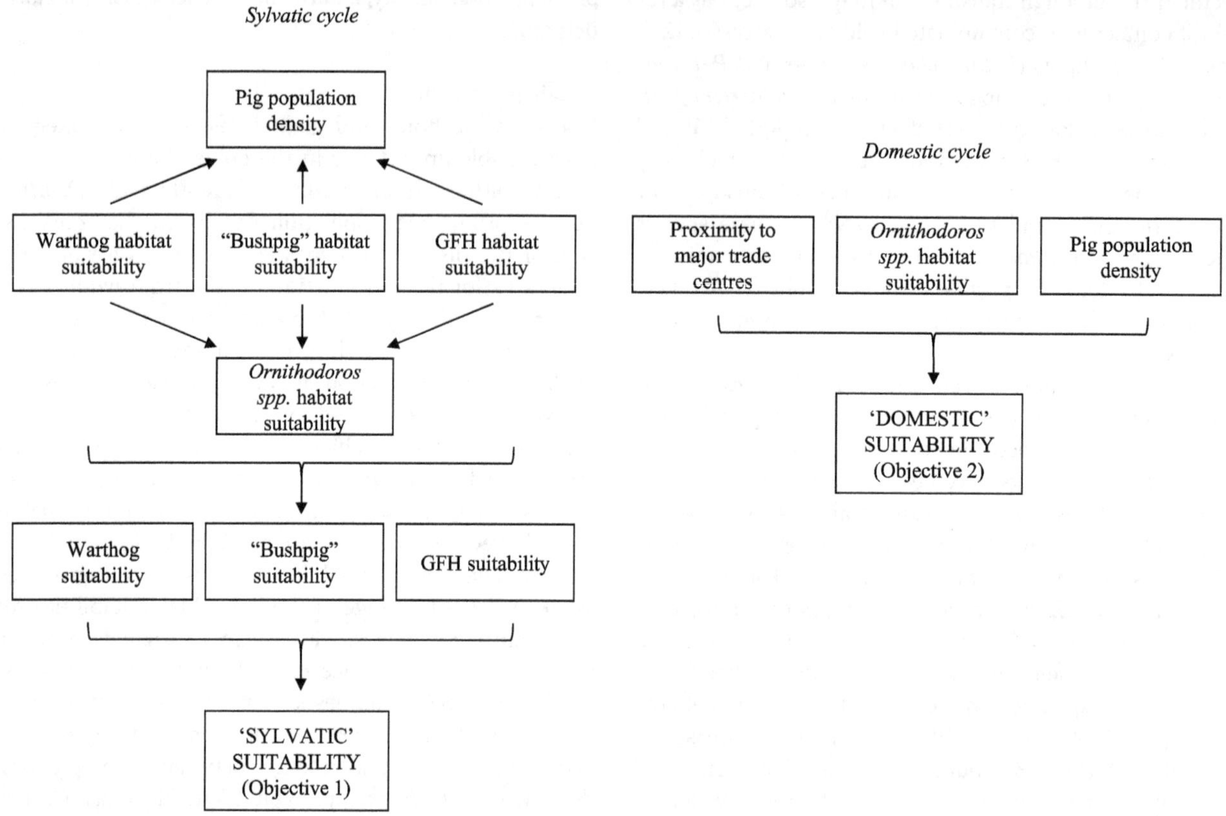

Figure 1 Framework for the MCDA procedure.

Excel (@Risk for Excel, Version 5.5., Palisade Corp., Newfield, NY). The distribution was defined on the basis of the expected minimum, most likely and maximum preference value for each pairwise comparison.

All pairwise comparisons were conducted by the lead author based on his own subjective assessment of the evidence available through literature review, and were reviewed with the co-authors who have all previously contributed peer-reviewed articles on aspects of the epidemiology of ASF in Africa. The final minimum, most likely, and maximum preference statements for each pairwise-comparison were those that were agreed by all authors.

Table 1 Preference statements and values used in pairwise-comparisons (after Saaty [35])

Value	Description
1	Equally important
2	Equal to moderately more important
3	Moderately more important
4	Moderately to strongly more important
5	Strongly more important
6	Strong to very strongly more important
7	Very strongly more important
8	Strongly to extremely more important
9	Extremely more important

Risk factor weights

In order to derive a weight for each suitability criterion that would correspond to its relative importance in relation to each objective, a comparison matrix was built using single values drawn from the distributions of pairwise comparisons. The resulting matrix was reciprocal, so that the pairwise-comparison for risk factor y and risk factor z was, $a_{yz} = a_{yz}^{-1}$ and all of its diagonal elements were unity, so that $a_{yz} = 1$ when $y = z$.

The preference values for each factor were summarised to derive a vector of weights by normalising the eigenvector associated with the maximum eigenvalue of the pairwise comparison matrix [38], so that:

$$a_{yz} = \frac{a_{yz}}{\sum_{y-1}^{1} a_{yz}} \text{ for all } z = 1, 2 \ldots .n.$$

and the specific weights for each factor were given by:

$$w_y = \hat{a}_{yz}$$

To prevent the generation of comparison matrices that could be considered inconsistent (i.e. in which the magnitude of the preference statement assigned to y vs. x and z vs. x was not consistent when comparing z vs. y), we assessed the overall consistency of each comparison matrix by calculating a 'consistency index' (CI) as the eigenvector of the normalised pairwise comparison matrix as:

$$CI = \frac{\gamma_{max} - p}{p - 1}$$

where γ_{max} is the largest eigenvalue that can be obtained once we have its associated eigenvector and p is the number of columns of the matrix [39]. The resultant matrix specific consistency index was then divided by a randomly generated consistency index to produce a 'consistency ratio' (CR). Comparisons were considered to be consistent if the CR was less than 0.1 based on the system defined by Saaty [37]. All comparison matrices in which the consistency ratio was 0.1 or greater were discarded. This process was repeated over multiple iterations, with comparison matrices populated by values drawn by Monte Carlo sampling from the Betapert distribution representing each pairwise-comparison, until a large number of consistent matrices and weights (at least 3000) were generated for each risk factor for each of the two objectives. The output was considered to represent the distribution of possible weights for each factor under consideration, given the authors' uncertainty in the factor's importance in relation to each objective.

The process was automated using the VBA programming language (Microsoft Corp) and implemented in Microsoft Excel (2010).

Producing spatial layers

Raster maps for the suitability criteria and constraints identified through the literature review were sourced and mapped in ArcMap 10 (ESRI, Redlands, CA). The source and structure of the spatial data used to represent suitability layers are given in Table 2. In the absence of data of sufficient accuracy to represent areas in which domestic pigs do not occur, a human population density of zero per km^2 (as defined by Landscan 2008, High Resolution Global Population Data Set, UT-Battelle, LLC, operator of Oak Ridge National Laboratory, US) was considered to provide the best evidence of areas in which domestic pigs cannot occur. This constraint layer and that representing the predicted home ranges of warthogs, the two bushpig species and giant forest hogs (as sourced from the African Mammals Databank (AMD) [40]), were converted into Boolean functions of 'suitable' and 'unsuitable' and assigned a value of 1 or 0, respectively.

Continuous values from each raster layer representing the suitability criteria (Table 2) and the Boolean constraints were extracted from each cell of a grid with a cell size 0.8 × 0.8 decimal degrees over the whole of mainland Africa and exported directly into Microsoft Excel, resulting in a dataset consisting of approximately 360,000 individual data points for each of the criteria. Suitability values were standardised to a common monotonic linear scale between 0 and 1 using the maximum score procedure [39], so that for linearly increasing criteria:

$$x'_{ij} = {}^{x_{ij}}/_{x_{jmax}}$$

And for linearly decreasing criteria:

$$x'_{ij} = 1 - {}^{x_{ij}}/_{x_{jmax}}$$

Where x_{ij} is the raw score for criterion j and x_{jmax} represents the point at which its contribution to predictions of suitability becomes zero: all values above x_{jmax}

Table 2 Data and standardisation approaches to derive suitability layers for the MCDA procedure

Suitability criterion	Source	Type	Standardisation		Shape
			x_{jmin}	x_{jmax}	
Warthog habitat suitability	African mammals databank (http://www.gisbau.uniroma1.it/amd/)	Continuous probability surface (habitat suitability)	1	RiskUniform (35,50)[1]	Linear decreasing[2]
Bushpig (*P. porcus*) habitat suitability	African mammals databank	Continuous probability surface (habitat suitability)	1	RiskUniform (10,37)[1]	Linear decreasing[2]
Bushpig (*P. larvatus*) habitat suitability	African mammals databank	Continuous probability surface (habitat suitability)	1	RiskUniform(11,26)[1]	Linear decreasing[2]
Giant forest hog habitat suitability	African mammals databank	Continuous probability surface (habitat suitability)	1	RiskUniform (11,40)[1]	Linear decreasing[2]
Pig population density	FAO GLW (http://www.fao.org/ag/AGAInfo/resources/en/glw/GLW_dens.html)	Predicted density surface pigs/km^2 (adjusted to match FAOSTAT 2005 national totals)	0	RiskUniform (1,14)[1]	Linear increasing
Ornithodoros spp. habitat suitability	Unpublished data (Vial and Estrada-Pena)	Continuous probability surface (habitat suitability)	10	100	Linear increasing
Travel time to market centres >20,000	Harvest Choice (http://harvestchoice.org/products/data)	Raster describing travel time (hrs)	0	RiskUniform (15,30)[1]	Linear decreasing

[1]Lower and upper bounds of the distribution defined by the 90th and 99th percentile of values for Africa within area defined by model constraints; [2]Values describe the Mahalanobis distance from ideal habitat suitability: suitability decreases as distance increases (see [40] for full details).

were assigned a value of 1 for criteria that increased linearly or 0 for criteria that decreased linearly. Where uncertainty existed in the appropriate value of, x_{jmax} a uniform distribution was defined using @risk in which maximum and minimum values for x_{jmax} were described by the 99th and 90th percentile of the distribution of values of each variable within the areas defined as suitable within the constraints for each cycle (Table 2).

Cartographic modelling

In order to derive an estimate of suitability, *S*, for each sampled point *i* in relation to each objective, the standardised suitability values and the weight for each criterion derived from the pairwise-comparison procedure (*w*) were combined using weighted linear combination (WLC) [39], so that:

$$S = \sum w_j x_{ij} c_i$$

where c_i represents constraint layers coded as 1 or 0 to describe suitability or unsuitability, respectively.

To incorporate the full range of possible combinations of *w* for each criterion, as well as the uncertainty associated with the standardisation of suitability layers, the process was repeated over 3000 iterations, with a specific weight combination randomly selected by Monte Carlo sampling for each iteration. Hence, each sampled point was associated with 3000 possible estimates of suitability (*S*) for each objective based on the linear combination of values of *x*. Three thousand iterations were used to allow the incorporation of the full range of weights (*w*) generated through the iterative pairwise comparison procedure (n = 3000).

The mean value and the 5th and 95th percentiles were extracted from the resulting distributions and exported to ArcMap where point values were converted directly to a continuous raster surface for the visual presentation of results.

To enable formal comparisons of the geographic coverage of areas of predicted suitability for persistence as part of either cycle, we defined a fixed suitability threshold of 0.5 on a 0 to 1 scale [41]. The total land surface area with suitability predictions above this threshold for the whole of Africa and for each of the UN sub-regions of Africa (Northern, Western, Central, Eastern, and Southern Africa) was calculated using the zonal statistics tool in ArcMap and the Lambert Azimuthal Equal Area projection.

Validation

ASF outbreak report data from 2005 to September 2012 for mainland Africa were downloaded from the World Animal Health organisation WAHID system (OIE, 2012). When geographic co-ordinates for the location of a reported outbreak were not provided but a location name was given, 'Fuzzy Gazetteer' (isodp.hof-university.de/fuzzyg) was used to select the most likely co-ordinates for the location of the outbreak.

Validation was performed on the mean suitability estimate for sylvatic cycles, domestic cycles, and a combination of the two. Given the non-independence of predictions for each objective (which were defined using some of the same criteria but with different weightings applied), the combined suitability estimate was derived by combining the mean value for each cycle using an ordered approach where the highest value for either objective was used to define the value at each pixel.

A partial ROC analysis was implemented on the combined suitability estimates and the mean estimates for each cycle using the Partial-ROC tool developed by Barve [42]. Only suitability estimates from countries in which outbreaks had been reported to the OIE were used for validation. The partial ROC is a plot of sensitivity (proportion of correctly predicted disease cases) against the proportion of study area predicted as being suitable for disease occurrence. Hence, the approach does not rely on absence data, which are difficult to generate for ASF for much of Africa, where animal disease surveillance systems are often inadequate. Moreover, the approach allows for the inclusion of a user generated error term (*E*) to account for the amount of error admissible along the true-positives axis (the omission error) [43]. The latitude and longitude describing the geographical location of ASF outbreaks reported to the OIE is typically given at one or two decimal places, and represents the focus of an outbreak that can cover a wide geographic area: the validation dataset can therefore be expected to contain substantial amounts of geo-referencing based error that could contribute to omission error.

The partial ROC output is the ratio of the area under the curve (AUC) of the restricted ROC curve (i.e. the region where the omission error is less than *E*) against the AUC of the restricted null model. Bootstrapping to evaluate the statistical significance of the AUC ratios was performed by resampling 50 % of test points 1000 times from the pool of outbreak data, as described by Peterson et al. [43]. The value of *E* was set at 20 % to represent the likely high levels of geo-referencing error present in the validation set.

Results

Multi-criteria decision analysis

Criteria weights

Objective 1 The pairwise-comparisons used for objective 1 are shown in Table 3 and the resulting weightings for each criterion in Table 4.

Table 3 Minimum, most likely and maximum values for the pairwise comparison of criteria for objective 1

Pairwise comparison*	Min	Most likely	Max
Warthog habitat suitability vs. Pig population density	1	5	9
Ornithodoros. spp. habitat suitability vs. Pig population density	1	3	9
Ornithodoros. spp. habitat suitability vs. Warthog habitat suitability	1	1	5
Bushpig habitat suitability vs. Pig population density	1	5	9
Ornithodoros. spp. habitat suitability vs. Pig population density	1/9	1/5	1/3
Ornithodoros. spp. habitat suitability vs. Bushpig habitat suitability	1/9	1/7	1/5
Giant forest hog (GFH) habitat suitability vs. Pig population density	1	5	9
Ornithodoros. spp. habitat suitability vs. Pig population density	1/9	1/7	1/5
Ornithodoros. spp. habitat suitability vs. GFH habitat suitability	1/9	1/9	1/7
Warthogs vs. Bushpigs	1	4	7
GFHs vs. Bushpigs	1/9	1/5	1/3
GFHs vs. Warthogs	1/9	1/9	1/7

*Minimum, most likely and maximum values defined based of the comparison of the importance of the first criterion in relation to the second for the objective under consideration using the preference statements in Table 1.

The bushpigs and giant forest hogs show a similar pattern of suitability weightings, with habitat suitability considered to be the most important factor in determining the suitability of an area for repeated introduction of ASF from these species, followed by pig density with relatively minor contributions from tick habitat suitability. Tick habitat suitability was considered to be substantially more important in the suitability of an area for sustained transmission of ASF to domestic pigs from warthogs.

The preference values used to describe the general importance of each wild suid species in acting as a reservoir of ASF for domestic pigs are also shown in Table 3, and the associated criterion weights in Table 4. Warthogs were considered to be the most important reservoir species for ASF for domestic pigs, followed by the bushpigs. Giant forest hogs were considered to be comparatively unimportant.

Objective 2 The preference statements from the pairwise estimation of the relative importance of each criterion in relation to objective 2 and the associated weightings are presented in Table 5 and Table 6, respectively. Pig population density was considered to be the most important factor influencing the sustained spread of ASF within domestic pig populations, with proximity to market centres and tick habitat suitability making smaller contributions.

Cartographic modelling

Objective 1 Areas with the highest estimated suitability for repeated introduction of ASF into domestic pig populations from sylvatic reservoirs were predicted in East and Central sub-Saharan Africa, with sustained sylvatic

Table 4 Distributional estimates of weights for criteria for objective 1 derived from the pairwise comparisons in Table 3 (see text)

	Criteria	Mean	5th percentile	95th percentile
	Warthog habitat suitability	0.40	0.30	0.48
Warthog	Pig population density	0.11	0.076	0.16
	Ornithodoros. spp. habitat suitability	0.49	0.41	0.59
	Bushpig habitat suitability	0.63	0.54	0.71
Bushpig	Pig population density	0.29	0.22	0.38
	Ornithodoros. spp. habitat suitability	0.077	0.066	0.089
	GFH habitat suitability	0.64	0.57	0.69
GFH	Pig population density	0.30	0.26	0.37
	Ornithodoros. spp. habitat suitability	0.060	0.055	0.066
	Warthog	0.66	0.57	0.73
Wild suids	Bushpig	0.27	0.20	0.36
	Giant forest hog	0.067	0.059	0.076

Table 5 Minimum, most likely and maximum values for the pairwise comparison of criteria for objective 2

Pairwise comparison*	Min	Most likely	Max
Ornithodoros. spp. habitat suitability vs. Pig population density	1/7	1/5	1/3
Proximity to market centres vs. Pig population density	1/5	1/3	1
Proximity to market centres vs. *Ornithodoros.* spp. habitat suitability	3	5	7

*Minimum, most likely and maximum values defined based of the comparison of the importance of the first criterion in relation to the second for the objective under consideration using the preference statements in Table 1.

transmission appearing to be relatively unlikely in West Africa, as well as the vast majority of northern and south-western Africa (Figure 2 and Table 7).

The southern Democratic Republic of Congo (DRC), Burundi, Rwanda, eastern Zambia, Malawi, Tanzania, parts of Kenya, Uganda, Zimbabwe, Mozambique and the north-east of South Africa all appear to have areas of relatively high potential suitability for repeated introduction of ASF to domestic pigs from sylvatic cycles.

Objective 2 Areas with apparently high suitability for cycles involving sustained spread of ASF within domestic pig population pathways can be found in all regions of Africa excluding Northern Africa (Figure 3 and Table 7). Countries with the highest suitability for sustained spread within domestic pig populations were predicted to be in South Africa, Malawi, Nigeria, Angola, Cameroon, Burkina Faso, Benin, Togo, Guinea-Bissau, Rwanda and Burundi, as well as smaller parts of Uganda and the DRC.

Validation

A total of 252 primary ASF outbreak reports from 20 countries were identified. The combined suitability estimates showed a very high degree of visual agreement with the outbreaks reported to the OIE (Figure 4). The average partial ROC AUC ratio for the combined sylvatic and domestic suitability estimate was 1.28 (range 1.20 – 1.36), where 0 of 1000 iterations resulted in a ROC AUC ratio ≤1, suggesting a consistently good degree of model predictability for the reported ASF outbreaks. The average AUC ratio when considering mean domestic suitability alone was 1.46 (range 1.30 – 1.62) and was 1.08 (range 1.01 – 1.14) for sylvatic cycles.

Discussion

To our knowledge, this is the first attempt to predict the spatial distribution of ASF in Africa using a standardised approach. The combined suitability estimates derived from the MCDA procedure reveal a good degree of agreement with the distribution of cases reported to the OIE between 2005 and 2012, although the number of officially reported ASF cases are likely to represent only a small proportion of those that actually occur across Africa, particularly in areas in which the disease is endemic. The predicted distribution of areas with high suitability for repeated introduction of ASF from wildlife reservoirs and for sustained transmission within pig populations also supports the anecdotal distribution of sylvatic and domestic pig cycles identified by a number of authors [1,2,5,44].

Outputs from the MCDA procedure suggest that most of western, south-western, and west-central Africa are relatively unsuitable for repeated introduction of ASF from wildlife reservoirs. African swine fever is endemic or approaching a situation of endemicity in several countries in these areas, including Nigeria [45], Senegal [31], Guinea Bissau [46], and Angola [47]. There are areas of widespread suitability for domestic ASF transmission in these countries, and it is likely that the persistence of ASF in such areas is the result of sustained domestic pig transmission cycles, without the need for repeated introduction from wildlife reservoirs [5,20].

Countries that are predicted to have widespread suitability for repeated introduction from sylvatic reservoirs are Tanzania, Zimbabwe, and Malawi. The southern DRC, eastern parts of Zambia, and smaller areas of Uganda, Kenya, Angola, Botswana, South Africa, Burundi, Rwanda and Mozambique also appear to be highly suitable for

Table 6 Distributional estimates of weights for criteria for objective 2 derived from the pairwise comparisons in Table 5 (see text)

Risk factor	Mean	5th percentile	95th percentile
Pig population density	0.56	0.49	0.63
Proximity to market centres	0.35	0.28	0.41
Ornithodoros. spp. habitat suitability	0.093	0.078	0.11

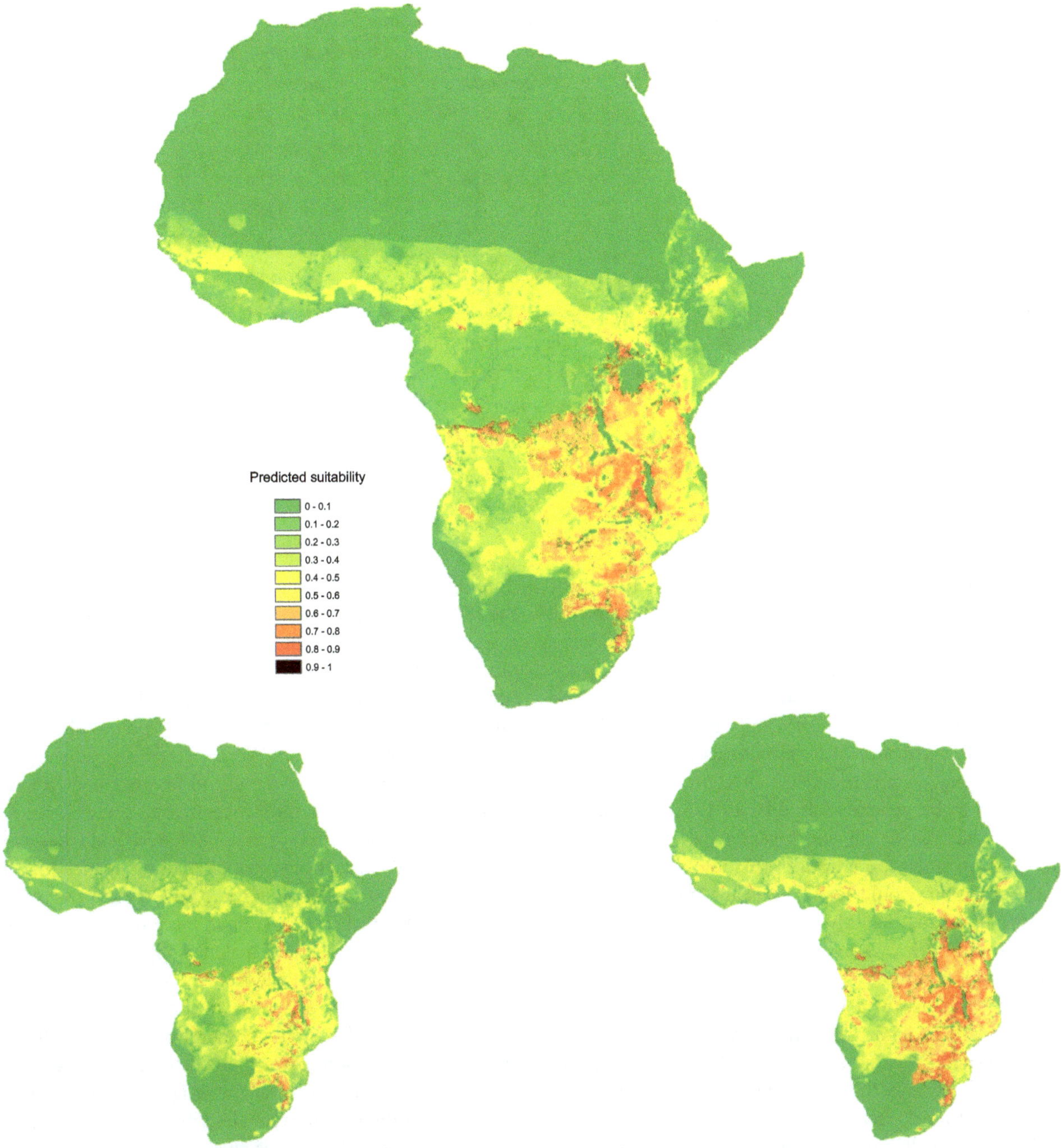

Figure 2 Suitability for ASF persistence as part of sylvatic cycles (5th percentile (left); average (middle); 95th percentile (right)).

ASF transmission associated with sylvatic cycles. Despite this apparently high suitability, the majority of recent ASF outbreaks in these regions are likely to have been caused by the movement of pigs and their products rather than sylvatic spill over [48-50]. We also predict that all of these countries, except Botswana, have a widespread distribution of areas of apparent high suitability for sustained transmission as part of domestic pig cycles. This is particularly the case in Angola, Malawi, Uganda, South Africa and the western DRC. The potential importance of transmission as part of domestic rather than sylvatic cycles in these areas, and continental Africa as a whole, is supported by the considerably higher predictive ability (based on average AUC ratio) of domestic suitability estimates for all areas in which ASF outbreaks have been reported compared to the combined suitability estimates and those for

Table 7 Total predicted land area above a 0.5 suitability threshold for the distributional estimates (5th percentile, mean and 95 % percentile) for each transmission cycle in the UN sub-regions of Africa

	Region	Sub-region land area (Km^2)	Land area predicted above 0.5 threshold (Km^2 (% of total))		
			5th percentile	Mean	95th percentile
Sylvatic	Western Africa	60 x 10^5	56 x 10^2 **(0.09)**	81 x 10^3 **(1.3)**	25 x 10^4 **(4.2)**
	Central Africa	66 x 10^5	61 x 10^4 **(9.3)**	87 x 10^4 **(13.2)**	13 x 10^5 **(20.2)**
	Southern Africa	27 x 10^5	22 x 10^4 **(8.3)**	31 x 10^4 **(11.5)**	40 x 10^4 **(14.9)**
	Eastern Africa	58 x 10^5	14 x 10^5 **(23.7)**	20 x 10^5 **(34.9)**	25 x 10^5 **(44.0)**
	Northern Africa	82 x 10^5	12 x 10^3 **(0.14)**	39 x 10^3 **(0.48)**	96 x 10^3 **(1.2)**
	Total	29 x 10^6	22 x 10^5 **(7.6)**	33 x 10^5 **(11.3)**	46 x 10^5 **(15.7)**
Domestic	Western Africa	60 x 10^5	26 x 10^4 **(4.3)**	47 x 10^4 **(7.9)**	81 x 10^4 **(13.4)**
	Central Africa	66 x 10^5	28 x 10^4 **(4.2)**	50 x 10^4 **(7.7)**	80 x 10^4 **(12.2)**
	Southern Africa	27 x 10^5	88 x 10^3 **(3.3)**	18 x 10^4 **(6.8)**	37 x 10^4 **(14.0)**
	Eastern Africa	58 x 10^5	11 x 10^4 **(1.9)**	30 x 10^4 **(5.2)**	71 x 10^4 **(12.3)**
	Northern Africa	82 x 10^5	64 x 10^2 **(0.08)**	42 x 10^3 **(0.51)**	20 x 10^4 **(2.4)**
	Total	29 x 10^6	74 x 10^4 **(2.5)**	15 x 10^5 **(5.1)**	30 x 10^5 **(10.0)**

sylvatic cycles alone. However, sporadic introduction from wildlife reservoirs should not be ignored as potential risk in such areas [44,51]. Indeed, although bushpigs were given a moderate weight in this study, recent work implicated *P. larvatus* as a possible source of ASF infection for domestic pigs living in close proximity to a National park in Kenya [52]. African swine fever viruses isolated from warthogs living on a cattle ranch in central Kenya were also shown to be genetically similar to those causing recent outbreaks in Kenya and Uganda [53]. Hence, it is quite possible that sporadic introduction of ASFV from sylvatic reservoirs could lead to onward transmission via domestic cycles, particularly in those areas of Central, East and Southern Africa where we predict high suitability for both transmission routes.

Through the use of a stochastic approach, this study has attempted to incorporate uncertainty into several of the key decision making steps in the MCDA procedure, and particularly into the assignment of relative importance scores to risk factor layers. The BetaPert distribution has been widely used for modelling expert opinion [54], and allowed us to incorporate the uncertainty that existed in our subjective assessment of the available evidence. To our knowledge, this is the first example of the formal introduction of stochasticity into a spatial MCDA in the area of disease or health mapping. Such a step is particularly important in the knowledge-driven mapping of diseases such as ASF where, in the absence of quantitative epidemiological studies, the contribution of several putative risk factors is unclear [14,16] and, as in this study, a highly subjective approach is used to assess this contribution. The overall geographic range of suitability for repeated transmission of ASFV as part of the domestic or sylvatic cycle was generally the same across the distribution of estimates. However, the application of a somewhat arbitrary (but commonly used [41]) threshold of 0.5 to dichotomise the output into unsuitable and suitable reveals the extent and impact of our uncertainty on the percentage coverage of areas of potential suitability for either cycle.

Pairwise-comparison is a method that has been applied widely to assess the importance of one factor over another in a decision-making process [38,55], and has been used previously for disease mapping using spatial MCDM [16,17]. An important issue in the pairwise-comparison procedure is that matrices are often inconsistent, potentially leading to senseless decision making [56]. Through the use of an iterative approach, in which the pairwise-comparison matrix is populated by values drawn at random from a distribution defining each pairwise-comparison, it is likely that the frequency of inconsistency in the construction of the matrix and resulting estimation of factor weights was increased in this study. Although the rule described by Saaty [37] was used to combat such inconsistency, the validity of the 10 % cut-off in the resultant consistency ratio has been questioned [57]. Kwiesielewicz and Uden [58] showed that a matrix that passes a consistency test successfully may still be contradictory. Hence, it is acknowledged that, on the basis of the stochastic approach adopted, some of the allocated weights selected from the distributional ranges used may have been the result of inconsistent comparisons. However, given that the resultant risk maps are the summarised estimates of a large number of independent weight combinations, the impact of any such inconsistency is likely to be small.

It is important that outputs from knowledge-driven risk mapping are interpreted in the light of the methodology

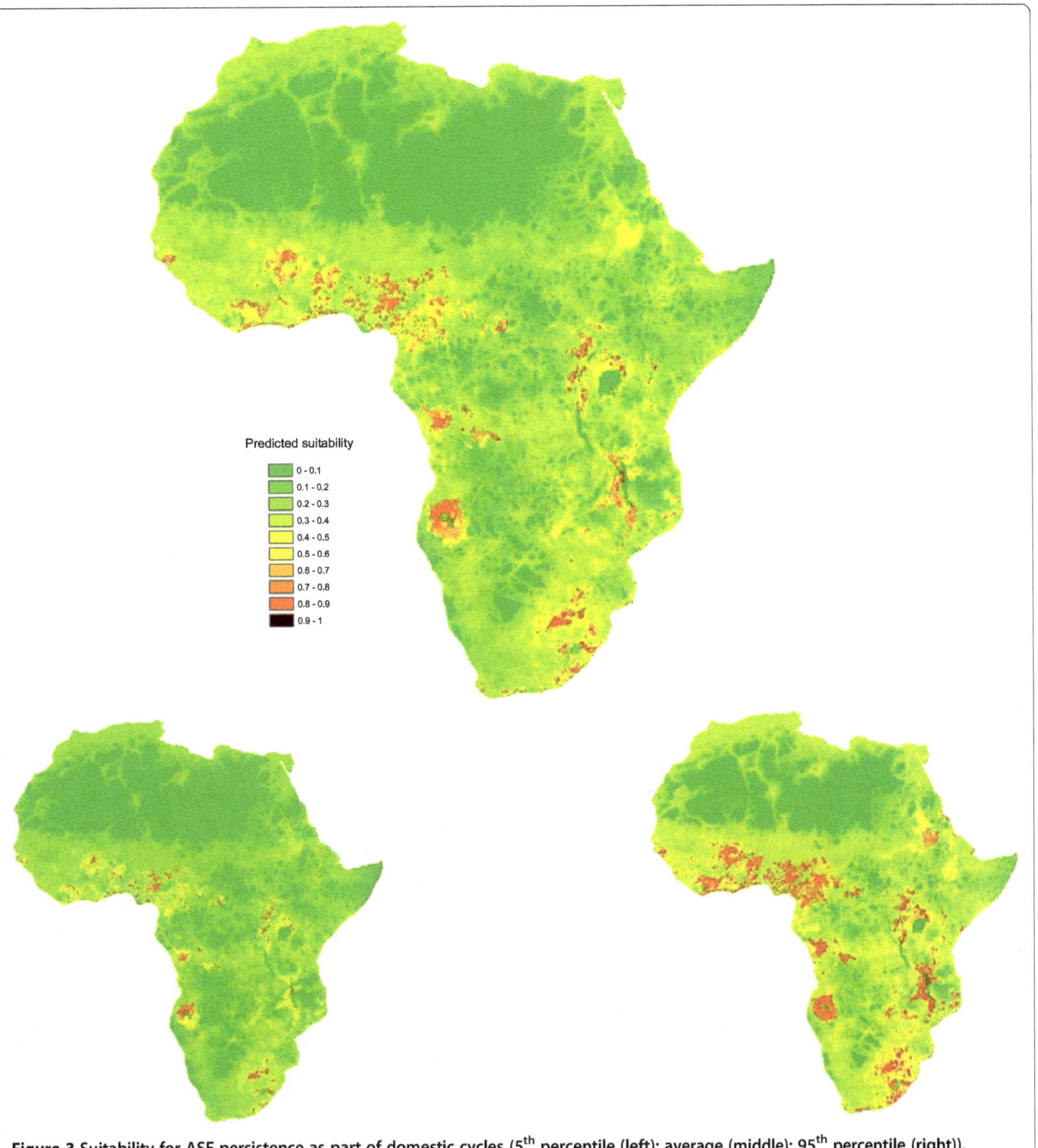

Figure 3 Suitability for ASF persistence as part of domestic cycles (5th percentile (left); average (middle); 95th percentile (right)).

adopted, which remains highly subjective and combines data sources of variable quality, most of which originated from internet-based data repositories. Moreover, the approach can only incorporate those risk factors that can be mapped. Trade of pigs and their products is likely to be a major mechanism by which ASFV spreads within and between regions [1]. The movement of middle-men between farms, for example, has been reported as an important risk factor in the spread of ASFV in Africa [8], but such activities cannot be mapped directly in the absence of spatial data describing such movements. Proximity to major market centres was used as a proxy for this, and other such trade-related activities, but the use of such a variable for this purpose cannot be expected to capture the local scale

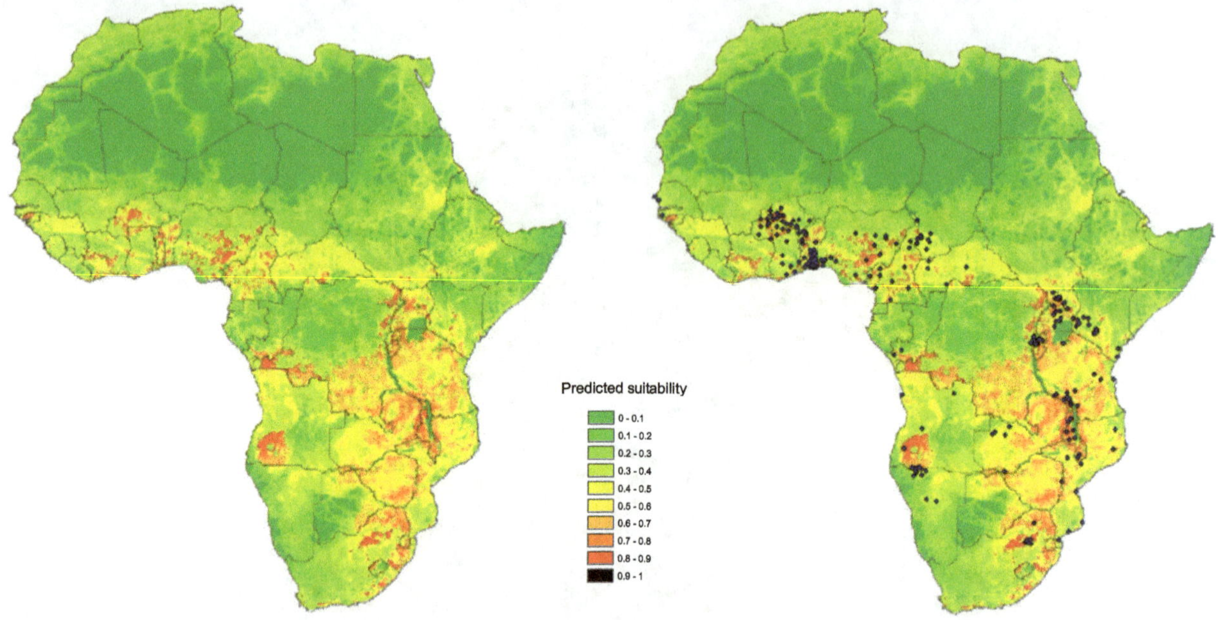

Figure 4 Combined estimates of mean suitability for ASF endemicity in domestic pig populations, with location of ASF outbreaks between 2005 and 2012 overlaid (right).

variability in the movement of animals and contaminated people, equipment and products that may contribute to virus spread.

The MCDA approach relies on knowledge that already exists: to date, there have been few quantitative epidemiological studies of ASF in Africa, and whilst MCDA provides a useful framework with which to aggregate the work that has been conducted, it remains limited by the scope of the available evidence. Given the limited consensus on risk factors for ASF in the literature, our model used limited number of criteria: as additional studies on the epidemiology of ASF in Africa are conducted, the criteria to describe ASF risk and in particular the perceived relative importance of these criteria, could be expected to change [20].

Moreover, this study is an interpretation of the existing knowledge and relationships between these risk factors by the authors only, since no other experts were consulted. Whilst we attempted to limit the potential impact of our subjective assessments through modelling the relative importance of criterion using probability distributions, a different set of experts may have chosen different minimum, most likely and maximum values for the BetaBert distributions, and thus derived somewhat different suitability estimates. The predictions from this work should be should be interpreted accordingly, but it would be reasonable to expect, given the current state of knowledge on ASF in Africa, that another set of experts' average suitability estimates using the same set of criteria would be likely to fall between the 5th and 95th percentiles of our own.

Conclusion

This study used a limited number of known or hypothesised risk factors for ASF and our own subjective assessment of the importance of those risk factors to predict the distribution of ASF persistence via sylvatic and domestic transmission cycles in Africa. The suitability predictions derived are not intended to be interpreted as definitive, instead, they provide a 'best guess' estimate based on the currently available evidence, and our own interpretation of that evidence. With these limitations in mind, outputs from this study indicate that areas of high suitability for transmission as part of domestic cycles occur throughout sub-Saharan Africa. Areas of sylvatic suitability are restricted to Central, East and Southern Africa, but commonly overlap areas of suitability for domestic cycles. Hence, whilst domestic transmission of ASF is likely to be the major means by which the disease persists throughout sub-Saharan Africa, and should probably continue to be the focus of disease control and prevention efforts, the continued potential for spill over from wildlife reservoirs should not be ignored.

Abbreviations

AMD: African Mammals Databank; AUC: Area under the curve; ASF: African swine fever; ASFV: African swine fever virus; CI: Consistency index; CR: Consistency ratio; DRC: Democratic Republic of Congo; GFH: Giant Forest

Hog; GIS: Geographic information system; MCDA: Multi-criteria decision analysis; OIE: World Organisation for Animal Health; ROC: Receiver operating characteristic; WAHID: World Animal Health Information Database; WLC: Weighted linear combination.

Competing interests
No author has any competing interest to declare.

Authors' contributions
WAdeG, SC, BW and DUP designed the study. WAdeG performed data analysis as part of the study. All authors contributed to the development of risk factor weightings. All authors made contributions to the conception, design, and revision of the manuscript. All authors read and approved the final manuscript.

Acknowledgements
This work was funded by the ASFRISK project; "Evaluating and controlling the risk of African swine fever in the EU" (EC, FP7-KBBE-2007-1, Project #211691). The funder had no role in study design, data collection and analysis, decision to publish, or preparation of the manuscript. We thank Kim Stevens for discussions on methodology.

Author details
[1]The Royal Veterinary College, Hawkshead Lane, Hatfield, Hertfordshire AL9 7TA, UK. [2]Centre International de Recherche Agronomique pour le Developpement, Montpellier, France. [3]Current address: Centre for Immunity, Infection and Evolution (CIIE), Ashworth Laboratories, University of Edinburgh, Edinburgh, UK. [4]Current address: EpiX Analytics, 1643 Spruce Street, Boulder, CO 80302, USA.

References
1. Costard S, Wieland B, de Glanville W, Jori F, Rowlands R, Vosloo W, Roger F, Pfeiffer DU, Dixon LK: **African swine fever: how can global spread be prevented?** *Philos Trans R Soc Lond B Biol Sci* 2009, **364**:2683–2696.
2. Penrith ML, Vosloo W: **Review of African swine fever: transmission, spread and control.** *J S Afr Vet Assoc* 2009, **80**:58–62.
3. el Hicheri K, Gomez-Tejedor C, Penrith ML, Davies G, Douati A, Edoukou GJ, Wojciechowski K: **The 1996 epizootic of African swine fever in the Ivory Coast.** *Rev - Off Int Epizoot* 1998, **17**:660–673.
4. Roger F, Ratovonjato J, Vola P, Uilenber G: **Ornithodoros porcinus ticks, bushpigs, and African swine fever in Madagascar.** *Exp Appl Acarol* 2001, **25**:263–269.
5. Jori F, Bastos ADS: **Role of wild suids in the epidemiology of African swine fever.** *Ecohealth* 2009, **6**:296–310.
6. Babalobi OO, Olugasa BO, Oluwayelu DO, Ijagbone IF, Ayoade GO, Agbede SA: **Analysis and evaluation of mortality losses of the 2001 African swine fever outbreak, Ibadan, Nigeria.** *Trop Anim Health Prod* 2007, **39**:533–542.
7. Costard S, Mur L, Lubroth J, Sánchez-Vizcaíno JM, Pfeiffer DU: **Epidemiology of African swine fever virus.** *Virus Res* 2013, **173**:191–197.
8. Olugasa BO, Ijagbone IF: **Pattern of spread of African swine fever in south-western Nigeria, 1997–2005.** *Vet Ital* 2007, **43**:621–628.
9. Blanton JD, Manangan A, Manangan J, Hanlon CA, Slate D, Rupprecht CE: **Development of a GIS-based, real-time Internet mapping tool for rabies surveillance.** *Int J Health Geogr* 2006, **5**:47.
10. Clements ACA, Pfeiffer DU: **Emerging viral zoonoses: frameworks for spatial and spatiotemporal risk assessment and resource planning.** *Vet J* 2009, **182**:21–30.
11. Elnaiem D-EA, Schorscher J, Bendall A, Obsomer V, Osman ME, Mekkawi AM, Connor SJ, Ashford RW, Thomson MC: **Risk mapping of visceral leishmaniasis: the role of local variation in rainfall and altitude on the presence and incidence of kala-azar in eastern Sudan.** *Am J Trop Med Hyg* 2003, **68**:10–17.
12. Haque U, Magalhães RJS, Reid HL, Clements ACA, Ahmed SM, Islam A, Yamamoto T, Haque R, Glass GE: **Spatial prediction of malaria prevalence in an endemic area of Bangladesh.** *Malaria J* 2010, **9**:120.
13. Ortiz-Pelaez A, Pfeiffer DU, Tempia S, Otieno FT, Aden HH, Costagli R: **Risk mapping of Rinderpest sero-prevalence in Central and Southern Somalia based on spatial and network risk factors.** *BMC Vet Res* 2010, **6**:22.
14. Clements ACA, Pfeiffer DU, Martin V: **Application of knowledge-driven spatial modelling approaches and uncertainty management to a study of Rift Valley fever in Africa.** *Int J Health Geogr* 2006, **5**:57.
15. Stevens KB, Gilbert M, Pfeiffer DU: **Modeling habitat suitability for occurrence of highly pathogenic avian influenza virus H5N1 in domestic poultry in Asia: a spatial multicriteria decision analysis approach.** *Spat Spatiotemporal Epidemiol* 2013, **4**:1–14.
16. Stevens KB, Pfeiffer DU: **Spatial modelling of disease using data- and knowledge-driven approaches.** *Spat Spatiotemporal Epidemiol* 2011, **2**:125–133.
17. Hongoh V, Hoen AG, Aenishaenslin C, Waaub J-P, Bélanger D, Michel P, Lyme-MCDA Consortium: **Spatially explicit multi-criteria decision analysis for managing vector-borne diseases.** *Int J Health Geogr* 2011, **10**:70.
18. Symeonakis E, Robinson T, Drake N: **GIS and multiple-criteria evaluation for the optimisation of tsetse fly eradication programmes.** *Environ Monit Assess* 2007, **124**:89–103.
19. Store R, Kangas J: **Integrating spatial multi-criteria evaluation and expert knowledge for GIS-based habitat suitability modelling.** *Landsc Urban Plann* 2001, **55**:79–93.
20. Jori F, Vial L, Penrith ML, Pérez-Sánchez R, Etter E, Albina E, Michaud V, Roger F: **Review of the sylvatic cycle of African swine fever in sub-Saharan Africa and the Indian ocean.** *Virus Res* 2013, **173**:212–227.
21. Thomson GR: **The epidemiology of African swine fever: the role of free-living hosts in Africa.** *Onderstepoort J Vet Res* 1985, **52**:201–209.
22. Thomson GR, Gainaru MD, Van Dellen AF: **Experimental infection of warthogs (Phacochoerus aethiopicus) with African swine fever virus.** *Onderstepoort J Vet Res* 1980, **47**:19–22.
23. McCall PJ, Hume JCC, Motshegwa K, Pignatelli P, Talbert A, Kisinza W: **Does tick-borne relapsing fever have an animal reservoir in East Africa?** *Vector Borne Zoonotic Dis* 2007, **7**:659–666.
24. Rennie L, Wilkinson PJ, Mellor PS: **Transovarial transmission of African swine fever virus in the argasid tick Ornithodoros moubata.** *Med Vet Entomol* 2001, **15**:140–146.
25. Wardley RC, De M, Andrade C, Black DN, De Castro Portugal FL, Enjuanes L, Hess WR, Mebus C, Ordas A, Rutili D, Sanchez Vizcaino J, Vigario JD, Wilkinson PJ, Moura Nunes JF, Thomson G: **African swine fever virus.** *Arch Virol* 1983, **76**:73–90.
26. Pérez-Sánchez R, Astigarraga A, Oleaga-Pérez A, Encinas-Grandes A: **Relationship between the persistence of African swine fever and the distribution of Ornithodoros erraticus in the province of Salamanca, Spain.** *Vet Rec* 1994, **135**:207–209.
27. Plowright W, Parker J, Pierce MA: **African Swine fever virus in ticks (*Ornithodorus moutaba*) collected from animal burrows in Tanzania.** *Nature* 1969, **221**:1071–1073.
28. Theiler G, Robinson BN: **Tick survey (Part VIII) Checklists of ticks recorded from the Belgian Congo and Ruanda Urundi, from Angola and Northern Rhodesia.** *Onderstepoort J Vet Res* 1954, **26**:447–461.
29. Van der Merwe S: **Some remarks on the 'tampans' of the *Ornithodoros moubata* complex in Southern Africa.** *Zool Anz* 1968, **181**:280–289.
30. Haresnape JM, Mamu FD: **The distribution of ticks of the Ornithodoros moubata complex (Ixodoidea: Argasidae) in Malawi, and its relation to African swine fever epizootiology.** *J Hyg (Lond)* 1986, **96**:535–544.
31. Vial L, Wieland B, Jori F, Etter E, Dixon L, Roger F: **African swine fever virus DNA in soft ticks, Senegal.** *Emerg Infect Dis* 2007, **13**:1928–1931.
32. Gulenkin VM, Korennoy FI, Karaulov AK, Dudnikov SA: **Cartographical analysis of African swine fever outbreaks in the territory of the Russian Federation and computer modeling of the basic reproduction ratio.** *Prev Vet Med* 2011, **102**:167–174.
33. Allepuz A, Saez M, Alba A, Napp S, Casal J: **Exploratory spatial analysis of Aujeszky's disease during four phases of the eradication programme in Catalonia, Spain (2003–2007).** *Prev Vet Med* 2008, **86**:164–175.
34. Poljak Z, Dewey CE, Martin SW, Christensen J, Carman S, Friendship RM: **Prevalence of and risk factors for influenza in southern Ontario swine herds in 2001 and 2003.** *Can J Vet Res* 2008, **72**:7–17.
35. Rhyan JC, Spraker TR: **Emergence of diseases from wildlife reservoirs.** *Vet Pathol* 2010, **47**:34–39.
36. Fasina FO, Agbaje M, Ajani FL, Talabi OA, Lazarus DD, Gallardo C, Thompson PN, Bastos ADS: **Risk factors for farm-level African swine fever infection in major pig-producing areas in Nigeria, 1997–2011.** *Prev Vet Med* 2012, **107**:65–75.
37. Saaty TL: *The Analytic Hierarchy Process.* New York: McGraw-Hill; 1980.
38. Boroushaki S, Malczewski J: **Implementing an extension of the analytical hierarchy process using ordered weighted averaging operators with fuzzy quantifiers in ArcGIS.** *Comput Geosci* 2008, **34**:399–410.

39. Malczewski J: *GIS and Multicriteria Decision Analysis*. New York: John Wiley and Sons; 1999.
40. Boitani L, Corsi F, De Biase A, Carranza I, Ravagli M, Reggiani G, Sinibaldi I, Trapanese P: *AMD African mammals databank. A databank for conservation and management of the African mammals*. Roma: Instituto di Ecologia Applicata: Report to the Directorate General for Development (GDVIII/A/1) of the European Commission; 1999.
41. Liu C, Berry P, Dawson T, Pearson R: **Selecting thresholds of occurrence in the prediction of species distributions.** *Ecography* 2005, **28:**385–393.
42. Barve N: *Tool for Partial-ROC*. Biodiversity Institute: Version 1. Lawrence, KS; 2008. Available: http://kuscholarworks.ku.edu/dspace/handle/1808/10059.
43. Peterson AT, Papeş M, Soberón J: **Rethinking receiver operating characteristic analysis applications in ecological niche modeling.** *Ecol Model* 2008, **213:**63–72.
44. Penrith ML, Vosloo W, Jori F, Bastos ADS: **African swine fever virus eradication in Africa.** *Virus Res* 2013, **173:**228–246.
45. Otesile EB, Ajuwape AT, Odemuyiwa SO, Akpavie SO, Olaifa AK, Odaibo GN, Olaleye DO, Adetosoye AI: **Field and experimental investigations of an outbreak of African swine fever in Nigeria.** *Revue d'élevage et de médecine vétérinaire des pays tropicaux* 2005, **58:**21–26.
46. Penrith ML, Bastos ADS, Thomson GR, Wilkinson PJ: *Epidemiology of African Swine Fever in West Africa*. Melborne, Australia: Proceedings of the 16th Biennial Congress of the International Pig Veterinary Society; 2000:560.
47. Plowright W, Thomson GR: **African Swine Fever**. In *Infectious Diseases of Livestock, with Special Reference to Southern Africa*. Edited by Coetzer JAW, Thomson GR, Tustin RC. Cape Town: Oxford University Press; 1994.
48. Atuhaire DK, Ochwo S, Afayoa M, Mwiine FN, Kokas I, Arinaitwe E, Ademun-Okurut RA, Okuni JB, Nanteza A, Ayebazibwe C, Okedi L, Olaho-Mukani W, Ojok L: **Epidemiological Overview of African Swine Fever in Uganda (2001–2012).** *J Vet Med* 2013:. doi:10.1155/2013/94963847.
49. Gallardo C, Ademun AR, Nieto R, Nantima N, Arias M, Martín E, Pelayo V, Bishop RP: **Genotyping of African swine fever virus (ASFV) isolates associated with disease outbreaks in Uganda in 2007.** *Afr J Biotechnol* 2011, **10:**3488–3497.
50. Misinzo G, Kasanga CJ, Mpelumbe-Ngeleja C, Masambu J, Kitambi A, Van Doorsselaere J: **African swine fever virus, Tanzania, 2010–2012.** *Emerg Infect Dis* 2012, **18:**2081–2083.
51. Lubisi BA, Bastos ADS, Dwarka RM, Vosloo W: **Molecular epidemiology of African swine fever in East Africa.** *Arch Virol* 2005, **150:**2439–2452.
52. Okoth E, Gallardo C, Macharia JM, Omore A, Pelayo V, Bulimo DW, Arias M, Kitala P, Baboon K, Lekolol I, Mijele D, Bishop RP: **Comparison of African swine fever virus prevalence and risk in two contrasting pig-farming systems in South-west and Central Kenya.** *Prev Vet Med* 2013, **1:**198–205.
53. Gallardo C, Okoth E, Pelayo V, Anchuelo R, Martín E, Simón A, Llorente A, Nieto R, Soler A, Martín R, Arias M, Bishop RP: **African swine fever viruses with two different genotypes, both of which occur in domestic pigs, are associated with ticks and adult warthogs, respectively, at a single geographical site.** *J Gen Virol* 2011, **92:**432–444.
54. Vose D: *Risk Analysis: a Quantitative Guide*. 3rd edition. Chichester, West Sussex: John Wiley and Sons; 2008.
55. Vaidya OS, Kumar S: **Analytic hierarchy process: an overview of applications.** *Eur J Oper Res* 2006, **169:**1–29.
56. Bozóki S, Rapcsák T: **On Saaty's and Koczkodaj's inconsistencies of pairwise comparison matrices.** *J Glob Optim* 2007, **42:**157–175.
57. Koczkodaj WW: **A new definition of consistency of pairwise comparisons.** *Math Comput Model* 1993, **18:**79–84.
58. Kwiesielewicz M, van Uden E: **Inconsistent and contradictory judgements in pairwise comparison method in the AHP.** *Comput OR* 2004, **31:**713–719.

23

Confirmation that "*Brachyspira hampsonii*" clade I (Canadian strain 30599) causes mucohemorrhagic diarrhea and colitis in experimentally infected pigs

Matheus O Costa[1], Janet E Hill[1], Champika Fernando[1], Hollie D Lemieux[2], Susan E Detmer[3], Joseph E Rubin[1] and John C S Harding[2*]

Abstract

Background: "*Brachyspira hampsonii*", discovered in North America in 2010 associated with dysentery-like illness, is an economically relevant swine pathogen resulting in decreased feed efficiency and increased morbidity, mortality and medication usage. "*B. hampsonii*" clade II strain 30446 has been shown to be causally associated with mucohemorrhagic diarrhea and colitis. Our objectives were to determine if "*Brachyspira hampsonii*" clade I strain 30599 is pathogenic to pigs, and to evaluate the relative diagnostic performance of three *ante mortem* sampling methodologies (direct PCR on feces, PCR on rectal GenoTube Livestock swabs, *Brachyspira* culture from rectal swabs). Five-week old pigs were intragastrically inoculated thrice with 10^8 genomic equivalents "*B. hampsonii*" (n = 12), or served as sham controls (n = 6). Feces were sampled and consistency assessed daily. Necropsies were performed 24 h after peak clinical signs.

Results: One pig died due to unrelated illness. Nine of 11 inoculated pigs, but no controls, developed mucoid or mucohemorrhagic diarrhea (MHD). Characteristic lesions of swine dysentery were observed in large intestine. "*B. hampsonii*" strain 30599 DNA was detected by qPCR in feces of all inoculated pigs for up to 6 days prior to the onset of MHD. The organism was isolated from the feces and colons of pigs demonstrating MHD, but not from controls. *B. intermedia* was isolated from inoculated pigs without MHD, and from 5 of 6 controls.

Conclusions: We conclude that "*Brachyspira hampsonii*" clade I strain 30599 is pathogenic and causes mucohemorrhagic diarrhea and colitis in susceptible pigs. Moreover, the three sampling methodologies performed similarly. GenoTube Livestock, a forensic swab designed to preserve DNA during shipping is a useful tool especially in settings where timely transport of diagnostic samples is challenging.

Keywords: "*Brachyspira hampsonii*", Swine dysentery, Mucohemorrhagic, Bloody, Diarrhea, Colitis, Pig, Porcine

Background

The first published description of swine dysentery (SD) appeared in 1921, although the causative agent was unknown at the time [1]. In 1971, *Treponema hyodysenteriae* (later renamed *Brachyspira hyodysenteriae*) was identified as the pathogen responsible for the syndrome [2,3]. Until the early 1990's, SD was considered a major production-limiting disease in North American commercial swine farms. Since the mid-2000's, swine producers and veterinarians have observed the re-emergence of mucohemorrhagic diarrhea (MHD) and colitis in commercial farms [4-7]. North American diagnostic laboratories observed an increase in the number of cases of *Brachyspira hyodysenteriae* diarrhea submitted, as well as cases associated with "atypical" *Brachyspira* spp. [8]. Further characterization of these atypical isolates led to the description of a novel *Brachyspira* species, provisionally named "*Brachyspira hampsonii*". It has been proposed that this new species is comprised of two

* Correspondence: John.Harding@usask.ca
[2]Department of Large Animal Clinical Sciences, University of Saskatchewan, Saskatoon, SK, Canada
Full list of author information is available at the end of the article

different phylogenetic clades, sharing 96% sequence identity in the NADH oxidase (*nox*) gene sequence [9].

Mucohemorrhagic diarrhea and colitis, indistinguishable from SD has been experimentally reproduced in pigs with "*B. hampsonii*" clade II isolates from Canada and the United States [10,11]. Burrough *et al.* has also reproduced SD experimentally in mice [12] and in pigs [11] using strongly β-hemolytic strains initially identified as *B. intermedia* based on PCR [13], which have since been confirmed to be "*B. hampsonii*" clade I [14]. These data suggests that clade I is pathogenic to pigs, but further studies are required to confirm this, evaluate additional strains and to characterize the disease including patterns of shedding.

The first Canadian diagnosis of "*B. hampsonii*" clade I was in November 2011 from grow-finish pigs with bloody, mucoid diarrhea. This was a unique event, since all previous "*B. hampsonii*" cases diagnosed by our laboratory were of clade II. The isolate recovered from this diagnostic case was designated "30599". Since its first diagnosis in Canada, "*B. hampsonii*" clade I (strain 30599) has been identified, isolated or both, in the absence of other *Brachyspira* spp., in feces or tissues from 39 cases of diarrhea from 15 farms in western Canada. Given the distance between farms and diagnostic laboratories in western Canada, this may be an underestimate of the number of farms affected by the organism. One of the main obstacles to obtaining high quality diagnostic samples and reliable results is the transit time required to ship samples to a diagnostic laboratory [15,16]. For PCR based diagnostics, sample quality may be improved by immediate preservation of target DNA in the sample and controlling the growth of opportunistic organisms. A forensic swab (GenoTube Livestock; Prionics, Switzerland) capable of rapidly drying the sample and providing minimal DNA loss after long-term storage without refrigeration may be a potential tool for aiding the diagnosis of infectious diseases by PCR in biologic samples shipped long distances to diagnostic laboratories.

The objectives of this study were to determine the pathogenicity of "*Brachyspira hampsonii*" clade I (strain 30599) when inoculated in naïve pigs, and to investigate the performance of GenoTube Livestock swabs for *ante mortem* sampling of pigs for PCR-based detection of "*Brachyspira hampsonii*" clade I. In order to accomplish these primary objectives, we also developed and validated a PCR assay for the detection and quantification of "*Brachyspira hampsonii*" clade I (strain 30599).

Methods

This work was approved by the University of Saskatchewan's Animal Research Ethics Board and adhered to the Canadian Council on Animal Care guidelines for humane animal use (permit #20110038) and ARRIVE Guidelines (Animal Research: Reporting In Vivo Experiments; Additional file 1).

Source of "*B. hampsonii*" strain 30599 inoculum

"*B. hampsonii*" clade I strain 30599 was isolated from a pig with mucoid diarrhea in Alberta, Canada in November, 2011. PCR for *B. hyodysenteriae* [13], *B. pilosicoli* [10] and "*B. hampsonii*" clade II [10] performed on case tissues returned negative results. Sections of small and large intestines tested negative for *Salmonella* (culture on brilliant green agar following enrichment with selenite broth), *Lawsonia intracellularis* (PCR) [17], and porcine circovirus type 2 (PCV2, immunohistochemistry) [18] at the Prairie Diagnostic Service Inc. (PDS), Saskatoon, SK. Culture of colon tissue on selective media resulted in areas of strong β-hemolysis, which were sub-cultured to obtain an isolate. Sequencing of the *nox*, *cpn*60 and 16S rRNA genes from this isolate demonstrated that it was similar to, but phylogenetically distinct from "*B. hampsonii*" clade II. Whole genome sequencing of the isolate was performed (NCBI BioProject PRJNA188379) and confirmed its affiliation with what has recently been proposed as clade I of "*B. hampsonii*" [9].

Experimental inoculation

The experimental inoculation was performed as described previously ("Pure Broth Culture Inoculation" in [10]). Briefly, 18 five-week old pigs (16 male, 2 inadvertently female) were obtained from a commercial farm in Saskatchewan, Canada. No history of MHD or previous diagnosis of *Brachyspira* spp. associated diarrhea was reported, and fecal samples collected from nursery (n = 20) and grow-finish (n = 10) pigs prior to the commencement of the study tested negative for *Brachyspira* spp. by culture and species-specific qPCR for *B. hyodysenteriae*, *B. pilosicoli* and "*B. hampsonii*" (data not shown). Upon arrival at the Animal Care Unit at the University of Saskatchewan, the pigs were allocated randomly to control (CTRL, n = 6) and inoculated (INOC, n = 12) groups housed in separate rooms with 3 or 2 pigs per pen, respectively. Group sizes were based on results of past experiments and provided an experimental power of 0.83 based on the assumptions that 8/12 INOC and 0/6 CTRL pigs would develop MHD and alpha = 0.05. One female pig was assigned to each group. Pigs were acclimated to their new diet and room environment for 7 days prior to inoculation, and were offered *ad libitum* water and commercially prepared, non-medicated, pelleted starter diet (Whole Earth Pig Starter, Federated Cooperative Ltd., Saskatoon, Canada) formulated with less than 15% soybean meal for the duration of the experiment.

Pigs were sedated with 8 mg/kg azaperone IM (Stresnil, Vetoquinol Canada Inc., Lavaltrie, Quebec) then inoculated by gastric tube on three consecutive days (day (D) 0, 1 and 2). INOC received 10 mL of frozen JBS broth containing 6.10×10^8 (D0), 4.14×10^8 (D1) and 4.24×10^8 (D2) genome equivalents of *"B. hampsonii"* strain 30599, followed by 40 mL of PBS (0.1 M, pH 7). CTRL received 10 ml of sterile JBS broth followed by 40 mL of PBS. For both groups, feed was removed 16 h prior to inoculation to increase gastric motility.

Feces and rectal swabs were collected on day −8, −5, −2 and 0 prior to inoculation, and daily thereafter until the end of the experiment. Fecal consistency was scored daily as: 0 = formed, normal; 1 = soft, wet cement consistency; 2 = runny or watery diarrhea; 3 = mucoid diarrhea; 4 = mucohemorrhagic diarrhea. Daily clinical assessment was performed on all pigs. Rectal temperature, responsiveness to external stimuli (e.g. the presence of researcher in the pen) and skin colour were recorded. Body weight was measured on D0 and D8. INOC pigs were humanely euthanized by cranial captive bolt and exsanguination approximately 24 hours after the development of mucoid or mucohemorrhagic diarrhea. INOC pigs that did not demonstrate MHD were euthanized on D13; CTRL pigs on D14.

Pathological assessments

A complete necropsy was performed and the gastrointestinal tract was completely removed from stomach to rectum, including mesenteric lymph nodes. Special attention was paid to the cecum and spiral colon which was completely linearized and divided into thirds (proximal, apex and distal). The mucosal surfaces of the large intestines were assessed for the presence of characteristic lesions of SD including hyperemia, congestion, edema, necrosis, fibrin and mucus by a single pathologist (SED). A blinded histologic evaluation of colon and cecum was performed by the same pathologist. Tissue samples were fixed in 10% buffered formalin for 24 hours and paraffin embedded. All microsectioned tissues were stained with Hematoxylin-Eosin (H&E) and a serial section of the spiral colon was also Warthin-Faulkner (WF) silver stained. Lesions in the spiral colon and cecum were scored based on the severity of the inflammation and necrosis: 0 = no lesions; 1 = minimal to mild necrosis of superficial enterocytes with minimal inflammatory infiltrates; 2 = moderate necrosis and attenuation of enterocytes with mild to moderate inflammatory infiltrates; 3 = severe necrosis (erosion or ulceration present) with moderate inflammatory infiltrates predominantly consisting of neutrophils. The presence of *Brachyspira*-like organisms was also scored from 0 to 3 in WF stained sections: 0 = no spirochetes observed; 0.5 = a single gland contained a few spirochetes; 1 = small numbers of spirochetes in multiple glands; 2 = many spirochetes within several glands; 3 = many spirochetes forming thick mats in numerous glands.

Microbiological assessments

Gastrointestinal tissues collected at termination were screened for the presence of other relevant swine enteric pathogens, including *Lawsonia intracellularis* (PCR, ileum), porcine circovirus type 2 (PCV2, immunohistochemistry, ileum and mesenteric lymph node) and *Salmonella* spp. (culture, ileum). All methods were the same as described above. PRRSv IgG antibody and RNA concentration were measured by ELISA (IDEXX PRRS X3, IDEXX Laboratories Inc., Westbrook, ME) and PCR (Tetracore Inc., Rockville, MD), respectively, at PDS in sera collected on D0 and at termination.

Quantification of *"B. hampsonii"* clade I strain 30599

Details on the development and validation of the strain-specific qPCR assay are given in the Results. DNA for PCR was extracted from feces and colon tissue using the QIAmp DNA stool mini kit (Qiagen Inc., Toronto, ON), and from cultured bacteria and colon tissue using DNEasy blood and tissue kit (Qiagen Inc.). SYBR green real-time qPCR detection of *"B. hampsonii"* strain 30599 was performed on a Bio-Rad MyiQ thermocycler in reactions containing 1× SYBR Green Supermix (Bio-Rad Laboratories (Canada) Ltd., Mississauga, ON), 400 nM each primer JH0436 (5'-AAA GTG CCA CAG GCA ATG TA-3') and JH0437 (5'-TGC AAG ATT AGA CGG AGC AA-3')) and 2 μL of template DNA, in a final volume of 25 μL. All qPCR reactions were run on a plate containing a no-template control and a standard curve composed of target-containing plasmids at concentrations of 10^0 to 10^7 copies/reaction. All reactions were performed in duplicate. Thermocycling parameters included an initial denaturation (95°C for 3 min.), followed by 40 cycles of 95°C for 15 sec., 63°C for 15 sec., 72°C for 15 sec., and a final extension at 72°C for 5 min. A dissociation curve was subsequently performed for 81 cycles at 0.5°C increments from 55°C to 95°C. Fluorescent signals were measured every cycle at the end of the annealing step and continuously during the dissociation curve data collection. All resulting data was analyzed using iQ5 Optical System Software (Bio-Rad Laboratories (Canada) Ltd., Mississauga, ON).

Brachyspira culture

Isolation of *Brachyspira* spp. was performed on BJ agar from feces and colonic mucosa, as previously described [10]. Presence of *Brachyspira* growth in zones of β-hemolysis was confirmed by dark-field microscopy, and genus-specific PCR targeting the *nox* gene [19] followed by DNA sequencing using the amplification primers.

Comparison of *ante mortem* sampling techniques

Three *ante mortem* sampling and detection methods were chosen for comparison: rectal swabs (CultureSwab

Liquid Stuart, BD Canada, Mississauga, ON) for culture on selective agar, qPCR on DNA extracted from fecal samples (200 mg samples, QIAmp DNA stool mini kit, Qiagen Inc.), and qPCR on DNA extracted from GenoTube swabs. Samples were collected D-8, D-5, D-2 and D0 prior to inoculation, and every other day thereafter to D12 in INOC pigs. Targeted sampling was employed in order to sample pigs with different fecal scores. On each day, samples were simultaneously collected from pigs with no diarrhea (n = 2), pigs with "wet-cement" or watery diarrhea (n = 2) and pigs with mucoid and mucohemorrhagic diarrhea (n = 2). If one or more category was not observed at the time of collection, pigs with the closest available fecal score on that day were sampled. The pigs from which samples were collected were blocked by pen.

To simulate a field situation where samples would be transported to the diagnostic laboratory over 24 h, culture swabs and feces were refrigerated at 4°C (to mimic shipment with ice packs), while GenoTube swabs were stored at room temperature for 24 h prior to processing. GenoTube swabs were expressed into 1.4 mL lysis buffer (buffer ASL, QIAmp DNA stool mini kit, Qiagen Inc., Toronto, ON) in a 2 mL microcentrifuge tube by pressing the swab head against the inside wall of the tube while twisting. To ensure consistent sample expression, swabs were turned exactly ten times each (5 clockwise and 5 counter clockwise). Following expression, extraction proceeded according to the kit instructions. DNA extracts (2 μL each) from feces and GenoTube swabs were used as a template for *"B. hampsonii"* clade I specific qPCR analysis. Culture swabs were used to inoculate BJ agar plates.

Statistical analysis

Statistical analysis was performed using SPSS v19.0 (SPSS Inc., Chicago, IL) or Stata v13 (StatCorp, College Station, TX). Group differences in the number of pigs demonstrating MHD (fecal consistency score 4) was compared using a Fisher's exact test. The same test was used to compare the presence or absence of specific gastrointestinal lesions based on gross and histopathological assessments. Continuous variables including average daily gain (ADG) and the concentration of *"B. hampsonii"* strain 30599 DNA detected by qPCR were non-parametrically distributed and compared between groups using a Kruskal-Wallis Analysis of Variance. Spirochete scores in colon were compared with a Mann–Whitney U test. To compare the severity of gross lesions among proximal, apex and distal colon segments, a Wilcoxon matched-pairs signed-rank test was used after assigning negative, mild, moderate and severe lesion scores as 0, 1, 2, 3 respectively. For all analyses, $P < 0.05$ was considered as statistically significant.

Results

Development of *"B. hampsonii"* clade I strain 30599 specific SYBR green PCR assay

A strain-specific, SYBR green quantitative real time PCR assay was developed to quantify *"B. hampsonii"* strain 30599 DNA. Primers JH0436 (5′-AAA GTG CCA CAG GCA ATG TA-3′) and JH0437 (5′-TGC AAG ATT AGA CGG AGC AA-3′) were designed to target a 176 bp region within a predicted open reading frame in the *"B. hampsonii"* strain 30599 genome encoding a hypothetical protein (Genbank accession WP_008726773). The target region lies within an approximately 15.8 kb region of the genome identified as being unique to strain 30599 in a comparison of the whole genome sequences of clade I strain 30599 (BioProject PRJNA187424) and clade II strain 30446 (BioProject PRJNA169353). The target sequence has no significant sequence identity to *"B. hampsonii"* clade II strain 30446, and is only 90% identical at the nucleotide level to a sequence within the genome of *B. intermedia* PWS/A (ATCC 51140^T). No other significant sequence identities to other *Brachyspira* species were identified.

An optimal annealing temperature of 63°C was determined, and a linear standard curve was obtained over a range of 10^0 to 10^7 target copies per PCR reaction using a ten-fold dilution series of cloned target amplicon in plasmid pGEM T Easy as template.

Analytical specificity was determined initially by applying the primers to genomic DNA from *B. hyodysenteriae* ATCC 27164^T, *B. pilosicoli* ATCC 51139^T, *B. intermedia* ATCC 51140^T, *B. innocens* ATCC 29796^T, *B. murdochii* ATCC 51284^T, and *"B. hampsonii"* clade II strain 30446. No amplification was detected from any template other than *"B. hampsonii"* clade I strain 30599. Further validation of the analytical specificity of the *"B. hampsonii"* strain 30599 specific qPCR involved its application to fecal samples from previous clinical cases determined to be positive for *"B. hampsonii"* strain 30599 by amplification and sequencing of the *nox* gene using previously published primers (n = 25) [19], and fecal samples from healthy pigs from the source farm that were confirmed negative for *Brachyspira* by the same method (n = 30). All (30/30) of the negative samples were found negative by the strain specific qPCR, and 24 of 25 of the positive samples were found positive by the strain specific qPCR, demonstrating significant agreement between the methods.

Acclimation period

Brachyspira culture was performed on all pigs on four days during the pre-inoculation acclimation period. *B. intermedia* (97% *nox* gene sequence identity over 810 bp to *B. intermedia* ATCC 51140^T) was isolated from one INOC and one CTRL pig on D-2, and from one INOC on D0. *"B. pulli"* (98% nucleotide identity over 848 bp of *nox* to strain

AN304/04) was isolated from one INOC on D-2 and D0. *"B. pulli"* is the provisional name for a spirochete originally identified in birds [20], which has recently also been isolated from pigs [21]. One CTRL had watery diarrhea on D-8 and D-7, immediately after arrival in the animal care facility, but *Brachyspira* was not isolated, and normal feces were observed during all other days pre-inoculation.

Clinical observations

One INOC pig presented with tachypnea and dyspnea on D3 and D4, and for welfare reasons was euthanized and necropsied on D5. Necropsy findings indicated aspiration of feed at the tracheal bifurcation. Data from this pig were removed from all analyses.

Post-inoculation fecal scores for INOC pigs are summarized in Figure 1. Eight of 11 INOC pigs developed MHD (score 4) (Figure 2), and one INOC developed mucoid diarrhea (#22, score 3). Of the two remaining INOC pigs, one (#19) remained healthy throughout the study, and one (#670) had fecal consistency typical of wet cement (score 1) on four post-inoculation days. To distinguish these from the nine diarrheic INOC pigs, they

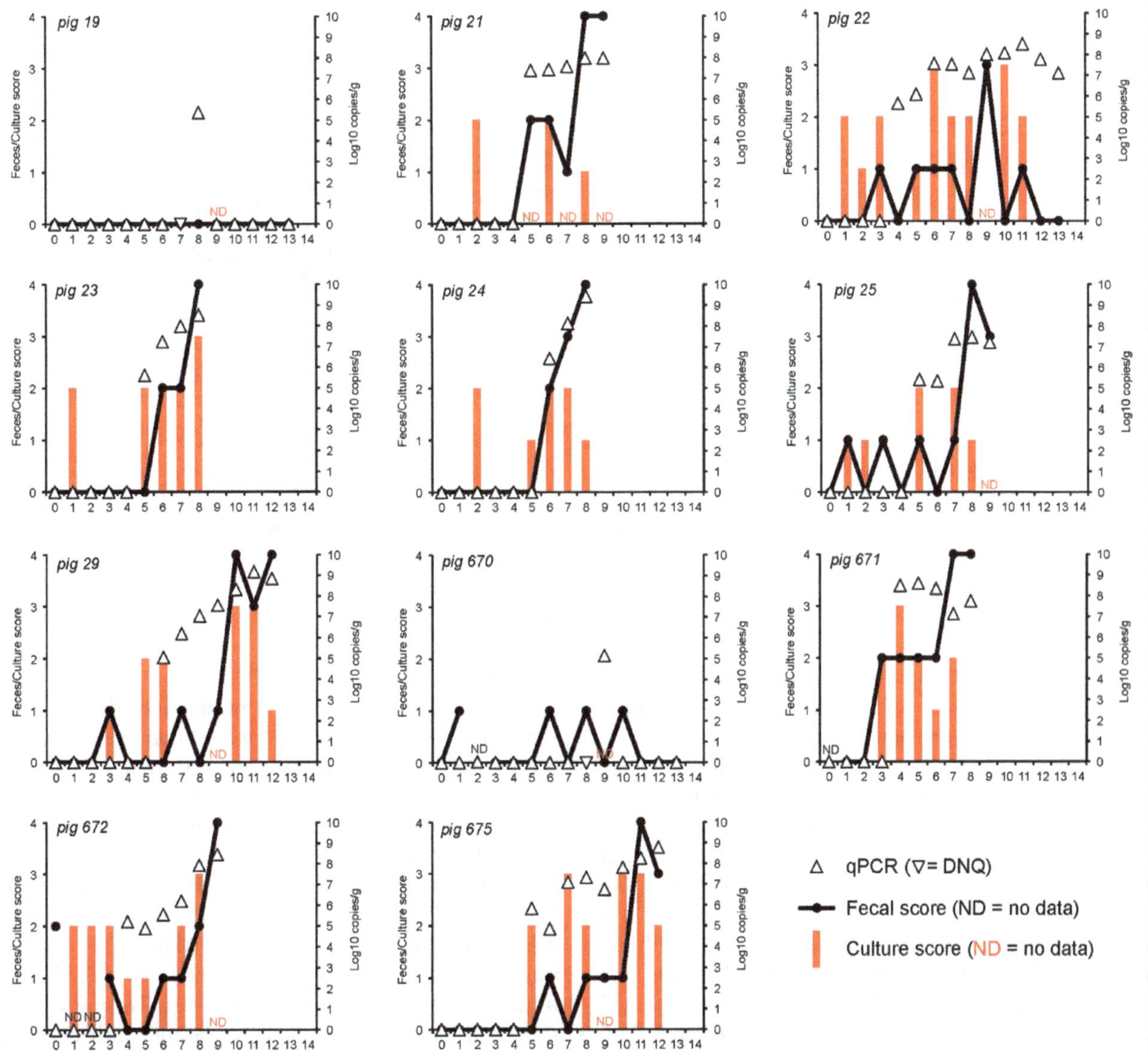

Figure 1 Fecal consistency scores, culture results and fecal concentration of *"Brachyspira hampsonii"* strain 30599 following inoculation. Fecal consistency scores (line, left ordinate: 0 = formed, normal; 1 = soft, wet cement consistency; 2 = runny or watery; 3 = mucoid diarrhea; or 4 = bloody diarrhea), semi-quantitative fecal culture score (red bars, left ordinate: 0 = negative; 1 = less than 10 colonies/1° streak; 2 = less than 10 colonies/2° streak; 3 = less than 10 colonies/3°streak; 4 = less than 10 colonies/4° streak), and strain 30599 DNA concentration in feces (triangles, right ordinate; upside down triangles indicate DNQ) are shown. Days post-inoculation are shown on the abscissa. ND = no data. Pig IDs are indicated in the upper left corner of each panel.

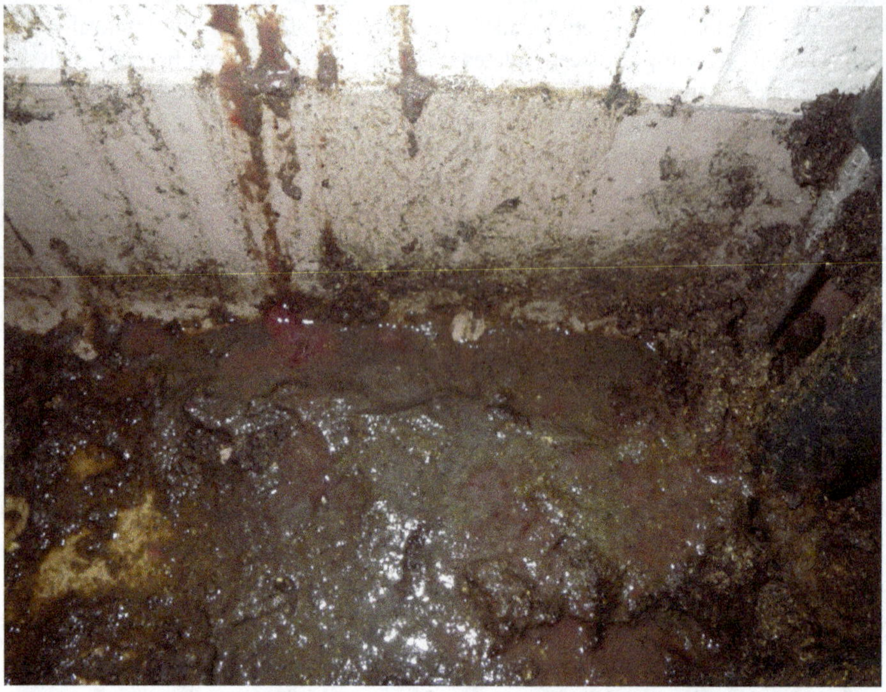

Figure 2 Mucohemorrhagic diarrhea. Accumulation of loose and runny feces with mucus and frank blood. Pig #675, 11 days post inoculation, day of first observation of mucohemorrhagic diarrhea, 7th day of *"B. hampsonii"* strain 30599 shedding, feces culture positive (3+ strongly beta-hemolytic *"B. hampsonii"* strain 30599) on this day, 1.86×10^8 strain 30599 genomic equivalents/g. In inoculated pigs the severity of bloody diarrhea ranged from that containing a few flecks of blood to diffusely hemorrhagic with copious blood and mucus as shown.

are referred to as "INOC (without MHD)". No CTRL pig demonstrated mucoid or bloody diarrhea after sham inoculation, although one had fecal consistency typical of wet cement (score 1) on D6 and D9, and one had runny diarrhea (score 2) on D4 and wet cement consistency on D8, but was normal on all other days. Mucohemorrhagic diarrhea was significantly more frequent in INOC than in CTRL pigs ($P = 0.002$).

On D0, one INOC pig (#672) unexpectedly presented with runny diarrhea and fecal samples were submitted for routine aerobic and anaerobic culture to PDS. The sample was negative for *Salmonella* spp. but *E. coli.* was isolated. PCR results indicated that the *E.coli* isolate was positive for virulence factors AIDA-I and STb. Fecal consistency from this pig scored 0 or 1 until D8, then progressed to MHD by D9. The median number of days from first inoculation to the demonstration of mucoid or mucohemorrhagic diarrhea in INOC was 8, with the shortest and longest incubation periods at 7 and 11 days respectively. The onset of MHD was generally acute with affected pigs progressing from relatively normal feces (score 0 or 1) to MHD within 2.4 days (range 1–4) (Figure 1).

Average daily gain between D0 and D8 was numerically decreased in INOC (359 ± 143 g/day) compared to CTRL (413 ± 123 g/day), but did not differ significantly between groups.

Serum from blood collected on D0 and at termination was PRRSv PCR and ELISA negative. Intestinal tissue samples collected at termination tested negative for *Salmonella* sp., *Lawsonia intracellularis* and PCV2 by culture or PCR.

Brachyspira shedding patterns

Brachyspira spp. isolates were recovered from feces from 10 of 11 INOC pigs between D0 and D4. This was likely associated with pass-through of the inoculation dose. Eight of 11 were culture positive for *"B. hampsonii"* strain 30599 solely, two of 11 for *B. intermedia*, one of 11 for *"B. hampsonii"* strain 30599 and *B. pulli* on different days (Figure 1). Between D5 and termination, *"B. hampsonii"* strain 30599 was consistently isolated in the feces and from the colon of all INOC pigs that developed MHD (Figure 1). *B. intermedia* was isolated from the feces and colon of the two INOC pigs without MHD. *B. intermedia* was also isolated sporadically from the feces of 5 of 6 and from terminal colon in 3 of 6 CTRL pigs. The presence of *B. intermedia* in feces was not associated with diarrhea. Inadvertently, an issue with the culture vessel on D9 resulted in negative cultures from all pigs. Culture positive isolates confirmed as *"B. hampsonii"* strain 30599 had 99-100% sequence identity to the inoculum based on sequencing of the *nox* gene. Any minor differences in sequence are most likely explained by

PCR artefact since the Taq DNA polymerase used was not a proofreading enzyme.

Quantifiable levels of *"B. hampsonii"* strain 30599 were detected by qPCR beginning D4 in 11 of 11 INOC pigs (Figure 1). *"B. hampsonii"* strain 30559 was not detected in CTRL pigs. In INOC pigs without MHD, quantifiable levels were detected on a single day in each pig (D8 or D9). In INOC pigs with MHD, quantifiable levels of *"B. hampsonii"* strain 30599 were detected over multiple consecutive days preceding euthanasia. On average, quantifiable levels were detected for four days prior to the onset of MHD (range 2 to 6). The average concentration of *"B. hampsonii"* strain 30599 across all days in INOC pigs with MHD was 8.05 (log 10 genomic equivalents/gram of feces).

Between D1 and D4, *"B. hampsonii"* strain 30599 was isolated by culture in 15 fecal samples of INOC pigs with MHD. In these same samples, the organism was detected by PCR 13 times. Of these, 3 samples had quantifiable levels of DNA whereas the remaining 10 had detectable but non-quantifiable levels (i.e. beyond the lower limit of the linear portion of the standard curve). From D5 to termination, *"B. hampsonii"* strain 30599 was isolated by culture in 37 fecal samples of INOC pigs with MHD, whereas DNA was detected in the same samples 41 times, always at quantifiable levels. These data indicate that PCR and culture had similar overall detection frequencies.

Pathological findings

A summary of gross pathological findings is presented in Table 1. Gross lesions in INOC pigs were confined to the large intestine, cecum and rectum. Cecum and rectum of INOC pigs displayed mild mucosal lesions, characterized as hyperemia associated with mucoid and fibrinous exudation. No lesions were observed in CTRL or in the small intestine of INOC pigs. In the two INOC without MHD, no lesions were observed in the proximal, apex or distal spiral colon; however, mild hyperemia of cecal mucosa was noted in one of these two pigs. Of the nine INOC with MHD, characteristic gross lesions of swine dysentery were observed consistently in spiral colon and cecum (Table 1). These lesions ranged in severity from mild, mucosal edema and hyperemia to severe, multifocal to coalescing, mucosal congestion with mucofibrinous exudate and focal areas of necrosis (Figure 3). In proximal, apex and distal spiral colon, gross lesions were significantly more frequent in INOC than in CTRL ($P < 0.05$ for all). In rectum, gross lesions were significantly more frequent in INOC with MHD than in CTRL ($P = 0.04$). Typhlitis was not a remarkable finding in INOC pigs, and lesion frequency did not differ between INOC and CTRL groups in this study. These results are contrary to previous descriptions of infections with *B. hyodysenteriae* or *"B. hampsonii"* clades I and II [2,10,11,22]. In INOC pigs with MHD, gross lesions were significantly more severe in the proximal and apex regions of the colon than in the distal colon ($P < 0.01$).

The frequency and severity of histopathologic findings were consistent with clinical signs and macroscopic lesions (Table 1). A thick layer of mucus and neutrophils (Figure 4) was observed on the colonic mucosa in all but one INOC pig. The nine of eleven pigs with positive cultures had histologic scores of 2 to 3 in the colon. By contrast, five of six CTRL pigs demonstrated mats of

Table 1 Comparison of gross and histopathological lesion frequency in CTRL and INOC groups

	P value				
Description	**CTRL (n = 6)**	**INOC (n = 11)**	**INOC (with MHD) (n = 9)**	**INOC vs. CTRL**	**INOC (with MHD) vs. CTRL**
Gross pathology frequency*					
Proximal colon	1/6	8/11	8/9	0.04	0.01
Apex colon	0/6	9/11	9/9	<0.01	<0.001
Distal colon	0/6	7/11	7/9	0.02	<0.01
Cecum	1/6	6/11	5/9	ns	ns
Rectum	0/6	5/11	5/9	0.08	0.04
Histopathologic lesion frequency**					
Colonic inflammation	0/6	9/11	9/9	<0.01	<0.001
Colonic necrosis	0/6	9/11	9/9	<0.01	<0.001
Cecal inflammation	0/6	6/11	6/9	0.04	0.001
Cecal necrosis	0/6	3/11	3/9	ns	0.02
Colonic spirochetes	0/6	8/11	8/9	<0.01	0.001

*Gross lesions include mucosal edema, hyperemia, congestion, with multifocal to diffuse mucofibrinonecrotic exudate.
**Histopathological lesions and colonic spirochete scores graded 0 to 3 reflecting negative, mild, moderate and severe inflammation or necrosis. Scores greater than 1 were considered lesional.

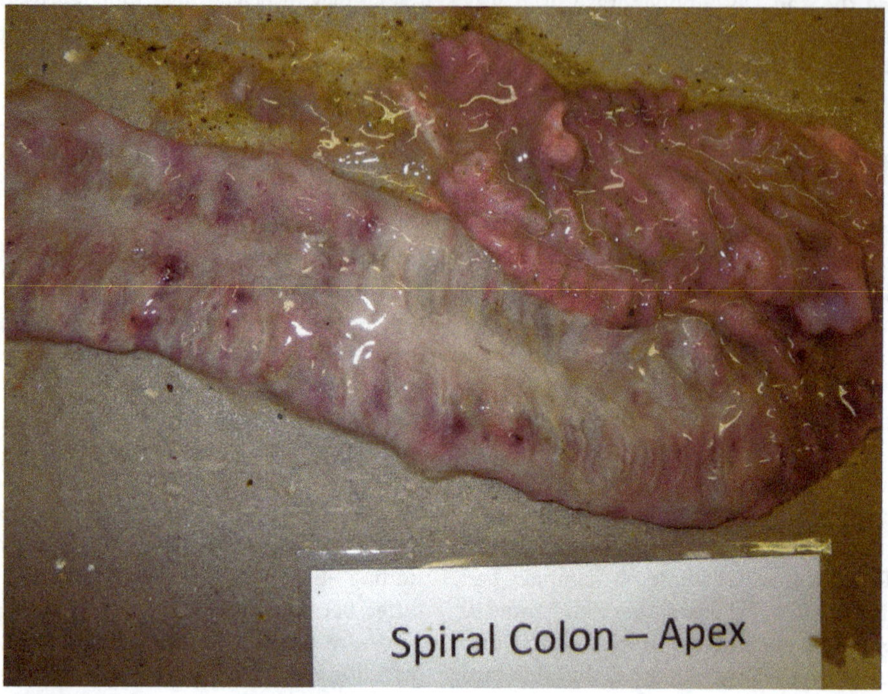

Figure 3 Mucohemorrhagic colitis. Congested mucosal surface of apex region of the spiral colon with thick layer of mucus and fibrin and occasional foci of haemorrhage. Pig #29, 12 days post inoculation, 48 hours post onset of mucohemorrhagic diarrhea.

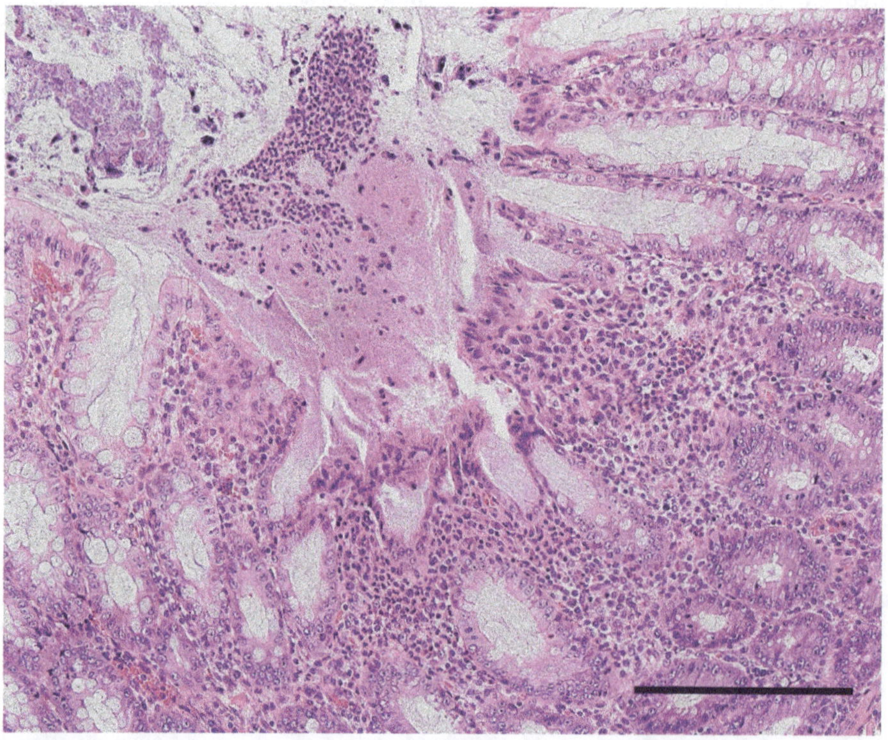

Figure 4 *Brachyspira* colitis. In a section of proximal colon (Pig #671) there is a focal area of epithelial necrosis surrounded in the lamina propria by a mixed inflammatory infiltrate composed primarily of degenerate neutrophils, and covered by a thick mat of mucous containing degenerate neutrophils, necrotic epithelial cells, and bacterial colonies. Hematoxylin and Eosin. Bar = 200 μm.

Gram-negative rod-shaped bacteria with minimal to no mucus (histologic score of 1). The presence of inflammation and superficial necrosis in the colon and cecum was higher in INOC than CTRL pigs (Table 1), as were numbers of spirochetes visualized in colon using silver staining (Table 1, Figure 5). Inflammation and necrosis were more severe in colon than cecum ($P < 0.01$).

Evaluation of *ante mortem* sampling techniques

One-hundred and sixty-five samples (55 GenoTube swabs, 55 culture swabs, 55 fecal samples) were collected. Since there were no diarrheic pigs on the majority of sampling days, 78% of samples (43/55) were obtained from pigs with normal feces (score 0 or 1), whereas 9% (5/55) originated from pigs with loose to watery feces (score 2) and 13% (7/55) from pigs with mucoid or mucohemorrhagic diarrhea (score 3 or 4). Forty-two percent (23/55) of the fecal samples were collected prior to inoculation.

Culture on BJ media followed by sequencing of the *nox* gene was set as the diagnostic gold standard for detection of *"B. hampsonii"* clade I strain 30599. A comparison of detection rate of *"B. hampsonii"* strain 30599 across the three *ante mortem* sampling methodologies is shown in Figure 6. Only 12 samples were collected from pigs with runny, mucoid or mucohemorrhagic diarrhea (score >1). Two of these were negative by culture, two were negative by GenoTube PCR, and one was negative by PCR of fecal DNA extracts. Both PCR methodologies detected *"B. hampsonii"* strain 30599 in all samples of mucoid and mucohemorrhagic diarrhea (score 3 or 4). On the other hand, one sample of mucohemorrhagic diarrhea collected on D8 was negative by culture, but positive by both PCR methodologies. This sample had 5.07×10^7 genome equivalents/g of feces based on qPCR. While this dataset is small, biased towards negative test results, and limited to a single experiment, the results suggest these assays have similar detection capabilities.

Discussion

The results of this experiment confirm that *"B. hampsonii"* clade I strain 30599 is pathogenic in susceptible pigs, and results in clinical disease indistinguishable from swine dysentery associated with *B. hyodysenteriae* and *"B. hampsonii"* clade II. This finding is relevant for pork producers in Canada and elsewhere whose herds experience mucohemorrhagic diarrhea. To our knowledge this is the first report of experimental reproduction of disease associated with Canadian strain 30599. Moreover, a previous report from Burrough *et al.* [11] pre-dated our present understanding based on *nox* sequences, that the strongly β-hemolyic strains of *B. intermedia* (KC35, EB106) used in these experiments were in fact *"B. hampsonii"* clade I. We hope the present research

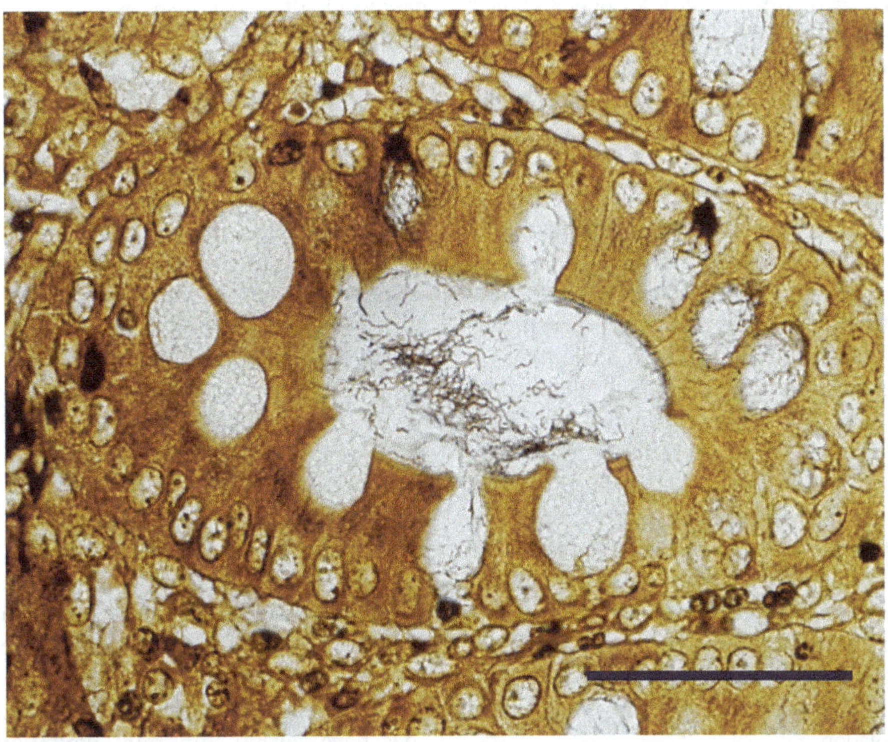

Figure 5 *Brachyspira* colitis. In the same section of proximal colon as Figure 4, the tubular mucous-secreting glands contain large numbers of long, thin spiral-shaped bacteria. Warthin-Faulkner. Bar = 100 μm.

A

GenoTube/qPCR \ Culture	+	-	
+	14	3	17
-	3	35	38
	17	38	

B

Feces/qPCR \ Culture	+	-	
+	15	3	18
-	2	35	37
	17	38	

Figure 6 Comparison of detection of "*B. hampsonii*" strain 30599 by qPCR on DNA extracts from feces or GenoTube swabs, or culture on selective media. Contingency tables show the numbers of samples determined to be positive or negative for "*B. hampsonii*" strain 30599 by **(A)** culture or qPCR on DNA extracts from GenoTube forensic swabs, and **(B)** culture or qPCR on DNA extracts from fecal samples.

will help to clarify any potential confusion that may exist regarding the pathogenicity of this organism.

A second substantial deliverable of this research is the first description of a novel quantitative PCR assay specific for "*B. hampsonii*" clade I. Based on a discriminating region of the genome, this SYBR-based PCR assay enables quantification, and does not cross react with other known *Brachyspira* species including "*B. hampsonii*" clade II.

Three *Brachyspira* species are capable of causing bloody diarrhea: *B. hyodysenteriae*, "*B. hampsonii*" clades I and II, and "*B. suanatina*". *B. hyodysenteriae* is globally distributed, while "*B. suanatina*" is reported only in Europe. Although "*B. hampsonii*" was discovered and mainly recognized in North America, isolations of clade I in Europe have been reported recently. One report details the isolation from two gilts that were imported from the Czech Republic to Belgium with soft watery feces within dilated large intestines [14]. The second account describes the isolation from a group of 17 grower pigs demonstrating mild to moderate diarrhea imported from Belgium to Germany [23]. A third study described the first finding of "*B. hampsonii*" from feces of birds, more specifically graylag geese and mallards in northwestern Spain [24].

In the present study, the onset of mucoid or mucohemorrhagic diarrhea in INOC pigs occurred within 7–11 days of inoculation, and was preceded by the fecal shedding of high levels (10^5 to 10^8 genomic equivalents/gram of feces) of "*B. hampsonii*" strain 30599 for up to 6 days. The prevalence of MHD was similar to that observed in the "*B. hampsonii*" clade II strain 30446 experimental reproduction [10] that used a similar animal model. It must be noted that this animal model does not require the feeding of 100% soybean meal prior to inoculation although a 16-hour period of fasting to enhance gastric motility is performed prior to each inoculation.

Swine dysentery is a multifactorial disease, with clinical expression dependent on individual host factors such as the gut microbiota [25], environmental conditions including diet composition [26,27], and presence of a virulent organism. Interestingly, two challenged pigs did not develop diarrhea and from both, *B. intermedia* was isolated in feces and in colonic tissue collected at termination. *B. intermedia* is generally accepted to be a gut commensal and non-pathogenic to pigs [28-30]. Whether or not it played a role in preventing the development of diarrhea in these pigs is not known, but *B. intermedia* was also isolated in five control pigs, suggesting it was a normal inhabitant of the pigs used in this study. A wide range of *Brachyspira* species can be isolated from healthy pigs from commercial farms [31] and are presumed to contribute to the commensal microbiota. The isolation of species other than that contained in the inoculum should therefore not be unexpected.

One pig (#22) developed a mucoid diarrhea with no evidence of blood prior to recovery over several days. This differed from pigs experimentally inoculated with "*B. hampsonii*" clade II, where 100% of the animals that displayed diarrhea progressed to blood-stained feces within 8 days of inoculation [10]. Field veterinarians, upon submission of diagnostic samples in western Canada, have often communicated variation in clinical presentation, particularly diarrhea associated with "*B. hampsonii*" clade I. We have further studies underway to help improve the understanding of the disease pathogenesis, and potential differences in pathogenic mechanisms associated with the pathogenic *Brachyspira* species.

Inoculated pigs with diarrhea had numerically lower ADG compared to non-challenged controls. However, due to study design limitations, experimental power was low and we could not investigate long-term effects of "*B. hampsonii*" clade I on the ADG of pigs. There are numerous reasons why ADG may be chronically depressed in surviving pigs, including any potential effects of "*B. hampsonii*" on the colonic mucosa and microbiota. These are relevant issues for the swine industry that are certainly worthy of future research.

The performance of qPCR on DNA extracted from GenoTube swabs was found to be comparable to qPCR on DNA extracted from feces, or culture. Rectal swabs are an easy and quick tool, enabling efficient sampling of large numbers of pigs, with minimal stress to the pigs and collectors. Moreover, a large percentage of laboratory errors occur during the pre-analytical phase of diagnosis, prior to samples arriving at the diagnostic laboratory [15,32]. This, and the fact that GenoTube swabs preserve DNA eliminating the need for refrigeration, makes it a practical, yet reliable methodology for sampling pigs with *Brachyspira*-associated diarrhea. However, the methodology does have several important limitations including the inability to isolate by culture. In addition, the use of rectal swabs precludes the ability to quantify target DNA in feces. Quantification may be important diagnostically since *"B. hampsonii"* clade I or II can be detected at low concentration (<10^5 genomic equivalents/gram) in healthy, non-diarrheic weaner or finisher pigs, whereas levels greater than 10^5 genomic equivalents/gram of feces or tissues [4].

Conclusions

In summary, recent reports describing the emergence of *"Brachyspira hampsonii"* in North America and Europe provide evidence of the importance of this pathogen for the global pork industry. Results of this study confirm the pathogenicity of a Canadian *"B. hampsonii"* clade I strain 30599 and describe the course of disease following experimental challenge. We confirmed that strain 30599 caused mucohemorrhagic diarrhea indistinguishable from swine dysentery associated with *B. hyodysenteriae* or *"B. hampsonii"* clade II strain 30446. All pigs with bloody diarrhea were both qPCR and culture positive. Gross pathology and histopathology revealed characteristic lesions that were more severe in the proximal and apex regions of the colon, than the distal colon. Testing for other relevant pathogens, including PRRSv, *L. intracellularis*, PCV2 and *Salmonella* sp. were negative. Additionally, we evaluated several *ante mortem* sampling techniques and confirmed that a forensic swab, GenoTube Livestock, designed to preserve DNA during shipping may be a useful tool for diagnostic and surveillance projects, especially in settings where timely transport of diagnostic samples is challenging. Further evaluation of GenoTube swabs in field situations that do not require *Brachyspira* isolation and DNA quantification is warranted.

Abbreviations

ADG: Average daily gain; Bp: Base pair; CTRL: Group serving as control; D: Day; H & E: Hematoxylin and Eosin stain; INOC: Treatment group inoculated with *"B. hampsonii"* clade I strain 30599; MHD: Mucohemorrhagic diarrhea; PCR: Polymerase chain reaction; PCV2: Porcine circovirus type 2; PDS: Prairie Diagnostic Services, Inc., Saskatoon, Canada; PRRSv: Porcine reproductive and respiratory syndrome virus; SD: Swine dysentery; WF: Warthin Faulkner silver stain.

Competing interests

The University of Saskatchewan has intellectual property applications pertaining to the *"B. hampsonii"* clade II Canadian type strain (*Brachyspira* sp. sask30446) titled: "Diagnostic Method for Colitis" (PTC CA/2011/000828) submitted in July 2011 and "Isolated *Brachyspira* and methods and compositions for expanding and isolating *Brachyspira*" (PCT WO/2013/010260) submitted in July 2012. Both are published and available online at: http://patentscope.wipo.int. JCSH, JER and JEH are named co-inventors. This does not alter the authors' adherence to all policies pertaining to publication, interpretation of results, or sharing of materials and reagents.

Authors' contributions

In vivo work was conducted by HDL, MOC and JCSH. *"Brachyspira hampsonii"* strain 305996 was initially isolated and propagated for the trial by JER. Laboratory work was conducted by CF, HDL and JEH. MOC evaluated the *ante mortem* sample methodologies. SED performed pathological assessments. JEH and JCSH are Principal Investigators. All authors read and approved the final manuscript.

Acknowledgements

Funding for this research was provided by generous contributions of the Canadian Swine Health Board. The GenoTube Livestock swabs were generously donated by Prionics, Switzerland.

Author details

[1]Department of Veterinary Microbiology, University of Saskatchewan, 52 Campus Dr., S7N 5B4 Saskatoon, SK, Canada. [2]Department of Large Animal Clinical Sciences, University of Saskatchewan, Saskatoon, SK, Canada. [3]Department of Veterinary Pathology, University of Saskatchewan, Saskatoon, SK, Canada.

References

1. Whiting RA, Doyle LP, Spray RS: **Swine dysentery.** *Purdue Univ Agric Experiment Station Bull* 1921, **257:**1–15.
2. Harris DL, Glock RD, Christensen CR, Kinyon JM: **Inoculation of pigs with *Treponema hyodysenteriae* (new species) and reproduction of the disease.** *Vet Med Small Anim Clinic* 1972, **67**(1):61–64.
3. Taylor DJ, Alexander TJL: **The production of dysentery in swine by feeding cultures containing a spirochaete.** *Br Vet J* 1971, **127**(11):58–61.
4. Harding JCS, Chirino-Trejo M, Fernando C, Jacobson M, Forster Z, Hill JE: **Detection of a novel *Brachyspira* species associated with haemorrhagic and necrotizing colitis.** In *Proceedings of the Carlos Pijoan Symposium on Swine Dysentery, 38th Allen D Leman Swine Conference; St. Paul, MN*; 2011:27–32.
5. Harding JSC, Fernando C, Rubin J, Hill JE: **Emergence of mucohaemorrhagic diarrhea associated with *"B. hampsonii"* in western Canada.** In *Proceedings of the 6th Colonic Spirochaetal Infections of Animals and Humans.* Guildford, UK: University of Surrey; 2013:61.
6. Harding JCS, Chirino-Trejo M, Fernando C, Jacobson M, Forster Z, Hill JE: **Detection of a novel *Brachyspira* species associated with haemorrhagic and necrotizing colitis.** In *Proceedings of the Int Pig Vet Soc Congr.* Vancouver, Canada: IPVS 2010; 2010:740.
7. Schwartz K: ***Brachyspira*: what is happening in Iowa and why.** In *Proceedings of the West Can Assoc Swine Vet Conf.* Saskatoon, SK: WCASV; 2011:25–33.
8. Clothier KA, Kinyon JM, Frana TS, Naberhaus N, Bower L, Strait EL, Schwartz K: **Species characterization and minimum inhibitory concentration patterns of *Brachyspira* species isolates from swine with clinical disease.** *J Vet Diagnost Invest* 2011, **23**(6):1140–1145.
9. Chander Y, Primus A, Oliveira S, Gebhart CJ: **Phenotypic and molecular characterization of a novel strongly hemolytic *Brachyspira* species, provisionally designated *"Brachyspira hampsonii"*.** *J Vet Diagn Invest* 2012, **24**(5):903–910.
10. Rubin JE, Costa MO, Hill JE, Kittrel HE, Fernando C, Huang Y, O'Connor B, Harding JCS: **Reproduction of mucohaemorrhagic diarrhea, colitis and shedding indistinguishable from swine dysentery following experimental inoculation with *"Brachyspira hampsonii"* strain 30446.** *PLoS ONE* 2013, **8**(2):e57146.
11. Burrough ER, Strait EL, Kinyon JM, Bower LP, Madson DM, Wilberts BL, Schwartz KJ, Frana TS, Songer JG: **Comparative virulence of clinical *Brachyspira* spp. isolates in inoculated pigs.** *J Vet Diagn Invest* 2012, **24**(6):1025–1034.
12. Burrough E, Strait E, Kinyon J, Bower L, Madson D, Schwartz K, Frana T, Songer JG: **Comparison of atypical *Brachyspira* spp. clinical isolates and classic strains in a mouse model of swine dysentery.** *Vet Microbiol* 2012, **160**(3/4):387–394.
13. Song Y, Hampson DJ: **Development of a multiplex qPCR for detection and quantitation of pathogenic intestinal spirochaetes in the faeces of pigs and chickens.** *Vet Microbiol* 2009, **137**(1/2):129–136.
14. Mahu M, De Jong E, De Pauw N, Vande Maele L, Vandenbroucke V, Vandersmissen T, Miry C, Pasmans F, Haesebrouck F, Martel A, Boyen F: **First isolation of *"Brachyspira hampsonii"* from pigs in Europe.** *Vet Rec* 2014, **174:**47. doi:10.1136/vr.101868.

15. Bonini P, Plebani M, Ceriotti F, Rubboli F: **Errors in laboratory medicine.** *Clin Chem* 2002, **48**(5):691–698.
16. Waldmann KH, Wendt M, Amtsberg G: **[Diagnostic examinations of *Brachyspira* species and therapeutic strategy in swine dysentery] Untersuchungen zur *Brachyspira*-Diagnostik und Behandlungsstrategie bei der Schweinedysenterie.** *Dtsch Tierarztl Wochenschr* 2000, **107**(12):486–489.
17. Jones GF, Ward GE, Murtaugh MP, Lin G, Gebhart CJ: **Enhanced detection of intracellular organism of swine proliferative enteritis, ileal symbiont intracellularis, in feces by polymerase chain reaction.** *J Clin Microbiol* 1993, **31**(10):2611–2615.
18. Harding JCS, Baker CD, Tumber A, McIntosh KA, Parker SE, Middleton DM, Hill JE, Ellis JA, Krakowka S: **Porcine circovirus-2 DNA concentration distinguishes wasting from nonwasting pigs and is correlated with lesion distribution, severity, and nucleocapsid staining intensity.** *J Vet Diagnost Invest* 2008, **20**(3):274–282.
19. Rohde J, Rothkamp A, Gerlach GF: **Differentiation of porcine *Brachyspira* species by a novel nox PCR-based restriction fragment length polymorphism analysis.** *J Clin Microbiol* 2002, **40**(7):2598–2600.
20. Stephens CP, Hampson D: **Prevalence and disease association of intestinal spirochaetes in chickens in eastern Australia.** *Avian Pathol* 2010, **28**(5):447–454.
21. Osorio J, Carvajal A, Naharro G, Rubio P, La T, Phillips ND, Hampson DJ: **Identification of weakly haemolytic *Brachyspira* isolates recovered from pigs with diarrhoea in Spain and Portugal and comparison with results from other countries.** *Res Vet Sci* 2013, **95**(3):861–869.
22. Jensen TK, Christensen AS, Boye M: ***Brachyspira murdochii* colitis in pigs.** *Vet Pathol* 2010, **47**(2):334–338.
23. Rohde J, Habighorst-Blome K, Seehusen F: **"*Brachyspira hampsonii*" clade I isolated from Belgian pigs imported to Germany.** *Vet Microbiol* 2014, **168**(2/4):432–435.
24. Martínez-Lobo FJ, Hidalgo Á, García M, Argüello H, Naharro G, Carvajal A, Rubio P: **First Identification of "*Brachyspira hampsonii*" in Wild European Waterfowl.** *PLoS ONE* 2013, **8**(12):e82626.
25. Durmic Z, Pethick DW, Pluske JR, Hampson DJ: **Changes in bacterial populations in the colon of pigs fed different sources of dietary fibre, and the development of swine dysentery after experimental infection.** *J Appl Microbiol* 1998, **85**:3.
26. Pluske JR, Pethick DW, Durmic Z, Hampson DJ, Mullan BP: *Non-Starch Polysaccharides in Pig Diets and their Influence on Intestinal Microflora, Digestive Physiology and Enteric Disease.* Nottingham, UK: Nottingham University Press; 2001.
27. Hansen CF, Phillips ND, La T, Hernandez A, Mansfield J, Kim JC, Mullan BP, Hampson DJ, Pluske JR: **Diets containing inulin but not lupins help to prevent swine dysentery in experimentally challenged pigs.** *J Anim Sci* 2010, **88**:10.
28. Fellstrom C, Gunnarsson A: **Phenotypical characterisation of intestinal spirochaetes isolated from pigs.** *Res Vet Sci* 1995, **59**(1):1–4.
29. Komarek V, Maderner A, Spergser J, Weissenbock H: **Infections with weakly haemolytic *Brachyspira* species in pigs with miscellaneous chronic diseases.** *Vet Microbiol* 2009, **134**(3/4):311–317.
30. Hampson DJ, Fellstrom C, Thomson JR: **Swine Dysentery.** In *Diseases of Swine.* 9th edition. Edited by Straw BE, Zimmerman JJ, D'Allaire SD, Taylor DJ. Ames, IA: Blackwell Publishing; 2006:785–805.
31. Patterson AH, Rubin JE, Fernando C, Costa MO, Harding JCS, Hill JE: **Fecal shedding of *Brachyspira* spp. on a farrow-to-finish swine farm with a clinical history of " *Brachyspira hampsonii*"-associated colitis.** *BMC Vet Res* 2013, **9**:137. doi:10.1186/1746-6148-1189-1137.
32. Plebani M, Carraro P: **Mistakes in a stat laboratory: types and frequency.** *Clin Chem* 1997, **43**(8 Pt 1):1348–1351.

24

Sero-prevalence and risk factors associated with African swine fever on pig farms in southwest Nigeria

Emmanuel Jolaoluwa Awosanya[1,2*], Babasola Olugasa[1], Gabriel Ogundipe[1] and Yrjo Tapio Grohn[2]

Abstract

Background: African swine fever (ASF) is one of the major setbacks to development of the pig industry in Nigeria. It is enzootic in southwest Nigeria. We determined the sero-prevalence and factors associated with ASF among-herd seropositivity in 144 pig farms in six States from southwest Nigeria during the dry and rainy seasons using indirect Enzyme Linked Immunosorbent Assay (ELISA) for ASF IgG antibodies. An interviewer-administered questionnaire was used to collect information on demography, environmental and management factors. We performed descriptive statistics, and univariate and multivariable analyses to determine the among-herd sero-prevalence of ASF and its associated factors.

Results: The overall herd sero-prevalence of ASF was 28 % (95 % Confidence interval (95 % CI) 21 – 36); it was significantly higher ($P < 0.05$) in the dry season (54 %; 95 % CI 37 – 70) than the rainy season (18 %; 95 % CI 11 – 27). In the univariate analysis, having a quarantine/ isolation unit within 100 m radius of a regular pig pen (OR = 3.3; 95 % CI 1.3 – 8.9), external source of replacement stock (OR = 3.2; 95 % CI 1.3 – 8.3) and dry season (OR = 5.3; 95 % CI 2.2 – 12.7) were risk factors for ASF among-herd seropositivity. In the multivariable logistic regression, there was interaction between season and herd size. Our final model included season, source of replacement stock, herd size and interaction between herd size and season. Herds with an external source of replacement always had higher ASF sero-prevalence compared with herds with an internal source. The herd size effect varied between seasons.

Conclusions: The ASF herd level sero-prevalence in southwest Nigeria was higher in pig herds with an external source of replacement stock and in the dry season. The effect of season of the year the samples were taken on ASF seropositivity was modified by herd size. We encourage strict compliance with biosecurity measures, especially using an internal source of replacement stock and measures that minimize movement on pig farms in southwest Nigeria, in order to enhance ASF free farms.

Keywords: Sero-prevalence, African swine fever, Pigs, Season, Management, Transmission, Southwest Nigeria

Background

African swine fever (ASF) is a highly contagious and fatal viral disease of pigs caused by a DNA virus of the *Asfarviridae* family. It is a trans-boundary animal disease, defined as a disease of significant economic, trade and/or food security importance for a considerable number of countries, which can easily spread across national borders and reach epidemic proportions and for which control and management, including exclusion, require international co-operation [1].

Globally, the ASF virus is present in Africa, Italy (Sardinia), Georgia, Latvia, Poland, Ukraine, Russia (Moscow) and some Caribbean countries, with an increasing risk of spreading to ASF-free countries in Europe and America [2, 3]. African swine fever is the main threat to the pig industry in Africa because of the heavy losses incurred by pig farmers [4, 5] when it strikes, with mortality approaching 100 % [4].

Three epidemiological cycles have been recognized: the sylvatic [6], domestic [7], and sylvatic and domestic cycle [4, 8]. In Africa, all three have been reported; however, in

* Correspondence: emmafisayo@yahoo.com
[1]Department of Veterinary Public Health and Preventive Medicine, Faculty of Veterinary Medicine, University of Ibadan, Ibadan, Oyo State, Nigeria
[2]Department of Population Medicine and Diagnostic Sciences, College of Veterinary Medicine, Cornell University, Ithaca, NY 14853, USA

Nigeria only the domestic cycle which maintains the ASF virus within domestic pigs is most recognized and reported [7] despite reports on detection of ASF virus in river hogs [9].

In Nigeria, the first ASF outbreak was reported in 1973 and subsequently in 1997, 1998 and 2001 [10–12]. Since the outbreak in 1997, there have been reported confirmed and unconfirmed sporadic outbreaks of ASF. African swine fever is enzootic in Nigeria [13, 14].

The pig industry in Nigeria can be classified into small holder farms – farms having fewer than 50 pigs in the herd at any point in time; medium holder farms – farms having from 50 to 100 pigs in the herd at any point in time and large holder farms – farms with over 100 pigs in the herd at any point in time. The pig farming industry in Nigeria has its largest presence in the southwest of Nigeria, with fewer high pig density areas in other geo-political zones in the country. Farming activities occur throughout the whole year with increased activities during festive periods in December. The pig production system in southwest Nigeria is predominantly confined within pig pens. The ASF scourge has however adversely affected the bustling and rising activities in this industry since the outbreak in 1997 [5]. Efforts have been made by the various State Governments through farm extension services in educating the farmers on biosecurity measures since that outbreak.

Several researchers have made efforts in contributing to the understanding of the dynamics of transmission, control and what will hopefully lead to its eventual eradication in Nigeria. Economic losses to farmers consequent to ASF scourge [5], molecular epidemiological description of the circulating strain of ASF virus in Nigeria [15, 16], surveillance of the ASF virus in both domestic and wild pig populations especially during the periods of outbreaks [9, 14, 17, 18], geographical and spatial spread of the ASF infection [19, 20] and identification of risk factors during ASF outbreaks at farm level [19] have been reported.

There had been a 5-year gap (2007–2012) between the last sero-monitoring of the ASF virus in southwest Nigeria [14]. Previous work on assessment of risk factors considered an outbreak situation; however, ASF has assumed a new enzootic status – the implication of this is that most infected farms are at subclinical level. Thus, factors responsible for the enzootic status of ASF in Nigeria are poorly elucidated.

This paper therefore attempts to address the above identified gaps of ASF herd level sero-status and unknown risk factors for ASF sero-positivity in an enzootic situation by assessing the current sero-status of pigs among herd ASF sero-prevalence and their associated factors in southwest Nigeria.

Results

Demography

Of 144 respondents, 108 (75 %; 95 % CI 67 – 82) were males; their mean age was 49.2 ± 14.6 years. Most of the respondents (64 %; 95 % CI 55 – 72) had tertiary education; 53 % (95 % CI 44 – 61) practiced pig farming as their only source of livelihood. The median year of practice was 7 years (Range: 1 – 36 years). Most of the farms (81 %; 95 % CI 73 – 87) were established after the last report of an ASF outbreak in 2001; the range was from 1949 to 2013. All the pig herds were raised in strict pen confinement. The median number of pigs in the herd was 45 (Range: 2 – 567). The median age of the pigs sampled was 8 months (Range: 1 – 72 months). The majority of the breeds were crosses, mainly large whites. The previous year average mortality ranged from 0 to 99 pigs: most of the pig herds (80 %; 95 % CI 72 – 86) had average mortality within 0 to 12 pigs. Only 6 (4 %; 95 % CI 2 – 9) of the pig herds had a reported history of ASF outbreak. Most of the farmers (91 %, 95 % CI 85 – 95) had access to potable water on the farm.

ASF seropositivity

The overall herd sero-prevalence of ASF was 28 % (95 % CI 21 – 36), (40 of 144). Lagos had the lowest sero-prevalence (13 %; 95 % CI 4 – 30) while Ogun had the highest value of 57 % (95 % CI 37 – 75); there was a significant difference ($p < 0.05$) in the sero-prevalence of ASF between Lagos and Ogun States (Table 1). The sero-prevalence of ASF was higher (18 %; 95 % CI 12 – 24) in older stock (more than 12 months old) than in the younger stock (10 %; 95 % CI 7 – 13); this was significant at $p = 0.01$. The herd sero-prevalence was highest (31 %; 95 % CI 21 – 43) in small pig herds (less than 50 pigs) and lowest (21 %; 95 % CI 10 – 37) in medium herds (51 – 100 pigs); however, the difference was not significant. There was a significant difference ($p < 0.05$) in the sero-prevalence during the dry season (54 %; 95 % CI 37 – 70) and rainy season (18 %; 95 % CI 11 – 27). Overall individual crude prevalence was 78 of 657 (12 %; 95 % CI 10 – 15). Overall individual prevalence adjusted by weight of total population size was 11.2 %.

Herd level associated environmental and management factors to ASF seropositivity

In the univariate analysis, the presence of a quarantine or isolation unit within 100 m radius of the regular pig pen (OR = 3.3; 95 % CI 1.3 – 8.9), season of the year the samples were taken (OR = 5.3; 95 % CI 2.2 – 12.7) and source of replacement stock (OR = 3.2; 95 % CI 1.3 – 8.3) were significantly associated with ASF sero-positivity (Table 1); however, the presence of pig farms within 1 km radius of another farm, having slaughter

Table 1 Factors associated with pig herd level African swine fever seropositivity of 144 pig herds in southwest Nigeria, 2013

Variables	Seropositive n = 40 (%)	Seronegative n = 104 (%)	OR (95 % CI)[a]	P Value
State Location				
Lagos	4 (10)	27 (26)	Ref	
Ondo	4 (10)	16 (15)	1.7 (0.3; 10.3)	0.76
Ekiti	4 (10)	13 (12.5)	2.1 (0.3; 12.9)	0.58
Osun	5 (12.5)	19 (18)	1.8 (0.3; 10.1)	0.67
Oyo	6 (15)	16 (15)	2.5 (0.5; 13.9)	0.34
Ogun	17 (42.5)	13 (12.5)	8.8 (2.2; 41.8)	0.001
Total No. of pigs on farm				
Large holder farms (101 – 567)	7 (17.5)	19 (18)	Ref	
Medium holder farms (51 – 100)	8 (20)	30 (29)	0.7 (0.2; 2.8)	0.80
Small holder farms (<= 50)	25 (62.5)	55 (53)	1.2 (0.4; 3.9)	0.88
Season				
Dry	21 (52.5)	18 (17)	5.3 (2.2; 12.7)	0.00
Rainy	19 (47.5)	86 (83)		
Having slaughter slabs within 1 km radius of the farm				
Yes	5 (12.5)	23 (22)	0.5 (0.1; 1.5)	0.28
No	35 (87.5)	81 (78)		
Having rubbish heap within 1 km radius of the farm				
Yes	29 (72.5)	64 (61.5)	1.6 (0.7; 4.1)	0.30
No	11 (27.5)	40 (38.5)		
Having a quarantine/isolation unit within 100 m radius of the regular pen				
Yes	13 (32.5)	13 (12.5)	3.3 (1.3; 8.9)	0.01
No	27 (67.5)	91 (87.5)		
Farm workers having designated working clothes				
Yes	28 (70)	85 (82)	0.5 (0.2; 1.3)	0.19
No	12 (30)	19 (18)		
Taking of shower/bath at work				
Yes	26 (65)	52 (50)	1.9 (0.8; 4.3)	0.15
No	14 (35)	52 (50)		
Lending out of service boars				
Yes	8 (20)	33 (32)	0.5 (0.2; 1.4)	0.23
No	32 (80)	71 (68)		
Daily cleaning of pen floor				
Yes	36 (90)	95 (91)	0.9 (0.2; 4.0)	1.00
No	4 (10)	9 (19)		
Daily disinfection of pen floor				
Yes	8 (20)	25 (24)	0.8 (0.3; 2.1)	0.78
No	32 (80)	79 (76)		
Daily cleaning of working utensils				
Yes	28 (70)	71 (68)	1.1 (0.4; 2.6)	1.00
No	12 (30)	33 (32)		

Table 1 Factors associated with pig herd level African swine fever seropositivity of 144 pig herds in southwest Nigeria, 2013 (Continued)

Daily disinfection of working utensils				
Yes	9 (22.5)	21 (20)	1.1 (0.4; 3.0)	0.92
No	31 (77.5)	83 (80)		
Snacking or eating while working				
Yes	10 (25)	19 (18)	1.5 (0.6; 3.8)	0.50
No	30 (75)	85 (82)		
Wearing of work clothes outside of farm				
Yes	8 (20)	15 (14)	1.5 (0.5; 4.2)	0.56
No	32 (80)	89 (86)		
Source of replacement stock				
External source	31 (62.5)	54 (52)	3.2 (1.3; 8.3)	0.01
Internal source	9 (37.5)	50 (48)		
Feeding of swill				
Yes	22 (55)	59 (57)	0.9 (0.4; 2.1)	1.00
No	18 (45)	45 (43)		
Having carcass disposal or burying site within 1 km radius of farm				
Yes	27 (67.5)	59 (57)	1.6 (0.7; 3.7)	0.32
No	13 (32.5)	45 (43)		
Presence of nearby pig farms (within 1 km radius)				
Yes	21 (52.5)	59 (57)	0.8 (0.4; 1.9)	0.79
No	19 (47.5)	45 (43)		
Sharing of farm workers among fellow farmers				
Yes	4 (10)	13 (12.5)	0.8 (0.2; 2.8)	0.93
No	36 (90)	91 (87.5)		
Sharing of working utensils among fellow farmers				
Yes	3 (7.5)	5 (5)	1.6 (0.2; 8.7)	0.78
No	37 (92.5)	99 (95)		
Farm workers having a designated work footwear				
Yes	27 (67.5)	77 (74)	0.7 (0.3; 1.8)	0.56
No	13 (32.5)	27 (26)		

[a]Odds ratio (95 % Confidence interval)

slabs or abattoir within 1 km radius of the farm, having rubbish heap or carcass disposal site within 1 km radius of the farm and presence of other animals or livestock within 100 m radius of the regular pig pen were not significantly associated with ASF seropositivity.

In the multivariable logistic regression adjusting for other covariates that were significant at $P < 0.20$ and biologically plausible ones, there was an interaction between herd size and season of the year the samples were taken. Source of restocking was a significant (OR = 2.7; 95 % CI 1.1 – 6.7) predictor for ASF herd level seropositivity. The final model included 4 predictors: season of the year the samples were taken, source of replacement stock, herd size and interaction between herd size and season of the year the samples were taken (Table 2). These were statistically significant in estimating ASF seropositivity (– 2 log-likelihood = 142.4; Goodness of fit = 0.97; $\chi 2 = 20.2$; $p = 0.0005$). The model correctly classified 76.5 % of the cases.

Compliance with standard biosecurity measures

Overall average compliance with standard biosecurity measures was 61 % (95 % CI 59 – 63). Of the 144 pig herds, only 5 (3.5 %; 95 % CI 1 – 8) had functional foot dip, 113 (78.5 %; 95 % CI 71 – 85) had farm designated working clothes, 57 (40 %; 95 % CI 32 – 48) had routine pest control, 3 (2 %; 95 % CI 0 – 6) reported presence of ticks on pigs, 81 (56 %; 95 % CI 48 – 64) fed swill to their animals, 30 (21 %; 95 % CI 15 – 28) disinfected

Table 2 Unconditional Logistic Regression of factors associated with African swine fever seropositivity of 144 pig herds with herd size as a continuous variable in southwest Nigeria, 2013

Variables	DF	β	Standard Error	Wald Chi-Square	OR[b]	95% Wald CI[c]	P-value
Intercept	1	−1.60	0.51	9.98			0.00
[a]Season (Dry/Rainy)	1	0.58	0.59	0.96			0.33
Source (External/Internal)	1	0.98	0.47	4.38	2.7	1.1; 6.7	0.04
[a]Herd size	1	−0.01	0.01	2.61			0.11
Season*Herd size	1	0.02	0.01	4.22			0.04

[a]Due to interactions between season of the year and herd size, odds ratio were not expressed because they depend on the individual value of both variables
[b]Odds ratio
[c]Confidence interval
*Interaction term

their working utensils daily, 33 (23 %; 95 % CI 16 – 31) disinfected the pen floor daily, 17 (12 %; 95 % CI 7 – 18) shared farm attendants with other pig farmers, 8 (5.5 %; 95 % CI 2 – 11) shared working utensils with other pig farmers, 41 (28.5 %; 95 % CI 21 – 37) either gave or took service boars, and 23 (16 %; 95 % CI 10 – 23) of the respondents wore their farm working clothes outside of their premises. None of these factors was significantly ($p < 0.05$) associated with ASF among herd seropositivity.

Frequency of identified ASF related signs by respondents as occurring on the farm

The most common ASF related signs identified by the respondents were weakness or unwillingness of the pigs to stand (31 %; 95 % CI 23 – 39), followed by abortion (30 %; 95 % CI 23 – 38); the least common was reddening of ear and snout (7 %; 95 % CI 3 – 12). Reddening of ear and snout, however, was the only ASF related sign identified by the respondents that was significantly ($p = 0.005$) associated with ASF sero-positivity.

Discussion

Our modeling indicated that source of replacement stock and season of the year the samples were taken are important determinants of ASF herd seropositivity in southwest Nigeria. However, the effect of season of the year the samples were taken on ASF herd seropositivity was modified by herd size. Herds with an external source of replacement always had higher ASF sero-prevalence compared with those with an internal source. This could be due to higher risk of introduction of an asymptomatic carrier into the herd at purchase. The spread of the ASF virus has been associated with asymptomatic carriers [21]. Introduction of ASF into a free area *via* movements of infected pigs has also been implicated in trans-boundary spread [4]. The higher ASF sero-prevalence in herds with an external source of replacement stock is also suggestive of a higher level of compromise in the bio-exclusion and bio-containment efforts, possibly due to more frequent human and vehicular movements in herds with external source of replacement stock [4].

The logistic regression technique allowed us to calculate the risk of ASF seropositivity as a function of the determinants in the final model using the formula: Prevalence (seropositive) $= 1/1 + e^{-[\alpha + Season*\beta 1 + Source*\beta 2 + Herdsize*\beta 3 + Season*Herdsize*\beta 4]}$. To demonstrate the interaction effect of season of the year the samples were taken and herd size we calculated the risk of ASF seropositivity for dry season and internal source of replacement, dry season and external source of replacement, rainy season and external source of replacement, and rainy season and internal source of replacement (Fig. 1). The risk of ASF seropositivity was always higher in farms with an external source of replacement stock than an internal source. Among herds with an external source of replacement the risk of ASF seropositivity was higher in the dry season than in the rainy season. Among herds with an internal source of replacement the risk of ASF seropositivity was higher in small and medium farms during the dry season than in the rainy; there was no difference in large herds. The risk decreased faster in the dry season with increasing herd size in farms with an internal source of replacement stock. The risk also increased faster in the rainy season with increasing herd size in farms with an external source of replacement stock (*i.e.*, the herd size effect was not constant between seasons). These ASF risk dynamics in pig herds in southwest Nigeria bring a new dimension to the understanding of the ASF epidemiological cycle and its enzootic status in the region. A second model considered herd size as a categorical variable; here there was no interaction between herd size and season. The likelihood of having an ASF seropositive pig herd increased by five and three times during the dry season and for farms with an external source of replacement stock respectively.

In our model, preponderance of susceptible pigs arising from increased restocking in the rainy season, especially in large herds, could explain the faster change in the risk of ASF seropositivity in the rainy season with increasing herd size in farms with an external source of replacement. The rapid reduction in ASF risk in the dry season with increasing herd size in farms with an internal source of replacement could also be explained from the above standpoint because most pig farmers dispose of their

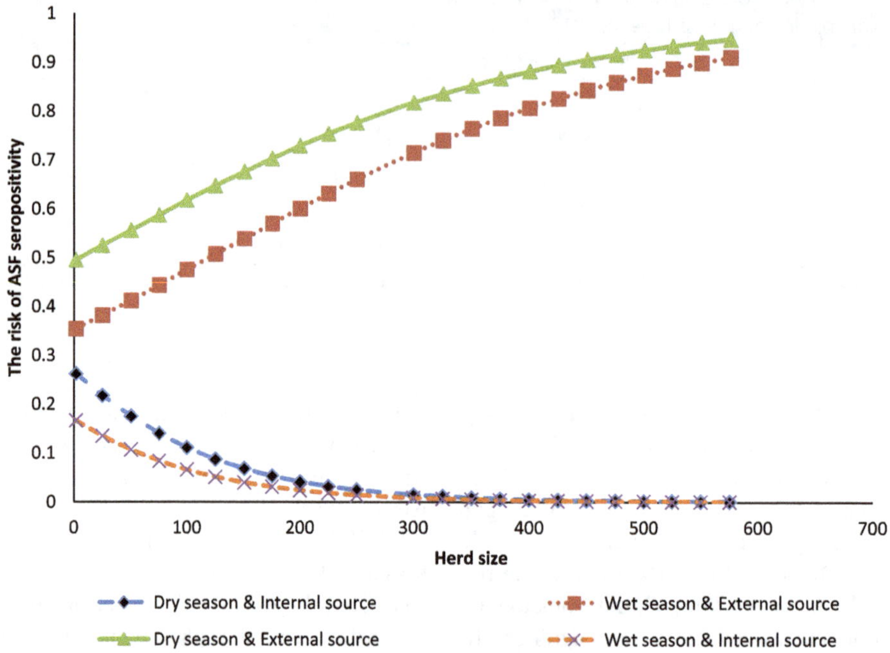

Fig. 1 The risk of African swine fever (ASF) seropositivity in dry and wet seasons in 144 pig herds with external and internal source of replacement stock in southwest Nigeria, 2013. The risk is calculated based on the logistic regression model in Table 2. The risk of ASF seropositivity was always higher in the dry than in the rainy season and in farms with an external source of replacement stock than an internal source. The risk decreased faster in the dry season with increasing herd size in farms with an internal source of replacement stock. The risk also increased faster in the rainy season with increasing herd size in farms with an external source of replacement stock

finisher stock in the dry season [22, 23]. Herd size has been associated with pig diseases [24, 25]. The higher ASF sero-prevalence in the dry season could be due to the presence of other factors that favor the prevalence and maintenance of ASF aside from restocking. The significant association between season of the year the samples were taken and source of replacement stock with ASF herd seropositivity in this study is similar to the findings of Atuhaire *et al.* [22] in a 12-year epidemiological overview of ASF in Uganda.

Numbers of movements of pigs and pig products increase in the dry season, resulting from increased trading demands during the festive period in December. Moreover, farmers have a higher propensity to dispose of mature pigs during this period because of feed scarcity and meeting of domestic (family) needs which is always on the increase during the dry season [22, 23]. Local and international trading in pigs and pig products has been associated with ASF outbreaks [2, 4, 22, 26].

Magali [27] reported insignificant but higher prevalence of ASFV in ticks during the dry than rainy season in South Africa. Although only 2 % of our respondents reported seeing ticks and their presence was not significantly associated with seropositivity in this study, this might have been under reported because of observational bias by the farmers. Thus, the role of ticks in the epidemiology of ASF in Nigeria may require further studies. Ticks play a major role in the sylvatic cycle of ASF transmission in East and Southern Africa [6], and in transmission between the sylvatic cycle and domestic pigs [4].

Another possibility could be that after infection consequent to introduction of an asymptomatic carrier by purchase in the rainy season in pig farms with an external source of replacement, the disease takes a chronic or subacute course and thus the higher sero-prevalence in the dry season. African swine fever viral infection has been reported to persist for a long time in the blood [28]. These disease dynamics may support the enzootic status of ASF in pig herds in southwest Nigeria.

In the univariate analysis, the presence of a quarantine or isolation unit within 100 m radius of the regular pig pen was significantly positively associated with ASF seropositivity. This underscores the importance of proper location of the quarantine or isolation units in order to achieve their intended purpose of biosecurity. The proximity of such units to other operational units like farrowing, fattening *etc.* could actually be a risk for having ASF seropositive farms. It is recommended that siting of the quarantine/isolation unit should not be less than 100 m from the regular pig pen [29], which is a challenge to most small holder farms in southwest Nigeria because of inadequate space due to land tenure system and financial constraints. However, when we tested the association between having quarantine/isolation unit within 100 m of the regular pig pen and ASF herd seropositivity controlling for other covariates the association was no longer significant. The effect poor siting of quarantine or isolation unit could have on herd seropositivity is, however, noteworthy.

In our study, we did not find a significant effect of environmental factors such as presence of pig farms within 1 km radius of another farm, having slaughter slabs or abattoir within 1 km radius of the farm, having rubbish heap or carcass disposal site within 1 km radius of the farm and presence of other animals or livestock within 100 m radius of the regular pig pen on ASF seropositivity. However, Fasina *et al.* [30] showed some of these factors like presence of an abattoir in a pig farming community and presence of an infected pig farm in the neighborhood to be significantly associated with ASF outbreaks. This difference could be due to the effects of environmental factors on ASF virus (ASFV) maintenance becoming insidious as the occurrence of ASF became enzootic.

We reported an overall herd ASF sero-prevalence of 28 %; this is significantly lower than the value (93 %) reported 5 years ago by Olugasa [14] across the same geographical region. The significant difference in our study sero-prevalence estimate of 28 % and the previous sero-prevalence of 93 % by Olugasa [14] which was used to determine our sample size would have slightly widened our set margin of error; however, our study sero-prevalence estimate is still within a 7 % margin of error of the population true sero-prevalence. All the other States except Ogun had a marked decline in their herd ASF sero-prevalence when compared with a 5-year value reported by Olugasa [14]. This indicates some improvement in the control measures by the Governments at all levels to eradicate the disease. The ASF herd sero-prevalence in Ogun is highest and almost stable, followed by Oyo: the high sero-prevalence in these States since the outbreak in 1997 could be because both States had international borders. Ogun was the first State in Nigeria to experience the outbreak of ASF in 1997 which spread through trans-border trade from the Republic of Benin [31]. Movement of pigs and pig products across borders from infected areas has been reported to be positively correlated with ASF seropositivity and outbreaks [4, 32]. The herd sero-prevalence is higher in small pig herds than in larger pig herds, though not significantly so; this may be due to difficulty in adhering to strict biosecurity by small holder farms or possibly less attention to simple biosecurity measures than on big farms. Moreover, the sero-prevalence of ASF is significantly higher in older stock than younger stock; this could be because restriction of movement to sections of the herds containing young pigs is greater than for older ones. It could also be that older stock had a longer time to develop antibodies to the ASF virus than younger stock, or possibly due to long persistence of ASF antibodies for a period of time after exposure [28]. There could also exist differences in ASFV transmission rates among the various age groups. Olugasa [14] also reported differences in sero-prevalence of ASF among various age groups.

Biosecurity is defined as the implementation of measures that reduce the risk of the introduction and spread of disease agents; it requires the adoption of a set of attitudes and behaviors by people to reduce risk in all activities involving domestic, captive/exotic and wild animals and their products [33]. There was no significant difference in the level of compliance with some of the biosecurity measures between seropositive and seronegative herds in our study population; however, Fasina *et al.* [30] reported significant associations between food and water control, separation/isolation of sick pigs, washing and disinfection of farm equipment and tools, consultations or visits by veterinarians/paraveterinarians, pest/rodent control, and sharing farm tools and equipment and ASF outbreaks in Nigerian farms.

With the understanding that ASF is enzootic in Nigeria, one would expect to see less apparent signs of peracute or acute forms of ASF, but rather, more of the subacute, chronic or subclinical forms. Farmers in this study reported noticing weakness or unwillingness of the pigs to stand (31 %), followed by abortion (30 %); the least common sign was reddening of the ear and snout (7 %). Reddening of the ear and snout, however, was the only ASF related sign identified by the respondents that was significantly ($p = 0.005$) associated with ASF seropositivity. There is no sign, however, that is pathognomonic to ASF. The implication of this is that the ability of the farmers to recognize such associated signs could assist early detection of an infection. However, the challenge with early detection is the non-willingness to report by the farmers. Farmers may not report because the adjudged compensation by the Government, if any, is non-commensurate. Early detection and reporting is critical to ASF control and eradication [34].

Pig farmers in Nigeria are mostly males, in their mid-50s (mean 49.2 ± 14.6 years) and most had tertiary education. More than half of the population of pig farmers studied had pig farming as their main source of livelihood. This indicates the importance of the farming sector and the socioeconomic impact adverse effects of disease such as ASF could have on livelihood. The pig sector appears to be recovering after the devastation caused by the ASF outbreak in 1997, which sent the majority of farmers out of business. Most of the farmers raised their pigs in strict pen confinement; greater risk of ASF seropositivity has been linked with free range pigs [32, 35, 36].

This study may be limited by information bias which is common to questionnaire administration, as respondents may give favoring or biased responses and not their actual practice. We mitigated this by triangulating – we designed the questionnaire in such a way that certain questions were deliberately repeated in different ways. We also envisaged interviewer bias and we reduced this by the training of the interviewers used in this study. These limitations were taken into consideration in the interpretation of the data.

Conclusions

Our findings indicate that ASF herd level sero-prevalence in southwest Nigeria was higher in pig herds with an external source of replacement stock than an internal source; and in the dry season than in the rainy season. The effect of season of the year the samples were taken on ASF seropositivity was modified by herd size. The observed increase in ASF risk in the rainy season with increasing herd size in pig herds with an external source of replacement and observed decrease in ASF risk in the dry season with increasing herd size in pig herds with an internal source of replacement suggest that large herds are at greater risk of ASF infection *via* introduction of an asymptomatic pig than through other indirect means such as fomites, movement of vehicles and personnel. We recommend strict compliance with biosecurity measures, especially using an internal source of replacement stock and measures that minimize movement on pig farms. The associations between ASF herd level sero-prevalence and source of replacement stock and the effect of herd size on season of the year the samples were taken have implications for the understanding of ASF transmission and application in the disease modeling and in development of a suitable control and eradication strategy for ASF in Nigeria. The role of ticks either on pigs or in pens in the enzootic status of ASF in Nigeria will be an area for further investigation.

Methods

Study locations

The study area included six States – Lagos, Ogun, Oyo, Osun, Ondo and Ekiti (Fig. 2). The choice of the States was informed by the large presence of pig farming

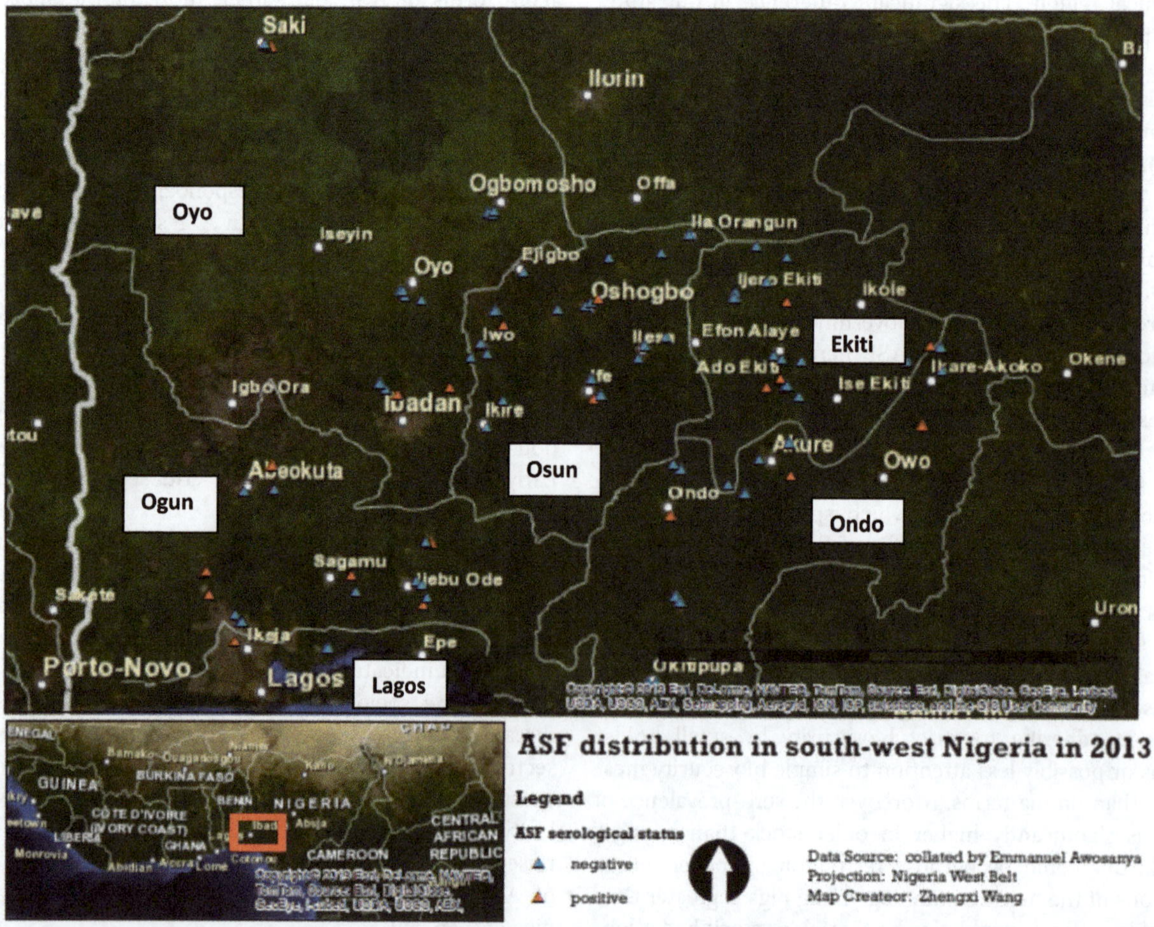

Fig. 2 Geographical spread of 144 pig herds surveyed for African swine fever (ASF) seropositivity in southwest Nigeria in 2013. Random distribution of the pig herds is shown

activities in these States and having reported outbreaks of ASF and the present enzootic status of those States. Each of the States has three senatorial districts and varying local government areas (LGAs). Pig farms from these senatorial districts and LGAs were included.

The study areas have varying sizes of pig populations: Lagos (approximately half a million pigs), Ogun (approximately half a million pigs), Oyo (approximately three hundred thousand pigs), Osun (approximately two hundred thousand pigs), Ondo (approximately a hundred thousand pigs) and Ekiti (approximately a hundred thousand pigs) [37].

Of the studied States only Ogun and Oyo have international borders with Benin Republic while Lagos is a coastal city. The location of Nigeria in Africa is shown in the inset (bottom left) in Fig. 2.

Study design, sample size and sampling

We conducted a cross sectional study on pig farms across the six States in southwest Nigeria from November 2012 to August 2013.

A total sample size of 657 pigs from 144 pig farms were used for the study. We approached this by using the formula below [38]:

$$n = \frac{Z^2 p(1-p) * D}{E^2}$$

Where Z is the reliability coefficient put at 1.96 at a 95 % confidence interval and E is the margin of error at 5 %. Based on previous studies we powered the study to detect among herd sero-prevalence (p) of 92.9 % [14]. This gave a minimum sample size of 101 farms. We adjusted for clustering by using the formula $D = 1 + (b-1)\rho$ [39], where D is the design effect, b is the average number of samples per cluster and ρ is the intra-cluster correlation coefficient. We decided to sample an average of four pigs per farm ($b = 4$), about 10 % of the pig population on the farm. An intra-cluster correlation coefficient of $\rho = 0.13$ was assumed based on an earlier study [40]. This gave us a D of 1.4. We multiplied the cluster design effect (1.4) by the earlier calculated sample size of 101 farms to arrive at a total of 141 farms. In all, a total of 144 farms and 657 pigs were sampled.

We used simple random sampling to select pig farms from a list of registered pig farms in Lagos (150) and Ogun States (124). However, for the remaining four States without a register, we used simple random sampling to select between two and four local government areas from the existing three senatorial districts in the States. At least one pig farm was chosen from each selected local government area and a total of at least six pig farms were chosen from each of the three senatorial districts. Randomness was verified using geospatial analysis by determining spatial autocorrelation (Global Moran's I) in ArcMap version 10.2. A minimum of 20 pig farms were selected from each State except Lagos and Ogun (30 pig farms) where there is a larger presence of piggery activities and Ekiti (17 pig farms) where we had fewer pig farms. The pigs were selected using stratified sampling (piglets (weaners and growers less than or equal to 12 months old) and adult pigs (sow and boars more than 12 months old)). Equal allocation was adopted. An average of four pigs per farm was sampled.

Data collection

Blood collection and Laboratory analysis

We obtained venous blood (3 – 5mls) samples from the cranial vena-cava of selected pigs. They were collected into plain tubes and transported in ice packs to the laboratory. Sera were properly labeled and stored at −20 °C until used in batches. We conducted the Indirect Enzyme Linked Immunosorbent Assay – ELISA – [41] test using the ASF kit (SVANOVIR® Sweden) to screen the pigs' sera for ASF IgG antibodies at the Immunology laboratory, Veterinary Public Health and Preventive Medicine, University of Ibadan, Nigeria. The test kit had sensitivity and specificity of 100 % and 92.5 % respectively and can detect antibodies from day seven post infection. The samples were collected from different farms during the dry (December to March) and rainy (June and July) seasons [42] in order to detect seasonal variation. Herd sero-prevalence was determined. We defined herds as seropositive if at least one pig was seropositive in the ELISA test. We also determined the overall individual crude prevalence and adjusted it by the weight of the total population size. This was achieved by dividing the individual herd size by the total population size and multiplying by the proportion that were positive in the samples taken from each farm. The sum of the adjusted proportions multiplied by 100 gave the overall individual adjusted prevalence.

Questionnaire design and administration

A pre-tested (pre-testing was done using seven pig farmers from two locations not included in the study areas) structured, interviewer-administered questionnaire was used to obtain data on demography, environmental and management factors, bio-security measures and ASF related signs. The questionnaires, containing 38 questions, were administered on farms where samples were obtained. A respondent was someone who was actively involved in the daily activities of the farm and was not necessarily the farm owner.

Statistical analysis

We conducted descriptive statistics and univariate analysis using SAS version 9.3 [43]. We determined the odds ratio and statistical significance between seropositive and seronegative pig farms using Fisher's exact test for discrete variables at the 95 % confidence level. Multivariable unconditional logistic regression was used to determine predictors for ASF seropositivity controlling for other covariates at $P < 0.20$ and biologically plausible ones such as feeding of swill, lending out boars for breeding and herd size. We tested for collinearity among predictors using the Chi square test for binomial variables. We also tested for interactions between selected variables. We used Akaike's information criterion in selecting the variables. A forward selection method was used. The goodness of fit of the model was tested using the Pearson goodness of fit test. In the final models, only variables or interactions that were found to significantly affect the outcome at $P < 0.05$, and corresponding lower-order interactions terms whether significant or not, were retained. We determined the overall average compliance with standard biosecurity measures by calculating the average compliance level of the 15 internal biosecurity measures (bio-management) considered.

Ethical considerations

This study was carried out in compliance with the guidelines of the Animal Ethics Committee of the Faculty of Veterinary Medicine, University of Ibadan, Nigeria. Informed consent was obtained from all participating pig farm owners.

Competing interests

The authors declare that they have no competing interests.

Authors' contributions

EJA conceived and designed the study, acquired, analyzed, and interpreted the data, drafted and revised the article. BO designed the study, revised and edited the drafted article. GO designed the study, revised and edited the drafted article. YTG analyzed the data, revised and edited the drafted article. All the authors have read and approved the final version of the manuscript.

Authors' information

EJA (DVM, MVPH, MPH) is a junior faculty member and doctoral student at the Department of Veterinary Public Health and Preventive Medicine, University of Ibadan, Ibadan, Nigeria and a Fulbright scholar at the Department of Population Medicine and Diagnostic Sciences, College of Veterinary Medicine, Cornell University, Ithaca, New York, USA. BO (DVM, PhD) is a senior lecturer and Principal Investigator at the Centre for Control and Prevention of Zoonoses, Department of Veterinary Public Health and Preventive Medicine, University of Ibadan, Ibadan, Nigeria. GO (DVM, PhD) is a Professor at the Department of Veterinary Public Health and Preventive Medicine, University of Ibadan, Ibadan, Nigeria. YTG (DVM, PhD) is a Professor at the Department of Population Medicine and Diagnostic Sciences, College of Veterinary Medicine, Cornell University, Ithaca, New York, USA.

Acknowledgements

The authors wish to acknowledge the financial support of Nigeria Science and Technology Education Post-Basic (STEP-B) Project (Cr: 4304-UNI) - Innovators of tomorrow Research and Technology Development grant. We also appreciate the co-operation of the Pig farmers' association in southwest Nigeria and the technical assistance of the various States' Ministry of Agriculture and Livestock resources and/or rural development and cooperatives and Zhengxi Wang for creating the map.

References

1. Food Agricultural Organization of the United Nations (FAO). Recognizing African swine fever. A field manual. FAO Animal Health Manual 2000. http://www.fao.org/docrep/004/x8060e/x8060e00.htm. Accessed on 4 Dec., 2013.
2. Sánchez-Vizcaíno JM, Mur L, Martínez-López B. African swine fever (ASF): five years around Europe. Vet Microbiol. 2013;165(1–2):45–50.
3. World Organization for Animal Health (OIE). Disease Distribution Maps 2014 and 2015 – Disease Information. 2015. http://www.oie.int/wahis_2/public/wahid.php/countrymapinteractive. Accessed on 30 March, 2015.
4. Costard S, Wieland B, de Glanville W, Jori F, Rowlands R, Vosloo W, et al. African swine fever: how can global spread be prevented? Phil Trans R Soc B. 2009;364(1530):2683–96.
5. Babalobi OO, Olugasa BO, Oluwayelu DO, Ijagbone IF, Ayoade GO, Agbede SA. Analysis and evaluation of mortality losses of the 2001 African swine fever outbreak, Ibadan, Nigeria. Trop Anim Health Prod. 2007;39:533–42.
6. Plowright W, Thomson GR, Neser JA. African swine fever. In: Coetzer JAW, Thomson GR, Tutsin RC, editors. Infectious diseases of livestock, with special reference to southern Africa. 1st ed. Cape Town, South Africa: Oxford University Press; 1994. p. 567–99.
7. Sánchez-Vizcaíno JM, Arias M. African swine fever. In: Zimmerman J, Kar-riker LA, Ramirez A, Schwartz KJ, Stevenson GW, editors. Diseases of swine. Iowa, United States of America: John Wiley & Sons; 2012. p. 396–404.
8. Boinas FS, Wilson AJ, Hutchings GH, Martins C, Dixon LJ. The persistence of African swine fever virus in field-infected Ornithodoros erraticus during the ASF endemic period in Portugal. PLoS ONE. 2011;6:e20383.
9. Luther NJ, Majiyagbe KA, Shamaki D, Lombin LH, Antiabong JF, Bitrus Y, et al. Detection of African swine fever virus genomic DNA in a Nigerian Red River hog (*Potamochoerus porcus*). Vet Rec. 2007;160:58–9.
10. Babalobi OO, Ayoade GO, Olugasa BO, Oluwayelu DO, Oyedela O. Differential diagnosis of a swine epizootic of unknown aetiology in Ibadan, Oyo State, Nigeria. IJVM. 2003;58(2/3):86–9.
11. Food Agricultural Organization of the United Nations (FAO). African swine fever in West Africa: Togo, Senegal, Gambia and Guinea-Bissau. [French] Mission report from 1 to 16 June 1998. (1998a) Available from: http://www.fao.org/docrep/field/382969.htm. Accessed on 25 March, 2012.
12. Food Agricultural Organization of the United Nations (FAO). African swine fever in Nigeria hits rural poor. News & Highlights. December 1998. (1998d) Available from: http://www.fao.org/NEWS/1998/981201-e.htm. Accessed on 25 March, 2012.
13. Sánchez-Vizcaíno JM, Martínez-López B, Martínez-Avilés M, Martins C, Boinas F, Vial L, et al. African Swine Fever. Scientific report submitted to EFSA 2009: 1–141
14. Olugasa BO. Serological evidence of African swine fever virus infection in commercial pig herds in southwest Nigeria. Afr J Livest Ext. 2007;5:61–6.
15. Owolodun OA, Bastos ADS, Antiabong JF, Ogedengbe ME, Ekong PS, Yakubu B. Molecular characterization of African fever viruses from Nigeria (2003 – 2006) recovers multiple virus variants and reaffirms CVR epidemiological utility. Virus Genes. 2010;41:361–8.
16. Odemuyiwa SO, Adebayo IA, Ammerlaan W, Ajuwape ATP, Alaka OO, Oyedele OI, et al. An outbreak of African swine fever in Nigeria: virus isolation and molecular characterization of the *VP72* gene of a first isolate from West Africa. Virus Genes. 2000;20:139–42.
17. Owolodun OA, Obishakin ET, Ekong PS, Yakubu B. Investigation of African swine fever in slaughtered pigs, Plateau state, Nigeria, 2004–2006. Trop Anim Health Prod. 2010;42(8):1605–10.
18. Fasina FO, Shamaki D, Makinde AA, Lombin LH, Lazarus DD, Rufai SA, et al. Surveillance for African swine fever in Nigeria, 2006–2009. Transbound Emerg Dis. 2010;57(4):244–53.
19. Owolodun OA, Yakubu B, Antiabong JF, Ogedengbe OE, Luka PD, John Audu B, et al. Spatio-temporal dynamics of African swine fever outbreaks in Nigeria, 2002–2007. Transbound Emerg Dis. 2010;57(5):330–9.
20. Olugasa BO, Ijagbone IF. Pattern of spread of African swine fever in south-western Nigeria, 1997–2005. Vet Ital. 2007;43(3):621–8.
21. Sánchez-Vizcaíno JM, Mur L, Martínez-López B. African swine fever: an epidemiological update. Transbound Emerg Dis. 2012;59(1):27–35.
22. Atuhaire DK, Ochwo S, Afayoa M, Mwiine FN, Kokas I, Arinaitwe E, et al. Epidemiological Overview of African swine fever in Uganda (2001–2012). J. Vet. Med. 2013, Article ID 949638, 9 pages http://dx.doi.org/10.1155/2013/949638.
23. Cocks P, Abila R, Bouchot A, Benigno C, Morzaria S, Inthavong P, et al. FAO ADB and OIE SEAFMD Study on Cross Border movement and market chains of large ruminants and pigs in the Greater Mekong Sub Region. Thailand: Bangkok; 2009. p. 1–63.

24. Boklund A, Alban I, Mortensen S, Houe H. Biosecurity in 116 Danish fattening swine herds: descriptive results and factor analysis. Prev Vet Med. 2004;66:49–62.
25. Gardner IA, Willeberg P, Mousing J. Empirical and theoretical evidence for herd size as a risk factor for swine diseases. Anim Health Res Rev. 2002;3:43–55.
26. Food Agricultural Organization of the United Nations (FAO). FAO takes a close look at the pig Sector in Eastern Europe to better understand the threats of African Swine fever. EMPRES Watch 2010. http://www.fao.org/docrep/012/ak755e/ak755e00.pdf. Accessed on 4 Dec., 2013.
27. Magali Jacquier. Occurrence, Distribution and Characterisation of African Swine Fever Virus (ASFV) in the Tick *Ornithodoros porcinus* in the Kruger National Park. *BFA SEMINAR SERIES* NO. 32 Held at Ulwazi Institute, Suburbs, Bulawayo, on 17 September 2004. (2004) http://www.biodiversityfoundation.org/documents/s32.pdf Accessed 2 Dec., 2013.
28. Carrillo C, Borca MV, Afonso CL, Onisk DV, Rock DL. Long-term persistent infection of swine monocytes/macrophages with African swine fever virus. J Virol. 1994;68:580–3.
29. Barcelo J, Marco E. On farm biosecurity. In: Proceedings of the 15th International Pig Veterinary Society Congress. 1998. p. 129–33.
30. Fasina FO, Agbaje M, Ajani FL, Talabi OA, Lazarus DD, Gallardo C, et al. Risk factors for farm-level African swine fever infection in major pig-producing areas in Nigeria, 1997–2011. Prev Vet Med. 2012;107:65–75.
31. Otesile EB, Ajuwape ATP, Odemuyiwa SO, Akpavie SO, Olaifa AK, Odaibo GN, et al. Field and Experimental Investigations of an Outbreak of African Swine Fever in Nigeria. Revue Élev Méd vét Pays trop. 2005;58(1–2):21–6.
32. Penrith ML, Vosloo W. Review of African swine fever: transmission, spread and control. J S Afr Vet Assoc. 2009;80(2):58–62.
33. Food Agricultural Organization of the United Nations (FAO). Biosecurity for Highly pathogenic Avian Influenza – issues and options. 2008. http://www.fao.org/docrep/011/i0359e/i0359e00.pdf Accessed on 4 Dec., 2013.
34. Sánchez-Vizcaíno JM. Early detection and contingency plans for African swine fever. Compedium of technical items presented to the OIE World Assembly of Delegates and to OIE Regional Commissions 2010, 129-168.
35. Mannelli A, Sotgia S, Patta C, Sarria A, Madrau P, Sanna L, et al. Effect of husbandry methods on seropositivity to African swine fever virus in Sardinia swine herds. Prev Vet Med. 1997;32:235–41.
36. Muhanguzi D, Lutwama V, Mwiine FN. Factors that influence pig production in Central Uganda—case study of Nangabo Sub-County, Wakiso district. Vet World. 2012;5(6):346–51.
37. Federal Department of Livestock (FDL) Nigeria. Report on study and mapping of poultry farming systems and pig production areas by support for the Integrated National Action Plan on Animal and Human Influenza (SPINAP) Project in Nigeria. Official document (2010).
38. Thrusfield M. What sample size should be selected? In: Veterinary Epidemiology. 3rd ed. UK: Blackwell Publishing Limited; 2007. p. 232–8.
39. Bennett S, Woods T, Liyanage WM, Smith DL. A simplified general method for cluster-sample surveys of health in developing countries. World Health Stat Q. 1991;44:98–106.
40. Otte MJ, Gumm ID. Intra-cluster correlation coefficients of 20 infections calculated from the results of cluster-sample surveys. Prev Vet Med. 1997;31:147–50.
41. Arias M, Sánchez-Vizcaíno JM. Manual de diagnóstico serológico de la peste porcina africana. Monografías INIA. 1992;83:5–44.
42. Ade-Ajayi JF, Falola TO, Hamilton A, Kirk-Greene M, Udo RK. Nigeria - Britannica academic edition. 2010 http://www.britannica.com Accessed on 2 Dec., 2013.
43. Statistical Analysis System (SAS) Institute Inc. *SAS/STAT® 9.3* User's Guide. Cary, NC: SAS Institute Inc. 2011. http://support.sas.com/documentation/cdl/en/statug/63962/HTML/default/viewer.htm Accessed on 2 Dec., 2013

Permissions

All chapters in this book were first published in VR, by BioMed Central; hereby published with permission under the Creative Commons Attribution License or equivalent. Every chapter published in this book has been scrutinized by our experts. Their significance has been extensively debated. The topics covered herein carry significant findings which will fuel the growth of the discipline. They may even be implemented as practical applications or may be referred to as a beginning point for another development.

The contributors of this book come from diverse backgrounds, making this book a truly international effort. This book will bring forth new frontiers with its revolutionizing research information and detailed analysis of the nascent developments around the world.

We would like to thank all the contributing authors for lending their expertise to make the book truly unique. They have played a crucial role in the development of this book. Without their invaluable contributions this book wouldn't have been possible. They have made vital efforts to compile up to date information on the varied aspects of this subject to make this book a valuable addition to the collection of many professionals and students.

This book was conceptualized with the vision of imparting up-to-date information and advanced data in this field. To ensure the same, a matchless editorial board was set up. Every individual on the board went through rigorous rounds of assessment to prove their worth. After which they invested a large part of their time researching and compiling the most relevant data for our readers.

The editorial board has been involved in producing this book since its inception. They have spent rigorous hours researching and exploring the diverse topics which have resulted in the successful publishing of this book. They have passed on their knowledge of decades through this book. To expedite this challenging task, the publisher supported the team at every step. A small team of assistant editors was also appointed to further simplify the editing procedure and attain best results for the readers.

Apart from the editorial board, the designing team has also invested a significant amount of their time in understanding the subject and creating the most relevant covers. They scrutinized every image to scout for the most suitable representation of the subject and create an appropriate cover for the book.

The publishing team has been an ardent support to the editorial, designing and production team. Their endless efforts to recruit the best for this project, has resulted in the accomplishment of this book. They are a veteran in the field of academics and their pool of knowledge is as vast as their experience in printing. Their expertise and guidance has proved useful at every step. Their uncompromising quality standards have made this book an exceptional effort. Their encouragement from time to time has been an inspiration for everyone.

The publisher and the editorial board hope that this book will prove to be a valuable piece of knowledge for researchers, students, practitioners and scholars across the globe.

List of Contributors

Christian P. Bertholle, Ellen Meijer, Arjan Stegeman and Arie van Nes
Department of Farm Animal Health, Faculty of Veterinary Medicine, Utrecht University, Yalelaan 7, NL-3584 CL Utrecht, The Netherlands

P. René van Weeren
Department of Equine Sciences, Faculty of Veterinary Medicine, Utrecht University, Yalelaan 112-114, NL-3584 CM Utrecht, The Netherlands

Willem Back
Department of Equine Sciences, Faculty of Veterinary Medicine, Utrecht University, Yalelaan 112-114, NL-3584 CM Utrecht, The Netherlands
Department of Surgery and Anaesthesia of Domestic Animals, Ghent University, 17 Salisburylaan 133, B-9820 Merelbeke, Belgium

Kimberlee L. Baker, Jianqiang Zhang, Chong Wang and Derald J. Holtkamp
Department of Veterinary Diagnostic and Production Animal Medicine, Iowa State University College of Veterinary Medicine, 1809 S Riverside Dr, Ames, IA, USA

Locke A. Karriker and Alejandro Ramirez
Department of Veterinary Diagnostic and Production Animal Medicine, Iowa State University College of Veterinary Medicine, 1809 S Riverside Dr, Ames, IA, USA
Swine Medicine Education Center, Iowa State University College of Veterinary Medicine, 1809 S Riverside Dr, Ames, IA, USA

Paul R. Thomas
AMVC Management Services, 1786 190th St, Audubon, IA, USA
Swine Medicine Education Center, Iowa State University College of Veterinary Medicine, 1809 S Riverside Dr, Ames, IA, USA

Domenico Ventrella, Francesco Dondi, Francesca Barone, Federica Serafini, Alberto Elmi, Massimo Giunti, Noemi Romagnoli, Monica Forni and Maria L. Bacci
Department of Veterinary Medical Sciences, Alma Mater Studiorum, University of Bologna, Via Tolara di Sopra 50, 40064 Ozzano dell'Emilia, BO, Italy

Hsin-Yi Weng
Department of Comparative Pathobiology, Purdue University, 625 Harrison Street, West Lafayette, IN 47907, USA

Shankar Yadav
Department of Comparative Pathobiology, Purdue University, 625 Harrison Street, West Lafayette, IN 47907, USA
Plum Island Animal Disease Center Research Participation Program (ORISE fellow), Orient Point, NY 11957, USA

Taofeng Du, Yunpeng Shi, Shuqi Xiao, Na Li, Qin Zhao, Angke Zhang, Yuchen Nan, Yang Mu, Yani Sun, Chunyan Wu and En-Min Zhou
Department of Preventive Veterinary Medicine, College of Veterinary Medicine, Northwest A&F University, Yangling, Shaanxi 712100, China
Experimental Station of Veterinary Pharmacology and Veterinary Biotechnology, Ministry of Agriculture, Yangling, Shaanxi 712100, China

Hongtao Zhang
Department of Pathology and Lab Medicine, University of Pennsylvania Perelman School of Medicine, 3620 Hamilton Walk, Philadelphia, PA 19104, USA

Yicheng Zhao, Li Yao and Chunbo Teng
College of Life Science, Northeast Forestry University, Harbin, China
College of Animal Sciences, Jilin University, Changchun, China

Hongsheng Ouyang and Tiedong Wang
College of Animal Sciences, Jilin University, Changchun, China

Bo Liu
College of Animal Sciences, Jilin University, Changchun, China
College of Veterinary Medicine, Inner Mongolia Agricultural University, Hohhot, China

Enrico Giacomini, Sara Gasparrini, Massimiliano Lazzaro, Federico Scali, Maria Beatrice Boniotti and Giovanni Loris Alborali
Istituto Zooprofilattico Sperimentale della Lombardia e dell'Emilia Romagna Experimental Zooprophylactic Institute of Lombardy and Emilia Romagna "Bruno Ubertini", Via Bianchi 7/9, 25124 Brescia, Italy

Attilio Corradi
Department of Veterinary Sciences, University of Parma, Parma, Italy

Paolo Pasquali
Istituto Superiore di Sanità, Rome, Italy
FAO Reference Center for Veterinary Public Health, Rome, Italy

Sara Amirpour Haredasht, Kyuyoung Lee and Beatriz Martínez-López
Center for Animal Disease Modeling and Surveillance (CADMS), Department of Medicine & Epidemiology, School Veterinary Medicine, University of California, 2108 Tupper Hall, one Shields Avenue, Davis, California 95616, USA

Dale Polson
Boehringer-Ingelheim Vetmedica Inc, Saint Joseph, Missouri, USA

Rodger Main and Derald Holtkamp
Department of Veterinary Diagnostic and Production Animal Medicine, College of Veterinary Medicine, Iowa State University, Ames, USA

Sergio Ghidini, Emanuela Zanardi, Pierluigi Aldo Di Ciccio and Adriana Ianieri
Department of Food and Drug, Parma University, Via Del Taglio, 10, 43126 Parma, Italy

Silvio Borrello and Sarah Guizzardi
Italian Ministry of Health, Via Giorgio Ribotta, 5, 00144 Rome, Italy

Giancarlo Belluzi
Italian Ministry of Health, Viale Tanara 31/A, 43100 Parma (PR), Italy

Cheryl M. T. Dvorak, Suzanne R. Stone and Michael P. Murtaugh
Department of Veterinary and Biomedical Sciences, University of Minnesota, 1971 Commonwealth Ave, St. Paul, MN 55108, USA

Zeynep Akkutay-Yoldar
Department of Veterinary and Biomedical Sciences, University of Minnesota, 1971 Commonwealth Ave, St. Paul, MN 55108, USA
Department of Virology, Ankara University, Faculty of Veterinary Medicine, Diskapi, 06110 Ankara, Turkey

Steven J. P. Tousignant
Swine Vet Center P.A., 1608 S. Minnesota Ave, St. Peter, MN 56082, USA

A. Vannucci
Department of Veterinary Population Medicine, University of Minnesota, 1365 Gortner Ave, St. Paul, MN 55108, USA

Silvia Martínez-Miró, Marina Ramón, Fuensanta Hernández, Josefa Madrid and Juan Orengo
Department of Animal Production, Campus of Excellence Mare Nostrum, Universidad de Murcia, 30100 Murcia, Spain

Silvia Martínez-Subiela, Fernando Tecles, Damián Escribano and José Joaquín Cerón
Department of Animal Medicine and Surgery, Campus of Excellence Mare Nostrum, Universidad de Murcia, 30100 Murcia, Spain

Xavier Manteca
Department of Animal and Food Science, Universitat Autònoma de Barcelona, 08193 Bellaterra, Barcelona, Spain

Salah Uddin Khan, Terri L. O'Sullivan, Zvonimir Poljak and Amy L. Greer
Department of Population Medicine, Ontario Veterinary College, University of Guelph, Guelph, ON, Canada

Janet Alsop
Ontario Ministry of Agriculture, Food and Rural Affairs, Guelph, ON, Canada

Yinchu Zhu, Wenyang Dong, Jiale Ma, Lvfeng Yuan, Hassan M. A. Hejair, Zihao Pan, Guangjin Liu and Huochun Yao
College of Veterinary Medicine, Nanjing Agricultural University, Nanjing 210095, China
Key Lab of Animal Bacteriology, Ministry of Agriculture, Nanjing Agricultural University, Nanjing 210095, China

Rachel Madera, Lihua Wang, Karen Lleellish, Amy Galliher-Beckley and Jishu Shi
Department of Anatomy and Physiology, Kansas State University, Manhattan, KS 66506, USA

Yulia Burakova
Department of Anatomy and Physiology, Kansas State University, Manhattan, KS 66506, USA
Department of Chemical Engineering, Kansas State University, Manhattan, KS 66506, USA

Wenjie Gong
Department of Anatomy and Physiology, Kansas State University, Manhattan, KS 66506, USA
Institute of Military Veterinary Medicine, Academy of Military Medical Sciences, Changchun, China

Jerome Nietfeld, Jamie Henningson and Jianfa Bai
Department of Diagnostic Medicine and Pathobiology, Kansas State University, Manhattan, KS 66506, USA

Kaimin Jia and Ping Li
Department of Chemistry, Kansas State University, Manhattan, KS 66506, USA

John Schlup
Department of Chemical Engineering, Kansas State University, Manhattan, KS 66506, USA

Changchun Tu
Institute of Military Veterinary Medicine, Academy of Military Medical Sciences, Changchun, China

Scott McVey
United States Department of Agriculture, Agricultural Research Service, Arthropod Borne Animal Disease Research Unit, Manhattan, KS 66502, USA

Małgorzata Pomorska-Mól, Arkadiusz Dors, Krzysztof Kwit, Ewelina Czyżewska-Dors and Zygmunt Pejsak
Department of Swine Diseases, National Veterinary Research Institute, Partyzantów 57, 24-100 Pulawy, Poland

Nobuhiro Takemae and Yuko Uchida
Influenza and Prion Diseases Research Center, National Institute of Animal Health, NARO, Ibaraki, Japan
Thailand-Japan Zoonotic Diseases Collaboration Center, Bangkok, Thailand

Takehiko Saito
Influenza and Prion Diseases Research Center, National Institute of Animal Health, NARO, Ibaraki, Japan
Thailand-Japan Zoonotic Diseases Collaboration Center, Bangkok, Thailand
United Graduate School of Veterinary Sciences, Gifu University, Gifu, Japan

Yugo Shobugawa and Reiko Saito
Division of International Health, Graduate School of Medical and Dental Sciences, Niigata University, Niigata, Japan

Phuong Thanh Nguyen, Phuong Duy Thai, Duy Thanh Nguyen, Dung Kim Nguyen, Thi Quynh Anh Le, Phan Truong Hua and Hung Van Vo
Department of Animal Health, Center for Veterinary Diagnostics, Regional Animal Health Office No. 6, Ho Chi Minh City, Vietnam

Tung Nguyen, Tien Ngoc Nguyen and Diep Thi Nguyen
Department of Animal Health, Epidemiology Division, Hanoi, Vietnam

Thanh Long To, Tho Dang Nguyen, Hoa Thi Do and Dang Hoang Nguyen
Department of Animal Health, National Centre for Veterinary Diagnostics, Hanoi, Vietnam

Weijie Bai, Zhijia Wang, Pu Sun, Jing Zhang, Huifang Bao, Yimei Cao, Yanyan Chang, Zaixin Liu, Dong Li and Zengjun Lu
State Key Laboratory of Veterinary Etiologic Biology, Lanzhou Veterinary Research Institute, Chinese Academy of Agricultural Sciences, Lanzhou 730046, Gansu, China

Jinqiu Zhang, Yu Lu, Bihua Deng, Fang Lv, Yanhong Zhao and Jibo Hou
National Research Center for Veterinary Vaccine Engineering and Technology of China, Jiangsu Academy of Agricultural Sciences, Nanjing 210014, China

Jinfeng Miao
College of Veterinary Medicine, Nanjing Agricultural University, Nanjing 210095, China

Xiangan Han and Chan Ding
Shanghai Veterinary Research Institute, Chinese Academy of Agricultural Sciences, Shanghai 200241, China

Fernando Núñez-Hernández, Fernando Rodríguez and José I. Núñez
Institut de Recerca i Tecnologia Agroalimentàries (IRTA)-Centre de Recerca en Sanitat Animal (CReSA), Campus de la Universitat Autònoma de Barcelona, Bellaterra, Barcelona, Spain

Gonzalo Vera
Centre de Recerca en Agrigenòmica (CRAG), Consorci CSIC-IRTA-UAB-UB, Bellaterra, Barcelona, Spain

Armand Sánchez
Centre de Recerca en Agrigenòmica (CRAG), Consorci CSIC-IRTA-UAB-UB, Bellaterra, Barcelona, Spain
Departament de Ciència Animal i dels Aliments, Universitat Autònoma de Barcelona (UAB), Bellaterra, Barcelona, Spain

Edyta Mikuła, Jerzy Radecki and Hanna Radecka
Institute of Animal Reproduction and Food Research of Polish Academy of Sciences, Tuwima 10, 10-748 Olsztyn, Poland

Cristiane Erdmann Silva
Universidade Estadual de Ponta Grossa - UEPG, Setor de Ciências Exatas e da Terra, Departamento de Química, Av. Carlos Cavalcanti, 4748, CEP 84030-900, Ponta Grossa/PR, Brazil

Edyta Kopera
Institute of Biochemistry and Biophysics of Polish Academy of Sciences, Pawińskiego 5a, 02-106 Warsaw, Poland
Research and Development Center, Olimp Laboratories, Pustynia, Dębica, Poland

Konrad Zdanowski
Institute of Biochemistry and Biophysics of Polish Academy of Sciences, Pawińskiego 5a, 02-106 Warsaw, Poland
Institute of Chemistry, University of Natural Sciences and Humanities, 3 Maja 54, 08-110 Siedlce, Poland

Huixing Lin, Hong Zhou and Lu Gao
MOE Joint International Research Laboratory of Animal Health and Food Safety, College of Veterinary Medicine, Nanjing Agricultural University, Nanjing 210095, China

Hongjie Fan
MOE Joint International Research Laboratory of Animal Health and Food Safety, College of Veterinary Medicine, Nanjing Agricultural University, Nanjing 210095, China
Jiangsu Co-Innovation Center for the Prevention and Control of Important Animal Infectious Diseases and Zoonoses, Yangzhou University, Yangzhou 225009, China

Bin Li and Kongwang He
Institute of Veterinary Medicine, Jiangsu Academy of Agricultural Sciences, Nanjing 210014, China

Index

S

T

V